Pharmacognosy

An Indian Perspective

Pharmacognosy
An Indian Perspective

K. Mangathayaru
Department of Pharmacognosy
Faculty of Pharmacy
Sri Ramachandra University
Chennai, Tamil Nadu

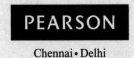

PEARSON

Chennai • Delhi

Assistant Editor—Acquisitions: R. Dheepika
Editor—Production: C. Purushothaman

ISBN 978-81-317-9726-6

First Impression

Published by Dorling Kindersley (India) Pvt. Ltd, licensees of Pearson Education in South Asia.

Head Office: 7th Floor, Knowledge Boulevard, A-8(A), Sector 62, Noida 201 309, UP, India.
Registered Office: 11 Community Centre, Panchsheel Park, New Delhi 110 017, India.

Compositor: Chennai Publishing Services, Chennai
Printed in India by Pushp Print Servicses

Dedicated to my Guru

Sadhguru Jaggi Vasudev

His Grace thus propels me…

Contents

Foreword   xi

Preface   xiii

1. Pharmacognosy—An Introduction   1
History of Pharmacognosy—1
Lessons from Research on Medicinal Plants—12
Focus of Pharmacognosy—29
Conclusion—30
Review Questions   31

2. Age-Old Indian Medical Wisdom—Ayurveda   32
Introduction—32
History, Growth and Development of Ayurvedic Medicine—34
The Basis of Ayurvedic Therapeutics—37
Ayurvedic *Materia Medica*—49
The Best of Ayurveda and its Influence Over Other Medical Systems—52
Revival and Current Status—56
Conclusion—57
Review Questions   58

3. Worldwide Trade in Herbal Products   59
Introduction—59
Trade in Plant-Based Products—60
Hurdles to the Development of Medicinal Plant Trade—63
Sources of Plant Material—64
Categories of Medicinal Plant-Derived Products Traded—66
Global Trade in Some Individual Plant Drugs—80
Conclusion—118
Review Questions   119

4. Herbal Drug Regulatory Affairs — 120

Introduction—120
Milestones in Herbal Drug Regulation—121
Specific Objectives of Herbal Drug Regulation—123
Current Status of Herbal Drug Regulatory Affairs—124
Conclusion—148
Review Questions 148

5. Herbal Institutes and Industries Working on Medicinal Plants in India — 150

Introduction—150
Global Volume of Herbal Drug Trade – India's Concern—151
India's Advantage—152
India's Initiatives—153
Central Governmental Establishments—155
State Level Governmental and Non-Governmental Organizations—176
Commercial Herbal Drug Industry—195
Conclusion—197
Review Questions 197

6. Quality Control and Standardization of Herbal Drugs — 198

Introduction—198
Standardization of Herbal Drugs—199
Important Parameters for the Quality Control of Herbal Drugs—200
Conclusion—216
Review Questions 216

7. Phytochemical Analysis—An Introduction — 218

Introduction—218
Some General Principles of Phytochemical Analysis—219
Extraction, Isolation, and Identification of Some Phytochemical Classes—221
Applications of Chromatography to Phytochemical Analysis—245
Conclusion—254
Review Questions 254

8. Plant-Derived Pure Drugs — 256

Introduction—256
Isolation, Identification and Estimation of Selected Plant-Derived Pure Drugs—257
Conclusion—306
Review Questions 306

9. Traditional Herbal Drugs   307

Introduction—307
Salient Features of Some Medicinal Herbs—309
Conclusion—333
Review Questions 334

10. Herbal Cosmetics   335

Introduction—335
Trade in Herbal Cosmetics—336
Indian Market—337
Herbals in Cosmetics—338
Importance of Herbals in Hair and Skin Care Products—340
Conclusion—363
Review Questions 363

11. Plant Biotechnology   364

Introduction—364
Milestones in the History of Plant-Tissue Culture—365
Scope of Plant-Tissue Culture Techniques—368
Media Requirements for Plant-Tissue Culture—371
Plant Growth Regulators—373
Types of Cultures—374
Plant Cell Immobilization—377
Bio Transformation—378
Transgenic Plants and Their Applications—381
Secondary Metabolite Production in Plant-Tissue Culture Systems—385
Conclusion—389
Review Questions 390

12. Intellectual Property Rights—Traditional Knowledge and Plant Drugs   391

Introduction—391
Events in History that Led to IP Regime—392
Recent International Developments in IP Arena—393
TRIPS Agreement—395
Controversies Surrounding TRIPS Agreement—399
Indian Patent Law—401
Issues Pertaining to Herbal Drug Patenting—406
Conclusion—414
Review Questions 415

13. Zoo Pharmacognosy—A Rediscovery?   416

Introduction—416
Some Interesting Facts Revealed by Observation and Research on Animals—417
Animal Self-Medication—Some Specific Reports—419
Animal Self-Medication—Implications for Humans—425
Conclusion—426
Review Questions   427

Bibliography   429
Index   447

Foreword

Pharmacognosy, an important segment of the pharmaceutical sciences, is concerned with the study of new drugs derived from plant, animal and mineral sources. It includes identification of lead molecules in herbal medicines, and development of pharmaceutical aids, colours, flavours, fragrances, pesticides etc. It has contributed a great deal for human welfare in the form of new drug discovery for the treatment of various ailments. The author Dr K. Mangathayaru, after extensive review of literature in the field of pharmacognosy, has presented the subject from a distinctive Indian context. The concepts of complimentary and alternative medicine and the usage of plants as drugs have been lucidly illustrated with the help of examples. The book has essential chapters on World Trade in Herbal Products and Regulatory Affairs, which are highly current in the present scenario. A unique feature of the book is the chapter that deals in detail with institutes/organizations involved in the research of herbal medicines, including non-governmental organizations. There is also a vital chapter to address the problem of safety and efficacy of herbal medicines. Detailed information on the exploitation of plants for the development of herbal cosmetics has been aptly provided. The book gives an insight into the latest development in pharmacognosy, especially plant biotechnology, zoo pharmacognosy and patents related to plant based products.

I congratulate Dr K. Mangathayaru for her sincere efforts in bringing out this book. The book is original in its approach and highly explanatory, while being a useful compilation of information for the students of pharmacy and professionals in the pharmaceutical and herbal drug industry. Those involved in herbal medicines and those engaged in the trade of medicinal plants and related products also stand to be benefited by the book.

Prof. Ciddi Veeresham
University College of Pharmaceutical Sciences
Kakatiya University, Warangal

Preface

This book, in conformance with the newly proposed AICTE syllabus, has been designed to be a course book on pharmacognosy for eighth semester B.Pharm. students. I have shaped this book out of my teaching notes for final-year B.Pharm. and M.Pharm. classes. Backed by a sound experience of teaching and research, a penchant for going from the basics, motivation from several spirited students and deference for unsophisticated knowledge, I have delved into the roots of natural drug knowledge in our country and laid bare the essence of the subject for the student's benefit.

Against the backdrop of current revival of global interest in traditional drugs, the rationale behind holistic drug administration is being explored and even espoused by modern science. Global research is trying to decipher the intricacies of drug administration in Ayurveda. Thus, while cutting-edge science continues to validate our medical wisdom, it is unfortunate that students of pharmacy in this country are largely ignorant of the depth of medicinal plant knowledge that we possess. Tutelage in pharmacognosy begins with the coinage of the word 'pharmacognosy' by Seidler and takes off from there. Students, however, learn such conventional curriculum on the subject disjointedly from the recently introduced topics on indigenous medical systems. It is ironic that while our students memorize several Latin words and their meanings just because modern drug dispensing got these root words from Galenical pharmacy, they are not even aware of the connotation of essential Sanskrit words like *rasa*, *guna*, *prabhava*, *vipaka* and so on, that are salient for understanding the basis of Ayurvedic drug selection. As with most other concepts, we appear to be waiting for approval to come from the West for re-introduction of the fundamentals of holistic medicine in our country.

India's rich traditional knowledge on herbal drugs caught worldwide attention when we fought against patent infringement on our traditional medicinal herbs, neem and turmeric. Despite such wealth of information on herbal drugs and the vantage position India holds to become the world leader in herbal drug trade, our students inadvertently continue to learn the subject as it was propounded to us by our Western brethren. I am sure many pharmacognosists will share with me the urgent need not only to impart the subject to our students with focus on its ancient roots in this subcontinent, but also to give them an insight into the depth of systematic medical knowledge that was ours.

Pharmacognosy – An Indian Perspective brings to the fore the Indian resource for the subject in terms of both materials and methods. The thirteen chapters covering the target syllabus also include a chapter on the current status of herbal drug regulatory affairs across selected countries, a special chapter on IP rights on herbal drugs and traditional knowledge and a chapter on zoo pharmacognosy.

With the seamless advancement of science into unexplored aspects of life, modern medicine is trying to tap into the potential of time-tested traditional concepts of health maintenance. A panoramic study of pharmacognosy is the need of the hour and I am sure that this book is a modest step in the right direction. Comments and feedback on the contents of this book are welcome. I may be contacted at kvmanga@yahoo.com

ACKNOWLEDGEMENTS

Words are insufficient to articulate my profound gratitude to Sadhguru Jaggi Vasudev for the interest evinced on the book. I humbly dedicate the book to Him as I bask in His boundless grace.

I am beholden to many who have supported me in the making of this book. I thank our Chancellor, Sri V. R. Venkatachalam, and the management, Sri Ramachandra University (SRU), for providing the needed academic milieu and support. I am obliged to our Dean of Faculties, Dr. K. V. Somasundaram, for enthusing me to go ahead with this task. I reiterate my thanks to all my colleagues and non-teaching staff at the department of pharmacy, SRU, for their cheer and friendship. My students, past and present, have been the incitement for me to seek more. I thank them all.

I express my gratitude to Dr K. Anandan, Assistant Director-in-Charge, Central Research Institute for Siddha, Arumbakkam, Chennai, for his thought-provoking insights on drug administration basics in indigenous systems. I am indebted to my teacher Prof. Ciddi Veeresham, Principal and Head, University College of Pharmaceutical Sciences, Kakatiya University, Warangal, for writing the foreword for the book. I am grateful to Maa Vaama and Dr Satchi A. Surendran of Isha Foundation, Coimbatore, for their support.

My salutations to the many researchers the world over, whose research contributions serve to validate traditional knowledge, granting it the long withheld recognition.

I thank my publisher, Pearson Education, for bringing out this book. I am grateful to the reviewers who took the time to review it. I appreciate the efforts of R. Dheepika, Pearson Education, whose professional follow-up right from the book proposal stage and useful inputs from the publisher's perspective helped me immensely to shape the book to its present form. I am thankful to C. Purushothaman, and his team for meticulously striving to bring this book out in time.

I owe it all to my loving family, my husband K. V. Krishna, my father Sri. V. K. Chary and daughters Kavya and Shreya, who have all been my source of strength.

The countless hours of writing and research that went into the making of this book have all been a transforming experience for me.

I thank the Omniscient Presence for making it all happen.

K. Mangathayaru

1

Pharmacognosy—An Introduction

CHAPTER OBJECTIVES

History of Pharmacognosy

Lessons from Research on
Medicinal Plants

Focus of Pharmacognosy

Pharmacognosy is the study of drugs derived from natural sources namely of plant, animal or mineral origin. Also defined as the study of crude drugs, pharmacognosy according to the American Society of Pharmacognosy is 'the study of the physical, chemical, biochemical and biological properties of drugs, drug substances or potential drugs of natural origin as well as search for new drugs from natural sources'.

The word pharmacognosy is derived from the Greek words *pharmakon* (remedy/magic spell/poison) and *gnosis* (knowledge). The term was first used as 'pharmacognosis' by the Austrian physician J.A. Schmidt in his work '*Lehrbuch der Materia Medica*' in 1811 and by C.A. Seydler—a medical student, as title for his dissertation '*Analectica Pharmacognostia*' in 1815.

At the beginning of the 20th century, pharmacognosy was used to define the branch of medicine dealing with drugs in their crude or unprepared form. Crude drugs are the dried, unprepared material of plant, animal or mineral origin used for medicine. The study of these materials under the name of *pharmacognosie* was first developed in German-speaking areas of Europe, while others used the older term *materia medica* taken from the works of Galen and Dioscorides.

HISTORY OF PHARMACOGNOSY

The use of natural materials for healing is possibly as old as mankind with the oldest evidence dating back to the Neanderthal era (70,000 BC) found in Shanidar Cave of Iraq. People on all continents have used hundreds of indigenous plants for treatment of ailments since prehistoric times. This knowledge could have arisen out of observing lower animals in disease and by trial and error. Thus the use of plants as medicine predates written human history. A fundamental difficulty of studying ancient history is that recorded histories cannot document the entirety of human events and only a fraction of these documents have survived to the present day.

Furthermore the reliability of information obtained from these surviving records must be considered. It is also essential to take into account the bias of each historian.

Going by written records, the study of herbs dates back to about 5,000 years to the Sumerians, who have described well-established medicinal uses of plants like laurel, caraway and thyme. Ancient Egyptian medicine of 1,000 BC is known to have used garlic, opium, castor oil, coriander, mint and indigo for medicine and the Old Testament also mentions cultivation of herbs including mandrake, vetch, wheat, barley and rye. Ancient medical documents like *Ebers Papyrus* (1500 BC) and the *Kahun Medical Papyrus* have recorded the use of several commonly used herbs by ancient Egyptians.

Herbal Medicine Tradition of India

India has a very strong tradition of use of natural materials as drugs. The oldest written records of an even ancient oral tradition, namely the Vedas, mention the virtues of several hundreds of herbs. Many herbs and minerals used in Ayurveda since centuries earlier were later described in written form by ancient herbalists such as Charaka and Sushruta during the first millennium BC. The Sushruta Samhita attributed to Sushruta in the 6th century BC describes 700 medicinal plants, 64 preparations from mineral sources and 57 preparations based on animal sources. Likewise the Charaka Samhita (1500–400 AD) provides an exhaustive description of around 600 plants with information on methods of collecting plants, classifying, combining, processing, their applications in specific stages and conditions, incompatibilities, contra-indications and information regarding poisons. There are approximately 1,800 botanical species mentioned in the classical Ayurvedic literature and around 8,000 species in folklore literature.

Ayurveda has a unique way of understanding plants. Unlike in western science, plant classification and nomenclature serve different purposes. The nomenclature of Ayurveda is not the binomial system that has been adopted by modern botany. Many names refer to a single plant and single name is used to denote many plants. A particular plant species may have a group of synonyms ranging from 1 to 50. Each of these names focuses on a special aspect of the plant and thus provides a comprehensive picture of the various aspects of the plant including its morphology, ecological factors, therapeutic parts, seasonal characters, qualities, biological actions and uses. This naming system was primarily designed to help a physician select a plant for medicinal purposes rather than to establish its taxonomical character. Thus plant nomenclature used in Ayurveda is a therapeutic nomenclature, based on a polynomial system of naming. Dravyaguna vijnana is the special branch of Ayurveda that elaborates the qualities and biological actions of several natural products of human consumption. Root (*moola*), bark (*valcra*), heart wood (*koshti*), secretions (*niryasaha*), stalk (*naalika*), extracted juice (*ras*), tender leaves (*mrdu patra*), alkali (*ksharaha*), latex (*niryasa*), fruit (*phalam*), flower (*pushpam*), ash (*bhasma*), oil (*taila*), thorn (*kantaka*), leaves (patra), leaf buds (*patra-mukula*), tubers (*kandaha*), sprouts (*ankuraha*), pedicle (*manjari*), petals (*dalam*), stamen (*pankesara*), seed (*beejam*) and whole plant (*gulma*) are the plant parts used in Ayurveda.

There are a good number of classic medical texts and manuscripts that deal with plants. These are largely treatises, compendiums, lexicons, critical commentaries and texts on specific areas like pharmacy, paediatrics, etc. Apart from major treatises like Charaka Samhita, Sushruta Samhita and Ashtanga Hridaya written before 1st century BC, several other treatises dating back to before this period include Harita Samhita, Bhela Samhita, Kashyap Samhita, which are not available in complete form. During medieval period or between the 8th and 15th century there have been many works written in the field of Ayurvedic pharmacology or 'dravya guna' (quality of drugs) as it is called in Sanskrit. A good number of nighantus were coined during this period. These were appendices to the ancient samhitas and contained synonyms, qualities of drugs and the condition in which they are to be used. Vyakhyas are critical commentaries on treatises and also carry elaborate references to plants.

The vast literature reserve thus indicates that the understanding of natural resources in the traditional pharmacopoeia had been quite dynamic. This knowledge was updated from time to time with the addition of newer drugs and removal of obscure ones. For example, rare drugs such as *soma* with supposedly celestial powers mentioned in the Sushruta Samhita were later dropped by Vagbhata, the author of Ashtanga Hridaya (600 AD) possibly because of non-availability of plants due to difficulties in accessing them. Plants whose therapeutic properties were newly identified were incorporated. There has been a gradual increase in the number of plants starting from Rig Veda to the nighantus. A number of drugs were introduced from other parts of the world through trade and foreign contacts. For instance spices, aromatics and other drugs like Hingu (asafoetida), Kesar (saffron) and Madhuka (licorice) were imported. Exotic plants like brinjal, green chillies, potato, tapioca, pineapple, tea and coffee have been studied based on Ayurvedic parameters and incorporated into literature only in the last few centuries.

Also Indian alchemy was well ahead of its times with the usage of mercury, sulphur, mica, arsenic, magnetic iron, antimony, zinc, iron pyrites and ferrous sulphate being used for medicinal purpose. A range of natural products apart from plants and minerals including exotic animal products made out of human skull, animal bones, bodily secretions, horns, hides, etc. were used in the amelioration of ailments both in humans and animals.

Chinese Use of Herbs as Drugs

The first Chinese herbal book, the *Shennong Ben Cao Jing*, compiled during the Han Dynasty but dating back to a much earlier period, possibly 2700 BC, lists 365 medicinal plants and their uses. Succeeding generations augmented on the *Shennong Ben Cao Jing*, as in the *Yaoxing Lun* (Treatise on the Nature of Medicinal Herbs), a 7th century Tang Dynasty treatise on herbal medicine. The *Huangdi neijing*, the most important classic in the history of Chinese medicine, had an enormous influence on medical thought in later centuries. It records the dialogues between a Chinese Emperor and some of his sage physicians on medical issues. While the emperor's questions encompass every possible aspect of diagnostics, pathology, acupuncture, and moxibustion, including both theory and practice, the sage teachers give detailed explanation of each topic.

Greek Herbal Tradition

The earliest source of Greek medical knowledge is Homer. Two epic poems attributed to him, belonging to 8th century BC, mention treatment of injuries of wounded warriors. *De Historia Plantarum* and *De Causis Plantarum* by Theophrastus (340 BC) and Dioscorides's *De Materia Medica* (78 AD) with several recipes same as the *Ebers Papyrus* contain approximately 80% plant medicines, 10% mineral- and 10% animal-derived drugs. While *De Historia Plantarum* founded the science of Botany and was considered important for herbalists and botanists of later centuries, Dioscorides's compendium of more than 500 plants remained in Europe an authoritative reference into 17th century. Pliny's natural history (60 AD) lists about 1,000 plants of Roman period and Galen's (130–200 AD) principles of preparing and compounding medicines ruled the western world for 1,500 years and his name is associated with galenicals, a class of pharmaceuticals compounded by mechanical means. Greek and Roman medical practices as preserved in the writings of Hippocrates and—especially—Galen provided the pattern for later western medicine.

Usage of Herbs as Medicines in Rest of Europe

In early medieval Europe, monasteries tended to become local centres of medical knowledge, and their herb gardens provided the raw materials for simple treatment of common disorders. Herbalists used to wander and provide herbal remedies to the sick and needy. Particularly well-known herbalists of medieval Europe were the so-called wise-women, who prescribed herbal remedies often along with spells and enchantments. However with the wave of missionary movement in the late Middle Ages such women who were knowledgeable in herblore became targets of the witch hysteria. One of the most famous women in the herbal tradition was Hildegard of Bingen, a 12th century Benedictine nun who wrote a medical text called *Causes and Cures*.

Herbal Tradition in the Medieval Islamic World

Medical schools known as Bimaristan began to appear from the 9th century in the medieval Islamic world among Persians and Arabs and they were generally more advanced than those in medieval Europe at the time. As a trading culture, the Arab travellers had access to medical knowledge and plant material from distant places such as India and China. Herbals, medical texts and translations of the classics of antiquity filtered in from east and west. Charaka Samhita and Sushruta Samhita from India were translated into Arabic during the Abbasid of Caliphate (750 AD). Botanists and physicians from the Islamic world significantly expanded on the earlier knowledge of *materia medica*. For example, Al-Dinawari described more than 637 plant drugs in the 9th century and Ibn al-Baitar described more than 1,400 different plants, foods and drugs in the 13th century.

Avicenna's *The Canon of Medicine* (1025 AD) lists 800 tested drugs, plants and minerals, and the healing properties of herbs including nutmeg, senna, sandalwood, rhubarb, myrrh, cinnamon and rosewater are discussed in it. Its Latin translation of the 12th century was a text book of European medical institutes for long. In it Avicenna expresses his indebtedness to Indian doctors and quotes verbatim from Ayurvedic treatises. Baghdad was an important centre for Arab herbalism, as was Al-Andalus between 800 and 1400.

With numerous drugs and spices entering the Arabic world, the flourishing Islamic civilization saw the development of newer and sophisticated palatable medicines, which required elaborate preparation. The specialists who engaged in this were the occupational forerunners of today's pharmacists.

In European countries exposed to Arabian influence such as Spain and southern Italy public pharmacies began to appear. In 1240 Frederick II of Hohenstaufen, who was Emperor of

Germany as well as King of Sicily, codified the responsibilities and the practice of Pharmacy as separate from those of Medicine.

The Book of Simples, authored by Abulcasis (936–1013) of Cordoba is an important source for later European herbals, while the *Corpus of Simples*, by Ibn al-Baitar (1197–1248) of Malaga is the most complete Arab herbal, which introduced 200 healing herbs including tamarind, aconite and nux vomica. Other pharmacopoeia books include those written by Abu-Rayhan Biruni in the 11th century and Ibn Zuhr (Avenzoar) in the 12th century (printed in 1491). The origins of clinical pharmacology also date back to the Middle Ages in Avicenna's *The Canon of Medicine*, Peter of Spain's *Commentary on Isaac*, and John of St Amand's *Commentary on the Antedotary of Nicholas*. The continuing importance of herbs for centuries after the Middle Ages is indicated by the hundreds of herbals published after the invention of printing in the 15th century. Theophrastus's *Historia Plantarum* was one of the first books to be printed, but Dioscorides's *De Materia Medica*, Avicenna's *Canon of Medicine* and Avenzoar's *Pharmacopoeia* were not far behind.

The 15th, 16th and 17th centuries were considered the great age of herbals, as many works on herbals began appearing for the first time in English and other languages rather than in Greek or Latin. The anonymous *Grete Herball* of 1526 was the first herbal to be published in English. *The Herball or General History of Plants* (1597) by John Gerard and *The English Physician Enlarged* (1653) by Nicholas Culpeper are among the other best known herbals in English.

Anglo-Saxon Leechcraft (512–1154)

Herbarium Apuleius (480–1050), one of the most copied manuscripts with uses of over 100 herbs, and the Leech Book of Bald are some of the Herbals of 'Leech' craft—the collective English word for medical practitioners. Some of the earliest herbals known are listed below:

1. *Ornus Sanitatus* (1491) by an unknown author, having many wood cut illustrations copied from an older German work known the *Herbarius Zu Teutsch,* was used in England during much of 16th century as the standard textbook of medicine. It contains quotations from the writings of Arabian (Rhazes and Avicenna), Greek (Dioscorides and Galen) and Roman (Pliny and Cato) authors.
2. *De Historia Stirpium* (1542) by Leonhart Fuchs contains illustrated plant descriptions for the correct identification of plants arranged alphabetically under their Latin names.
3. *A New Herbal* (1551) by William Turner has a scientific account of plants used as 'simples' (plants as drugs in their unprocessed form).
4. Materia Medica (1839) by Pereiras was an encyclopedic collection of information on all available details of actions and descriptions of the then existing drugs of plant, mineral and animal origin.

Era of Pure Drugs

The second millennium in Europe however saw the beginning of a slow erosion of the pre-eminent position held by plants as sources of therapeutic effects. This began with the 'Black death' due to plague and syphilis that raged through Europe, which the then dominant Four Element (referring to the four humors) medical system seemed powerless to stop. A century later Paracelsus (1493–1541), an itinerant Swiss surgeon, with his introduction of active chemical drugs such as arsenic, copper sulphate, iron, mercury and sulphur became an important advocate of chemically prepared drugs. These were accepted even though they had toxic effects because of the urgent need to treat syphilis. Eventually as the efficacy of some of these drugs became known, they entered professional medical practice. This preparation of medicines was an important milestone in the history of pharmacy in the western world. Through the 16th, 17th and 18th centuries subsequent rapid advances in Chemistry made it a separate profession. Isolation of some opium alkaloids in the early 19th century was a key event in the development of modern pharmacy. This was because, it showed that isolated compounds could have the same activity as the crude drug from which they were isolated. This paved the way for introduction of pure compounds for treatment, the corner stone of current modern western medicine.

For a period of about 300 years a small minority of practising pharmacists made significant investigations into the chemistry of drugs, and along the way isolated many drugs used even today and contributed much to the general chemical knowledge.

William Withering (1741–1799) discovered the use of Digitalis from preparations popularly given by an old 'witch' (woman herbalist) doctor for dropsy. Later in 1875 digitoxin, the active fraction of Foxglove, was isolated and its chemical structure identified in 1928. Although the advent of new diuretics and vasodilators has added to the repertoire of heart medicines, there is still no alternative to digitalis for the first line treatment of fast atrial fibrillation.

The great expansion in the knowledge of chemistry in the 19th century, much extended the herbal pharmacopoeia that had previously been established. Building on the work of Lavoisier, chemists throughout Europe refined and extended the techniques of chemical analysis. Acetic acid synthesis by Kolbe in 1845 and methane synthesis by Berthelot in 1856 saw the beginnings of organic chemistry.

Pharmacognosy, which until then dealt with medicinal products of plant, animal or mineral origin in their crude state, was taken over by physiological chemistry. The focus shifted from finding new medicaments from the vast world of plants to finding active principles that accounted for their pharmacological properties.

Earlier isolation of morphine from opium by German apothecary Friedrich Wilhelm Adam Serturner (1783–1841), emetine from Ipecac in 1817 and quinine and cinchonine from Cinchona in 1820 by P.J. Pelletier (1788–1842) and J.B. Caventou (1795–1877), strychnine and brucine from nux vomica in 1818 paved the way for modern phytochemistry, and this was followed by the isolation of several active principles from plant drugs each of which began to get added to the arsenal of pure drugs.

Not only were these pure drugs rapidly adopted by physicians because their potency was assured, but their existence also allowed physiologists to administer drugs accurately during their research, which became the wellspring of modern pharmacology.

Thus commercialization of herbal single ingredients became more apparent and plant drugs popularly used as drugs in several indigenous medical systems began to be screened for newer drugs with enormous success. Reserpine the anti-hypertensive and tranquillizer isolated from *Sarpagandha* or *Rauwolfia serpentina* indicated in Ayurveda for paralysis and insanity, ephedrine the bronchodilator from Ma-Huang of Chinese medicine prescribed for inflammatory conditions, narcotics codeine and morphine from opium are some such drugs isolated from plants of ethnomedical usage. Niemann isolated cocaine in 1860 and the active ingredient, physostigmine, from the Calabar bean in 1864. As a result of these discoveries and the progress made in organic chemistry, the pharmaceutical industry came into being at the end of the 19th century.

In the past two centuries, modern methods of isolation and pharmacological screening have yielded numerous such purified compounds which have proven to be indispensable to modern medicine. These include atropine, bulbocapnine, cocaine, codeine, colchicines, ephedrine, hyoscyamine, ipecac, morphine, papaverine, physostigmine, picrotoxin, pilocarpine, pseudoephedrine, quinidine, reserpine, scopolamine, strychnine and d-tubocurarine.

Parallel developments in related fields namely the invention of the microscope by Zacharias Jansen in 1595, visualization of cells by Robert Hooke in 1665, Joseph Lister's theory of antisepsis, Louis Pasteur's identification of microbial origin of disease were followed by significant advances in medicine and chemistry.

The synthesis of urea in 1828 by German Chemist Friedrich Wöhler from ammonium cyanate gave birth to synthetic organic chemistry. This synthesis of organic molecules, a radical new direction in chemistry combined with more traditional analytical approaches revolutionized chemistry leading to a deep understanding of the fundamental principles of chemical structure and reactivity. The beginning of synthetic medicinal chemistry was made in Germany with the synthesis of chloral hydrate in 1869. This was followed by several others: to name a few, paraldehyde in 1882, sulphone in 1888, phenacetin in 1889 and aspirin in 1899.

Likewise, outstanding work of Paul Ehrlich, discovery of penicillin from fungal source by Alexander Fleming, discovery of sulpha drugs, etc. began adding to the ever-growing arsenal of newer drugs from various sources including plants, microbes and chemical synthesis.

As chemical methods became more prevalent in medical practice, pharmacists were forced to learn new methods of preparation and manipulation. The volume of chemical discoveries made by pharmacists is enormous.

The knowledge related to drugs having become unwieldy with different distinct areas of expertise, the study of medicinal substances which were no longer only plant derived became subdivided into the following areas to be pursued exclusively:

- Pharmaceutical chemistry—including the theory and fundamentals of scientific chemistry with emphasis on chemical substances of medicinal importance.
- Pharmacy or Pharmaceutics—concerned with the modes of treatment of chemicals or crude drugs in the preparation of galenicals and medicines in forms suitable for administration.
- Pharmacology—study of biological effect of drugs on organisms.
- Pharmacognosy—the objective study of crude drugs of animal, vegetable and mineral origin treated scientifically, which meant the study of their structural, physical, chemical and sensory characters including their history, cultivation and collection and other processing they undergo between the supplier and manufacturer.

As can be seen, since *pharmacognosy* is the starting point of all these specializations, it is considered the *mother of other facets of pharmaceutical sciences*.

Herbs as Sources of Drugs: Recent Decline and Current Renaissance

Before 1900 most drugs in orthodox medicine too were plant-derived pure chemicals as against unprocessed plant-based formulations and preparations in other traditional medical streams. Pharmacists dominated the investigation of botanical drugs during the 1700s and 1800s. Interested physicians, pharmacists documented the sources of different plant drugs, making considerable contribution to the nascent science of botany. Combining this proficiency with their skills in manipulative chemistry they continued their search for drugs from medicinal plants.

Despite the successful isolation of several therapeutically useful molecules from plants, there was a setback in the study of plant-derived drugs especially towards the mid-1900s against the backdrop of the following:

- The search was for pure, crystalline chemicals that could be measured accurately and identified chemically. Search, separation, characterization and identification of scores of chemicals contained in plant drugs were both laborious and uneconomical.

- Advances in synthetic chemistry enabled cost-effective total synthesis of several plant-derived drugs like caffeine, theophylline, theobromine, ephedrine, pseudo-ephedrine, emetine, papaverine, levodopa, salicylic acid and tetrahydrocannabinol.

- Several classic plant-derived drugs lost much ground to synthetic competitors. For example, emetine lost its position as an amoebicidal to metronidazole and related nitroimidazoles, and the use of theophylline as a bronchodilator has declined considerably since the arrival of long-acting β_2-adrenergic agonists.

- Antibiotics represented the greatest single contribution of modern drug therapy. Their successful large-scale production resulted in the effective control of several human microbial pathogens that had previously caused incapacitation or death.

- New classes of therapeutic agents, such as corticosteroids, tranquillizers, antidepressants, anti-hypertensives, radioactive isotopes and oral contraceptives were introduced.

- Successful eradication of diseases like small pox through immunization, generation of therapeutic proteins such as human insulin, human growth hormone via genetic manipulation of microbes.

- Generation of several pharmaceutical microbial products such as dextrans, organic acids, vitamins, amino acids, therapeutic enzymes like streptokinase, etc.

- Impressive advances in imaging and other diagnostic equipment including analytical and spectroscopic instrumentation aided quicker disease diagnosis.

The pharmacy which served as an outpost for the relief of suffering and the treatment of minor ailments came to hold preventatives and cures for serious disease. *Interest in studying indigenous medicine as a source of new drugs thus waned on account of the availability of several feasible alternatives for the generation of the needed drugs or so it appeared!*

There has however been an unexpected turnaround. Traditional systems of medicine have become a topic of global importance during the last two decades and the use of traditional medicine has gained popularity. It has not only continued to be used for primary health care of the poor in developing countries, but has also been used in countries where conventional medicine is predominant in the national health care system. Although conventional medicine (CM) is available in these countries, phytomedicines have often maintained popularity for historical and cultural reasons. Concurrently people in developed countries have also begun to turn to alternative therapies including herbal drugs. In these countries popular use of herbal drugs is fuelled by concerns about adverse effects of chemical drugs, questioning of approaches and assumptions of allopathic medicine and greater public access to health information. Today many reasons are given for the resurgence of holistic traditional medicine (Figure 1.1):

- Loss of faith in conventional science as its products have led to reckless exploitation of the environment, depletion of ozone, drug misuse and iatrogenesis.

| Escalating global disease burden – few effective cures for most diseases |

| Conventional Medicine (CM) largely palliative – handling only symptoms |

| Failure of CM to address the patient as a whole as opposed to its view of a patient as collection of organ systems each attended by 'specialists' |

| 'Management only' approach of CM to lifestyle disorders that are assuming epidemic proportions |

| Prohibitive cost of medical care beyond the reach of poor |

| Loss of faith in conventional science whose products are destroying our environment, resources and health |

| Greater access to information and better political freedom has empowered the common man to see through the fallacies and prejudices of 'modern science' |

| Better exposure to 'safer' traditional healing practices due to greater transmigration of people across continents |

Figure 1.1 Resurgence of interest in traditional drugs—possible reasons

- CM has failed to meet continuously rising medical expectations and it seems to have succeeded only in identifying all the major disorders for which there is no easy cure.
- Longer life expectancy has brought with it increased risks of developing chronic debilitating diseases. There is no doubt that CM will probably never fully conquer such old age-related disorders such as bronchitis, arthritis, rheumatism, heart disease, back pain and hypertension. Since these degenerative chronic diseases of old age simply do not respond well even to the most modern treatments, many of these are even considered normal consequences of ageing.
- Aside from the successful 'treatment' of infectious diseases, CM is largely palliative attending only to the symptoms. Diseases like diabetes, hypertension, asthma, arthritis, etc. are

only 'managed' with drugs enabling the patients a better quality of life. There seem not many diseases that can be cured with CM.

- Even with over usage of antibiotics for infections, resurgence of infections with strains that are resistant to many antibiotics is a major challenge to reckon with.
- Rising costs of medical care have neither helped promote efficient use of all the major advancements in medical technology nor have they given better attention to the patient.
- The profit-driven motive of drug designing just to capture a fraction of established markets have led to the addition of more and more 'me too' drugs which really do not promise important therapeutic gains.
- Because of lack of patent protection, pharmaceutical companies are not willing to produce certain natural molecules or even drugs meant for a very small population of sufferers such as orphan diseases.
- Fragmentation of medical knowledge with ever-increasing specialties and super specialties does not seem to address the patient as a whole, leave alone his ailment. Instead of being seen as real persons, patients are merely seen as 'problems' or interesting 'cases' to solve.
- CM's prime concern is the disease, not in the least its origination, prevention, healing or general overall wellness. Its main focus is disease and human organ systems rather than health and its maintenance.
- Increased trade relations, better transportation, greater economic well-being, better political freedom, better communication and transmigration of people across continents have enabled greater interaction and exposure to the holistic nature of traditional medical practices through contacts with migrants who have carried drugs and success stories along with them.
- Traditional therapies appear to offer gentler means of managing chronic debilitating diseases than CM. Some of the best-known evidence for efficacy of a herbal product besides *Artemisia annua* for the treatment of malaria concerns the use of *Mucuna pruriens* for Parkinsonism. Patients express far fewer side effects than when treated with the standard drug levodopa.

A recent survey showed that 78% of patients living with HIV/AIDS in the United States use some form of traditional therapy. Out-of-pocket expenditure for such complementary and alternative medicine is estimated at US$ 2700 million. In Australia, Canada and United Kingdom it is US$ 80, 2400 and 2300 million respectively. Though many of the theories on which alternative therapies are based are not in accord with current medical concepts, many of these therapies have become popular and are in demand by the world populace and these need to be understood by all health practitioners.

It looks like we have reached a state of diminishing returns in CM. There is absolutely no doubt that CM has enabled better health care through the last century. Human life expectancy is greatly enhanced, infantile and maternal mortality at child birth is greatly reduced. CM is best for the management of acute care and definitely one cannot do without the sophisticated instrument-enabled disease diagnosis of today.

However global disease burden is greatly increased due to several factors namely explosive population growth, shedding of traditional dietary habits, massive urbanization, uncontrollable pollution, fast-paced mechanical lifestyle, competitive work ethics, fast-growing consumerism, changing social habits, economy-driven societal needs, etc. While CM is not able to grapple with the skyrocketing proportions of lifestyle-related disorders world over, there are ever-increasing newer diseases, sudden epidemics of infectious viral diseases that seem to strike almost anywhere and everywhere. Overall we seem to be going from one health crisis to another with not many drugs or treatment options to be considered before hundreds of lives are claimed.

What Seems to Have Gone Astray? The Possible Factors

Though science has been a fantastic tool for developing conveniences in our life it is threatening the very existence of this planet. On retrospection it becomes sufficiently clear that scientific progress-enabled modern medical achievements are largely the result of a 'one-sided' approach to nature and its ways. When we look at the epistemological basis of traditional systems world over it is clear that their knowledge systems had a different understanding of nature and its workings. Western scientific paradigms were seen as superior to indigenous paradigms, and what the world faces today is the result of this partisan way of looking at what accounts for 'knowledge'.

Despite the demonstrable historical success in using indigenous knowledge systems to guide drug discovery, there has been considerable resistance to incorporation of information from such knowledge systems into modern programmes of drug discovery. Supremacy of western culture over all other cultures is a deep theme in most of the western world. Since western medicine was regarded as *prima facie* evidence of the intellectual and cultural superiority of western culture, indigenous medicine was consciously denigrated by western academics particularly during the period of colonial expansion. This led to the caricature of indigenous healing practices as superstition. Such denigration by the colonial powers and their academic institutions was incredibly destructive of traditional medical knowledge. In most developing countries the medical infrastructure has been patterned almost entirely after western models. In many countries it even became illegal to practice traditional medicine. Only in the last decade have several nations, including China, Nigeria, Mexico and Thailand, attempted to incorporate traditional medicine into their primary health care systems.

Western science examines studies, interprets, writes about indigenous cultures but never grants them a fundamental role in education and it would never permit them to displace science from the central role it now assumes. Though traditional drugs and guidance of traditional healers was sought in identifying new drugs, no credit is bestowed upon them. They are merely referred to as 'anonymous' informants. Nobody knows the name of the old traditional healer from Shropshire who led William Withering to his discovery of the use of Digitalis. Also there is greater resistance in crediting any scientific discovery if it is not from the west. Though variolation (inoculation of small pox obtained from diseased pustules from patients recovering from the disease) was practised extensively in India and China since ancient times, Edward Jenner, an English country doctor who made similar observations as late as 1750 is referred to as the 'Father of Immunology'. Similarly, fumigating the place of surgery with neem and bdellium leaves prior to surgery was an age old practice predating 1,000 BC in India—which has a strong and enviable medical tradition of surgical practices—Joseph Lister is credited with the discovery of the theory of antisepsis.

As a result of this strong cultural superiority of the west and its nascent antipathy to traditional medical practices, western science remains largely ignorant of indigenous science.

Today for whatever reasons it is no longer possible to impose any medical system on the populace. What works and what is needed becomes the obvious choice. The increasing public demand for traditional medicine has led to considerable interest among policy makers, health administrators and medical doctors in the possibilities of bringing together traditional and modern medicine.

This global resurgence of interest in traditional medicine has been formally acknowledged by the World Health Organization (WHO), which in its traditional medicine strategy 2002–2005 has framed policies to integrate TM/CM with national health care systems. As a part of the strategy to reduce financial burden on developing countries which spend 40–50% of their total health budget on drugs, *WHO currently encourages, recommends and promotes the inclusion of herbal drugs in national health care programmes* because such drugs are easily available at a price within the reach of common man and as such are time tested, and thus considered to be much safer than modern synthetic drugs. Today the global market for herbal products is estimated to be around US$ 62 billion and growing at the rate of 15–20% annually.

LESSONS FROM RESEARCH ON MEDICINAL PLANTS

Concurrent with the resurgence of interest in herb-based therapies and drugs, research efforts centred on plant drugs the past half century offer interesting insights into their uniqueness. A look at these shall help us understand better the factors that culminated in the renewed interest towards plant-derived drugs.

Higher plants are solar-powered biochemical factories which manufacture what they need to survive from air, water and minerals. Many species of higher plants biosynthesize and accumulate extractable organic substances in quantities sufficient to be economically useful. Natural substances are employed either directly or indirectly by a large number of industries and phytochemicals figure prominently in several of these.

Plant Secondary Metabolites—Better Candidate Drugs?

Plant-derived organic compounds may be classified as either primary or secondary metabolites (SMs). Macromolecules such as structural and functional proteins and informational biopolymers such as nucleic acids are generally excluded from this classification. Primary metabolites (PMs) are widely distributed in virtually all organisms in different forms for storage and are also needed for general growth and physiological development, because of their role in primary cell metabolism. Several PMs are being harvested from higher plants since earliest times. Vegetable oils, fatty acids used in soap and detergent making, sucrose, starch, pectin, hydrocolloid gums and cotton are some of these used as industrial raw materials, foods or food additives. Rarely are PMs used as intermediates in the manufacture of semi-synthetic pharmaceutical products.

SMs are biosynthetically derived from primary metabolites, but are more limited in distribution in the plant kingdom, usually being restricted to a particular taxonomic group. Since they are not nutritive and not directly essential for growth, they have no obvious role in the plant primary or mainstream metabolism.

There have been a number of studies to investigate the physicochemical parameters of SM in recent years, and it has been concluded that

- 'Libraries', or collections of these substances, tend to afford a higher degree of 'drug-likeness' when compared to compounds in either synthetic or combinatorial 'libraries'
- Produced by living systems, SMs are subject to transport and diffusion at the cellular level. They are thus capable of modulating protein-protein interactions and therefore can affect cellular processes that may be modified in disease states.
- Compared to synthetic compounds, plant SMs have more protonated amine and free hydroxyl functionalities and more single bonds, with a greater number of fused rings containing more chiral centres.
- They also differ from synthetic products in the average number of halogen, nitrogen, oxygen and sulphur atoms, in addition to their steric complexity.
- They play ecologically significant roles in how plants deal with their environment and are therefore important in their ultimate survival. Plant SMs serve as pollinator attractants or represent chemical adaptations to environmental stress, or they may serve as defensive, protective or offensive chemicals against other higher plants.
- As they serve to combat infectious diseases, aid in weed aggressiveness and discourage herbivores and herbivory, they are by definition biologically/physiologically active compounds.
- SMs being metabolically expensive to produce and accumulate, they are present in plants in much smaller quantities than are PMs.
- Unlike PMs they are biosynthesized in specialized cell types and at distinct developmental stages, making their extraction, isolation and purification difficult.
- Due to their powerful biological activity, they are also economically important as pharmaceuticals, flavours, fragrances, pesticides, etc. Steroidal sapogenins and cardioactive glycosides, alkaloids including anti-cancer *Catharanthus* alkaloids, cocaine, colchicine, opium alkaloids, physostigmine, pilocarpine, quinine, quinidine, reserpine and d-tubocurarine are a few examples.
- Other SMs are being used in limited quantities as pharmacological tools to study various biochemical processes such as phorbol-type diterpenoid esters from croton oil and from lattices of various species of Euphorbia—potent irritant and carcinogens useful in the study of chemical carcinogenesis.

The Chiral Benefit of Natural Compounds

It is to be noted that except for inorganic salts and a few low molecular organic substances, the majority of molecules in living systems—both in plants and animals are chiral. Although these molecules can exist as a number of stereoisomers, almost invariably only one stereoisomer is found in nature. Thus nature is inherently chiral with the building blocks of life namely amino acids, nucleotides and sugars being chiral and they exist in nature in enantiomerically pure forms.

Because the interactions between molecules in living systems take place in a chiral environment, a molecule and its enantiomer will elicit a different physiological response when compared to the same molecule's diastereomer. Thus while α-glucose is metabolically active in living systems its isomer β-glucose is non-assimilable; (+)-epinephrine is a less active adrenergic than (−)-epinephrine.

Today it is known that S-thalidomide is a sedative while its R isomer is teratogenic. The thalidomide catastrophe of the 1960s could have been prevented by marketing its 's' form instead of the racemic drug. When a chemical substance containing a centre of symmetry such as thalidomide is synthesized in the lab, this generally yields a racemate that is a mixture of both enantiomers in equal amounts. Thus commercially available synthetic drugs are racemic and today we know now that this has clinical implications as enantiomers can show important differences in pharmacodynamic and pharmacokinetic behaviour.

It has been shown in a review of 1,522 pharmaceutical substances discovered in the 1960s and 1970s that out of 1,096 synthetics, 422 had an asymmetry centre and as many as 370 of these were not used as enantiomers. In contrast, 424 of the 426 natural and semi-synthetic drugs had an optically active carbon atom and only 2 were not used as enantiomers. This illustrates the selectivity and stereospecificity of natural compounds which is a clear advantage over synthetics.

- Plant SMs often have complex stereostructures with many chiral centres, which may be essential for biological activity. Hence many of these complex biomolecules cannot be synthesized economically on a commercial basis in enantiomerically pure forms. Vincristine, vinblastine and azadirachtin are a few examples.

- Thus SMs are generally recognized to afford a source of small and complex organic molecules of outstanding chemical diversity, which are highly relevant to the contemporary drug discovery process.

- Plant kingdom can thus provide us with unique chemical structures that are unlikely to be synthesized *de novo* on a commercial scale. Anti-cancer drug paclitaxel containing 11 chiral centres with 248 possible diastereomeric forms is a classic example.

- Several SMs often serve additionally as chemical models or templates for the design and total synthesis of new drug entities—e.g., d-tubocurarine for atracurium besylate, visnadin for sodium cromoglycate, podophyllotoxin for etoposide and artemisinin for artemether.

Statistics on Plant Drug Usage

Today natural products and their derivatives represent about 50% of all drugs in clinical use with higher plant-derived natural products representing approximately 25% of the total.

In a review article, Newman et al from the National Cancer Institute pointed out that from 1982 to 2002, approximately 28% of the new chemical entities in western medicine were either natural products per se or derived from natural products. Thus of 1,031 new chemical entities over this 22-year period, 5% were unmodified natural products, and 23% were semi-synthetic agents based on natural product lead compounds. An additional 14% of the synthetic compounds were designed based on knowledge of a natural product 'pharmacophore'.

Further in the 13th revision of the WHO Model List of Essential Medicines, of approximately 300 drugs considered necessary for the practice of medicine, approximately 210 are smaller molecular agents. Of these, more than 40 are unmodified natural products, 25 are semi-synthetic drugs based on natural product prototypes, and more than 70 are either synthetic drugs based on natural product prototype molecules or synthetic mimics of natural products.

Though some plant drugs were replaced by synthetic equivalents, several of them have been studied in recent years to evaluate new uses and/or new dosage forms, providing at least a new therapeutic or investigational impetus in several cases, as can be seen from the examples below:

- Antimalarial quinine is also shown to relieve frequency of nocturnal cramps at an oral dose of 200–300 mg at bedtime.
- Transdermal scopolamine a drug introduced for motion sickness in 1980s is found to be equally effective in the reduction of nausea and vomiting after ear surgery.
- *Cannabis sativa* is the source herb of psychoactive cannabinoids. New synthetic cannabinoids are under development, which have anti-emetic effects without psychotropic activity.
- Apart from its therapeutic utility in asthma, theophylline is also shown to have anti-inflammatory actions at low serum concentrations of $</= 10$ mg/L and may also be used in acute life-threatening asthma attacks to reduce the need for mechanical ventilation.
- Though the use of the cinchona alkaloid quinine as an antimalarial declined with introduction of synthetic antimalarial agents such as chloroquine and mefloquine, its use has been re-established due to the widespread emergence of chloroquine-resistant and multiple drug-resistant strains of malarial parasites. It is being considered to be the drug of choice for several chloroquine-resistant malaria due to *Plasmodium falciparum*.

Lessons From Biotechnology-Aided Drug Discovery/Production

In the era of drug design by chemical synthesis aided by computational and combinatorial techniques, emphasis on the screening of natural products for new drugs by pharmaceutical companies decreased with greater reliance being placed on screening large 'libraries' or collections of synthetic compounds. Natural product extracts have been regarded by some as being incompatible with modern rapid screening techniques and the successful market development of a natural product derived drug as being too time consuming. Also taking out patents on natural compounds is usually more difficult than it is for synthetic substances. With the introduction of newer drugs obtained increasingly through biotechnological processes, it appeared that natural products no longer had any significant role in new drug development.

Advances in cell and molecular biology and the resultant biotechnological breakthroughs have brought about profound repercussions in all aspects of life sciences. Plant cell culture is one such biotechnological tool of growing plant cells, tissues or organs isolated from the mother plant on artificial media. It is an experimental technique through which a mass of cells is produced from the ex-plant tissue. Being unaffected by changes in environmental conditions, studies on production of useful metabolites by plant cell culture have been carried out on an increasing scale since the end of 1950s. Though their results stimulated recent studies on the industrial application of this technology, there are several hurdles to be overcome before successful utilization of this technology and not many drugs are being commercially produced this way today.

Similarly genetic engineering and recombinant DNA technology has made available novel therapeutic enzymes and human therapeutic proteins for the mitigation of several deficiency disorders. Likewise genetic engineering of bacteria or yeast to produce the complex SMs naturally biosynthesized by certain plant species is a difficult task because of the nature of SM biosynthesis. This is because SMs, unlike simple proteins, are not the products of single genes. Instead, they are often complex biomolecules, generally the end products of long, multistep, enzymatically catalysed reaction cascades, i.e., complex biosynthetic pathways involving multiple gene products. It would therefore be a difficult task to assemble and transfer all of the necessary biosynthetic machinery into a foreign microorganism and have it functional to achieve the desired biosynthesis. The greatest long-term potential of genetic engineering and related rDNA-based technologies lies not in the direct production of plant proteins, but in the improvement of the efficiency of the biosynthetic machinery of those plant cells producing extractable plant metabolites of interest. Therefore it is not a simple task to manipulate and genetically engineer plant cells at this level of organization and complexity.

A Fresh New Perspective to Pharmacology

On occasion, a natural product lead compound may help elucidate a new mechanism of interaction with a biological target for a disease state under investigation. Natural products may serve to provide molecular inspiration in certain therapeutic areas for which there are only a limited number of synthetic lead compounds.

Thus natural product research can make substantial contributions to drug innovation by presenting us with novel mechanism of action, such as stabilization of cellular microtubules by paclitaxel or the topoisomerase-I inhibiting activity of camptothecin. Similarly yohimbine derived from yohimbe bark and structurally related to reserpine, unlike classic α-antagonists like phentolamine and phenoxybenzamine, is much more active at presynaptic α_2-adrenoreceptors than at post synaptic vascular α_1-adrenoreceptors. This selectivity makes it a useful pharmacological probe for studying adrenergic innervation.

Remarkably even crude herbal preparations can find a useful niche as pharmacological research tools. While the therapeutic role of ipecacuanha as an emetic in drug poisonings has declined, emesis induced by this herb still has a niche as a useful model for testing the therapeutic activity of new anti-emetic drugs.

Ginseng is an herb, the pharmacological activity of whose extracts and constituents has given a new perspective to drug-activity correlation. The spectrum of activities associated with this herb and its constituents are quite inconsistent with the unidimensional activity patterns so far attributed to drugs. An ancient and time-honoured drug in Chinese medicine, the roots of *Panax quinquefolius* or ginseng is one of the major botanical drugs of US foreign trade. Containing a complex mixture of steroidal and pentacyclic triterpenoid saponins, the drug acts 'favourably' on metabolism, central nervous system (CNS) and endocrine secretions. Thoroughly studied by modern methods of analysis, it is also constituted of groups of high molecular weight polysaccharides and acetylenic compounds and D group vitamins in addition to the major saponins. A baffling array of activities ranging from hypoglycaemic, anti-ulcer, immunomodulatory, anti-tumour to hypotensive effects are reported for its constituents. Employed in Asia for the treatment of anaemia, diabetes, gastritis, sexual impotence, insomnia, neurasthenia, etc., arising from old age, it is also an extremely popular remedy in the recent years in the west for improvement of stamina, concentration, resistance to stress and to disease. The drug is described as an 'adaptogenic' since it helps the body adapt to stress in general. The refreshingly new activity profile of this drug has given new research impetus to drugs like ashwagandha used for similar indications in Indian traditional medicine.

As modern science begins to appreciate the complexities of living systems, it is rediscovering principles that may be consistent with oriental insights. For example the medicinal properties of water, its ability to rid the body of disease-permeating factors through a unique residual memory effect has been extensively explained in the verses of Atharvana Veda. These references have been discounted as an extrapolation of the solvent properties of water. However today the concept of water memory proposed by Jacques Benveniste, a French immunologist, though not consistent with currently accepted scientific laws, is published in *Nature*. This work has gained support from a section of the scientific community open to paranormal claims. With further experimentation it is possible that this claim may be proven right thereby scientifically validating the references in Atharvana Veda.

Multicomponent Herbals Versus Single Chemical Entities

The early years of the 21st century appeared opportune for renewed efforts to be made in regard to the discovery of new SMs and prototype biologically active compounds from animals, fungi, microorganisms and plants of both terrestrial and marine origin. Despite huge investments in combinatorial chemistry and natural product drug discovery, there have been disappointing numbers of single chemical entities being introduced as drugs in recent years. An unfortunate sequel to the introduction of new drugs at the end of a long-drawn pre-approval testing period following huge investments is the rapidity with which they are withdrawn from the market on grounds of new evidence of toxicity.

Concurrently, the last three decades have seen widespread use of herbal drugs with renewed popularity of phytomedicines world over. Herbal remedies are prescription products in Germany and several other countries of Western Europe. During the last decade, there has been a large influx of botanical products into community pharmacy practice and health food stores in the United States as a result of the Dietary Supplement Health and Education Act in 1994. A parallel increased interest in herbal remedies has occurred in Europe, Canada and Australia, in part because of an overall greater awareness of complementary and alternative therapies. This has opened a new door of research inquiry for natural product scientists world over.

- Some of the most popular and widely sold phytomedicines such as Indian gooseberry (*Emblica officinalis*), turmeric (*Curcuma longa*), ashwagandha (*Withania somnifera*), ginseng (*Panax quinquefolius*), valerian (*Valeriana wallichii*), ginkgo (*Ginkgo biloba*), St. John's wort (*Hypericum perforatum*), etc., have considerable pharmacological and clinical evidence to support their use.
- These herbs are used in whole or as extracts in Ayurveda and traditional Chinese medicine (TCM). Combinations of herbs are fundamental to the philosophy of these systems and have been so used traditionally, much similar to the usage of multiple drugs for treating a single complaint such as hypertension, psychoses and cancer in CM. This applies also to single-plant extracts which are mixtures of several phytoconstituents.
- It is rather uncommon to find a pure molecule showing more activity than that shown by the parent extract. Since the individual molecules may not be sufficiently active to achieve the desired effect, most efforts in plant research are unable to reach a critical stage of identification of a prospective biomolecule and its final development to an effective drug.

- Today it is accepted that unlike compounds approved as single-chemical drugs, combinations of plant SMs are responsible for the physiological effects of herbal medicines. For example both the terpene lactone (e.g. Ginkgolide B) and flavonoid glycoside constituents of *Ginkgo biloba* leaves are regarded as being necessary for mediation of the symptoms of peripheral vascular disease, for which this phytomedicine is used in Europe.

- Thus attempts are not being made to isolate individual components from popular herbal remedies of long-time history of usage that are sold as standardized extracts. In several cases, the single active ingredient is either not known (St. John's wort) or is unstable (ginger).

- Thorough phytochemical analysis of several herbal remedies has failed to yield a single active ingredient if not a novel chemical entity. Such an analysis has revealed them to be mixtures of well-known groups of compounds, such as polyphenols (myrobalans), polysaccharides (ginseng, gymnema, aconite, dioscorea), simple organic acids (garcinia), flavonoids (*Pterocarpus marsupium*), steroids (ficus, ginseng, m*Momordica charantia*), etc. Thus the main active ingredients of even such drugs as St. John's wort (*Hypericum perforatum*) are still under discussion.

- This has opened up understanding of the concept of 'Synergism' to explain the efficacy and superiority of single herbs and polyherbals over single chemical entities.

- Synergy broadly means a beneficial interaction of the constituents of a single herb or a polyherbal mixture resulting in greater combined effect than would be expected from a consideration of individual contributions of each of the constituents. The interaction between the component constituents may involve a potentiation of therapeutic effects or an attenuation of toxicity or side effects within the preparation. The effect may be truly synergistic or additive.

- Generally a substantial decrease in toxicity levels is observed when whole plant extracts are compared with individual molecules derived from a plant even when used in the same proportion as found in the whole plant.

- Medical herbalists today insist that better results are obtained with whole plant extracts rather than with isolated compounds.

- Plants being subjected to selection pressure have, over millions of years, developed optimal chemical defences to resist threats such as radiation, reactive oxygen species and microbial attack in order to survive. The multicomponent composition of herbs thus simultaneously addresses effectively the causative factors of multifactorial human diseases better than single pure drugs.

- The benefits of multicomponent drugs may reside not only in enhancing therapeutic action through bioavailability improvement, but also in permitting the use of lower doses.

- Diseases are caused by a multiplicity of factors and complications rather than due to a single gene, receptor, enzyme or protein resulting in both visible and invisible symptoms. Illustrations of failed drugs that target a single protein and ignore a sophisticated network system of disease processes are numerous. Allelochemicals of a single plant can have complementary and overlapping activities on human physiology thus bringing relief.

- For example the side effects of ephedrine are not usually found with an extract of the herb Ephedra. Likewise initially whole extracts of *Rauwolfia* root were used clinically for their anti-hypertensive effects. The growing dominance of the reductionist model of reducing the extract to its active component however pushed chemists to isolate reserpine and use it as a drug. Relatively an effective and safe anti-hypertensive when combined with a thiazide diuretic, reserpine has been unjustly discarded from drug use, on grounds of adverse effects actually associated with the drug at doses higher than required to cause a hypotensive effect. The whole extract was safe and had better overall efficacy as a hypertensive and a calming sedative effect owing to synergism between the alkaloids and other constituents of *Rauwolfia*.

- Synergistic enhancement of activity has been reported with multiple herb combinations of several drugs of Ayurveda, TCM and European herbalism.
- Further research to demonstrate synergy and polyvalent action in phytomedicines has reported the attenuation of toxicity effect of herbs such as liquorice in polyherbals. Its detoxifying effect is due to an unspecified interaction of the non-glycyrrhizin components of liquorice during intestinal absorption. This reduces the bioavailability of glycyrrhizin as well as the actives of other drugs such as aconitine of aconite, etc.
- But then piperine of pepper is demonstrated to be a bioavailability enhancer of other drugs, probably as a result of its potent inhibitor effect on drug metabolism. Its inclusion in Ayurvedic drugs such as 'trikatu' is possibly to reduce the needed dosage of other drugs critical for activity.
- Synergy is implicated in the anti-ulcer effect of ginger widely used for its anti-emetic, anti-ulcer effect. A range of chemically unstable compounds probably acting synergistically are responsible for its anti-ulcer activity.
- Likewise it has been demonstrated that the anxiolytic effect of tetrahydrocannabinol, the main psychoactive ingredient of cannabis, is beneficially modulated by the psychoactive cannabidiol also present in it, thus producing an overall relaxant effect by the resin drug.
- It has been established that the physiological activity of herbs is the resultant effect of a variety of constituents interacting with each other synergistically, additively or modulatorily.
- Evidence such as decreased microbial resistance to antibiotics with herbal drug co-administration is accumulating to demonstrate clearly the therapeutic benefits of poly pharmacy.
- The age old wisdom of the benefits of using whole plant extracts over single drugs in traditional medicine has now been elevated in status from being a 'superstition' to 'science' in the understanding of modern medicine.

Pharmaceutical researchers recognize the concept of drug synergism but note that clinical trials may be used to investigate the efficacy of a particular herbal preparation. It is today conventional practice to use cocktails of chemotherapeutic agents for better treatment of cancer and AIDS. Whatever may be the mechanism involved, understanding the polyvalent action of herbal remedies is very essential towards developing methods of standardization.

Standardization of Herbal Drugs

Need for quality control

The methods of quality control of pure drugs, either plant derived or synthetic, is today well established with standards covering authenticity, general quality, purity and assay. The situation regarding the quality of numerous herbal drugs used by manufacturers or sold directly to the public is by no means well established. From a conventional pharmacological perspective, herbal medicines taken in whole form cannot generally guarantee a consistent dosage or drug quality, since certain samples may contain more or less of a given ingredient. Quality control of even popular herbal remedies based on traditionally used formulae and methods is a challenge, especially because they are now mass produced in contrast to the one-to-one careful dispensing of these recipes by the physicians of yore. Then the obligation to quality was implicit with no external drivers or standards to be adhered to.

In the present times, the need for standardization is all the more imperative as herbal drug preparation has now moved from a small scale to mass production by stakeholders whose primary objective is mass salability and of course profit. Large-scale production of herbal drugs has only started in the last 100 years or so. Now that the commercialization of herbal medicine has happened, the onus of maintaining its quality is shared by all concerned with its development. Herbal market being poorly regulated in many countries, the assurance of safety, quality and efficacy of herbal products has become an important issue.

Herbs different from pure drugs

Because of their natural diversity it is not possible to describe all herbs and herbal products as a single entity. The herbal raw material is prone to a lot of variation due to several factors, the important ones being the identity of the plants, seasonal variation, the ecotypic, genotypic and chemotypic variations, drying and storage conditions and the presence of xenobiotics. Unlike pure drugs, herbal drugs are complex mixtures of constituents of a single herb or several of them. It is therefore much more difficult to characterize such complex mixtures than a pure compound. Hence standardizing herbal drugs using approaches developed for pure drugs is not going to work. Though the advancements in modern methods of analysis and the development of their application have made it possible to solve many of these problems, development of standards for plant-based drugs is a challenging task and needs innovative and creative approaches different from routine methods. There is an urgent need to ensure quality of the ever-expanding volume of herbals that manage to reach the market.

The WHO stresses the importance of the quantitative and qualitative methods of characterizing samples, quantification of biomarkers and/or chemical markers and the fingerprint profiles. These products should be free of adulteration; free of deliberately added non-authentic plant material which may be biologically active or inactive; other additives such as herbicides, pesticides, heavy metals and solvent residues; and also free of microbial and other biological contaminants. Methods of standardization should take into consideration all aspects that contribute to the quality of herbal drugs.

A number of official monographs for the standardization of botanicals have been developed in countries across the world. Monographs of plant materials of long-established commercial use are being developed similar to pure drugs. Research and evaluation of herbal medicines without a long history of usage or those which have not been previously researched should follow regulations of WHO's Research Guidelines for Evaluating the Safety and Efficacy of Herbal Medicines.

Other scientific challenges regarding herbal remedies are to establish more completely their dissolution, bioavailability and shelf life.

One of the first requirements in herbal drug development is the need to create a uniform product for controlled, double blind, cross over, placebo-controlled clinical trials.

Standardized herbals—approaches and drawbacks

1. One approach is the use of a specified ratio of raw materials to solvent. Since different specimens of even the same plant species may vary in chemical content, Thin Layer Chromatography (TLC) is sometimes used by growers to assess the content of their products before use.

   For this purpose although official standards are necessary to control the quality of the crude drugs used, their use does raise certain problems. To accommodate considerable variation that occurs between different batches of a natural product, it is necessary to set low standards which allow the use of commercial material available in any season. This results in the tendency of suppliers to reduce all of their material to the lowest requirement.

2. If the 'active principles' of an herbal remedy are known or can be discovered, these substances can act as reference standards, and their specified concentration levels can be quantified in chemical quality-control procedures, which are predominantly preformed by High Performance Liquid Chromatography (HPLC). The extract is prepared by adjusting to a high degree of concentration the active ingredient. Such extracts offer the opportunity to use herbs in a more specific way for specific predetermined therapeutic objectives. Ginkgo leaf standardized to 24% flavonglycosides is used to increase blood circulation especially to the brain instead of its more traditional use by the Chinese as a tonic for the lungs.

   Examples of active constituent extracts are ginkgo (24% flavonglycosides), milk thistle (80% silymarin), grape seed (95% polyphenols), turmeric (95% curcumin), saw palmetto (90% free fatty acids), green tea (60% catechins), cascara sagrada (20–30% anthraquinones), bilberry (25% anthocyanosides), pygeum (12% phytosterol), kava (30–40% kavalactones).

   This approach regulates a specific biochemical constituent to a level that may not be naturally found in the plant. Concentrating 95% curcuminoids, for instance, in a standardized turmeric extract creates a product that, while derived from the crude herb, is not expected to be naturally found concentrated at that level. This leaves only 5% of the other turmeric constituents with which the curcumin is combined thus displacing other constituents which may be responsible for the biological activity of the herb.

   One of the principal issues with extracts standardized to a high degree of concentration of an active ingredient is that they limit the range of the herb's influence. Well-known medicinal herbs such as turmeric, garcinia, milk thistle and commiphora have several indications. A complex range of chemicals gets excluded from these herbs as a consequence of standardizing them to a high concentration of specific active constituents, causing the herb to lose its more varied and diverse traditional functions.

   Thus turmeric extracts standardized to a high curcumin content cannot be used in the manner Ayurveda prescribes it, i.e., for promoting blood circulation and to improve digestion. This is because while turmeric is classified as a thermogenic drug-stimulating metabolism, standardized turmeric extract with 95% curcumin is more cooling and it is a more effective anti-inflammatory, but is not as effective a digestant or circulatory stimulant.

   In the case of certain herbs, the active ingredients are not found to be exclusively responsible for the activity. Other constituents are eventually identified to be more active biologically. Thus, promoting an herb as a standardized extract overlooks the spectrum of uses it covers. For e.g. milk thistle extract, though sold specifically as a hepatoprotective, is actually also indicated for promotion of pelvic blood circulation in dysmenorrhoea, amenorrhoea and irregular passive uterine haemorrhages.

3. Another method is standardization on a signal chemical. It may be a known active constituent or a marker compound not necessarily the active constituent but that which is satisfactorily measurable. Extracts standardized with respect to a marker chemical are not based on the concentration of an established active constituent. Instead they represent a specified amount of a specifically selected biochemical constituent, characteristic of the plant, so selected for positive identification or to create a higher degree of uniform potency. E.g. Feverfew, Ginseng (5–15% ginsenosides), brahmi (10% asiaticosides), liquorice (12% glycyrrhizin), green tea (20–50% polyphenols), Ephedra (6–8% ephedrine/pseudoephedrine), etc. Marker extracts that contain all constituents in a proportion similar to the herb retain more relationship to the traditional way herbs are used.

Issues with herbal drug standardization

While it is true that standardization attempts arose out of the need to deliver a quality-assured product, the situation has become all the more complex with the introduction of the so-called standardized herbal drugs.

- It is seen that 'standardized' herbals may not have the intended traditional functions attributed to the original formulae since they have now been strengthened with respect to a particular constituent for purposes of quality control.
- While a standardized extract can ensure that sufficient amounts of the herb's constituents (marker compounds?) are present to deliver an efficacious product, standardization presents herbs as medicines in a way that is fundamentally different from the way they were traditionally meant to be given.
- Standardization renders herbal drugs into 'phytopharmaceuticals', which are more drug-like forms rather than herbs used in the traditional sense. Once a herb is regarded as a phytopharmaceutical, it is a short stretch for it to be considered as just another drug.
- Many herbs sold as standardized extracts are not consistently standardized to one marker, because it is not clear which of the constituents are responsible for their therapeutic action. Nettle root is standardized by one company to 5% amino acids, by another to 8% sterols, and a third uses 35 ppm scopoline. Likewise Echinacea can be standardized to at least three different constituents (echinosides, polysaccharides and polybutylides) and each is used as a marker by different companies.
- According to Joerg Gruenwald one of the editors for the German Commission E Monographs—one of the standard books on medicinal herbs and plant products in the western world, only 5% of botanicals are standardized to the one and only known active constituent. A maximum of 10–15 botanicals have undergone well-controlled clinical trials and it is doubtful whether all of them will hold up to Food and Drug Administration (FDA) standards.
- Standardization cannot be equated with efficiency and potency. While they may offer no advantage in terms of efficacy over the use of more traditional high-quality herbal products, developing a truly standardized extract would require such tremendous technology that not only will smaller companies that can manufacture quality products due to lesser quantity requirements be pushed out of the picture, but the technology applied to botanicals also will increase prices dramatically.

- This means that using a quality non-analysed herb product might be just as well or even better than a standardized extract based on known active ingredients. Also it will be cheaper in cost and even the quality of herb used is likely to be superior because the manufacturer would be selecting herbs based more on quality than quantity.
- According to Dr. Rudolf Bauer, one of the leading botanical research scientists in Germany, the three primary reasons for the standardization of herbs into phytopharmaceutical drugs are as follows:

  1. To be regarded as rational drugs, they need to be standardized and pharmaceutical quality must be approved.
  2. For pharmacological, toxicological and clinical studies, the composition of the herbal drugs needs to be well documented to produce reproducible results.
  3. WHO has published guidelines to ensure reliability and repeatability of research on herbal medicines.

- Herbs, unlike chemical drugs, themselves are not patentable. However, a standardized product used for research is patentable for the process of extraction and standardization.
- The high cost of standardization and patentability instigates more commercial interest rather than a desire to heal or to understand herbal medicine. As a result it seems like the pharmaceutical industry, the medical establishment and the herbal industry are more interested in capitalizing on the union of herbal medicine and science by making it more acceptable within their paradigm rather than being interested in being transformed by holistic herbal medicine.
- The regulation of herbal drug quality is thus an area of controversy. Some herbalists opine that herbs of long history of use do not require the level of safety testing as pure drugs. Others favour legally enforced quality standards, safety testing and prescription by a qualified practitioner.
- Thus while herbalists call for a category of regulation for herbal products, some others believe it can be managed through reputation without government intervention at the same time agreeing to the need for more quality testing. Also the legal status of herbal drugs varies from country to country.
- Presently there are shortcomings in currently used standardization methods and a better way of standardization may be a biochemical standardization on the majority of active constituents.
- Many processes of standardization are not standardized. To truly standardize every variable concerning the growth, harvest and preparation of a plant must be controlled. The very many variables related to plants in terms of components, interactions and interdependencies make it impossible to control by merely controlling one or a limited number of active constituents.
- One of the premises of standardizing herbal drugs is that before the availability of standardized herbal extracts, most herbal products were inferior.
- Historically there have been highly sophisticated methods of herbal extraction and processing. They abound in folkloric, traditional Ayurvedic, Chinese and western herbal medicine.

- Some of these methods such as detoxification of aconite by preparing it with salt and/or long boiling decoction are the mainstay of TCM.

- Ayurvedic medicine employed many ingenuous and complex methods of extracting, concentrating and preparing herbs for specific conditions. In this regard, purified guggulsterones are traditionally extracted from crude guggul resin (*Commiphora mukul*) in a botanical decoction consisting of equal parts of chebulic myrobalan, embolic myrobalan and beleric myrobalan, a formula widely known in India as Triphala.

- Thus it is possible to guarantee optimal levels of all plant ingredients without laboratory analysis by paying attention to the right growing requirements of the plant, best stage for harvest, right time of the day optimum for yielding the highest levels of all known 'active' constituents. Other factors such as proper drying and storage are also required to be adhered to. All of this requires training and experience thus making herbal medicine both an art and science.

- For thousands of years herbalists have been using and prescribing herbs both singly as well as in complex formulas with utmost attention to quality. Considering that we know very little not only about the complex chemical compounds they are constituted of, but even less about their synergistic relationship to each other and how they affect therapeutic activity, there is no need to abandon the use of traditional formulas.

- Though standardized extracts can be based on many markers, apart from enhancing the cost of processed herbs, it has little relevance to clinical herbal practice. By the generation of such highly priced and heavily promoted prescription herbal drugs by large herbal drug manufacturers, there may be further devaluation of already demonstrated, quality non-chemically standardized products.

- At this point it is difficult to access the potency and efficacy of these artificially standardized herbal products over whole, non-standardized herbs. While they have very specific applications compared to commercial, non-analysed whole herbal products, they might not always be the best choice.

- Further studies to compare the effect of standardized biochemical extracts with whole herbs or traditional herbal formulations are much needed.

- Thus while high doses of herbs as standardized extracts have their place in modern herbal medicine, they should not displace the use of herbs in other forms.

Other issues related to quality of herbal drugs

Toxcity risks and adverse effects

Herbal medicine is not free from toxicity. A natural poison can kill as efficiently as a synthetic one. Many herbal remedies can cause harmful drug interactions when accidentally substituted or taken along with conventional medicines. Eg., Aristolochia fangchi when consumed as a substitute for an anti-density chinese herb has been reported to induce chronic nephropathy in women. Likewise St. John's wort products decrease plasma concentrations of several prescription drugs such as alprazolam, cyclosporine, dijoxin, oral contraceptions etc. This is because hyperforin in St. John's wort induces cytochrome P450 enzymes.

Common fruits like cranberry also interfere with this enzyme – critical to drug metabolism. This is a cause for concern when such fruits are taken along with many herbal drugs.

Herbal drugs in widespread use are also associated with adverse reactions. Eg., Chronic liquorice ingestion is attributed with potassium depletion.

The question of metals in traditional drugs

Metals and minerals are an important aspect of Siddha medicine—an ancient system of indigenous medicine practiced in south India. Formulations containing a significant proportion of heavy metals such as mercury, arsenic, copper, etc., have been prescribed since centuries with no reports of toxicity. Several such formulations are successfully used in the management of diseases such as cancer and AIDS. Concerns have been raised over their presence in these medicines. Siddha practitioners claim that the mode of preparation of the drug renders them non-toxic. Metals are claimed to be completely transformed into inert compounds or ores through a multistep processing involving extremely high temperatures before being prescribed as medicines. Several papers have reported experimental proof of non-toxicity of several such formulations. However questions remain about the safety of these preparations till appropriate methods of analysis can actually reveal the difference in the elemental nature of these metals post absorption in the body. This may be much similar to the current knowledge of the differences in the absorption, bioavailability and ability to be retained in bone tissue of different forms of calcium. The high heat and presence of other plant-based preparations (that could chelate) in the extract could be altering the very nature of the metals post processing. Innovative methods of elemental analysis of these preparations along with that of the raw material shall be supportive evidence that can substantiate the claims of safety of these drugs in animal experimentation.

Activity evaluation

- Biological evaluation is often the only method of evaluation in the case of herbals which have been evaluated based on certain physicochemical parameters only. Either the active ingredient is not known or is too unstable to be used as a marker.
- Evaluating traditional remedies biologically by modern standards is beset with a number of difficulties. Apart from the wide variation in the quantity of pharmacologically active substances in plants, many findings of therapeutic efficacy are more subjective than objective.
- The modern scientist has difficulty recognizing subjective experiences because no reliable methodology has been developed to measure and reproduce such experiences. Subjective experience is limited as senses vary in ability and reality for one is unreality for another. For example patients with osteoarthritis experienced substantial and highly significant improvement in pain and disability with no significant side effects with a certain herbal drug treatment. However since the radiological findings did not improve, there was no way for its efficacy to be scientifically recorded.
- Several herbs of proven therapeutic efficacy in traditional medicine wait to be understood, identified and introduced into mainstream modern herbal medicine, because of the inability to prove their therapeutic efficacy by modern methods of activity assessment.
- In the context of measurement of subjective aspects, using tools of quantitative, technical science to describe biologic and living systems' phenomenon one soon encounters limits. Usually artificial distinctions are imposed to reduce variables and to interpret non-linear events.

- There is therefore an urgent need to arrive at newer methods of bioactivity measurement, especially subjective phenomenon. This calls for lateral methods of devising with fresh approaches by collaborative efforts of specialists from modern medicine, traditional medicine, phytochemists, analytical chemists, biomedical engineers, etc.

Limited Scientific Study on Plants—Disappearing World Flora

- Plant kingdom has been a time-tested source of drugs, considering the fact that plant-derived natural products represent a large proportion of drugs in clinical use. Despite this, it is a fact that about 85% of the existing 250,000–500,000 species of higher plants have not been so far surveyed for biological activity.

- Despite spectacular advances in extraction technology, separation science, analytical instrumentation not much is known about the SM composition of most of the world's higher plants. 5–15% of plants that have been surveyed so far have been screened mostly for a single type of biological activity. Hence, plant SMs being genus or even species specific, a huge resource of undiscovered and potentially useful drugs are yet to receive scientific attention. For example, more than half of the plants in the tropics that contain most of the world's plant species have never been phytochemically studied. It is estimated that the chemistry of 99% of the plant species comprising the vast flora of the Brazilian rainforest remains unknown.

- This limited scientific study on higher plants is especially a serious concern considering the current rate of extinction and decimation of tropical floras and ecosystems.

- One of the first drug plants to be rendered extinct in the ancient world was Silphium (*Ferula* sp.), a birth-control agent highly valued by ancient Romans. Its employment as a contraceptive was so widespread that this difficult-to-cultivate plant no longer existed in the Mediterranean area or anywhere else, after 3rd century AD.

- Many unrecorded valuable medicinal plants like 'soma' mentioned by legendary Ayurvedic physicians such as Charaka have been unavailable ever since prehistoric times, so much so they are considered mythical plants.

- Climate change, increasing population making demands on land and resources, as well as commercial exploitation of the environment all play a part in this and result in loss of habitats.

- Today tropical rainforests are under threat of such habitat destruction. Several species endemic to biodiversity 'hotspot' areas—said to represent 44% of all vascular plant species and 35% of all vertebrate species in about 1.4% of the earth's surface—are threatened with extinction due to massive habitat loss.

- Some 400 medicinal plants including *Taxus* sp.ecie, *Hoodia* sp.ecie (e.g. *Hoodia gordonii* used as appetite suppressant in Namibia), many magnolia species (ancient genus under Magnoliaceae), crocus species (source of valuable saffron) have been identified as being at risk of extinction from over collection and deforestation as per a 2008 report from the Botanic Gardens Conservation International—a consortium representing botanic gardens across 120 countries.

- Global boom in exploiting plant resources for newer drugs has brought up several issues related to farming practices. For example, ginseng is being field farmed to produce enough ginseng to meet rising demand. Unlike wild-growth ginseng, field-raised ginseng is susceptible to fungus, making fungicide contamination of the drug a problem to be dealt with. Sandalwood, echinacea, black cohosh, which are to be collected from root/wood growth often in excess of 50 years, are now being collected from younger trees. It is not known if the same medicinal effect will be ensured in these.

- Not much time is left before the disappearing flora could be adequately catalogued and studied. We are losing out on the significant opportunity of surveying our plant resources for therapeutically useful compounds. The imminent extinction or increasing rarity of species is thus a loss of potential new drugs in the coming years.

- Another disturbing fallout of biodiversity erosion is the irretrievable loss of basic affordable or valuable medicines of local inhabitants and ethnic groups of these biodiversity regions.

- While disappearance of the world's biodiversity and habitats is a serious issue being realized world over, not much attention is being paid to the imminent loss of local traditional medical knowledge which may not last long.

- Apart from disturbance of ecosystems due to overexploitation and climate change, breakdown of traditional living patterns, urbanization and westernization of societies is leading to irretrievable loss of ethnomedical knowledge systems.

Conservation Efforts

Convention on biodiversity

Sustainable utilization of biodiversity, its conservation as well as those of associated knowledge systems is an urgent priority of action for the biodiversity-rich South Asian nations that are home to about 1/5th of the vascular plants of the world.

- Convention on Biodiversity (CBD) is a legally binding international treaty established in 1992, motivated by the recognition of the importance of conserving our natural biodiversity towards supporting human life. Developing national strategies for the conservation and sustainable utilization of biodiversity is its prime objective. This treaty was opened for signature at the Earth Summit in Rio de Janeiro in 1992 and entered into force in 1993.

- Other key objectives of CBD are ensuring conservation of biodiversity through sustainable utilization of its components and implementation of fair and equitable sharing of benefits arising from its use.

- These CBD objectives are ratified by 175 countries and concepts of sovereignty of states over their genetic resources, their obligation to facilitate access are within its framework. It also covers issues pertaining to measures and incentives for conservation and sustainable utilization of biodiversity.

- The United Nations Organization (UNO) has declared 2011–2020 as the decade of biodiversity. Global Strategy for Plant Conservation (GSPC) is a programme under CBD—a 16-point plan aimed at slowing plant extinction rate around the world by 2010.

Lessons from Research on Medicinal Plants

✓ Plant secondary metabolites have more drug like-ness and better modulate cellular processes affected by disease states.

✓ Their chirality is a clear advantage as interactions between molecules in living systems take place in a chiral environment.

✓ Plants are a treasure trove of amazingly complex molecules of outstanding chemical diversity that are NOT feasible for chemical synthesis on a commercial basis.

✓ Today natural products and their derivatives represent about 50% of all drugs in clinical use with higher plant-derived natural products representing approximately 25% of the total.

✓ Genetically manipulating plant cells to generate secondary metabolites is difficult as they are not products of single genes.

✓ Natural product research has unravelled novel action mechanisms and concepts that are redefining the erstwhile 'drug activity' equation.

✓ Multiconstituent herbs/extracts/polyherbals simultaneously and effectively address the causative factors of multifactorial human diseases better than pure single drugs.

✓ Attempts to prepare standardized herbal drugs using approaches applicable to pure drugs compromise on their intended traditional functions/biological activity thus discounting on their holism.

✓ Though relatively safe, herbal drugs can precipitate unwanted herb-drug interactions.

✓ Metal-based traditional drugs should be subjected to newer evaluation methods before being relinquished as toxic.

✓ Several herbs of proven therapeutic efficacy in traditional medicine wait to be understood, identified and introduced into mainstream modern herbal medicine, because of the inability to prove their therapeutic efficacy by modern methods of activity assessment.

✓ Natural biodiversity conservation efforts must be the urgent priority of all global and national policies.

- Within the framework of the convention are the concepts of the sovereignty of states over genetic resources and their obligation to facilitate access. The contracting parties are expected to establish measures for benefit sharing in the event of commercial utilization. This involves collaboration between the collector, the source country and the industrial partner.

Indian Initiative—National Biodiversity Strategy and Action Plan

- National Biodiversity Strategy and Action Plan (NBSAP) is the principal instrument of CBD at the national level. The goals and objectives of CBD are implemented through national laws, which integrate conservation initiatives of various bodies involving farmers, indigenous local communities, land owners, academia such as universities, botanical institutes, etc.

- A signatory to CBD, NBSAP is formulated by the Ministry of Environment and Forests and it has envisaged a comprehensive action plan for conserving biodiversity in India.

- It has recommended strong measures calling for huge reorientation of the process of economic development and governance of natural resources, such that the health of the environment and interests of biomass-dependent communities are protected.
- These recommendations are already being implemented in nine states, with the support of NGOs such as Kalpavriksh Environmental Action Group. The administration of this NGO is coordinated by the Biotech Consortium of India Ltd through 33 state level, 18 local level and 10 interstate level plans.
- The initiatives being implemented include the following:
  1. Building up scientific expertise and skilled human resource personnel in the areas of Biosystematics, Conservation Biology and medicinal plant resources.
  2. Newer agrotechnology development for medicinal plant cultivation at village level thereby generating employment.

FOCUS OF PHARMACOGNOSY

In the early 20th century, pharmacognosy was basically concerned with the description and identification of drugs both in the whole state and in powder form. Today the subject has expanded enormously into other areas. Botanical aspects being still of fundamental importance for pharmacopoeial identification and quality control purposes, currently microbes and even marine organisms are of pharmacognostical interest. It is an interdisciplinary subject incorporating phytochemistry, analytical chemistry, biochemistry, SM biogenesis, plant cell and tissue *in vitro* propagation, ecology, ethnobotany, microbiology and chemical taxonomy to name a few.

With the aforementioned changes in the global scenario with respect to the use of herbal drugs, the explosive growth of the herbal drug industry, the booming trade in plant-based raw materials and products, recognition of the scientific community of the need to integrate herb-based therapies and drugs into mainstream medicine, WHO's promotion of the same, escalating global disease burden driving the medical fraternity to look at indigenous medical knowledge systems are some of the factors that have hugely expanded the scope, focus and field of pharmacognosy.

Today Pharmacognosy includes the study of the following fields:

- Medical ethnobotany, the study of traditional use of plants for medicinal purposes;
- Ethnopharmacology, the study of the pharmacological qualities of traditional medicinal substances;
- Phytotherapy, the study of the medicinal use of plant extracts and traditional medicine therapeutics;
- Phytochemistry, the study of chemicals derived from plants (including the identification of new drug candidates derived from plant sources) including phytoanalytical chemistry;
- Zoopharmacognosy, the process by which animals self-medicate, by selecting and using plants, soils and insects to treat and prevent disease;
- Marine pharmacognosy, the study of chemicals derived from marine organisms;
- Medicinal plant biotechnology.

Skills to be acquired by a pharmacognosist are thus manifold with a variety of options to choose from depending on the area of focus.

CONCLUSION

The beginnings of pharmacognosy as a branch of science are claimed to have happened in the early 20th century in Europe, though there are written records of the use of natural materials for healing since antiquity in several places in the world. Whatever 'science' in the form of organized systematic knowledge that happened in the west is only considered as 'Conventional Science'. Rest of human progress is categorized as 'non-scientific', 'mythical belief systems' or 'superstition' till experimentation proves otherwise.

Traditional medicine with its unprocessed plant drugs and other natural materials which at one time was dismissed as 'non-scientific' is today much sought after by the common man and the scientific community: the former as a safe alternative that heals more than it harms, the latter as another source of 'newer' weapons that will fight the scourge of rising global disease burden. In the course of this search many of the erstwhile unscientific methods are today accepted and accommodated within science, which itself is being redefined in order to have a fresh look at all forms of knowledge.

The study of pharmacognosy appears to be at the axis of the wheel of change that has happened in medical sciences during the last century. Because of numerous technological advancements, it is now riding the high tide of global acceptance with extensive investigation of several natural drugs and therapies like never before.

It is true that there continues to be a steady stream of new natural product-derived drugs introduced for the treatment of many common human diseases. It is said that there is ample potential for much greater utilization of natural product-derived compounds in the treatment or prophylaxis of major worldwide scourges such as HIV/AIDS, tuberculosis, hepatitis-C and tropical diseases (inclusive of lymphatic filariasis, leishmaniasis and schistosomiasis). It is believed that the search for such agents may be enhanced by the availability of extensive libraries of taxonomically authenticated crude extracts of terrestrial and marine origin as well as pure SMs from microorganisms, plants and animals. This search could be better facilitated by technology-enabled options such as biocatalysis, combinatorial chemistry, combinatorial biogenesis, tissue culture and metabolic engineering. The high 'drug-like' ness of natural molecules bettered by such technically ingenious and expedient avenues by pharmacognosists are more likely to provide the much-needed newer drugs.

On the other hand as modern herbalists opine, transforming age-old drugs into 'phytopharmaceuticals' takes out the holistic, polyvalent or multidimensional approach of traditional medicine which is really its forte. What is needed is to evolve ways and means of looking at other forms of knowledge, such that these drugs become available to the populace in the form they were meant to be delivered. Such an effort requiring an interdisciplinary approach with innovative methods of assessment, the field of pharmacognosy is rapidly expanding in all possible directions.

Notwithstanding this the commercial aspects of the ethnopharmacological approach have aroused much controversy in recent years with regard to the intellectual property rights of the groups having the knowledge. Several international agreements, particularly the Rio Declaration and CBD of 1992 have concentrated on sharing with the source countries the benefits and profits that might arise from the development of new drugs based on ethnopharmacological leads. The effect that such measures might have on their patent rights and returns from investment have been considered closely by pharmaceutical companies and some have decided not to take the risks involved. Some other companies, however, have been willing to sign agreements aimed at sharing profits directly or making substantial payments to countries in exchange for access to their flora for testing purposes.

With the imminent threat to our natural resources, attempts at conserving our flora and fauna should be the immediate first step before aspiring to 'mine' for drugs of tomorrow from the disappearing wealth of our valuable plant resources.

REVIEW QUESTIONS

Essay Questions

1. Describe the factors that influenced the global resurgence of interest in herbal drugs.
2. Discuss the importance of herbal drug standardization. Outline the challenges faced.
3. Why is conservation of medicinal flora important? Discuss the national initiative coordinating conservation efforts.

Short Notes

1. History of use of plant drugs in India.
2. Suitability of plant secondary metabolites as therapeutic drugs.
3. Present focus of Pharmacognosy.
4. Merits of polyherbal drugs.
5. Herbal medicine—lessons learnt in pharmacology.

2 Age-Old Indian Medical Wisdom—Ayurveda

CHAPTER OBJECTIVES

Introduction

History, Growth and Development of
Ayurvedic Medicine

The Basis of Ayurvedic Therapeutics

Ayurvedic *Materia Medica*

The Best of Ayurveda and its Influence Over
Other Medical Systems

Revival and Current Status

INTRODUCTION

The world's major healing traditions are commonly categorized as Eastern, influenced by Asian-Pacific philosophy or Western, molded by Greco-Roman philosophy and later the scientific revolution of the 16th or 17th century. While modern medicine in the west has developed quite independent of religion, Eastern healing traditions that developed in the East before the Christian era are strongly and inextricably founded in the religious and philosophical thoughts of their cultures. While several indigenous healing traditions in the East have been preserved and are being practised today as discrete systems, Ayurvedic and Chinese medicine remain among the most heavily practised traditions in their respective regions. These two oldest extant and expounded systems of traditional medicine dating several thousand years into antiquity are relevant today for all people throughout the world.

It has been argued that Ayurveda is the basis for traditional Tibetan medicine, traditional Chinese medicine (TCM) and later Greek, Roman and Arabic (Unani) medicines. All these traditional healing methods share a common body-mind-spirit orientation, meaning that disease and health are the result of interaction of all three aspects of being.

Eastern Versus Western Medical Knowledge

Western medicine, in contrast, heavily delineates between mind and body, between doctor and patient and between healthy and diseased. Based on this philosophy of reductionism and mainly guided by science in which truth is derived from observation and empirically correct interpretation, faith – that which cannot be proven through scientific method – is seen as of lesser value (than knowledge gained by direct experience). While health is defined in the East as a unity of individual, environmental and societal factors, western definition of health though having recently moved towards encompassing physical, mental, social and spiritual arenas, still represents it as a separate entity and theories of pathology still drive mechanism perceptions of health disorders. While eastern healing traditions view illness to be caused by imbalances of patterns that should be in harmony, illness in modern western medicine is described by specific pathology caused by discrete foreign pollutants and often cured by another foreign element. Ayurveda was the first medical system to recognize the concept of individual mind-body types and the importance of the mind-body connection. The ancient Vedic culture in India took this concept of constitutional medicine to its highest development in the form of Ayurvedic medicine.

Ayurveda and its Validation

Ayurveda is one of the most ancient systems of medicine known today whose origin according to scholars of ancient Ayurvedic literature is around 6,000 BC. A complete medical system that has evolved over time integrating centuries of wisdom derived from experience, it is now undergoing a vigorous revival not only in the place of its birth, India, but also throughout the world. This holistic practice has a consistent and logical framework with detailed instructions for preservation of health and treatment of disease.

Considerable modern research has proven the efficacy of Ayurvedic treatment practices, with current research having demonstrated the effectiveness of Ayurvedic herbal preparations in conditions for which modern medicine has limited or no success. E.g., Animal studies have shown that *Withania somnifera* (Ashwagandha) can reverse the immunosuppression caused by cyclophosphamide, azathioprine and prednisolone and a 50% alcoholic extract of *Phyllanthus embelica* protects liver from paracetamol. The basic principles of this ancient tradition of health are so resonant of fundamental insights that are only now being developed in cutting edge science. Accumulation of considerable factual knowledge on cellular physiology in modern science has given sensitive modern biomedical research tools with which Ayurveda is being validated with surprising results.

Ayurvedic concepts developed with intuitive knowledge and tremendous insight into the working of the human system without the need for so-called sophisticated technology will hopefully be further validated with tomorrow's technological knowhow, thus gaining greater acceptance by the scientific community. Though Ayurvedic philosophy may strike the contemporary reader as unnecessarily complex for the conceptual territory it addresses, it is actually quite succinct and relevant to modern life. This time-tested healing practice has not got the deserved recognition primarily because of inability to evaluate Ayurvedic medicine by modern standards as the modern scientist has difficulty recognizing subjective experiences because no reliable methodology has been developed to measure and reproduce such experiences. Totally objective experience, completely disregarding the subjective and describing biologic and living systems' phenomena using tools of quantitative technical science may be wrong and even dangerous.

Ayurveda vis-a-vis Science?

It seems necessary to appreciate the historical fact that various knowledge systems have had their genesis and basic evolution in specific cultural spaces in time and hence are bound to be different in their expression. The key to appreciating cultural plurality is an acceptance of the fact that cultures are guided by their own way of looking at the world and acquiring knowledge from it. Modern science as we know it today is a product of European culture. Thus modern western medicine cannot be viewed as the only valid form of health care.

In this context there is no need to describe Ayurveda as a complete 'science' to affirm its universality because 'science' by its very definition being based on reason and deduction is subject to change. What is science yesterday is not so today. Classic examples of changing concepts are found in every arena of both basic and applied sciences. Physics once saw the Universe as purely physical, now it is deduced as being pure energy. Modern drugs introduced into medical practice after much scientific experimentation are withdrawn in haste in the light of further 'scientific proof' of toxicity.

If one defined science as an ongoing methodological study of the world in order to discern knowledge, then it must inherently evolve and expand over time. The definition of science should continue to expand, beyond objectivity, towards phenomena that have not yet been explicitly defined or successfully examined by scientific inquiry. Ayurveda is thus science that has not yet been examined. There is an urgent need for modern medicine to move beyond the older ethos of scientific method, thus shifting towards pluralism, enlarging and expanding into a deeper perspective of disease and health.

HISTORY, GROWTH AND DEVELOPMENT OF AYURVEDIC MEDICINE

The Lineage

The term Ayurveda is a combination of two Sanskrit words – 'Ayush' meaning health and longevity and 'Veda' meaning profound knowledge. Ayurvedic medicine originated in the early civilizations of India some 3000–6000 years ago. Reference to it in the form of verses is recorded in Vedas – the ancient religious and philosophical texts that are the oldest surviving literature in the world, making Ayurveda the oldest surviving healing system. According to legend (Figure 2.1) the origin of Ayurveda is stated to be a divine revelation of Brahma, the Lord of Creation, who passed it on to his son Dakshaprajapati and then through a succession of deities to Sage Bharadwaja – the first human exponent of Ayurveda. He in turn taught Ayurveda to a group of assembled sages, who then passed down different aspects of this knowledge to their students. Sage Bharadwaja taught Ayurveda to Punarvasu Atreya, who later formed the Atreya School of Physicians. Ascetic King Deodas Dhanwantri formed the Dhanwantri School of Surgeons. These two schools transformed Ayurveda into a scientifically verifiable and classifiable medical system.

Literature on Ayurveda

References to diseases, herbs and herbal cures can be seen in all the four Vedas. Atharvana Veda has many hymns eulogizing herbs. Aushadhi Sukta in Rig Veda is the oldest document available on medicinal plants in this region. Ayurvedic teachings were originally transmitted for thousands of years before being written down in melodious Sanskrit poetry. Ayurveda in its first recorded form is specifically called Atharvana Veda. The earliest scripts were written on palm and betula leaves. Being perishable the scripts were later written on stone and copper sheets (Table 2.1).

The depth of medical knowledge possessed by Ayurveda is reflected in the large number of medical manuscripts and the range of subjects they cover. Apart from knowledge of drugs, there

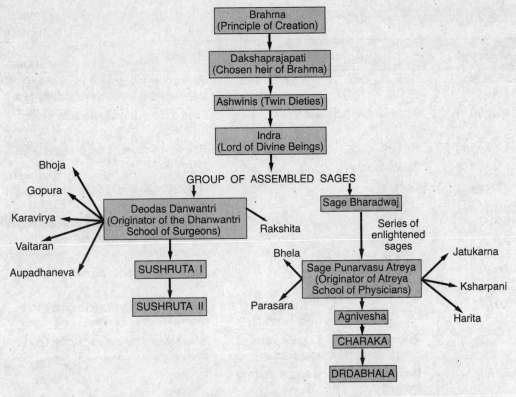

Figure 2.1 The lineage of Ayurveda

is extensive coverage of diagnostic methods, therapeutic techniques, surgery, specialized lines of treatment, physiological concepts as well as an understanding of the mind-body relationships.

This knowledge today lies scattered in several ancient manuscripts in oriental libraries and in private custody not only in India, but also in Sri Lanka, Nepal, Burma, Mongolia, China and Thailand as well as in the libraries of Western Europe and the United States. These are largely Samhitas (treatises), Samgrahas (compendiums), Nighantus (lexicons), Vyakhyas (critical commentaries) and texts on specific areas like pharmacy, paediatrics etc.

Major Treatises

Great exponents of the Atreya school of physicians were the six disciples of Sage Atreya – Agnivesha, Bhela, Jatukarna, Parasara, Harita and Ksharpani. Each of them wrote a comprehensive work on the practice of medicine. These works were passed on orally in the teacher-student lineage before being put down in text form. The knowledge was passed down through generations in the form of terse poetic verses which were easy to commit to memory and this was done *in-toto* till the dawn of written tradition. According to tradition, Ayurveda was first described in text form in Agnivesha Tantra. It was later redacted by *Charaka*. This incomplete task was later extended by 17 chapters in 8th C AD by Dridabhala which became the '*Charaka Samhita*'.

Table 2.1 Literature on Ayurveda

Chronology	Literature		Remarks
40,000 BC	Oushadha Sukti (Rig Veda)	Atharvana Veda	Passed down through generations orally as poetic verses to enable memorization *in-toto*
8,000 BC	Written on palm leaf manuscripts		Dawn of written language, redactions of oral material
4,000 – 2,000 BC	Rig Veda	Atharvana Veda	Rewritten on stone and copper sheets to retain in non-perishable form
1,500 BC	Agnivesha Samhita		
1,000 BC	Charaka		He redacted *Agnivesha Samhita* but incompletely
900 BC		Sushrutal	Compiled the oral tradition of surgical practices into *Shalya Tantra* – older version of *Sushruta Samhita*
400 AD	Dridabhala (Brhat tryi)		Added 17 chapters and completed *Charaka Samhita*
500 AD		Sushruta II (Brhat tryi)	Revised it by adding *Uttara Tantra* to complete *Sushruta Samhita*
	Vagbhatta – Ashtanga Sangraha, Ashtanga Hrdaya, Ashtanga Nighantu (Brhat tryi)		Succinct compilations of the teachings of both Charaka and Sushruta
700 AD	Madhava – Paryayaratna mala or Madhava Nidanam		Laghu tryi
1300 AD	Sarangadhara – Sarangadhara Samhita		
1500 AD	Bhava Mishra – Bhava Prakasha Nighantu		

Modern Christian view places Charaka Samhita at 1000 BC. However ancient oral tradition places Sage Atreya around 5000 BC and Rig Veda, the first Veda, at about 1500 BC.

Further each of the exponents of the school of surgeons namely Sushruta, Bhoja, Gopura, Karavirya, Aupadhaneva, Aurabhra, Vaitaran, Rakshita, etc., wrote a comprehensive work on the practice of surgery and midwifery. *Sushruta Samhita* – another early text of Ayurveda was written around the same period (6th C AD) by Sushruta the primary pupil of Dhanwantri. In his compilation, Sushruta, known as the father of ancient surgical practices, consolidated and complemented the teachings and surgical techniques of Dhanwantri with additional findings and observations related to topics ranging from obstetrics and orthopaedics to ophthalmology.

Later during the spread of Buddhism, there was an accelerated development in the practice of Ayurveda (600 –700 BCE). During this time several famous centres of medical learning – such as the Takshashila University in what is now Afghanistan – evolved that taught an apparently advanced knowledge of surgery and other specialities. This period, the *golden period of Ayurveda*, saw the development of newer and more effective therapies and medicines. Post Kalinga war, Emperor Ashoka, influenced by Buddhist teachings, banned bloodshed in his kingdom due to which many Ayurvedic practitioners left surgical intervention and evolved newer medical treatments. The practice of the accompanying surgery however slowly died out during this period. During the regime of Chandra Gupta Maurya (375–415 AD), Ayurveda was part of mainstream Indian medical techniques and continued to be so until the Mughal invasion and colonization by the British during which time it witnessed a drastic decline.

Other Works

Apart from the above mentioned major treatises, a few others dating back to the period between 1500 BC–7th century include *Harita Samhita*, *Bhela Samhita* and *Kasyapa Samhita*, which are not available in complete form. Between the 8th and 15th century, there have been many works written in the field of Ayurvedic pharmacology or *Dravya Guna*. These nighantus were appendices to the ancient samhitas and contain synonyms, qualities of drugs and the conditions in which they are to be used.

Critical commentaries on the classic treatises during this period are Ayurveda Dipika by Chakrapani Dutta (11th C AD) for *Charaka Samhita*, *Nyaya Chandrika* by Gayadasa (11th C AD) for *Sushruta Samhita*, *Nibandhasangraha* by Dalhana (12th C AD) for *Sushruta Samhita*, *Sarvanga Sundari* for *Astanga Sangraha* by Aruna Datta (13th C AD), *Sasilekha* by Indu for *Astanga Sangraha* (13th C AD) and *Tattva Pradipika* by Sivadas Sen for *Charaka Samhita*. Post 16th century saw works like *Bhavaprakasha Nighantu*, *Raja Nighantu*, *Sivakosa*, *Vaidyavatamsam* and *Dravyagunastakam* (17th C AD), *Rajavallabah Nighantu* (18th C AD) and *Nighantu Sangraham* (19th C AD).

Sushruta Samhita together with *Charaka Samhita* served as the textual material in the ancient universities of Takshashila and Nalanda. Both these are highly technical texts and many subsequent Ayurvedic scholars contributed to the store house of Ayurvedic literature, making it more accessible and comprehensible. Among such Ayurvedic scholars was Vagbhata (600 CE), author of the *Ashtanga Sangraha* and *Ashtanga Hrdaya*. The latter is a succinct compilation of the teachings of both *Charaka* and *Sushruta*.

The Greater and the Lesser Triad

Together the teachings of Charaka, Sushruta and Vagbhatta form the *Brhat Tryi*, the 'greater triad' of surviving texts that are the heart of Ayurvedic literature. Comparatively later texts namely *Madhava Nidanam* (700 CE), *Sarangadhara Samhita* (1300 CE) and the *Bhava Prakasa Nighantu* (1300 CE) form the *Laghu Tryi* or the 'lighter triad'. Besides these texts, there are many more highly respected Ayurvedic physicians including *Ayurveda Dipika* (1100 CE), *Bhaishyaja Ratnavali* (c.1700 CE) and *Yogaratnakara*. An important early text is the *Kasyapa Samhita*, which is concerned with the theory and practice of paediatric and obstetric disease (*Kaumara Bhrtya*). These later texts not only dealt with disease classifications but also had descriptions of properties of newer drugs introduced in the subcontinent.

THE BASIS OF AYURVEDIC THERAPEUTICS

Tracing Back to Samkhya Philosophy

The theoretical core of the practice of Ayurveda is allied with the four principle Vedas, the substance of which is carefully expounded in a six-pronged approach. These six limbs or *angas*, as they are called, refer to the six *Darshanas* or perceptions of the Vedas that explicate the philosophy of the Vedas in a rationalistic approach. They are Nyaya, Vaiseshika, Samkhya, Mimamsa, Yoga and Vedanta.

Ayurveda mainly draws to a large extent from the first three and to a lesser extent from the others. Thus the philosophical orientation of Ayurveda is through Samkhya, which is based on the theory of transformation. Propounded by Sage Kapila, it is derived from two Sanskrit words 'sat' (truth) and 'khya' (to know). It does not acknowledge a creator or an act of creation. It explains existence as a mutual relationship between two basic principles – *Purusha* and *Prakruti*.

The Genesis of Perception

According to Samkhya philosophy *Purusha* refers to an unmanifest cosmic consciousness, which is formless, colourless, choiceless and beyond attribute. Also referred to as the 'Grace' it does not take part in the manifestation of the universe and is eternal. Emanating from this Grace is *Prakruti* – the womb of all creation. It is a dynamic principle through which all forms of creation manifest by virtue of its three qualities or *gunas*. These qualities are *Sattwa* (pure consciousness), *Rajas* (transformation) and *Tamas* (inertia or non-transformable finality). They are in balance in the unmanifest precreative *Prakruti*. While *Sattwa* is the well spring of consciousness, dynamic *Rajas* is the basis of energetic transformation and *Tamas* represents the end product of transformation, i.e., stasis or inertia. Samkhya explains the universe as having evolved out of disequilibrium between the three qualities (*Trigunas*). Resulting subtle vibrations manifesting in this state of consciousness give rise to creation. From the thus manifest *Prakruti* arises '*Mahat*' or Buddhi – the cosmic intelligence and knowledge of universality that is within all. Due to further evolution, *Mahat* manifests itself as '*ahamkara*' the principle that fragments the universality into an individual sense of self (Figure 2.2).

The Six Expositional Perceptions of Vedas

✓ **Nyaya** – the closest Indian equivalent to anaytical philosophy, this darshana gives logical proofs for existence and considers 'perception, influence, comparison and testimony' as the only four sources of knowledge.

✓ **Vaiseshika** – an empiricist school of atomism, it conceives all objects of the physical universe to be reducible to certain basic atomic units and *Brahman* is regarded as the fundamental force that causes consciousness in these atoms. This approach accepts only two sources of valid knowledge – 'perception and inference'.

✓ **Samkhya** – a theoretical exposition of human nature, mind and matter analysing the manner of cooperation in a state of bondage.

✓ **Mimamsa** – an anti-ascetic and anti-mysticist exposition, it emphasizes unquestionable faith and focus on those aspects of Vedas that focus on spiritual connectivity, acknowledging centred understanding of Vedas much more than traditional ritualism.

✓ **Yoga** – the dynamics of the process of disentanglement of bondage of self unto universality.

✓ **Vedanta** – the most widely recognized dharshana, reiterates Brahman as the absolute reality and the rest of creation as an illusory power of *Brahman*. Liberation lies in realizing the oneness of the individual soul with that of the all-pervading *Brahman*.

Further under the influence of *rajoguna* from the *sattwic* aspect of *ahamkara* develops *manas* or mind i.e., further evolution. *Mahat, Ahamkara* and *Manas* are the inner organs of the human body (*Antahkaranas*) and are the receptacles of one's consciousness. Together called '*Chitta*' they impart direct awareness of self. The *ahamkara* shapes one's personality.

From further interplay of the trigunas arise external organs (*bahyakaranas*) – the five organs of knowledge (Gyanendriyas) – sense organs (nose, tongue, eye, skin and ear) and five organs of action (Karmendriyas) – hands, feet, genitals, anus and tongue.

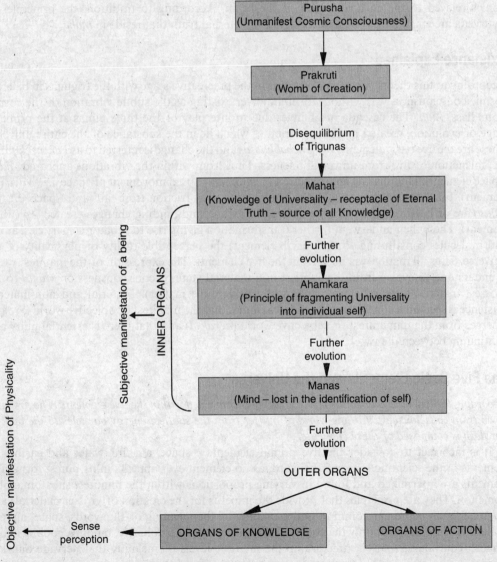

Figure 2.2 The Samkhya basis of existence

Predominance of *tamas* gravitates *ahamkara* towards generating the *sukshma bhootas* or the five subtle elements of perception (*tanmatras*), i.e., the five senses namely scent (*gandha*), flavour (*rasa*), form (*rupa*), consistency (*sparsha*) and sound (*sabda*) representing the essence of human sense perception. While the inner organs and outer organs under the control of *sattwa* and *rajoguna* belong to the realm of subjective manifestation of a being, the subtle elements under the control of *tamas* represent the objective manifestation or perception or physicality (reality).

The state of predominance of any of the three gunas has a formative influence on one's personality imprinting itself strongly on one's character. *Chitta* is the user of the Bahya karanas or outer organs. *Manas* or mind is the constant that links and coordinates activities between the conscious cortex and the subconscious hypothalamic region from where most outside information is relayed to the cortical region of the brain. According to tradition, the principles of Ayurveda are emanations of an unchanging and eternal truth that reside in *mahat*.

Existence Explained

According to this theory, when *Prakruti* was in the precreative stage with the trigunas in balance, cosmic consciousness was without form, however existing as the subtle vibration of the cosmic 'soundless' *Aum*. The cascade of changes due to interplay of the three gunas at the primeval stage of evolution, created five basic attributes which lie in the substance of the entire universe. These are the five basic elements or *Panchabhootas* and the change is referred to as *Pancheekarana*, i.e., formation of five from universal oneness. Thus from within the vibrations appeared *Akash* (space element). Dominant transformation or rajoguna caused movement of space, i.e., *Vayu* (air element). Further evolutionary change brought about by friction from 'air' and 'space' created *Tejas* (fire or heat element). Further cohesive bonding and binding changes created *Ap* (water element). These then underwent further transformation giving rise to subatomic particles, atoms and molecules constituting *Prithvi* (earth element) the perceptible reality or physicality of the universe. Thus all matter was born from the five elements. The expression of the manifest world is understood to evolve from the subtlest non-material state of consciousness or *Mahat* to the grossest material state of Prithvi (physically perceptible matter). Material and non-material existence is seen on a continuum. Samkhya assumes that the manifest or objective world (*vyakta*) emerges from the unmanifest or subjective world (*avyakta*) and that there is essential unity and continuum between the two.

The Five Basic Elements and the Universe

According to Ayurveda everything in the universe is contained within the five elements. The first step down from consciousness into the world of matter from the subtlest energy particles to the bulk of our flesh is composed of these elements.

It is incorrect to consider the five primal elements – space, air, fire, water and earth – as elements in the scientific sense of the word, as no element ever appears in its purest form. The elements are intermixed and found in varying proportions within the minutest subatomic phenomenon. They are principles that provide the impetus for the creation of grosser materials and do not literally represent common understanding of the meaning of the words, space, air, etc. Water for example is not only the chemical H_2O, it represents a cohesive, binding, cooling entity. English equivalents many a time cramp the multiple levels of meaning that pervade Sanskrit words.

Samkhya vis-à-vis Modern Theories on the Origin of Universe

Among the scores of modern theories that attempt to explain the origin of the universe, the popular big bang theory based on Sir Albert Einstein's theory of relativity and proposed by George Gamow conceives the universe as having started out as a very hot gas. Made up of neutrons it decayed into protons, electron and neutrinos. He and Ralph Alpher theorized in 1948 that all elements in the universe resulted from early thermonuclear action. The proposal of a very hot beginning for the universe by all big bang theories seems quite in agreement with the transformative changes that culminated in the formation of prithvi according to the ancient Samkhya perception of the origin of existence.

Panchamahabhootas and the Human Body

With an intuitive insight into the complexity of our origin, Ayurveda understands that the knowledge of the body is never complete, a truth that is painfully obvious to anyone who tries to keep abreast of the myriad developments and contradictory opinions of today's medical science. This merry-go-round of shifting phenomenon and perceptions is identified as a property of 'Samsara', which represents the inexorable law of change, which states that no subject or object ever remains completely static. Modern science though is based upon the systematic observation, experimentation and analysis of such shifting material existence (Samsara). Ayurveda states that the limits of human perception (including the technology that expands that awareness) are unconsciously guided by the principle of ahamkara, which represents the act of naming, identification and discrimination. It creates a vocabulary, a semantic description of a conditioned reality that lulls the scientist into believing in the idea of objectivity, that the individual self can somehow observe the machinations of Samsara without the perception itself being affected.

The Samkhya philosophy of creation that is at the core of Ayurveda perceives humans as microcosm – a universe within themselves – while the rest of the universe is the macrocosm and cosmic energy is manifest in all living and non-living things. According to this lucid physiological model, human body is thus a holographic representation of the microcosm and within our being and within our bodies exist all the clues and data we need to understand the universe.

Human Sensory Perception

The human body is thus a microcosm of nature and is essentially composed of the five basic elements (see box). In the context of perceptivity, while the Mahabhootas and thus the totality of corporeal existence by itself cannot be perceived objectively, their presence can be inferred by the manifestation of certain qualities. In other words the evolution of the Mahabhootas gives rise to the distinction of qualitative differences that can be objectively perceived.

The three gunas of Prakruti – the fundamental qualities – are present in all of the five elements or building blocks of existence, but disturbance of equilibrium results in the dominance of one or two gunas in each element imparting distinctive properties to each of them. By virtue of this quality they are perceived by the Tanmatras or sense organs, the first link in perceptivity. Thus sense perception closely corresponds to the five universal elements both conceptually and physiologically.

1. Sattwa predominates 'Akash' and it corresponds to sound perception since space is the medium through which sound travels as vibrations even according to modern science.

2. Rajas predominates '*Vayu*' and this according to Ayurveda is essential for touch perception, movement being vital for test of palpability or consistency.

3. Sattwa and Rajas are innate in '*Tejas*' and is associated with *visual* perception as light energy is the basis for vision.

4. Sattwa and Tamas are predominant in '*Ap*' corresponding to *taste* perception for which water and binding of taste receptors is a primary requirement.

5. Tamas is predominant in '*Prithvi*', which is responsible for *smell* or flavour perception. This is in agreement with the modern theory of 'no molecule – no flavour' referring to the actual locking of flavour molecules within smell receptors triggering a highly complex neurosensory apparatus enabling flavour perception.

In other words the five universal elements are directly related to human ability, both to perceive and to respond to the external environment.

Mahabhootas – Gurvadi gunas, the essence of Ayurvedic pharmacology

Matter is a mixture of five universal elements containing one or the other in a predominant ratio. According to Sushruta, all substances are derived from a combination of the five *bhootas* and a predominance of any one of them in a particular substance determines its character and this is at the heart of Ayurvedic pharmacology.

Apart from the predominant quality, each *Mahabhoota* is also attributed with other traits described in terms of 10 opposing pairs of qualities. These are the *Gurvadi gunas* or the associated qualities (Table 2.2). The *Gurvadi guna*s and their relationship to the five basic elements and five senses is shown in Table 2.3. Each of these is associated with a particular element and its opposite quality will be manifest in the element that has an opposing action or effect; e.g., *Prithvi* is associated with the quality of *guru* (heavy); the opposing quality of *laghu* is associated with *Vayu*. To some extent *prithvi* and *vayu* have opposing forms and actions. Each pair of opposites is only one specific dimension in interaction, however with each subsequent pair representing a contrasting dimension. By recognizing several different dimensions of interaction the result is a multidimensional model that explains the complexity of interactions that occur between the five basic elements.

The Five Basic Elements and the Human Body

✓ **Akash** is represented in the hollow spaces of the mouth, nose, gastrointestinal tract, abdomen, thorax, respiratory apparatus, capillaries, lymphatics, tissues and cells.

✓ **Vayu** exists as movement – as pulsation, expansion or contraction of the various organs. Bodily movement is controlled by the central nervous system, itself governed by Vayu.

✓ **Tejas** is the source of heat and light somatically present as metabolism, grey matter, vision, temperature, digestion and intelligence.

✓ **Ap** exists as secretions of the salivary and digestive glands and mucous membranes and within plasma and cytoplasm.

✓ **Prithvi** is the solid structures, i.e., bones, cartilage, nails, muscles, tendons, skin and hair.

Table 2.2 Gurvadi gunas – the 10 opposing pairs of qualities

Guru (heavy)	Laghu (light)
Manda (slow)	Tiksna (fast)
Sita (cold)	Usna (hot)
Snigdha (greasy)	Ruksa (dry)
Slaksna (smooth)	Khara (rough)
Sandra (solid)	Drava (fluid)
Mrdu (soft)	Kathina (hard)
Sthira (stable)	Cala (moving)
Suksma (subtle)	Sthula (obvious)
Visada (friction)	Picchila (slimy)

Italics – upakarmas

Table 2.3 Pancha Mahabhootas, Tanmatras and Gurvadi gunas

Basic Element	Sensory Perception	Associated Quality
Prithvi	Gandha	Guru, manda, sthira, kathina, sthula, sandra
Ap	Rasa	Sita, snigdha, mrdu, guru, drava, manda
Tejas	Rupa	Usna, laghu, tiksna, drava
Vayu	Sparsa	Laghu, ruksa, cala, visada, khara, suksma
Akasa	Sabda	Suksma, visada

Thus while *prithvi* displays the quality of *guru*, it is also considered to be *ruksa*. *Vayu* displays the opposing quality of *laghu*, but it is also *ruksa*. The relationship between *prithvi* and *vayu* is therefore complex, displaying both similar and opposing qualities.

While all 10 pairs of opposite qualities are generally considered in Ayurveda, for purposes of diagnosis and treatment, they are usually whittled down to three dominant dimensions of interactions that in large part guide the manifestation of all subsequent qualities, called *Upakarmas*. These form the basis of the six *Samana karmas* used in Ayurvedic therapeutics. They are *Guru* and *Laghu* (heavy and light), *Sita* and *Usna* (cool and hot) and *Snigdha* and *Ruksa* (greasy and dry). It is no coincidence that these correspond exactly to the full–empty, dark–light and wet–dry opposing triads or the three axes of balance of the Chinese Yin-Yang concept of existence.

The Tridoshas

Health is defined in Ayurveda as the soundness of body (*sharira*), mind (*manas*) and soul (*atma*). Each part of this tripod of life should receive equal attention as psychic influences strongly affect the body in health as well as in disease, a fact that is only recently being acknowledged in modern medical science. Modern medicine takes pride in its understanding of physiology thus emphasizing fragmentation, isolation and disunity in its study of human system, while according to Ayurveda, disease is seen as the result of disruption of the spontaneous flow of nature's intelligence within the physiology. Ayurvedic definition of health or *svasthya* provides a good illustration of the holistic nature of the knowledge system. It implies equilibrium of body tissues, physiological functions, excretory processes, the senses and the mind.

While western health sciences look to the physical body for their data, studying them as isolated parts, Ayurvedic medicine views the human body as groups of interrelated and interdependent structures and functions governed basically by three biological elements or biophysiological factors. These are the Tridoshas.

In perfect balance in the body *Vata*, *Pitta* and *Kapha* are the *Tridhatus* or the three root governing principles. *Dhatu* is derived from Sanskrit 'Dha' meaning that which nourishes and supports. *Dhatus* essentially sustain and nourish the body. In all living things – animals or plants – these constitute the basic functional units and are subject to influences both within and without. Within the constitutional limits of disease-free state, *dhatus* are not taken away from equilibrium enough to cause or trigger causative factors leading to disease. Since in their disequilibrium lies the root cause of all disease, they are called *Tridoshas* (*dosha* literally meaning a blemish).

Arogya (absence of disease) is the result of a balanced state of the *doshas* each of which has a specific *pramana* (quantity), *guna* (quality) and *karma* (action) in the body. Food habits and environmental factors that are contrary to the qualities of a particular dosha bring about its increase (*vriddhi*) or decrease (*ksaya*). Though both of these are considered abnormal (*vikruta*), it is the increase that causes major disturbances, while decrease typically causes only minor disturbances.

Vata, *Pitta* and *Kapha* correspond to *Vayu*, *Tejas* and *Ap* of the *Panchamahabhootas*. This is because *prithvi* and *akash* have no definite actions of their own and are not the direct cause of any disease. They function in association with the other three elements in the body. The terms *vata*, *pitta* and *kapha* (or *sleshma*) are derived respectively from the Sanskrit roots 'Va' meaning to move or to excite, 'Tap', to heat and 'Slis', to hold together. A right conception of these factors is the basis for a right understanding of the essence of Ayurveda.

Vata

According to *Charaka Samhita*, *vata* is the grossest manifestation of the *Panchabhautic vayu* or air element and is the motivating force which keeps everything going (read as moving). This subtle influence pervading everywhere governs all biological movement – breathing, blinking, muscle and joint movement, heart beat and all nerve and membrane contractions and expansions, as well as tremors and spasms. It also controls the psychological functions governing the emotions of fear and anxiety. Since all movement is determined by the dictates of space and (displacement of) air, vata is said to be governed by space and air. Though these two are neutral in temperament, physical body being dominant in *Prithvi* (perceivable physicality) and *Ap* (water and cohesion), together they create a solidifying influence and thus vata assumes a cold temperament in the body.

When *vata* is disturbed, the pervasive nature of *akasha* and the catabolic activity of *vayu* represent widespread degenerative changes in the body, characterized by a lightness (*laghu*) and dryness (*ruksa*) of the tissues, which in turn promotes roughness (*khara*) and friction (*visada*) in the body. These are the primary qualities of *vata* and the principal seat of residence of *vata* is colon and bladder, governing the regions of the body from the umbilicus downwards. *Charaka* considered *vata* to be the most important *dosha* as it gives a direct reflection of *prana-shakti* or life force in a living being.

Permeating throughout the body, depending on its functions in different parts of the body, it is subdivided into five types namely

1. *Prana vayu* – First and the most important of the five *vatas*, *prana* initiates and controls all binary functions in the body such as inspiration–expiration, stimulation–relaxation, contraction–expansion etc. It resides in the heart and attends to the regulation of cardiopulmonary activity, governs ingestion, chewing, swallowing and initiates expectoration, sneezing and belching.

2. *Apana vayu* – Located in the sacral plexus, primarily bladder and colon, it governs the functions of pelvic organs. Movement being downwards, it controls the activities of *prana* and *udana* by creating a negative pressure in the chest. All downward movement of excretory products, including menstrual blood, semen as also fetal expulsion, is under its influence.

3. *Samana vayu* – Residing in the umbilical region it governs digestion, assimilation and waste separation. It assesses or measures the metabolic needs of the body and guides the process of anabolism and catabolism. Under its influence thirst, hunger and satiety are facilitated.

4. *Udana vayu* – Residing in the vocal chords and tongue it governs expiration, sound and speech.

5. *Vyana vayu* – Though rooted in the heart, it circulates through the body as spiral currents moving like a wheel. It governs circulatory function, distribution of oxygen, nutrients and heat throughout the body through movement of bodily fluids like blood, lymph etc.

Pitta

It corresponds to metabolism of western physiology and is roughly synonymous to bodily fire. All metabolic processes in the organism are *pitta* mediated. Thereby it governs all metabolic transformation in the body involving digestion, absorption, assimilation, nutrition, temperature, skin colour, lustre of the eye, intelligence and understanding. Through it are aroused anger, hate and jealousy. Energy being the underlying requirement of all metabolic activity, fire is a component of *pitta*. Lack of it is represented by the quenching attribute of fire, which is water. Thus *pitta* is said to be constituted of *tejas* and *ap*. Due to catabolic action and heat generative activity of *tejas*, *pitta* is *laghu* and *tiksna*. The bonding and binding anabolic reactions of *Ap* impart *snigdha*, *drava* and *sara* properties to *pitta*. With these primary qualities, the seat of *pitta* is stomach, duodenum, liver and spleen, governing the area between the umbilicus and the diaphragm. Depending upon its location in the economy *pitta* is of five types of which the first two are grosser forms, while the others are the subtler ones.

1. *Pachaka agni* – Established in the stomach and duodenum it enables digestion of ingested food and guides the manifestation of all subsequent forms of energy resulting from digestion.

2. *Ranjaka agni* – Residing in the liver and spleen, it is associated with metabolism involved in the formation of blood, bile, semen etc.

3. *Bhrajaka agni* – Residing in the skin it is involved in bodily temperature regulation and imparts a natural glow to the skin.

4. *Sadhaka agni* – Situated in the heart, it drives away *tamas* from it enabling cardiac activities. Also it is instrumental in proper functioning of memory and intellect through its cerebral activities. Finest of all *pitta*s, *sadhaka agni* enables comprehension, cognition and sensory perception.

5. *Alochaka agni* – Exerting its functions on a subtle (*sukshma*) plane it enables metabolism associated with visual perception.

Kapha

Also called *Sleshma*, it is the formative, cohesive, cementing and cooling component lending firmness, stability, flexibility and calmness to the body. It aids anabolism and builds up tissues. Enabling mental strength, endurance and bodily resistance to diseases, *kapha* most strongly relates to the physical structure of the body. *Kapha* is the cooling element that keeps *vata* and *pitta* confined to their normal limits, in the absence of which the combustion going on in the human system will feed upon the constituent principles of the body. Restraining factor of fire being water and physical matter (water by taking up a lot of heat energy in latent form and food by utilizing bodily heat for digestion helps quench it), *pitta* is constituted of *Prithvi* and *Ap*, i.e., gross physicality and cooling cohesiveness. Thus food and water are the prime sources of *kapha* component in our system. Derived from the root word '*slis*' which means to embrace, *kapha* is *sthira*, *snigdha* and *picchila*. It combines solidity with substance to bind tissues together in a cooling embrace. *Kapha* is located primarily in lungs and heart and the governing areas are from the diaphragm upwards. Depending on the function and location, it is of five types.

1. *Avalambaka kapha* – Located in the chest within the pleura of the lungs and the pericardium of the heart, it lubricates bronchial passages and alveoli. It supports and protects the heart in the chest.

2. *Kledaka kapha* – Associated with mucus secretions of the gastrointestinal tract it protects underlying tissues of the stomach from the *usna* and *tiksna* nature of digestion. Moistening and liquefying ingested food this *kapha* lubricates and nourishes the digestive tract.

3. *Bodhaka kapha* – Present in the mouth as salivary secretions, it is specifically related to the function of taste.

4. *Tarpaka kapha* – Located in the head it appeases and cools sense organs, slows neural activity, induces relaxation and promotes contentment and emotional stability.

5. *Sleshaka kapha* – *sleshaka* means that which joins. Situated in the joints it provides lubrication.

The tridoshas thus control all biologic, psychological and physiopathologic functions of the body, mind and consciousness producing natural urges and individual tastes in food, flavour and temperature. They govern the maintenance and destruction of bodily tissues and the elimination of waste products. They are also responsible for psychological phenomena, including the emotions of fear, anger and greed as well as the highest order of emotions, understanding, compassion and love.

Having arisen from the five basic elements, the human body is thus postulated to be under the control of *tridoshas*. Ayurveda elucidates and investigates the causes through which *vata*, *pitta*, *kapha* which sustain life are transformed into the dynamics of disease.

Ayurvedic View of Disease Causation

The fundamental doctrines of Ayurveda describe the human system in terms of 3 *dosha*s that describe its principle of function, 7 *dhatu*s that describe the principle of structure and 3 *mala*s through which bodily impurities (physical and subtle) are eliminated. A balance of these doshas, good quality structural supports – the 7 *dhatu*s (*Ras* – plasma, *Rakta* – blood, *Mamsa* – muscles, *Meda* – fat, *Asthi* – bone and cartilage, *Majja* – bone marrow and *Shukra* – sex hormones and immunity) – and a certain character of excretions *mala*s (*Svet* – sweat, *Poorish* – faeces and *Mutra* – urine) are essential for maintaining health. Health is defined as the equilibrium between the *dosha*s, *dhatu*s and *mala*s. Such equilibrium is considered a natural consequence of living consciously and Ayurveda prescribed the ways and means of attaining this balance in terms of the various lifestyle choices.

When there is disruption to this equilibrium the result is *vikara* or disease. According to Ayurvedic pathology, *dosha* disturbance progressively leads to disease through various stages with discernable symptoms appearing only in the later stages. Sushruta observes that the relation between a disease and disturbed *vata, pitta* and *kapha* and the pathogenic factors which lie at the root of disease is not real but contingent. These morbific principles permeate the body without creating any discomfort, and it is only when they find distinct lodgement and centre in some bodily tissue that they become the factors exciting disease. Thus according to Ayurvedic pathology *dosha* disturbance progressively leads to disease through various stages, culminating in discernable symptoms.

According to the classical definition of Charaka, an individual may be regarded as healthy only when the tridoshas are in equilibrium. Life is considered a sacred path in Ayurveda, a ceaseless interaction between the internal environment (tridoshas) and the external environment or the sum of cosmic forces. To counteract external changes an individual may create a balance on internal forces by altering diet, lifestyle and behaviour.

Diagnosis and Treatment

Each individual is born with a particular *dosha* predominating his or her constitution that is determined at conception. Thus permutations of *vata, pitta* and *kapha* during fertilization determine his/her constitution or *Prakrti*. There are thus seven basic types of *Prakrti* namely *vata, pitta, kapha, vata-pitta, vata-kapha, pitta-kapha* and *vata-pitta-kapha*. These basic traits are also shaped by other important factors such as diet, lifestyle, behaviour, emotions and seasons. Depending on lifestyle choices, this predominant *dosha*, quite apart from genetics, age, environment and dietary factors may make an individual susceptible to a certain disease.

Ayurveda teaches that the origin of most diseases is found either in exogenous or endogenous *dosha* imbalance or an inherent or acquired weakness of the tissues. Therefore a successful treatment or prevention of disease consists of normalizing cellular functions through correcting any *dosha* imbalance or by improving inherent tissue vitality. It stresses on one's responsibility for one's well-being and emphasizes lifestyle behavioural modification procedures and biopurification procedures that strengthen the indigenous immune system. This innate ability of the body to bounce back to a healthy equilibrium is referred to as *Swabhavaparamavada*.

Unlike current medical science, the focus of Ayurveda is not as much about disease as it is about healthy living and maintenance of the same. Its tenets thus largely emphasize the different modalities of prevention of disease causation. Disease is considered a preventable consequence and the event of its occurrence is then dealt with – as a last resort through drugs and other options aimed at restoring the balance of the tridoshas.

In Ayurveda there is little emphasis on differentiation of disease states and it classifies only the causes of disease. It does not seek to understand the minutiae of the human body nor does it pretend to have an objective perspective. In contrast modern medicine because of fragmentation of knowledge is becoming increasingly specialized, so much so that today it is rare to find a medical doctor with skills in a variety of specialities. Ayurvedic physicians however traditionally worked with all kinds of disease in both genders, young and old and even treated domesticated animals. This was possible because this 'knowledge of life' comes from a deep understanding of the manifestation of a basic life principle and all the living bodies that arise from it as a natural consequence.

Disease is understood on the basis of relatively simple principles and thus it lays minimal stress on classification, disease nomenclature or even the complexity of pathological definitions. As such, it may seem perplexing fact that there are quite a few disease forms according to Ayurveda. In other words from an Ayurvedic perspective any disease is understood as disorientation of certain simple principles regarding the body as a whole and grasping the flux manifested in the doshas is the basis of identifying disease causation. A seemingly paradoxical outcome of this is the fact, however, that there could be as many diseases as there are people experiencing them, for, each state of illness arises from unique physical, emotional, mental and spiritual factors. Stated simply, as per Ayurveda, *disease forms are few, but disease types are limitless.*

Thus for example at the root of diabetes lies vitiation of *dosha* largely due to external factors aggravated by inherited debilitation of certain tissue systems. The innate *prakrti* of the individual determines the treatment protocol, as each type has a different prognosis and hence a different treatment strategy. Using the same example, diabetes in a *vata* individual has poor prognosis and spectrum of presenting features of the disease could be vascular derangement, neuritis, arthropathy, renal diseases, insomnia, hyperactivity etc. In a p*itta* constitution while the prognosis is intermediate, liver and cardiac complications could be the presenting features. Asthma and bronchitis will invariably be the associated complications in a *kapha* individual with diabetes for whom the prognosis is much better than the other two types. Thus drugs and dietary recommendations are also different for each of these types.

Medicinal therapy in Ayurveda is thus highly individualized. The choice and dose of medicine are influenced not only by disease but by the individual's constitution and the environmental conditions likely to affect that individual's *doshas.* Treatment in Ayurveda eradicates the illness from its roots thus minimizing the risk of relapses and side effects. It is beyond the scope and context of this book to go into the methodology of diagnosis and treatment in Ayurveda. However the details presented are meant to give a little 'peep through the window' into this vast knowledge.

The subject matter of Ayurveda thus goes on to enumerate the basic factors that affect *dosha*s and has elaborate clinical methodology to formulate a diagnosis based on an eight-pronged examination protocol including *nadi pariksha* or pulse diagnosis. A systematic diagnosis of a patient is expected to take into consideration a multiplicity of factors ranging from the status of the patient's various physiological states to inferences drawn based on the natural habitat in which the patient resides, his/her constitution (*prakrti*), mental state and dietary habits.

Further treatment strategy is through various modes of therapy depending on the patient's constitution as well as disease process. Modalities include dietary alterations, plant drugs, minerals, animal products, exercise, yoga, meditation, counselling and surgery.

Food as Nutrition and Medicine

According to Ayurveda, food is meant for nourishment and is to be consumed based on bodily needs rather than by the dictates of taste value of the eatable. Diet is considered a more significant modifier than even drugs, which are secondarily resorted to when dietary correction is insufficient. Thus food is to be consumed with awareness and choice and the right diet is the primeval requirement for a disease-free state.

Charaka Samhita asserts that 'when properly used even a poison becomes a good remedy and even food can become a poison if improperly used'. Mindless overindulgent food intake with little concern for its nutritional value is today acknowledged as the primary causative agent (thus a poison!) in numerous chronic ailments thus currently validating the medical wisdom of 'yester centuries'.

Ayurveda places great emphasis on diet, because proper assimilation of dietary constituents is essential for the maintenance of health and improper assimilation results in intermediary products of digestion with toxic properties called *ama*. Ayurveda stresses prevention of the formation and accumulation of *ama* through appropriate diet and the use of therapies to improve digestion. It also considers various dietary factors that trigger or eliminate certain diseases. Since dietary constituents are believed to influence drug action, Ayurveda also prescribes special diets or abstinence from specific regular food items.

AYURVEDIC *MATERIA MEDICA*

There are thousands of medicinal plant species found in the *materia medica* of Ayurveda, a tribute to the great biodiversity of the Indian subcontinent. Ayurveda has a unique way of understanding plants, with classic treatises like *Charaka Samhita* providing an exhaustive description of around 600 plants and their medicinal uses. It contains information on nomenclature, descriptions for identification, biological properties and action, habitat, regional specifications of substitutes and poisonous plants, methods of collecting plants, methods of classifying, combining and processing plant drugs.

Ayurveda has a long history of incorporating non-native plants into its *materia medica* such as Smilax chinensis (*madhusnuhi*) brought from China in the 16th century and later mentioned as a treatment for syphilis in the *Bhavaprakasha*. Drugs are admitted into the *materia medica* of Ayurveda only after they have been rigorously appraised in terms of their biological properties and systemic action. They are then classified into a therapeutic class and fixed into a set of formulations after specifications are provided for their processing and clinical application.

Charaka Samhita has expounded general principles of drug action based on five factors namely *rasa, guna, virya, vipaka* and *prabhava*.

1. *Dravya guna vignana* is the branch of Ayurveda concerned with the medicinal properties of food and medicine.
2. *Namarupa vignana* is a system of mnenonics providing a comprehensive picture of the naming and drug identification system adopted in Ayurveda.
3. *Yukti vignana* is concerned with application aspects and consists of
   - *Guna karma gnana* (actions and properties of drugs)
   - *Kalpana gnana* (pharmaceutical processing methods)

- *Samyakyogagnana* (incompatibilities, combinations and formulations)
- *Prayogagnana* (clinical applications).

Guna karma gnana concerned with the knowledge of properties and actions of drug substances is roughly equivalent to modern pharmacology. *Padartha* is any substance constituted like any other matter in the universe of a combination of all or some of the five universal elements. It is insentient, has no inherent quality and is devoid of consciousness. Conscious use of a *padartha* makes it a *dravya*. *Dravya*s are grouped into different ways in Ayurvedic literature based on their final therapeutic utility, effect upon the doshas, predominance of five universal elements etc.

According to *guna karma gnana*, medicinal virtue of any substance is described in terms of five essential attributes referred to as the *Pancha sheel* or five pillars of Ayurvedic pharmacology (Figure 2.3). These are *Rasa, Guna, Virya, Vipaka* and *Prabhava*.

Rasa refers to the sensory character of the dravya. Based on perception through the tongue a *dravya* could be categorized into six rasa types depending on the predominant taste it elicits. These are *madhur* (sweet), *lavana* (salt), *katu* (pungent), *kashaya* (astringent), *amla* (sour) and *tikta* (bitter). *Anurasas* are tastes that are difficult to ascertain or are tasted secondarily. They add to the overall activity of the *dravya* though weaker than the primary *rasa*. It is to be noted that

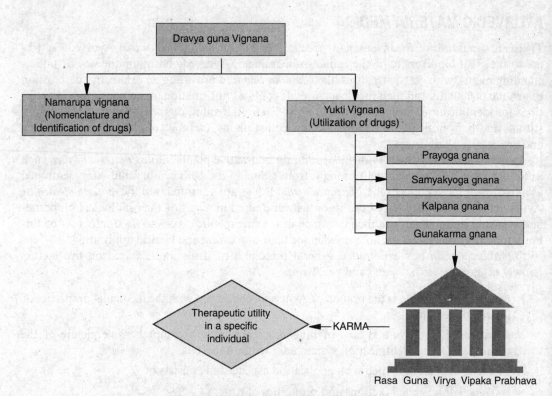

Figure 2.3. Ayurvedic principles of drug action

the classification of a *rasa* is not static due to changes occurring to the *dravya* over time, including processing and storage. E.g., ethanol extract (tincture) will add *katu rasa* to the overall *rasa* of the crude drug.

Guna refers to the *gurvadi guna* of the *dravya*. Depending on the relative preponderance of the five elements, each *dravya* is attributed with a set of these *guna*s. It can be detected from the *rasa* which is reflective of its *panchabhauti*c composition. It must be understood that each *rasa* is in general reflective of predominance of any of the five basic elements in the *dravya*. Though composed of all of the five elements, its *rasa* enables us to identify the predominant elements in the *dravya*. Thus each of the six *rasa*s is generated by a specific combination of two different *mahabhoota*s. E.g., *madhura* due to *jala* and *prithvi* (Table 2.3). Thus from the panchabhautic composition, the *guna* of the *dravya* is inferred. For example, a *dravya* with *madhura rasa* is of *snigdha guna* followed by *sita* and then *guru*. Likewise *lavana rasa dravya*s, being composed of *prithvi* and *agni,* are *guru* followed by *usna* and then *snigdha*.

Knowing that each *rasa* is composed of a particular combination of the five universal elements is a process of inference based on observation and experience recorded from innumerable *dravya guna*s. In other words taste perception helps ascertain the possible combination of the *gurvadi guna*s of a *dravya*.

Virya is the specific potency by which a *dravya* acts, based on its *guna*. Though each *dravya* is associated with a set of *gurvadi guna*s, the three primary *guna*s (*upakarma*s) which are preponderant in each *dravya* indicate its *Virya*. Or in other words the primary energetic or predominant *guna*s or qualities of a *dravya* refer to its *virya*. Thus *amalaki* fruit has a definite *amla rasa* (*ap* and *teja*) with *ap* being predominant. Hence its *virya* is *sita* and as a cooling remedy *amalaki* is used to treat *pitta*. Its *agni* constitution corrects digestion normalizing *agni*. Here the primary *ap* is predominant over *tejas*. Likewise *haritaki* fruit (*Terminalia chebula*) has a *kasaya rasa*. Of its *vayu* and *prithvi* composition *vayu* being the predominant primary attribute, its *virya* is *usna*. Thus the fruit hastens digestion at the same time countering the *sita virya* of *vata*.

Sometimes a drug is neutral in quality with neither of these being especially predominant. In this case the secondary or non-primary energetic attributes become the primary ones. The *virya* of the *dravya* is then ascertained based on these non-primary *guna*s. In general the degree of exceptional characteristics that a given *dravya* displays is often proportionate to its usefulness and such herbs that contain contradictory qualities are often a better choice in the treatment of complex disease states.

Vipaka refers to the systemic effect of the *dravya* post digestion. It describes in part where in the gastrointestinal tract the *dravya* will exert its activity and how it might affect the *dosha*s within their seats. Simply put, *vipaka* refers to the effect of the *dravya* upon the *dosha*s. Since not directly observable, it is inferred by observing its effect upon the body. According to Sushruta, *vipaka* of any *dravya* could be of either *guru* or *laghu* type. While the former increases *kapha* and decreases *vata* and *pitta*, the latter increases *pitta* and *vata* but decreases *kapha*. Charaka describes *vipaka* of a *dravya* to be of three types: *madhura vipaka* enhances *kapha* decreasing *pitta*; *amla vipaka* enhances *pitta*, decreasing *vata;* and *katu vipaka* enhances *vata*, decreasing *kapha*.

Prabhava is the actual physiological effect the *dravya* has in a specific disease state. More often than not *prabhava* refers to the tropism of a *dravya* to a specific ailment. Since it is not logically inferred from *rasa, virya, vipaka* of the *dravya*, Ayurveda calls it the inexplicable attribute, *achintya*. Because it is subject to numerous influences namely the individual's *prakrti*, age, diet, heredity, disease stage, etc., it cannot be rationalized within the conceptual framework of *dravyaguna* unlike *rasa*, *vipaka* and *virya* which are explicable (*chintya*), i.e., it is beyond inferential thought.

Two drugs having the same *rasa*, *virya*, *vipaka* may have a different *prabhava:* e.g., *Citraka* (Plumbago zeylanica) and *danti* (Baliospermum montanum) have identical *rasa*, *virya*, *vipaka*, but the latter is a strong purgative while the former is not. Thus *prabhava* describes how certain *dravya*s seem to display a specificity in action that cannot be matched by another herb which otherwise exhibits the same qualities.

Karma literally means action and refers to the specific therapeutic activity of a given *dravya* in a specific individual. Thus *rasa*, *guna*, *virya*, *vipaka* and *prabhava* are the qualitative indicators which guide in ascertaining the *guna karma* or actual therapeutic activity in a certain individual. While the latter is patient specific, the former listed qualities are *dravya* specific. There are approximately 150 types of pharmacological actions (*karma*s) listed in Ayurvedic literature. These are specific actions that the *dravya* could exert on the body through different combination of factors. E.g., *Langhana* (depletion), *Brhmana* (nourishing), *Vamana* (emesis), *Virecana* (purgation) etc.

The therapeutic effects of *dravya* on different physiological systems form the basis of Ayurvedic pharmacology. There are an estimated 50,000 herbal formulations in the traditional formulae of Ayurveda. Charaka Samhita discusses remedies for several diseases and lists specific drugs. These formulae get modified to suit local conditions by, for instance, substituting the non-principal component (*apradhana dravya*) with an equivalent either listed in the *Sastra*s or selected on the basis of the principle of *rasa*, *virya* etc. From time to time in tune with such an understanding, *Vaidya*s produce regional texts and manuals that set out recipes for drugs in any given area based on what is available and suitable to the requirements of that area.

Bhaisajya Vyakhyana under *Kalpana gnana* refers to the principles of pharmacy used in the preparation of a *dravya* into an *oushadi* or medicine. It is processed in a certain way to either remove impurities and toxins or to make the medicament more bioavailable etc. Multiplicity of techniques engaged involves the subject matter of *bhaisajya vyakhyana*. Compared to other medical systems Ayurvedic medicine maintains a relatively sophisticated dosing strategy, dependent upon a number of factors, including the disease being treated and the specific disease underlying the pathology.

THE BEST OF AYURVEDA AND ITS INFLUENCE OVER OTHER MEDICAL SYSTEMS

Ayurveda grew into a respected and widely used system of healing in India. Having influenced many of the other older traditional methods of healing including Tibetan, Chinese and Greek medicine, it is rightly considered as the 'Mother of healing sciences'. Every occidental and Asian civilization has borrowed Ayurvedic knowledge and applied it to their cultural context and medical system. Plastic surgery, acupuncture, disease classification, organization of medical schools – all stem from the Ayurvedic tradition. Further to the classic text period Ayurveda delineated eight specific branches:

1. *Kayachikitsa* – Medicine
2. *Shalya-tantra* – General surgery
3. *Shalakya-tantra* – Ophthalmology and Otorhinolaryngology
4. *Agada-tantra* – Toxicology and jurisprudence

5. *Rasayana* – Geriatrics
6. *Vajikarana* – Fertility and sterility
7. *Bhuta-vaidya* – Psychiatry
8. *Kaumarabritya* – Paediatrics, Obstetrics and Gynaecology

The fact that *kayachikitsa* or treatment with drugs was an evolved specialization is evident from the extensive Ayurvedic *materia medica* which represents full utilization of environmental resources. More than 600 drugs of animal, plant and mineral origin are used in Charaka Samhita and about 650 in Sushruta Samhita. At the beginning of the 20th century Paul Ehrlich introduced the western world to the concept of targeting drugs to the site of action. This concept was used in India since the teaching of Charaka who wrote among other texts, the *Adhisthana* in the 1st century AD, in which he described using drugs that have an affinity for specific tissues.

Surgery was at its best in the pre-Buddhist era with description of various operative techniques and procedures like abdominal operations for intestinal obstruction and removal of bladder stones; plastic surgery like rhinoplasty; operations for delivering the foetus; amputation of limbs, treatment of complicated fractures and dislocations; treatment of piles and fistula, cataracts and complicated ophthalmic operations; correction of strangulated hernia; intestinal perforations and visceral protrusions due to accidental injuries being described in the Sushruta Samhita.

Surgery was considered the best, quickest and generally the most successful method of treatment, as it involves total removal of the diseased part or morbid accumulation of *doshas; dhatus* and *malas* and gives the organism a better chance to acquire a new equilibrium by post-surgical medication to replenish removed tissues, fluids and secretions. A great variety of surgical accessories namely bandages, splints and plasters made of an assortment of materials like horse-mane, human hair, silk, vegetable oils, pulverized cereals as also surgical instruments including scalpels, razors, saws, probes, needles, hooks, forceps, pincers, hammers, tubular appliances, hollow hemispheres are described in the Sushruta Samhita. He describes 8 broad groups of surgical procedures, 101 different types of blunt surgical instruments and 24 types of sharp surgical instruments. Sushruta's classification of surgical instruments is considered complete in every respect even today.

Historical evidence of rhinoplasty practised as late as the 18th century indicates the technical expertise available and today it is actually being incorporated in modern plastic surgery. Earlier British physicians travelled to India to study rhinoplasty using a flap of skin from the forehead being performed by Indians. Reports on Indian rhinoplasty were published in the Gentleman's Magazine by 1794. Joseph Constantine Carpue spent 20 years in India studying local plastic surgery methods and he was able to perform the 'Indian' method of nose reconstruction in the western world by 1815.

The uncanny observations of Sushruta on the spread of infectious diseases through physical contact are an obvious forerunner to Joseph Lister's germ theory and antisepsis.

Ayurveda and Siddha

In the course of time, Ayurveda prevalent in the north supplemented itself and also enriched the Siddha system of medicine prevalent in the south. The latter's origin is attributed to sage Agasthya and ancient texts mention 18 Siddhars or seers of knowledge as the initial proponents of this system. The therapeutics of Siddha medicine, an ocean of knowledge by itself, consisted mainly of the use of metals, minerals and ores including mercury, arsenic, mica, magnetic iron, gold, silver, antimony etc. Well versed in alchemy, ancient Siddha practitioners knew the medicinal uses of metallic compounds and ores and were adept in the preparation of medicines from these which unlike vegetable drugs are not subject to decay and do not lose potency over time. These medicines administered in small doses and available at all seasons could be well preserved. According to Siddha percepts, which shared the same panchabhautic concept of the human body with Ayurveda, metal-based drugs could arrest the decay of the human body. This, the ancient forerunner of *Rasayana* therapy, possibly influenced the development of *Rasachikitsa* referring to the collection of treatment practices under the *Rasayana* or rejuvenative therapy of Ayurveda. It employed metals, their salts and alloys and also sulphurs. Works devoted to the preparation of inorganic and metallic remedies are among the most prolific and rewarding sources of knowledge of ancient Indian chemistry. The *Rasachikitsa* school of medicine has been a rival of Ayurveda in popularity and prestige during many centuries in the past especially in south India, eastern provinces and Sind. It survives to the present day as a living system of medicine and has absorbed many tenets of classic Ayurveda.

Ayurveda, Unani and Greek Medical Traditions

Since its inception Ayurveda has had global appeal. Its influence spread to other parts of the world, namely South East Asia as early as 1000 BC. Trade and cultural relations with Mesopotamia, Gulf countries and Persia as early as the 3rd millennium BC, attracted scholars from Tibet, China, Indo-China, Sri Lanka, Rome, Egypt, Afghanistan and Persia. They travelled to India to learn medical wisdom and the spirituality it sprang from.

During the Islamic period Ayurveda contributed to the development of Arabic medical sciences when translations of Ayurvedic texts were done in Persian (700 AD) and Arabic (800 AD). All the Abbasid Caliphs from Al-Mansur (754–773 AD) to Al-Mutawakkil (847–886 AD) were patrons of arts and sciences. The former, the second Abbasid caliph, received embassies from Sindh, one of which included some Indian *pandits* who presented him two Indian books on astronomy, The *Brahma Siddhanta* and the *Khandakhadyaka,* which by the orders of the Caliph were translated into Arabic by Ibrahim-al-Fazari (786–806 AD).

Yahya bin Khalid (805 AD) the vizier of Caliph Mahdi sent an Arab scholar to India to study and bring Indian drugs and spices. Manaka (Mankha or Minikya) proficient in Ayurveda with a sound knowledge of Indian and Persian languages was deputed as Chief of the Royal Hospital at Baghdad and translated several books from Sanskrit to Persian or Arabic language. Ibn Dhan (Dhanya or Dhanwantri) was an Indian *Vaidya* at Baghdad who at the behest of Yahya Bin Khalid rendered a few Sanskrit texts into Arabic. Saleh bin Behla a competent practitioner of Ayurveda is known to have cured Ibrahim bin Saleh of apoplexy after being declared dead by the Caliph's own physicians.

Maulana Shill Numani mentioned as Duban, a well-known Indian orientalist mentions in his scholarly monographs entitled Al- Mamun, the visit of several Indian scientists and experts of Ayurveda to impart Indian medical education and to render scientific books in Pehlavi language in the medical academy and translation Bureau of Jundishapur.

Rhazes (865–965 AD) and Avicenna (Ibn Sina 980–1037 AD) were Arabic medicine scholars who influenced global medical literature for a long time. The 'Canon of Medicine' written by Ibn Sina quotes Indian medical texts and has been used for centuries as an authoritative text on Unani medicine. It was translated into Latin in the 12th century AD and was a text book in European Medical Institutes for a long time.

Around 500 BC various Ayurvedic works spread to other parts of the world after being translated into Arabic. Several Ayurvedic texts were translated into Greek by Cnidos (300 BC). The medical historian Major wrote that after the conquest of Alexander the Great in the 4th century BC, contact with India was established and Indian medical science became part of Greek heritage.

The fact that Greeks followed the four-element theory of earth, air, fire and water and considered the four governing humours of the body as black bile, yellow bile, blood and phlegm is definitely no mere coincidence or serendipity. The Hippocratic method influenced by Ayurvedic medical thought through Arabic medical literature favoured dietary and life-style adjustments over drug use. Failure of these approaches led to drug preparation and administration. Greek literature mentions that Galen attempted to balance the humours of an ill individual by using drugs (polypharmaceutical preparations) of a supposedly contrary nature. This is starkly reminiscent of the adjustment of *dosha* imbalance through drugs in Ayurveda.

In 16th century Europe, Paracelsus, known as the father of modern western medicine, practised and propagated a system of medicine (involving minerals) which borrowed heavily from Ayurveda.

Ayurveda, Chinese and Tibetan Medicine

India was in contact with China even during the Kushana times (1 AD). Bahlika (now located in Afghanistan) was an important centre where traders from China, India and West Asia met and exchanged ideas and goods. India's contact with China was firmly established during the Gupta period with numerous scholars from China, Tibet and other Far Eastern countries travelling to India to study Buddhism and Ayurvedic medicine at the famed Nalanda University by 300 AD. Chinese scholars like Fahiyan, Ywan Chwang and Itsing were great cultural ambassadors between the two countries. They translated Ayurvedic texts into Tibetan and Chinese (Sharma 1992). The Bower Manuscript (named after its discoverer Lieutenant H. Bower) found in 1890 in Kuchar in eastern Turkestan, on the great caravan route to China indicates its writers to be Indian Buddhist monks. Thus not surprisingly Chinese medicine has several parallels with Ayurveda. Its *Yin* and *Yang* concept is comparable to Indian *Purusha* and *Prakriti*. So also are the five basic elements of both the systems.

With the translation of *Ashtanga Hrdaya* into Tibetan (Das 1992) in 8th C AD, Tibetan system of medicine was greatly influenced by Ayurveda while retaining its integral place with Buddhism. This trend of exportation of Indian medical literature which continued till early 19th century resulted in translation and preservation of a huge collection of Indian literature on various subjects like religion, sciences, arts, culture, language etc. 'Sowa-Rigpa' or the Amchi system of medicine – one of the oldest and well-documented medical traditions of the world popularly practised in Tibet, Mangolia, Bhutan, some parts of China, Nepal, Himalayan regions of India and a few parts of the former Soviet Union – is a classic example of an amalgamation of medical knowledge across countries. Thus the practice of Ayurveda flourished and spread to many other countries up to the Buddhist period. However it suffered a gradual decline due to serious Mughal incursions followed by the British rule.

That these systems were alive until the beginning of the 20th century is borne out by the 19th-century Ayurvedic studies recorded in *Nighantu*s of the Ayurvedic properties of exotic plants like tea, coffee, green chillies, brinjal, tomato, potato, pineapple, etc., which entered the Indian soil only in the last 200 years. *Bhava prakasha* written by Bhava Mishra in the 16th century mentions a syphilitic disease called *Firanga roga* (foreigner's disease) prevalent among the Portuguese who came to India for trade at that time. Foreign invasions also brought about destruction and loss of valuable medical texts. In the early 18th century, the British removed state patronage to Ayurveda and the East India Company closed all schools of Ayurvedic medicine to start its own medical college in Calcutta.

REVIVAL AND CURRENT STATUS

In the early 19th century however, there was a national awakening in India which promoted a revival in Ayurveda. A government committee was constituted in 1946 which made recommendations for Ayurvedic teaching, research and education. Education of Ayurveda has been regularized by the Central Council of Indian Medicine, an autonomous body established under a Parliamentary Act. Revival of this age-old science in post-independence India resulted in Ayurvedic medicine being widely practised and taught often in conjunction with western medicine. Currently Ayurveda is being taught throughout India in more than 200 Ayurvedic colleges (check current figures) and universities of which around 140 colleges have facilities for UG studies and 60 of them have PG teaching facilities. At present there are more than 4 lakh Ayurvedic practitioners in India. Most of the clinical research in Ayurveda is being performed as post doctoral thesis work at several reputed Ayurveda universities.

The Government of India has accorded equal status to Ayurvedic and modern medicine graduates. It has created a separate Directorate for Indigenous Systems of Medicine in the Ministry of Health from March 1995 in order to fully utilize the potential of Ayurveda and other alternate medical sciences in the National Health Programmes.

There has however been a 'lull' in the 20th century in terms of new applications in Ayurveda. Despite the existence of large amounts of readily usable reference materials there has been a dearth of knowledge expansion in these systems not because of medical inefficiency but more due to economic, cultural and political factors. There is an urgent need on the part of the Ayurvedic medical fraternity and Indian policy makers to enable serious research on the theoretical foundations of indigenous medicine, which is well underway in many western universities.

An important feature of the wealth of ancient scientific, medical and technological wisdom in this subcontinent is that its theories and principles are not meant to be reposed in a small number of experts, institutions or texts. These were instead created and shared by great men and women who in stark contrast to the current craving for authorship, ownership and patent rights made this available on a wider scale to even ordinary folk. Thus local health practices interacted and developed with traditional knowledge such that our folk tradition is a treasure trove of nutritional information about thousands of ecosystem-specific food resources in addition to plant drug know-how.

However in India in the last 200 years, the scientific, economic and political influence of western biomedicine has been overwhelming and has affected all sections of society including the tribals. Also large-scale westernization and loss of cultural values are fast leading to erosion of such commonly available medical knowledge. There is reduced use of home remedies, traditional diets and health customs and a declining interest in folk traditions even in villages thanks to the heavy promotion of western values and products through the omnipresent media. It is alarming to see that traditional medical knowledge is further marginalized due to the renewed political and economic effects of globalism, which in its current form, has its intellectual and philosophical roots in mainstream western cultures.

The western world however has taken great interest in Ayurveda in recent times. During the last few decades many original Ayurvedic Sanskrit texts have been translated into various European languages, including English. Countries that have taken up study of Ayurveda include Australia, Poland, Brazil, Pakistan, Russia, Bangladesh, Switzerland, Germany, Netherlands, Italy, South Africa, Sri Lanka, Japan, United Kingdom, Mauritius, Nepal, Venezuela and the United States. Today there is a new proliferation of Ayurvedic classes, schools and treatment centres in most major metropolitan areas. The Maharishi International University in Fair Field, Iowa, USA has set up an Ayurvedic college. It has Ayurvedic Medical Centers in 29 countries and has treated over 90,000 patients in the United States alone. This has greatly contributed to the current popularity of Ayurveda in the west. The number of books on Ayurveda has also increased with a steady stream of interesting titles expanding global awareness of this profound field of medicine.

Research institutes world over are today engaged in the study, research and promotion of Ayurvedic medicine. The fast growing number of these institutes in Europe, the United States and Australia are a standing testimony to the global awareness of the significance and realization of the need to tap the hidden potential of this ancient knowledge. Ayurveda is gradually entering mainstream health care, being adopted by medical doctors, naturopaths, chiropractors, herbalists, nutritionists etc. The concept of integrating the best of all treatment practices towards providing a safe, holistic and comprehensive medical care is considered a pertinent solution to the current global health crisis. It is thus time for the study of pharmacognosy in our country to include and pursue the immense knowledge reserve of Ayurveda by

- Initiating interdisciplinary research efforts across the fields of Ayurvedic medicine, pharmacognosy, phytoanalytical chemistry, phytotherapy etc.
- Developing newer methods of standardization of traditional dosage forms
- Exploring newer methods of measuring/reproducing subjective phenomenon
- Development of more sensitive biomedical research tools to evaluate the concepts of Ayurveda more effectively.

CONCLUSION

The 'mother of all healing sciences' – Ayurveda is a complete system that evolved over time integrating centuries of wisdom derived from experience. A striking characteristic of Indian traditional knowledge sourced right from the Vedas is the principle of amalgamation. No area of study, be it philosophy, medicine, astronomy, alchemy or architecture, is expounded to the exclusion of other inter-related disciplines. Thus an understanding in perspective of the nature of the mind (manas) – the origination of which has been the preoccupation of Indian philosophy for millennia – consciousness (chitta) and pure awareness (mahat) is very essential to understand their impact upon healthy living and causes of disease or disturbance to this normal state. Modern medical science's current stand that most chronic ailments are psychosomatic is a current day affirmation of an ancient knowledge in this sub-continent. Ousted from its legitimate pedestal at the heyday of western colonization and supremacy, today Ayurveda is undergoing a vigourous revival not only in the country of its origin – India, but also throughout the world. Global disease burden and acknowledgement of the limitations of modern medicine are driving the global search for more holistic and preventive health care access to all. The ancient tradition of Ayurveda is resonant of such fundamental insights that are only now being developed in cutting edge science and is hence being validated on modern lines. With the global awakening of the need to integrate the best of all medical systems each addressing the facet of its strength towards meeting the rising health care needs, pharmacognosy research in our country needs to be specifically geared to explore the potential drugs/treatment options Ayurveda has to offer in the coming years.

REVIEW QUESTIONS

Essay Questions

1. What are tridoshas? Describe their centrality to health and disease causation as conceived by Ayurveda.
2. Outline the principles of drug action as propounded by the Ayurvedic *materia medica*.
3. Discuss the significant contribution of Ayurveda to health and healing in it best days.

Short Notes

1. Literature on Ayurveda.
2. Panchamahabhootas and the human body.
3. Gurvadi gunas and Ayurvedic pharmacology.
4. Revival of interest in Ayurveda.
5. Principles of diagnosis and treatment in Ayurveda.

3

Worldwide Trade in Herbal Products

CHAPTER OBJECTIVES

Introduction

Trade in Plant-Based Products

Hurdles to the Development of Medicinal Plant Trade

Sources of Plant Material

Categories of Medicinal Plant-Derived Products Traded

Global Trade in Some Individual Plant Drugs

INTRODUCTION

Using plants for medicinal purposes has a long tradition dating back thousands of years in countries such as China and India. According to the World Health Organization (WHO) they still form the basis of traditional or indigenous health systems for majority of populations in most developing countries. Today in several parts of the world, there is growing credibility for traditional Chinese medicine (TCM), Ayurveda, Unani and also for complementary or alternative medicine utilized in industrialized countries. On account of several significant contributing factors herbal medicine, once discounted as superstitious/irrational medicine of native and ancient cultures, is emerging as a popular alternative and even supplement to modern medicine. In acknowledgement of the worldwide demand for holistic treatment practices, the WHO is encouraging, promoting and recommending its member countries to reintroduce time-tested medicinal plants and derivatives into primary health care, where modern medicine is unavailable as low-cost alternatives.

According to Food and Agriculture Organization of United Nations (FAO, UN), the last three decades have seen substantial growth in herb and herbal product markets across the world. There is a huge global market for plants used in the preparation of phytomedicines as used by traditional systems, homeopaths and herbalists. Such medicines are today available in pharmacies, supermarkets and health food outlets. To enable easier access, traders and crude drug suppliers have extended their market base by supplying medicinal plants, spices and plant extracts to food, flavour, fragrance and cosmetic industries. Today the herbal drug industry is thus a very fast growing sector in the international market. The fact that the global market for herbal products is affected by regional changes in regulatory or marketing strategies is illustrated by its impressive growth in the United States fuelled by passage of the Dietary Supplement Health and Education Act of 1994. Also the United States Food and Drug Administration (USFDA) has published draft guidelines for development of botanical medicines as drugs, reflecting a growing interest in the drug model for these products.

Rapidly rising exports of medicinal plants during the past decade attests to worldwide interest in these products as well as in traditional health systems; 30% of the drugs sold worldwide contain compounds derived from plant material and a far higher figure is associated to a great variety of medicines bought over the counter.

Higher plant products either unmodified or altered, account for 25% of all prescriptions in OECD countries and upto 60% of those in Eastern Europe. These include important therapeutic categories such as contraceptives, steroid and muscle relaxants, antimalarials (quinine and artemisinin), cardiotonics (digoxin) and anti-cancer drugs (Taxol, etoposide, vincristine/vinblastine). These drugs are not amenable to cost-effective total synthesis and require for their production reliable supplies of plant material. About 95 plant species are listed as sources of 121 clinically useful prescription drugs and many more are associated with a large number of OTC drugs. As per a WHO estimate, 80% of the population in developing countries depend on plant-based drugs for their health care needs and it predicts that in the coming decades, a similar percentage of the world population will rely on plant drugs.

TRADE IN PLANT-BASED PRODUCTS

According to the Secretariat of the Convention on Biological Diversity, global sales of herbal products totalled an estimated US $ 60 billion in 2002 and it is expected to get higher at 6.4 per cent average growth rate. This figure represents the world market for all plant-derived chemicals – pharmaceuticals, industrial ancillary products, pesticides, fragrances, flavours and colour ingredients.

As per the 1982 International Trade Classification (ITC) report, pharmaceutical applications of medicinal plant-derived products represented less than 20% of the total market for botanical products. *According to this report it is not possible to assess the volume of or value of trade in all botanicals that are used medicinally because trade statistics do not identify medicinal and other uses separately.*

Assessing all aspects of medicinal plant trade with certainty on a global level is difficult due to a number of reasons.

- Wide diversity of plants involved.
- Non-availability of accurate trade-related data on medicinal plants.
- Individual trade statistics of several hundred medicinal plants in commerce cannot be estimated as these are not itemized in national trade data. Only plants entering a country in very large quantities are listed individually.
- Available trade data does not distinguish between medicinal and other uses.
- Medicinal plants like liquorice have multiple uses ranging from flavouring a variety of products to stabilizing foam in fire extinguishers. This is in addition to its being used as an expectorant and anti-inflammatory.

- Products reported as medicinal plants include gums, spices, teas, infusions, insecticides and cosmetics.
- Essential oils such as mint oil, eucalyptus oil, cinnamon leaf oil etc. are used both in flavouring and as medicine.
- Large part of domestic trade is poorly classified and/or improperly recorded.
- Rising worldwide demand for medicinal plants has created a sustained and largely 'underground' trade in plant materials, most of which are collected in an unregulated manner.

According to Lewington (1993) the situation in medicinal plant trade is rather more complicated because of various levels of secrecy maintained by the traders and the complexity of the trade structure itself. According to ITC, medicinal plants come under Non-Wood Forest Products (NWFP) which are a heterogeneous group. Thus trade data based on compilation of items coded Standard International Trade Classification (SITC) 292.4, 292.41, 292.42 and 292.49 (Table 3.1) are indicative of products not only used for medicinal purposes but also as cosmetics, paints, dyes, insecticides and detergents. Of the over 3,000 botanical raw material species in global commerce the ITC report covers the most important exported natural products. Measuring the size of the sector is thus a challenge as there is no comprehensive and exhaustive listing of Hormonized Tariff Codes (HTCs) for Medicinal and Aromatic Plants (MAPs) and their extracts. For e.g., products under the SITC Revision 3 are classified into 10 sections, 67 divisions, 261 groups, 1,033 sub-groups; 720 sub-groups are further divided into 2,805 items providing 3,118 basic sub-groups. The SITC Rev 3 follows a 5-digit coding. Many countries are struggling with the lack of specificity of their tariff schedules and are looking to add more specific 8- and 10-digit codes for

Table 3.1 Plant-derived industrial products

S.No	Plant-Derived Product	Industrial Use
1	Essential oils	Perfumery, cosmetics, food, pharmaceuticals
2	Resins and balsams	Pharmaceutical aids besides other non-pharmaceutical uses
3	Fixed oils	Medicinal/nutritive/pharmaceutical aid
4	Fatty acids	Nutraceutical/soap/detergent making
5	Gums	Medicinal/non-medicinal
6	Condensed tannins	Medicinal/tanning
7	Saponins and surfactants	Chemical/pharmaceutical aids
8	Natural rubber	Rubber industry, automobile, aircraft, consumer products
9	Waxes	Pharmaceutical aid/other
10	Dyes	Edible/non-edible
11	Pesticides	Insecticides/herbicides/rodenticides
12	Industrial organic acids	Fine chemicals, textile, pharmaceutical and others
13	Cotton and other vegetable fibres	Textile, paper, pharmaceutical and others
14	Industrial starch	Textile, food, cement, paper and others
15	Food or food additives	Food, beverage and others

their most important botanical imports and exports. Even when national schedules of tariff codes are referenced by an enterprise, these lack the specificity to differentiate down to the botanical species level (using Latin binomials) and furthermore to the various processed forms of a species. In addition, natural botanical ingredients are not cohesively grouped within the current HTCs. A botanical ingredient may be classified by some exporters as a dried root or tuber, by others as a spice and by yet others as a medicinal substance.

Based on import statistics of medicinal plants for the period 1987–1991, world trade in medicinal plants on an average is US $853,000. Total value of world trade in medicinal plants during 1991 was around US $1.08 million.

- China is the biggest producer as well as exporter of medicinal plants, accounting for 30% of total world trade (by value) in 1991, followed by Korea, the United States, India and Chile.
- China with exports of over 12,000 tonnes per annum and India with some 32,000 tonnes per annum dominate the international markets. Singapore and Hong Kong are the main re-exporters of medicinal plants in Asia. Japan, the United States, Germany, France, Italy, Malaysia and Spain are the major markets.
- Hamburg is the world trading centre in medicinal plants.
- About 53 countries supply medicinal plants to Germany of which important ones are India, Argentina, former Yugoslavia, Greece, China, Poland, Egypt, Hungary, Czechoslovakia, Zaire, Albania, Netherlands and France.
- 400,000 tonnes of medicinal plants with an average market value of US $1 billion are imported into Europe from Africa and Asia.
- According to IUCN/WWF (IUCN-WWF, 1988) sources, the annual turnover of plant-derived pharmaceuticals industry in the United States is US $10 billion.
- North America is an important region for medicinal plant trade with retail sales of herbal medicine industry in 1994 at an estimated US $1.6 billion.
- There is a significant demand for medicinal plant material in North America which is a fast growing market. Eastern Europe and Asia supply most of its needs and in the last five years, demand in North America for Chinese medicine, Indian herbs and Latin American crude drugs is also significant.
- Traditional medicine is an important part of African culture and 80% of Africans rely on plant-based medicine.
- About 70% to 90% of the population in South Africa, Zambia, Nigeria, Mozambique, Ethiopia and Democratic Republic of Congo among others rely on traditional medicine for their health care.
- In South Africa on a national level 20,000 tonnes of medicinal plant materials are traded, corresponding in value to US $60 million.
- In Zambia, trade in traditional medicine is worth US $43 million per annum. Medicinal plant-based therapies also play a significant role in most Latin American countries. 70–80% of the population rely on such therapies and there is a lack of access to modern drugs in a significant part of Latin America.
- Developing countries with a long tradition of use of medicinal plants such as China, India, Republic of Korea, Thailand, Brazil and Chile are major exporting countries of plant raw materials.

- China and India are two of the world's largest markets for medicinal plants, but are not the largest traders. This is because markets in developed countries, especially Europe and the United States, are highly regulated and difficult to penetrate because of stringent test requirements for plant material by the pharmaceutical manufacturers of developed countries.

- As a result developing countries tend to export unprocessed or slightly processed materials, while developed countries undertake mass production of finished products thus becoming dominant exporters of finished products.

- Thus in absolute terms, developing and developed countries import similar values of medicinal plants. For e.g. 80% of Indian exports constitute raw materials, including dried plants, extracts and isolated ingredients, while finished herbal products mostly homeopathic and Ayurvedic medicines account for only 20%.

- Chief herbal drug importing countries by value are China, Hong Kong, United States, Japan and Germany. Germany is a leading importer and its pharmaceutical companies are major players in the world market.

Out of the global market of US $60 billion a year, as per an estimate in 1991, the herbal product market in European countries was about $ 6 billion, with Germany accounting for $ 3 billion, France $ 1.6 billion and Italy 0.6 billion while in other countries it was 0.8 billion. In 1996, the herbal product market in European countries was about $ 10 billion, in the United States $ 4 million, in India about $ 1.0 billion and in other countries $ 5 billion. In 1997 the European market alone reached $ 7 billion. The German market corresponds to about 50% of the European market, about $ 3.5 billion. This market is followed by France, $1.8 billion; Italy $ 700 million; the United Kingdom, $ 400 million; Spain 4 300 million; the Netherlands, about $ 100 million.

According to a 2009 study by BCC Research, the global market for botanical and plant derived drugs is expected to increase from $ 19.5 billion in 2008 to $32.9 billion in 2013, an annual growth rate of 11%. In terms of volume global exports and imports of medicinal plants has been increasing, although the total value has been declining, suggesting falling average unit prices.

HURDLES TO THE DEVELOPMENT OF MEDICINAL PLANT TRADE

International trade in medicinal plants is expanding with increasing market for plant materials that are used in health and medical products. Most developing countries endowed with vast resources of medicinal and aromatic plants have immense opportunity for utilizing this growing market value of these resources. Countries such as China, India and Sri Lanka have officially recognized the use of traditional medicines in their health care delivery systems. There are however hurdles to be overcome to fully capitalize upon the current growth opportunity. According to Tuley De Silva, Chemical Industries Branch, United Nations Industrial Development Organization (UNIDO), they are as follows:

1. Lack of information on the social and economic benefits that could be derived from the industrial utilization of medicinal plants. Except for the use of these plants for local health needs, not much information has been available on their market potential and trading possibilities. As a result, the real potential of these plants has not been fully explored.

2. Pressure on the natural resource is increasing for plants which are in greater demand, with serious implications in terms of long-term sustainability.

3. Legislation to control harvesting and trade of medicinal plants is inadequate and ineffective in its present form.

4. The share received by local producers and gatherers for raw plants being usually low and cost of production in organized cultivation being higher it is difficult to persuade communities to undertake organized cultivation.

5. The market for herbal products is very diverse throughout the world, with each region or country having its own prerequisites for bringing those products on the market.

6. Herbal product classification varies in different parts of the world. While herbals are classified as medicine in one country, they are categorized as food in another. Quality control procedures and hence regulation for both being different, no universal quality control standards are applicable to herbals.

7. Markets for herbal medicines in developed countries are highly regulated and difficult to penetrate. Thus several traditional drugs of proven safety and efficacy are not marketable in the western world. Decisions concerning marketability are not driven solely by proof of safety and efficacy. To be marketable a drug candidate must affect only one point on a biochemical pathway. Products that affect multiple points of the same pathway are unlikely to be marketed because only 'magic bullets' are viable in today's legal and economic environment.

8. Consistent and reliable volumes of unadulterated plant material of consistent quality are required for use in medicine and health care markets. Proper harvesting and post-harvesting treatment practices difficult to meet fully under wild harvesting conditions are constraints.

9. Several Least Developed Countries (LDC's) lack knowledge of their supply capabilities and few have the resources and institutional capability to advise on policy or the regulatory mechanism to provide consistent high-quality products.

10. These countries have limited knowledge of the herbs' medicinal properties beyond traditional knowledge and belief. This restricts their use and marketability even in local markets.

11. There is insufficient research on development of high-yielding varieties, quality control procedures are poor and R&D on product and process development is inadequate in these countries.

12. An issue of potentially major importance to all developing country exporters is intellectual property rights (IPR). Plants have been used in traditional medicines for centuries and hence cannot be protected by patents. They can be registered as individual or regional trade marks, with explicit rules of origin. Knowledge of IPR is limited in developing countries as is access to IPR systems. This issue is currently under discussion, debate and negotiation on a broader scale than for medicinal plants in the World Trade Organization (WTO).

SOURCES OF PLANT MATERIAL

The two sources of supply of medicinal plants are collection from the *wild* and *cultivated* material. In many traditions of medicine, wild harvested material is considered to have higher therapeutic benefits, and therefore commands a higher price.

Plant material sourced from the wild such as bark, leaves, fruits, herbs, flowers, wood or roots are collected from many locations including open pasture, waste agricultural lands, gardens, roadside and forest land. Sometimes they may be 'weeds' found in agricultural or waste land, or plants or plant parts found in horticultural areas. The bulk of the material traded, both domestically and internationally, is still wild harvested and only a very small number of species are cultivated. Although the major part of the wild harvested material is sourced from developing countries, a surprisingly high amount is also gathered in developed countries. For example, in the United States, an estimated 200 tonnes of *Echinacea angustifolia* is wild harvested annually and 220,589 pounds of ginseng were wild harvested in 1992. In France, more than 500 species were wild harvested during 1988–1989, including those used homeopathically.

A significant part of wild-harvested material now traded commercially, with very low prices being paid to gatherers, commercial plant gatherers often 'mine' the natural resource with no concern about its sustainability. Prices of medicinal plants collected from the wild tend to vary in a cyclic manner. Price cycles of 6 to 7 years are common as the availability of many plants goes from over supply to scarcity very quickly and then takes several years to return to normal. Of particular concern for the sustainability of the wild resource is the fact that many of the materials are roots of plants, which are the most difficult plant parts to harvest sustainably. Many countries do not have regulations controlling the collection of material from the wild. India has banned the export of several endangered wild species in the form of raw material, with no such restrictions however on the export of finished herbal products containing such species. Despite this, an estimated 95% of medicinal plants collected in India are gathered from the wild and the process of collection is said to be destructive. Equally a major part of the high-range Himalayan plants are wild harvested and many of these are close to extinction from over-harvesting or unskillful harvesting, e.g., *Nardostachys jatamansi, Aconitum* spp. An estimated 70–90% of medicinal plant material imported into Germany is wild harvested and only 50–100 species among these are currently propagated on a large scale.

In China the output of the area cultivated is estimated to be between 300,000 and 400,000 tonnes whilst in 1994 the total demand for medicinal plant material was 1,600,000 tonnes. This huge gap must be made up by wild harvested material. TCM tends to use the roots of plants, which are the most difficult plant parts to harvest sustainably.

According to Lewington (1993) it is difficult to ascertain the precise origin of medicinal plants entering world trade as traders are reluctant to reveal their sources. It is however certain that the vast majority of the medicinal plants come from wild sources. There are very few plants that are only collected from cultivated material such as *Catharanthus roseus, Chamomilla recutita, Cinchona* sps, *Digitalis lanata* and *D. purpurea, Duboisia* spp, *Mentha piperita, Papaverum somniferum* and *Plantago ovata.*

Quality control requirements for cultivated material are becoming increasingly important due to stringent drug regulations in many countries. With cultivated material being more suitable for large-scale use, countries such as Argentina, China, Hungary, India, Poland and Spain cultivating plant material on a large scale are now looking at more successful commercial cultivation to produce high-quality plant material to compete in a highly competitive international market.

Due to the high cost of cultivation, it is often done under contract and only those plant species used in large quantities or in the production of derivatives and isolates that require to pass critical standardization parameters are cultivated.

Globally the areas cultivated are limited because cultivated material bears higher production costs, must have secured land ownership or access and requires more expensive and sophisticated management expertise. Costs may be carried for long periods and the low prices of wild-harvested material make the returns for cultivation low in many cases. The very long supply chain between the farmers and primary collectors and specialized wholesale suppliers is the reason for the former receiving low prices for their products.

As collection from wild is still more common than cultivation, huge differences in the quality of materials occur. Amount of active ingredients vary depending on the region the plants are grown, plant parts collected, method of harvesting and their storage conditions. Adulteration of wild drugs is a common problem as there can be no guarantee over the uniformity of the raw material. According to Cunningham (1996) medicinal plant trade passes through the following main channels:

1. Trade at the national level is the first involving hundreds of species through regional medicinal plant markets.
2. Trade across national borders, however within continents, is the second. This informal trade channel consists of fewer numbers of species with many unfortunately being threatened. E.g. *Nardostachys* and *Valerian* being traded from Nepal to India.
3. More formal international export trade is level three in which several hundred species are traded in significant volumes.

Major part of the plant material is sold by trading companies who hold enormous stocks and also have facilities to undertake the quality controls required or raw material used in the production of drugs. They play an important role in the medicinal plant trade, partly because of the large quantities they purchase which enables them to more or less dictate the price. Such traders are also able to guarantee the supply of material of specified standard of quality at a fixed price. This price and quality guarantee is a major incentive to the end user, for whom cost, quality, reliability and flexibility are said to be the key requirements for purchasing pharmaceutical raw material. In addition there are brokers who engage in purchase and sale of plant material adding their commission. Having contacts at the purchasing level they do not stock material and have no warehousing facilities. Recently emerging are the ecological traders. According to Lange (1996), they source botanical material for use generally by the smaller herbal medicine/health product companies and alternate practitioners. Such traders generally deal with organically cultivated products and are more discerning/ethical in their purchasing approach. Having shorter sales routes involving fewer parties, they establish their own contacts in the source countries and purchase only raw material and not extracts.

CATEGORIES OF MEDICINAL PLANT-DERIVED PRODUCTS TRADED

Medicinal plant material is used by a large number of industries including pharmaceuticals, cosmetics, detergents, dyes, insecticides, foods and paints. Demand for medicinal plants is undoubtedly increasing in the medicinal and health-related sectors and this growth is fuelling an increase in both the number of species and volume of plant material being traded. It is estimated that some 10,000 plant species are used medicinally with only a relatively small number of species used in significant volume. Medicinal and aromatic plants are traded both as unprocessed plant material and as processed final products. Demand for a wide variety of species is increasing as these markets expand and new end uses are developed. Figure 3.1 depicts the various categories of medicinal plant-derived products commonly traded and their inter-relationship. Each of these groups has wide subsets of products and there is an overlap of categories with products belonging to either subset in many cases.

Plant Extracts

The use of galenicals or plant extracts directly for therapeutic purpose in modern medicine stems from the herbal remedies of the Middle Ages. In addition to this such extracts may provide the first

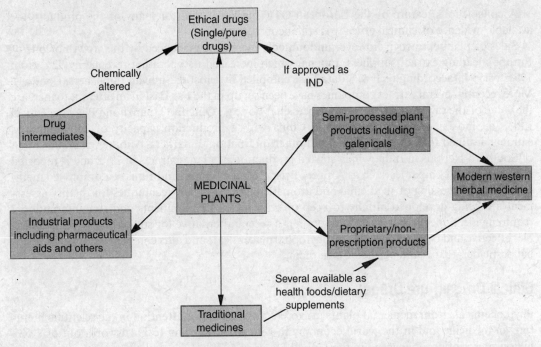

Figure 3.1. Medicinal plant products traded – their inter-relationship

stage in the isolation of active ingredients. With the resurgence of interest in herbal medicine several of these plant extracts have regained their popular usage as medicinals. Today a significant percentage of medicinal plant material is used to make plant extracts. This is carried out either by the end product manufacturer or by extract companies. The current trend of medicinal plant-based drug industry is to procure standardized extracts of plants as raw material. Plant extracts could be standardized fluid/solid extracts, powders or tinctures. Standardized extracts of many plants such as *Aloe* sps, *Atropa belladonna, Cassia angustifolia, Capsicum annum, Centella asiatica, Cephaelis ipecacuanha, Digitalis* sps, *Commiphora mukul, Panax ginseng,* etc., are widely used in health care.

An important factor behind the increasing use of standardized extracts is that they can be better incorporated into modern dosage forms and also standardization is considered necessary to achieve as much control in double blind studies as possible.

The following are the types of plant extracts or processed plant products in trade:

- Dried whole/plant parts size-reduced to form powders;
- Fluid extracts using different solvents resulting in tinctures, medicinal wines, syrups, liquid mixtures etc.;
- Solid extracts standardized and formulated or fractionated to yield concentrates of active ingredients or pure compounds.

Standardized plant extracts are sold as over-the-counter (OTC), non-prescription items. According to International Medical Statistics (IMS), half of the world expenditure on branded non-prescription herbal medicines in 1994 (US $11.9 billion) was spent in Europe. Such decoctions, tinctures and other galenicals form a part of many pharmacopoeias of the world.

A conspicuous feature of the European OTC market is that for many of the products, the available evidence of clinical efficacy is still inconclusive.

Sales of plant extracts is however undoubtedly increasing evidenced by the growth of one of Europe's leading extract suppliers, Indena, which increased its operating revenue by 92% from 1991 to 1994 (according to F & S data base compiled by Frost & Sullivan Publishers, London). More recently several extract companies have been set up in the Far East in an attempt to increase the value of the raw material through processing. For e.g., Qingdao Huanzhong Pharmaceutical Ltd is a Sino-Japanese joint venture in China with a production capacity of 240 tonnes of extracts destined for export to Japan and other international markets. Another example is that of Southern Herbals in India which started production of plant extracts in 1992 and is reported to be supplying companies such as Amgen, Bristol Meyer Squibb and Fujisawa. Improved methods for the processing of medicinal and aromatic plants and new techniques for quality assessment are being developed rapidly to keep up with recent developments and new international requirements. Super critical fluid extraction is a recent alternative for solvent extraction. It enables effective and quick processing of phytopharmaceuticals and aids complete removal of residual pesticides, toxins and surfactants in them.

Ethical Drugs (Pure Drugs)

Phytochemicals from medicinal plants are receiving ever greater attention in the scientific literature, in medicine and in the world economy in general. According to Farnsworth out of 1.532 billion prescriptions dispensed in the United States in 1973, 41.2% contained one or more constituents derived from plants. An analysis of such plant derived medicines used in prescription drugs during 1980's found that only 40 sps of higher plants are used as sources of drugs. This indicates the potential of identifying newer leads from plants considering the vast unexplored flora of the tropical rainforests. Natural product research guided by ethnopharmacological knowledge can make substantial contributions to drug innovation by providing novel chemical structures and /or mechanism of action.

Higher plants are the direct or indirect source of several modern medicines. While many erstwhile plant drugs have been replaced by better synthetic equivalents, newer plant-based molecules have gained new investigational or therapeutic status in recent years. Also a number of novel drug candidates such as taxoids, camptothecin, artemisinin have entered the drug markets following successful plant-based clinical research. The value of medicinal plants as a source of foreign exchange for developing countries depends on the use of those plants as raw materials in the pharmaceutical industry.

Production of pure phytopharmaceuticals used in modern medicine requires more processing stages and more sophisticated machinery. Such processing techniques are patent protected and even technology transfer through contractual agreements and payments may not be of much help unless there is a large local demand for such drugs. Drugs so produced are expensive due to limitations over the economy of scale of production and also because safety and pollution aspects related to these sophisticated processing techniques have to be considered. In addition to purified plant-derived drugs such as quinine, reserpine, digoxin, etc., there is an enormous market for crude herbal medicines such as extracts, powders and tinctures. In the developing countries, OTC remedies and 'ethical phytomedicines', which are toxicologically standardized and clinically defined crude drugs, are seen as a promising low-cost alternatives in primary health care.

Besides an impressive OTC market, there is also an enormous prescription market for herbal medicines in some western countries. In Germany alone, the annual sales of herbal drugs is

$2.5 billion with per capital spending of $37 on phyto medicines. Preparations from Ginkgo leaf are on the top of the best selling list. In 1995, German physicians ordered 254 million of defined daily doses of ginkgo mono preparations which corresponded to DM 425 million.

In the United States herbal medicines, vitamins and minerals are still a very small part of the entire medicine industry when compared to generic (64 billion in sales) and OTC (24 billions) drugs of modern medicine. However there are some botanicals approved as OTC drug ingredients and over a hundred botanicals either individually or in formulas are currently going through FDA's clinical trial process. The US FDA has just published draft guidelines for development of botanical medicines as drugs, reflecting a growing interest in the drug model for these products. Even before the document was published, there have been many companies and individuals that have submitted the Investigation New Drug Applications (INDs) and these are in process. The day the first IND is approved will be the turning point for the herbal drug industry as it would open the doors for the availability of herbal drugs as approved ethical drugs.

Intermediates for Drug Production

Certain plants are rich sources of intermediates used in the production of drugs. For e.g., plant saponins such as Dioscin (from Dioscorea tubers) can be extracted and altered chemically to produce sapogenins (diosgenin) required to manufacture medicinally important steroids. Steroidal saponins are of great pharmaceutical importance because of their relationship to compounds such as sex hormones, cortisone, diuretic steroids, vitamin D and cardiac glycosides. Some are used as starting material for the synthesis of these compounds. The primary processing of parts containing the intermediates could be carried out in the country of origin thus retaining some value of the resource material. For example, diosgenin and hecogenin (from Sisal) used in the production of steroids can be commercially produced in the countries of origin where there are steady supplies of sufficient raw materials. So far more than 4,000 plant species have been investigated resulting in the identification of some 30 naturally occurring steroid sapogenins many of which could provide valuable source materials for steroid compounds.

Traditional Medicines

Considerable volumes of plant material are used in traditional systems of medicine, particularly in Asia. China's total output of medicinal plants from both cultivated and wild-harvested sources is 1,600,000 tonnes. In comparison, that of Germany is relatively small at 40,000 tonnes. China is also a significant exporter of medicinal materials with export sales in 1993 reported at US $ 270 million although this figure includes plant, animal and mineral drugs. Ayurvedic and Unani herbs from India are also traded in large quantities and over a very wide geographical area. It is estimated that the total value of products from the entire Ayurvedic production in India is US $5.5 billion. The annual turnover from indigenous herbal medicines is about Rs.2,300 crores as against the pharmaceutical industry's turnover of Rs.14,500 crores. The export value of herbal drugs from India amounted to Rs. 32,603.83 lacs with a CAGR of 17.45 in 2008. Indian exports are largely to Bangladesh, Japan, Pakistan, Saudi Arabia, United States and United Arab Emirates. Major herbals exported from India is recent years are Isabgol, opium alkaloids, senna derivatives, vinca extract, cinchona alkaloids, ipecac root alkaloids, solasodine, diosgenin/16 DPA, menthol, gymnema and henna. PHARMEXCIL is the Pharmaceuticals Export Promotion Council of India governing exports of herbals and pharmaceuticals from India.

The age-old practice of the traditional practitioner dispensing his own medicines using simple but ingenious traditional methods is being gradually shifted to profit-oriented large-scale herbal drug manufacturing units. Today these medicines are produced industrially using improvised techniques with the technology available today. Traditional herbal medicinal products are characterized by the fact that their efficacy can neither be demonstrated by clinical studies nor by bibliographical data. Their efficacy may only be apparent from long-term traditional use and experience. Importance of traditional medicine in medicinal plant trade is highlighted by the WHO estimate that 80% of the population in developing countries rely on traditional medicine, primarily constituted of plant drugs, for their primary health care needs. In addition to ancient and renowned traditional systems such as Ayurveda, Unani and TCM, many less-documented systems of traditional medicine have been handed down from one generation to the next by word of mouth and are still being practised in many parts of the world. In addition to the traditional practitioners in developing countries, there are an increasing number of alternative medicine practitioners in the developed world.

It is estimated that some 10,000 plant species are used medicinally; most of these are used in traditional systems of medicine. However only a relatively small number of species is used in a significant volume. For e.g., in TCM 9,905 botanicals are used, but only an estimated 500 are commonly used.

Industrial Products

Phytochemicals are employed either directly or indirectly by a large number of industries including pharmaceutical, cosmetics, food, agrochemical and chemurgic industries. Economically important plants serve as irreplaceable sources of several industrial phytochemicals (exclusive of plant-derived products such as wood, cork, paper, etc., and whole plant-based foods such as whole grains, nuts, vegetables, fruits and spices). Table 3.1 lists them.

Essential Oils

Essential oils are highly volatile substances isolated by a physical process from an aromatic plant of a single botanical species. Such oils were called 'essential' because they were thought to represent the very essence of the odour and flavour of the plant. Aromatic plants include herbs, shrubs and trees of all sizes, and may be annual, biennial or perennial. The oil-accumulating organ or tissue varies between species and no single part of the plant is excluded from the list of organs which serve as oil stores.

An essential oil may contain up to several hundred chemical compounds and this complex mixture of compounds gives the oil its characteristic fragrance and flavour. They are isolated from plant parts by various methods such as distillation, solvent extraction, enfluerage (absorbing into fixed oils and fats), fractional distillation, head space techniques and extraction with liquid carbondioxide.

Distribution

Most volatile oil-bearing plants are found in the tropical world and cannot be easily grown in other geoclimatic regions. Whereas the commercially important volatile oil-bearing plants of the temperate and subtropical regions can easily be grown in the tropics.

Essential oil-bearing plants are spread over a wide range of families of both Angiosperms and Gymnosperms. A few families to which most of the commercially important aromatic plants belong are listed below:

Gymnosperms
- Pinaceae (from which turpentine oil, the world's largest essential oil in terms of volume produced, is obtained)
- Cupressaceae (cedarwood)

Angiosperms – Monocots
- Gramineae (lemongrass, citronella, vetiver)
- Zingiberaceae (ginger, turmeric, cardamom)

Angiosperms – Dicots
- Compositae (chamomile, davana, tarragon),
- Geraniaceae (geranium),
- Labiatae (mint, lavender, thyme, basil)
- Lauraceae (bay, cinnamon, camphor, Litsea)
- Myristicaceae (nutmeg, mace)
- Myrtaceae (eucalyptus, clove)
- Oleaceae (jasmine, lilac)
- Piperaceae (pepper)
- Rosaceae (rose)
- Rutaceae (citrus)
- Santalaceae (sandalwood)
- Umbelliferae (coriander, cumin, parsley)

Uses

Applications of aromatic plants and volatile oils extracted from them include

(i) direct culinary use: as fresh or dried herbs, spices and condiments;

(ii) perfumery, cosmetics and household and personal hygiene products either directly as major or minor ingredients or as raw materials for the extraction and/or synthesis of specific aroma chemicals;

(iii) food, drink and confectionery: as flavouring agents;

(iv) human and veterinary medicine: as components of pharmaceutical preparations;

(v) crop protection: as pesticides and insect repellents;

(vi) antibacterial and antifungal agents in a range of situations.

Furthermore, the requirements of essential oils for use in aromatherapy are increasing, creating a demand for organically produced exotic oils.

Trade

The first records of essential oils come from ancient India, Persia and Egypt. Both Greece and Rome conducted extensive trade in odoriferous oils with countries of the Orient (referring to erstwhile countries of Asia). The much-prized spices of India, China and the Indies served as the impetus for the advent of European traders to India. By the middle of the 18th century about 100 essential oils were introduced in Europe. Knowledge about their chemistry was added in the 1800s and 1900s. This led to their usage in foodstuffs, beverages and perfumes exceeding their use in medicine. These oils and their products have undergone various degrees of processing, extraction and alteration over the centuries.

Thus international trade in essential oils was one of the oldest known to history. The widespread use of aromatic plant products by consumers around the world and increasing international trade have been accompanied by attempts to identify new species of potential interest, to bring them into cultivation from the wild and to introduce them to distant locations away from their places of origin.

Aromatic substances of natural origin currently used by the pharmaceutical, perfumery, cosmetic and food industries are those derived from plants which have been cultivated for a long time and yet others are obtained from species which grow abundantly in the wild. Today the growing demand in industrialized countries for natural products in place of synthetic compounds has created a niche market for essential oils. The development of the essential oil industry is therefore important to many developing countries which have rich resources of raw materials or the climatic conditions for the initiation of crop-wise cultivation programmes. Though a lot of research has gone into synthetic substitutes for essential oils, the demand for natural oils has not declined. Essential oils are further processed or rectified to add value.

Based on the commercial value of produce, it has been estimated that developing countries and Eastern Europe together account for approximately two-thirds of the total world production of volatile oils. Among developing countries, the largest producers are China, India, Brazil, Morocco, Egypt, Indonesia and Turkey, these seven countries accounting for 85% of total production.

According to United Nations COMTRADE database, global imports of essential oils stood at US $2 billion in 2005. This increased by an average of 8% between 2000 and 2005 with no corresponding increase in volume. The top 10 importing countries in 2005 as listed by COMTRADE is given in Table 3.2. The fastest growing markets based on import spending between 2000 and 2005 included Vietnam (14% growth per annum), Poland (35%), Nigeria (16%), Turkey (25%), South Africa (14%), Indonesia (14%), Saudi Arabia (14%), India (19%), Spain (13%), Singapore (35%), Switzerland (14%) and Japan (13%).

Table 3.2 Top 10 essential oil importing countries

S.No.	Country	Essential Oil Import Value ($ million)
1.	USA	391
2.	France	199
3.	UK	175
4.	Japan	152
5.	Germany	117
6.	Switzerland	103
7.	Ireland	75
8.	China	65
9.	Singapore	61
10.	Spain	61

Source: COMTRADE database.

The world trade in essential oils and their products is thus vast and oils of major importance such as sandalwood, peppermint, lemongrass, patchouli, palmarosa, vetiver, geranium, clove, citronella and aniseed occupy a prominent position in the world market.

India with its wide agroclimatic zones is one of the few countries in the world with the exact requirements for the cultivation of scores of essential oil-bearing plants. There has been a spiralling growth in the production of essential oils making it an emerging agro-based industry in the country. Currently 30% of the fine chemicals used in perfumes and flavours come from essential oils. The estimated production of perfumery raw materials in India is around 5000 MT per annum valued at Rs 400 crores. About 3800 MT per annum valued at Rs. 100 crores is the total consumption of perfumery raw material in India. Out of this, the share of food, dental and pharmaceutical industries is 700 MT, with the rest being used for perfumery.

Essential oils currently produced in India are citronella oil, lemongrass, basil, mint, sandalwood, palmarosa, eucalyptus, cedar wood, vetiver and geranium. Rose oil, lavender, davana, oil of khus and ginger grass are produced in small quantities. Peppermint, spearmint and other mint oils constitute 68% of the total volume of production of essential oils in the country, with basil, citronella, eucalyptus, lemongrass, palmarosa, sandalwood and vetiver oils constituting the rest. Approximately 90% of the present requirement of essential oils in the country is met by indigenous production and 10% from imports. In 1950 our essential oil production was hardly 75–80 tonnes and now it has risen to 8,000 tonnes.

Within India the demand for essential oils is from consumer industry products that may be grouped under fragrance, flavours and aromatic chemicals. The annual growth rate of the pharmaceutical industry in terms of volume and value of aromatic chemicals consumed is 11% to 13%. Flavours, i.e., usage by processed food industry, particularly ice creams and confectionary items, is rapidly expanding. Fragrances used in toiletries and personal care products are an important sector with volume-wise use of essential oils in toiletries constituting 90% of all these products. The requirement of essential oils by consumer industries under flavour, fragrance and aroma chemicals are 60%, 20% and 20%, respectively.

India is the world leader in the production of mint oil with 5,000 tonnes of menthol valued at Rs 100 crores being produced annually. Around 40,000 hectares are under mint cultivation mainly in Uttar Pradesh, Punjab and Haryana, and to some extent in Bihar and Madhya Pradesh. Similarly citronella oil which we used to import earlier is now produced to the tune of 500 tonnes per annum. The export of essential oils during the year 1991–1992 has been 53.6 crores as against 40 crores during the year 1990–1991 thereby registering an increase of 37% over the previous year. According to an estimate of the Association of Essential Oil Manufacturers of India, with growth in export value of essential oils form Rs 50 crores in 1991–1992 to Rs 125 crores in 1995–1996, India ranks 14th in the world export trade.

Some important essential oils exported from India are ginger, sandalwood, lemongrass, jasmine, tuberose concentrate, cedarwood, clove, eucalyptus, palmarosa, patchouli, davana, coriander, dill, spearmint and rose. The major importers of essential oil from India are the United States, France, UK, Netherlands, former USSR, UAE, Saudi Arabia, Spain, Morocco, Germany, Australia, Korea, Taiwan and Pakistan.

Some of the oils produced in excess of their domestic demand are exported while a few like lavender, patchouli, clove, nutmeg, geranium, ylang ylang and rose oil are imported. Cultivation of these essential oil-bearing plants has started in India. The consumption of basil, sandalwood, cumin, dill and juniper oils are fully met out of local production.

In view of the burgeoning growth of the processed food, herbal formulations and cosmetics industry the demand prospects of essential oil industry is expected to grow substantially in the coming years.

Proprietary Non-Prescription Products (Herbs as Health Foods)

An ancient Siddha medicine dictum *'Unave marundhu, marundhe unavu'* which means food as medicine, medicine as food, well reinforces the importance of diet for disease-free living. This ancient wisdom of our country seems to be lost in the folds of history with the adoption of western medical system as the more superior health care provider for most of our populace. An ever increasing craze for anything western – consumer items, lifestyle and even food choices have resulted not only in loss of cultural and traditional values, but also in the abandonment of traditional diet patterns meticulously developed over the ages.

The wheel of time having gone a full circle, today the important role of diet in disease prevention is being increasingly realized in current scientific thinking. This is partly triggered by a global pandemic of lifestyle disorders, chiefly linked to excess/improper/reckless eating patterns in addition to other factors such as sedentary lifestyle and stress-filled work habits.

Diet-Disease Link – 'New' Evidence

Cross-cultural comparisons and epidemiological studies form the basis for understanding the role of dietary factors in disease etiology. Research activities of nutritionists and food scientists have historically run parallel to those of phytochemists, pharmacognocists and natural product chemists. While vitamins, minerals, aminoacids, carbohydrates and lipids are compounds of primary interest to food chemists, natural product chemistry focuses on compounds as potential sources of new pharmaceuticals and other industrial chemicals. An overlap of interests of food chemists and pharmacognocists resulted in the recognition that alkaloids, saponins, polyphenolics and other compounds have positive and complex roles in the physiological processes affecting human health. A growing body of epidemiological data linking diets high in plant foods with reduced incidence of chronic degenerative diseases such as non-insulin-dependant diabetes mellitus, cancer and coronary heart disease gave impetus for the convergence of interests of nutritionists and phytochemists. Thus the role of non-nutritive plant constituents consumed on a routine basis as normal mediators of health is recently recognized. There is now increasing interest in natural herbal home remedies, which have been effectively used for thousands of years for curing diseases and sustaining good health. Foods are now being examined intensively for added physiological benefits, which may reduce chronic disease risk or otherwise optimize health. Such a global awakening coupled with an ageing health-conscious population, changes in food regulations, numerous technological advances and a marketplace ripe for the introduction of health-promoting products, coalesced to create a trend for a category of products referred to as health foods, phytomedicines, dietary supplements, nutraceuticals, functional foods, fortified foods and organic foods.

Health Foods and Related Definitions

Health foods or functional foods have no universally accepted definition. *Functional foods are those whole, fortified, enriched or enhanced foods that provide health benefits beyond provision of essential nutrients such as vitamins and minerals.* They may do more than supply the macronutrients and micronutrients the body needs for normal biochemical reactions.

Functional foods have bioactive components that can potentially enhance health when eaten on a regular basis as part of a varied diet. The simplest examples of functional foods are fruits and vegetables. These not only offer life-essential vitamins and minerals, but also contain an array of phytochemicals that may fight certain diseases.

The concept was first developed in Japan in the 1980s when, faced with escalating health care costs, the Ministry of Health and Family Welfare initiated a regulatory system to approve certain foods with documented health benefits in hopes of improving the health of the nation's ageing population. These foods which are eligible to bear a special seal are now recognized as foods for specified health use (FOSHU). As of July 2002, nearly 300 food products had been granted FOSHU status in Japan.

Nutraceutical is a term used interchangeably with functional food. It refers *to those diet supplements that deliver a concentrated form of a presumed bioactive agent from a food, presented in a non-food matrix and used to enhance health in dosages that exceed those that could be obtained from normal food.*

Dietary supplements are defined as any product that is intended to supplement the diet and contains one or more of the following: vitamins, minerals, herbs or other botanicals, aminoacids and other dietary substances intended to supplement the diet by increasing the total dietary intake or as any concentrate, metabolite, constituent, extract or combination of these ingredients.

The term dietary supplement means products intended for ingestion in a form (tablet, capsule, powder, softgel, gelcap and liquid) that is not represented as conventional food or as the sole item of a meal or of diet and that are labelled as dietary supplements.

In view of the increasing awareness of the health benefits of plant-based diets and the general perception that plant-derived drugs provide better and safer health care than pure chemical drugs, there is a huge demand for these drug/dietary botanicals. Several medicinal plant-based formulations are today flooding the market in various forms such as tablets, capsules, gels, syrups etc. Depending on the local regulations they are available as drugs, health foods, dietary supplements, nutraceuticals etc. While some of them are direct adaptations of traditional recipes taken from classic medical treatises, many are new or research-based proprietary products developed according to the need of the medical condition they claim to cater to. For e.g., anti-obesity, hypolipidemic herbal drugs either single or in combination with other anti-oxidant/anti-inflammatory herbs are promoted for use in cardiovascular ailments. While such ad hoc new combinations seem appealing and marketable, safety and efficacy of such newer herbal cocktails are very much questionable and cannot be considered equivalent to time-tested traditional drugs. This is a cause of concern for regulating bodies world over especially in view of the ready availability of such concoctions under the name of herbal remedies, drugs, health supplements etc.

According to the Department of Health and Human Services, USA, diet plays a role in 5% to 10% of the leading causes of death, including coronary heart disease (CHD), certain types of cancer, stroke, diabetes type 2 and atherosclerosis. The dietary pattern that has been linked with major causes of death in developed countries is characterized as relatively high in total and saturated fat, cholesterol, sodium and refined sugars and relatively low in unsaturated fat, grains, legumes, fruits and vegetables. An accumulating body of research now suggests that consumption of certain foods or their associated physiologically active components may be linked to disease risk reduction. There are also many classes of physiologically active functional food ingredients of plant, animal or microbial origin with a great majority of them derived from plants.

Probiotics are a class of biologically active animal-derived components and defined as viable microorganisms that are beneficial to human health. Examples include *Lactobacillus acidophilus* and other strains of lactobacillus being incorporated into functional food products now on the market.

Prebiotics are non-digestible food ingredients that beneficially affect the host by selectively stimulating the growth and/or activity of one or a limited number of beneficial bacteria in the colon, thus improving host health. Synbiotics are mixtures of probiotics and prebiotics that beneficially affect the host by improving the survival and implantation of live microbial dietary supplements in the gastrointestinal tract, by selectively stimulating the growth and/or by activating the metabolism of one or a limited number of health-promoting bacteria, thus improving host welfare.

The Growing Market for Health Foods

Many herbs have health benefits and millions of people have already resorted to the use of herbal medicines with the conviction that these being natural are effective and safer than standard medicines. Herbal additives have begun to appear in conventional foods ranging from teas, juices, snack chips, energy bars, etc. The size of this tremendous market is not well understood. It is estimated by BCC research that the global market for functional food industry will reach 176.7 billion in 2013 with a current annual growth rate (CAGR) of 7.4%; specifically the functional food sector will experience 6.9% CAGR, the supplement sector will rise by 3.8% and the functional beverage sector will be the fastest growing segment with 10.8% CAGR.

In terms of reach of these products in different parts of the world, there are different routes to the consumer. According to a recent survey, the US functional food market is currently estimated to be approximately $18.5 billion. Here half of the consumers are buying their herbs from speciality food stores. On the other hand, in Europe, a much larger percentage goes through pharmacies or drug stores because of different regulations. In Japan over 50% are direct sales or multilevel marketing. In India too they are available at all levels as traditional/non-traditional herbal products on prescription and outside it. The market for foods positioned for their health benefits will continue to be strong for the next several decades given the consumer interest in self-care, aging demographics and increasing health care costs.

Reasons for the Growth of Health Food Market

Research results linking diet to disease reinforced by epidemiological studies establishing the same in several population studies of disease-free groups.

1. With a large ageing population in many countries, chronic diseases of ageing such as heart disease, cancer, osteoporosis, Alzheimer's disease and age-related macular degeneration are inevitable imposing an enormous stress on the cost of health care.
2. Several surveys have indicated that increasing numbers of consumers are taking greater responsibility for their own health and well-being and are increasingly turning to their diet to enable them to do so.
3. Consumer interest in self-care and dissatisfaction with the current health care system will continue to be a leading factor motivating consumer food-purchasing decisions.

4. Tendency of the consumers to view the 'kitchen cabinet' as the medicine cabinet is being identified as a leading phenomenon in the food industry.

Safety and Regulation

While on one side mounting evidence is demonstrating the benefits of health foods in disease prevention and health promotion, several safety concerns have been recently raised particularly with regard to the seemingly indiscriminate addition of botanicals to food. A plethora of cereals including rice, maize, wheat, jowar, and drinks, soups, teas, noodles and flours are being enhanced with botanicals, some of which may pose a risk to certain consumers. Several herbal products are prone to be contaminated with pesticides, heavy metals, etc., especially when the herbs used are through improper cultivation/collection practices. While many herbs are considered safe, some have hazardous side effects. Not much is known of the short-term and long-term benefits and risks of many herbs. Many are shown to be toxic and in some cases addition of small amounts of herbs, even those found in teas has serious effects.

Though herbs are being used like drugs for health-related benefits, they are not tightly regulated like drugs and other medications. Regulation of this category of products differs in different parts of the world. The availability of herbal products world over depends upon regional changes in regulatory strategies. In European countries herbal drugs are even prescribed and a lot of industrial standards are applied to those products. Still herbs unlike drugs are not standardized in terms of the same amount of active ingredient. A single herb can be standardized to different ingredients by different manufacturers. Also doses differ between products and from product to product. The active ingredient may vary depending on the plant part (flower, root, stem etc.), plant form (dried extract, tincture, tea) and plant species.

Thus the safety issues related to herbs are complex and the issue of herb-drug interaction has received increasing attention. Herbs may interact with prescription medications, OTC drugs, vitamins and minerals. For example, ginkgo taken with ibuprofen may lead to spontaneous/ excessive bleeding. High doses of garlic may enhance the effects and adverse effects of anticoagulant and anti-platelet drugs, including aspirin, clopidrogel, enoxaparin and others.

In the wake of such data there is growing concern about the sale of such foods enhanced with herbs such as St.John's wort, guarana, gotukola, ginseng, ginkgo, echinacea, kavakava and spirulina in the United States. Following the Government Accountability Office (GAO) report in 2000 that raised concerns about safety of certain functional foods – significant regulatory changes followed:

- Nutritional Labelling and Education Act of 1990 (NLEA) enabled the use of FDA pre-approved health claims that characterize the relationship of any food/food components to a disease/health condition.
- Dietary Supplement Health and Education Act of 1994 (DSHEA) regulates dietary supplements as foods (not food additives) defining them as vitamins, minerals, herbs or botanicals, aminoacids and other dietary substances for use by man to supplement the diet including concentrates, metabolites, constituents, extracts or any combination of the above.

As per US FDA herbs cannot claim to prevent, diagnose, treat or cure a condition or disease. This requires sound scientific evidence and significant scientific agreement. What counts as significant scientific agreement is outlined in a guidance document issued by the US FDA in 1999.

This would require the support of a body of consistent relevant evidence from well-designed clinical, epidemiological and laboratory studies and expert opinions from a body of independent scientists. Herbs may carry health-related claims about effects on the 'structure or function' of the body or 'general well-being' that may result from the product. Examples of structure/function claims include 'helps support a healthy immune system' for dietary supplements containing echinacea and 'maintains cholesterol levels that are already in the normal range' for a combination product containing fish oil, flaxseed oil and garlic. Manufacturers using structure/function claims must simply notify the FDA within 30 days of marketing the product that displays the claim. Each such claim must be accompanied by a disclaimer stating that the claim has not been evaluated by the FDA and the product is not intended to diagnose, treat, cure or prevent any disease. Structure/function claims may also appear on conventional foods without displaying the disclaimer that must appear on dietary supplements. When used on conventional foods, the claims must include an indication of how the nutrient in question affects the structure or function of the body. The DSEA has thus opened up a favourable regulatory environment for herbal products. This opportunity to make statements on food labels related to the health benefits of functional foods has resulted in major companies venturing into foods for the health and wellness market.

Health Foods and Disease Prevention

Foods in general provide us either taste/convenience benefits or nutrition/enhancement utility. Food habits in several traditionally established cultures world over were largely dictated by the need for nutrition and energy. Fruits, leaves and other plant parts were essential components of diet in these societies and apart from being an energy source, food thus also included consumption of a variety of plant secondary chemicals. These compounds were not only a part of dietary ecology, but may have become essential to physiological homeostasis.

Today it is being understood that organic molecules in the diet could be determinants of human gut morphology and without the inhibitory effects of various allelochemicals on rates of carbohydrate digestion, the human small intestine might not need to be as long as it currently is. Much later in the course of human evolution cooking and other processing techniques, guided by taste as a predominant determinant in food choices, largely decreased the ingestion of plant secondary compounds in the diet. Until recently few of the studies linking diet and disease considered ingested phytochemicals as positive agents in disease prevention.

Recognition that chronic diseases of industrial societies have a dietary basis has led to recommendations to reduce dietary fat and increase consumption of fibre, anti-oxidant vitamins and complex carbohydrates. This is diet higher in plant material and consequently closer to diets of traditional societies. The actions of plant secondary compounds in mediating lipid and carbohydrate metabolism suggest that physiological homeostasis could include both plant non-nutrients and fats in higher levels than currently recommended. Growing evidence for the role of non-nutrients such as those with anti-cholesterolemic activity, anti-oxidants and those mediating carbohydrate metabolism in physiological processes should be accessed not simply from a clinical perspective, but in relation to disease prevention.

Functional foods are viewed differently from the eastern and western perspectives. They are considered revolutionary and represent a rapidly growing segment of the food industry in the west. There is tight competition between the food and pharmaceutical companies to bring functional foods to the mass market. In the east on the other hand, functional foods have been a part of its culture for centuries. Ayurvedic and Siddha systems of medicine in India recognized the crucial role of food towards health maintenance as early as 10,000 B.C.E. From ancient times Indians and the Chinese have used foods for both preventive and therapeutic benefits, a view that is being currently recognized around the world. The current huge market for functional foods is dictated by economic benefits, as they give higher profitability margin compared to conventional foods. Developing countries have started to emerge as exporters to cater to increasing demand in the developed countries. Moreover demand for the modern functional foods is also growing in developing countries thanks to enhanced disease burden due to massive westernization and forgotten traditional food habits. This growing market presents a lucrative opportunity to develop domestic markets.

In India apart from CFTRI (Mysore) and NDRI (Karnal) not many public sector organizations are working on the R&D of functional foods. Functional food market in India is still in its infancy, but the demand for functional foods will continue to increase due to their specific health benefits. The government is therefore planning to invest US $21.5 billion in food processing industry in the next five years. Functional foods already available in the Indian market are largely copies of western food products. Instead of trying to copy these, more extensive study on traditional diets in various parts of the country will reintroduce time-tested healthy food items in our daily diet. Further modifications on these traditional foods in terms of enrichment with added botanicals or minerals will take care of problems of competition from traditional foods, patentability etc.

Health Food Categories

Overall health foods may be of three types.

1. Conventional foods with identified bioactive phytonutrient

With modern science better able to qualify the bioactivity of our foods, manufacturers 'call out' the compounds that confer health benefits. This 'call-out' marketing of food products currently constitutes the majority of health foods, e.g., whole wheat atta (flour). Here the manufacturer has called out the presence of wheat bran in the wheat flour that maintains gut health and reduces the risk of some types of cancers. Oats, soy, fish, garlic, flax seed, nuts are other examples.

2. Enriched/fortified/superfortified foods

Currently the second largest segment of functional products, these incorporate a beneficial bioactive compound into a health food, e.g., vitamins and minerals added as per RDA (or more) for that nutrient. E.g., breakfast cereals fortified with B vitamins, health drinks for children enriched with added vitamins and minerals, juices with calcium, infant formulas with iron, milk with vitamin D, etc.

3. Products engineered for bioactive benefit

The most significant emerging segment of functional products, these constitute products specifically altered with an added ingredient which is not a normal constituent of the health food. For example, rice for diabetics, polished rice grains are coated with anti-diabetic herb extracts and are meant to be cooked without the usual washing. Such rice products claim to counter the high glycemic index of rice. Other examples are tea with added powdered herbals, carbonated waters spiced with herbal extracts such as those from ginger, amla etc. Biscuits with whole nuts, added fibre and foods containing sugar alcohols in place of sugar (sweets for diabetics) are other examples. It is estimated that in the United States more than 250 botanicals often in the form of concentrated extracts are commonly added during food product manufacturing for flavour, fragrance or technical characteristics such as colouring, thickening or preservative activity. These are added as natural ingredient additives for many categories of food products including baked goods, canned goods, meat products, dairy products, candy, non-alcoholic beverages and alcoholic beverages.

Some Functional Food Components and Their Role in Disease Prevention

The simplest examples of functional foods are fruits, vegetables, whole grains and nuts. These offer life-essential vitamins and minerals and also an array of phytochemicals that may fight certain diseases. Most traditional diets incorporate a host of plant-derived articles under the guise of colouring or flavouring in effect actually adding a number of non-nutrient phytochemicals to the diet. Table 3.3 gives some identified classes of phytochemicals with functional health modifying effects present in foods with functional benefits. These are in addition to plants ingested in a number of other forms in various traditional diets.

GLOBAL TRADE IN SOME INDIVIDUAL PLANT DRUGS

Rauwolfia

One of the most important native medicinal plants of India, the crude drug consists of the air-dried roots and rhizomes of *Rauwolfia serpentina* Benth (Apocynaceae).

Synonymns

Rauwolfia trifoliata (Gaertn.)
Ophioxylon salutiferum Salisb.
Ophioxylon obversum Miq.
Ophioxylon serpeninum L.
Rauwolfia obversa Miq.

Common names

English: Indian snake root, rauwolfia
Sanskrit: Sarpagandha
Hindi: Chotachand
Tamil: Civanamelpodi
Telugu: Paatala garuda

Commercial Importance

An important component of traditional medicine in India, the drug is a source of hypotensive alkaloids, principal of which are reserpine, rescinnamine and ajmaline. First isolated from the roots in the early 1950s, it quickly became important in the treatment of hypertension and mental illness through its effect as a tranquillizer. Use has decreased in view of the reports of its adverse effects at doses higher than the hypotensive dose. It continues to be used in phytopharmaceutical preparations in India and elsewhere.

Table 3.3 Some functional food components and their role in disease prevention

Phytochemical Class	Sources	Pharmacological Effect/ Health Benefits	References
CAROTENOIDS			
1. β-carotene (pro-vitamin A carotenoid)	Carrots, pumpkin, sweet potato, capsicum, turnip leaves, musk melon, brown Indian hemp, bladder dock	This lipophilic anti-oxidant scavenges singlet oxygen, it can be made into vitamin A in the body – bolsters anti-oxidant defences	Giovannucci et al. (1995)
2. Lycopene (non–pro-vitamin A carotenoid)	Tomatoes, water melon, red/pink grape fruit (pomelo/sadaphal)	Potent anti-oxidant, more powerful scavenger of singlet oxygen. Beneficial in cancers of prostate, lung and stomach	Giovannucci (1999)
3. Lutein (yellow carotenoid – principal pigment of the macula of the eye)	Pumpkin, chilli, several Indian green leafy vegetables, cabbage, brinjal, vegetable oils such as mustard and palm oils	Neutralizes free radicals that can damage the eye, prevents photo oxidation and age-related macular degeneration or cataracts	Mares-Perlman et al. (2002)
4. Zeaxanthin (isomer of lutein, common carotenoid alcohol, animals derive zeaxanthin from a plant diet)	Capsicum, corn, saffron, most leafy green vegetables, spinach, garden peas	High dietary intake related to lower incidence of age-related macular degeneration	Mares-Perlman et al. (2002)
FLAVONOIDS			
1. Anthocyanins (water-soluble glycoside pigments that impart colour to flowers and other plant parts (over 5,000 different anthocyanins isolated from plants) – cyanidin, delphinidin, malvidin	Brinjal, black and blue berries, cherries, red grapes, jamun, oranges, red onion, mango, fig, olives, sweet potato, radish	Enhances cellular anti-oxidant defence, may contribute to maintenance of brain function	Edwards et al. (2000)
2. Flavanols (most abundant class of flavonoids, not attached with a sugar moiety) – catechins, epicatechins, epigallocatechins, procyanidin	Tea, cocoa, chocolate, apples, red grapes	Because of their chemical structures they easily oxidize themselves thus quenching free radicals, lower cholesterol, beneficial to heart health	Huang and Ferraro (1992)
3. Flavanones (the dominant flavonoid class of citrus fruits) – hesperitin, naringenin	Citrus fruits like orange, lemon	Neutralize free radicals, positive effects in the treatment of CVD, cancers, beneficial to bone health, lowers cholesterol	Morand et al. (2011)

(Continued)

Table 3.3 Continued

Phytochemical Class	Sources	Pharmacological Effect/ Health Benefits	References
4. Flavonols (found in outer layers of plants, they absorb UV light and act as sunscreen to plants; they are attached to a sugar) – quercetin, kaempferol, isorhamnetin, myricetin, robinetin	Cherry, tomato, onions, apples, tea, broccoli	Because of their chemical structures they easily oxidize themselves thus quenching free radicals, anti-mutagenic	Pratt (1992)
5. Proanthocyanidins (group of condensed flavanols)	Cranberries, cocoa, strawberries, grapes, wine, peanuts, cinnamon	May contribute to the maintenance of urinary tract health and heart health	Howell et al. (1998)
ISOTHIOCYANATES			
1. Allyl isothiocyanate, Sulforaphane (natural isothiocyanates produced by the enzymatic conversion of glucosinolates, also known as mustard oils)	Mustard, cauliflower, broccoli, cabbage, kale, moringa (drum stick)	Potent inducer of phase II detoxifying enzymes, accelerating inactivation of toxic substances and their elimination	Nakamura and Miyoshi (2006)
2. Sulphides and thiols (physiologically active organo sulphur compounds) – diallyl sulphide, allyl methyl trisulphide	Garlic, onions, leeks, spring onions	Reduce total cholesterol, protective in stomach cancer, may contribute to maintenance of heart health and healthy immune function	Qian et al. (2011)
GLUCOSINOLATES, INDOLES (sulphur-containing glycosides)	Cauliflower, cabbage, mustard, turnip, radish, moringa leaves	Anti-oxidant, anti-cancer, antibiotic properties, reduce risk of cancers of lung and alimentary tract	Fahey (2005)
PHENOLIC ACIDS/ PLANT POLYPHENOLICS (plant compounds of great structural diversity involved in diverse plant functions) – caffeic acid, ferulic acid, chlorogenic acid, carnasol, rosmarinic acid, curcumin	Apples, pears, prunes, citrus fruits, coffee, grapes, oats, cereals, soy beans, peas, chick peas	They affect diverse mammalian cell processes with anti-carcinogenic, anti-atherogenic implications; anti-oxidant, tumour-inhibiting activities, reduce platelet aggregation	Keevil et al. (2000)

PLANT STANOLS/STEROLS

1. Free stanols and sterols (naturally occurring substances found in plants, unlike cholesterol can only be obtained through dietary sources)	Corn, soy, wheat, many fruits, vegetables, nuts, seeds, cereals, legumes, vegetable oils	Reduce total and LDL cholesterol by preventing absorption from the small intestine, may reduce the risk of CHD	Katan et al. (2003)
2. Stanol/sterol esters	Fortified margarines (dalda?), beverages, table spreads	Reduce total and LDL cholesterol by trapping it in the gut, may reduce the risk of CHD	Katan et al. (2003)

PHYTOESTROGENS

1. Isoflavones (group of weakly estrogenic non-steroidal compounds widely occurring in plants) daidzein, genistein	Soy beans, psoralea, lupine and fava bean, kudzu, wheat, bengal gram, moong beans, chick peas, cherries, parsley, apples, alfalfa and red clover	Many contribute to maintenance of bone health, healthy brain and immune function, in women may contribute to maintenance of menopausal health	Doris et al. (1998)
2. Lignans (group of plant polyphenolics, estrogen-like chemicals) – pinoresinol, lariciresinol, matairesinol	Flax, rye, oil seeds such as linseed, millet, sesame and sunflower besides legumes, pulses, whole grains	May contribute to maintenance of heart health and healthy immune function	Murkies et al. (1998)

FATTY ACIDS

1. Monounsaturated fatty acids (MUFAs) – fatty acids with one double or triple bond per molecule	Almond oil, ground nut oil, sunflower oil, corn oil, sesame oil, whole milk products, olives, avocados, red meat, cashews	Promote insulin resistance, reduce LDL, may reduce risk of CHD	Satoshi et al. (2004)
2. Polyunsaturated fatty acids (PUFAs) – Omega-3 fatty acids (found in plant sources –body converts it to EPA and DHA)	Walnuts, flax, tung oil, poppy seed oil, leafy greens	A balance of both omega-3 and omega-6 fatty acids is ideal for health, boosts heart health and lowers triglycerides	Lovejoy (2002)
3. Polyunsaturated fatty acids (PUFAs) (omega-6 fattyacids, considered essential, found in animal sources, essential component of the phospholipids of cellular membranes especially of the brain and retina of the eye) – docasohexanoic acid, eicasohexanoic acid	Salmon, tuna, mackerel, sardines, herring and other fish oils	Stimulate skin and hair growth, maintain bone health, regulate metabolism and maintain the reproductive system.	Lovejoy (2002)

(Continued)

Table 3.3 Continued

Phytochemical Class	Sources	Pharmacological Effect/ Health Benefits	References
4. Conjugated linolenic acid (mixture of structurally similar forms of linolenic acids) – Cis-9, trans-11 octadecadi-enoic acid	Beef, lamb, some cheese	Anti-mutagenic, may decrease body fat and increase muscle mass, may contribute to maintenance of desirable body composition and healthy immune function	Balnkson et al. (2000)
DIETARY FIBRE (functional and total) – indigestible portion of plant foods called roughage			
1. Soluble fibre – prebiotic, found only in plants	Root tubers, almonds, raisins, lentils, split peas, barley, oats, beans (channa), brown rice, psyllium seed husk, apples	Readily fermented in the colon into gases and physiologically active byproducts, reduce total and LDL cholesterol, may reduce risk of CHD and some types of cancer	Park et al. (2011)
2. Insoluble fibre – found only in plants	Wheat bran, corn bran, fruit skins, beans, peas, potato skin, cauliflower	Change the nature of contents of gastroin-testinal tract and alter chemical and nutrient absorption, contribute to maintenance of a healthy digestive tract; may reduce some forms of cancer	Park et al. (2011)
3. Functional fibres (isolated fibre components of whole foods rich in fibre) – beta glucans, inulin, cellulose, maltodextrans, polydextrose	Oat bran, oat meal, oat flour, barley, rye, millet, pearl millet, ragi, corn	More and more foods being fortified with these functional fibres, but may not confer all the benefits of total or complete fibre obtained from natural foods	Khaw et al. (1987)
4. Whole grains	Barley, rye, millet, pearl millet, ragi, corn, wheat, brown rice	May reduce risk of CHD, lower cholesterol by binding it in the intestine	Jacobs et al. (1998)
NON-ANIMAL PROTEIN	Soy bean, chick peas, lentils, cashew, almonds, pistachios, pumpkin seeds, nuts, sprouts, green leafy vegetables	Plant protein is much healthier than protein from dairy and meat	Gertjan (2000)

Habit and Distribution

An erect, small, evergreen perennial semi-shrub growing upto 50 cm tall, the species is wide ranging in Asia and found in India, Bangladesh, Bhutan, China, Indonesia, Malaysia, Myanmar, Nepal, Pakistan, Sri Lanka, Thailand and Vietnam. It is found in almost all parts of India up to an altitude of 1000 m, and is more common in submontane regions of Himalayas and in the lower ranges of eastern and western ghats across states of Himachal Pradesh, Uttaranchal, Sikkim, Assam, Kerala, Orissa, Tamil Nadu, West Bengal, Bihar, Maharashtra and Andaman islands. Between Sirmor and Gorakhpur districts of Uttar Pradesh, the plant is frequently noticed in shady moist or sometimes swampy localities. In eastern localities in Bihar, north Bengal and Assam as well as in Khasi, Jantia and Garohills, the plant is encountered more numerously on the forest margins of mixed deciduous forests. Rauwolfia occurs more frequently in Goa, Coorg, North Canara and Shimoga districts of Karnataka and Palghat, Calicut and Trichur districts of Kerala. In Orissa, Andhra Pradesh and Madhya Pradesh, the areas comprising the catchment of river Godavari are the richest. The species is now considered 'endangered' in Karnataka, Kerala, Tamil Nadu and in central India.

Principal Constituents

The root and the root bark which constitute 40% to 60% of the whole root contain over 60 indole alkaloids, the most significant being reserpine, rescinnamine, deserpidine, reserpinine, serpinine, serpentine, ajmaline, ajmalicine, rauwolfinine and yohimbine. The root bark contains more than 90% of total alkaloids, which varies from 1.4–3% depending on location, season and soil conditions.

Harvest and Processing

The root system consists of a prominent tuberous soft tap root upto 6 cm in diameter when fresh and having a corky outer bark with longitudinal fissures. Generally roots and sometimes leaves are harvested. Roots are harvested during winter months for maximal alkaloidal content. The root is to be harvested 15–36 months after planting to obtain the optimum yield of alkaloid. The plant can be propagated from seeds, stem cuttings or root cuttings. Most of the produce is collected from the wild, however in view of the wild populations of the species being threatened efforts to cultivate it are underway in India and Nepal. It is cultivated on a small scale by the forest departments of Bihar, Assam and Meghalaya. Private growers have small areas under plantation in Uttaranchal, Karnataka and Kerala. Given the concerns regarding the status of the species, urgent attention is required to document the source and quantity of specimens in trade, both in the domestic and international markets and to develop mechanism to ensure that wild harvests and trade are maintained within sustainable levels.

Traditional Medicinal Uses

In India, rauwolfia has been employed for centuries in the treatment of various central nervous system (CNS) disorders, including anxiety states, maniacal behaviour associated with psychosis, schizophrenia, insanity, insomnia and epilepsy. Extracts of the roots are valued for the treatment of intestinal disorders and also as an anthelmintic: mixed with other plant extracts, they have been used in the treatment of cholera, colic and fever. The species is also used by traditional healers to treat snake bites, from which it possibly derived the name snake root. Several herbal formulations containing rauwolfia are manufactured in India. In Nepal traditional healers use the roots to treat hypertension, fever, mental disorders, depression and memory loss.

Uses

Rauwolfia is considered an important therapeutic option for patients with mild to moderate essential hypertension not improved by lifestyle changes. Rauwolfia alkaloids bind irreversibly to catecholamine storage granules in neurons, primarily those in the mid-brain autonomic centres and cells in the adrenal medulla, causing depletion of catecholamines and 5-HT from those granules. As a result there is a lessening of systemic sympathetic tone leading to reduction in blood pressure. This entirely central mechanism of action of reserpine has no direct effect on the heart or blood vessels.

Reserpine at a low dose (0.05–0.25 mg/day) in combination with a thiazide diuretic was the first therapeutic combination with reduced incidence of adverse effects such as chronic hypertension and stroke in large double-blind trials. The longer half-life and hence once-daily dosing of reserpine has been an added advantage. High-dose reserpine (0.5–1 mg/day), on the other hand, is associated with depression, Parkinsonism, impotence and peptic ulcer. Low-dose reserpine is extremely safe and less expensive than any synthetic antihypertensive drug. The whole plant is shown to have better overall efficacy than isolated reserpine.

Trade Details

India at one time had a monopoly on the supply of rauwolfia to the world market. It is among the top 178 medicinal plants considered to be in high volume trade and consumption with global demand for rauwolfia estimated in the early 1980s to be 100–150 tonnes annually. Today it is growing significantly with the widespread use of the species by several phytopharmaceutical companies worldwide. There is a great demand for the alkaloids as well as the raw drug in the international market.

India is the world's leading producer and consumer of rauwolfia root with estimated domestic consumption ranging from 200–500 tonnes. As per a 1993 FAO study 400–500 tonnes of roots are exploited annually mainly in India, Thailand, Bangladesh and Sri Lanka; 800 tonnes more are collected from wild sources in the western coast of Africa, mainly in Zaire, Mozambique and Rwanda, from where it is exported to Italy and West Germany.

According to data provided by the Ayurvedic Drug Manufacturers Association in Mumbai, India produced 800 tonnes of rauwolfia crude drugs in 1999 of which only 20% was used by India's Ayurvedic industry. A supply and demand study including rauwolfia commissioned by the Department of Indian Systems of Medicine and Homeopathy of the Indian Government and WHO, estimated demand for 2001–2002 as 423.6 tonnes and for 2004–2005 as 588.7 tonnes, much higher than earlier estimates. The market price during 1999–2000 was reported to be INR 150,000/tonne (US $3435/t). The current market price of rauwolfia in the world trade is INR 600–3000/kg (US $10–50/kg) depending on the quality.

The major trading centres for rauwolfia are Kolkata, Mumbai and Patna which in turn are supplied by a number of primary traders throughout the country. Over-collection of rauwolfia root earlier has significantly decreased supply and since 1997 there is no embargo on export of wild-harvested drug from India. India exports over 260 tonnes of extracts/formulations based on rauwolfia. The chief importing countries of rauwolfia from India are UK, Netherlands, Phillippines,

UAE, United States, Portugal and Singapore. Exporters other than India are Thailand, Zaire, Mozambique and Rwanda. Export of Rauwolfia from Nepal was banned in 1995.

Taxol

Taxol or paclitaxel is a diterpenoid pseudoalkaloid first obtained from the bark of North American Taxus species *Taxus brevifolia* Nutt (Pacific Yew). Family: Taxaceae

Common Names

English: Yew tree – Pacific yew, Himalayan yew
Hindi: Barmi, Talispatra

Commercial Importance

Leaves, twigs, bark and roots of Taxus species contain a unique class of diterpenoid alkaloids called taxanes that are a source of taxol, a chemotherapeutic drug used to treat a range of human cancers. Discovered by the US National Cancer Institute (NCI) in the bark of Pacific Yew, paclitaxel was brought to the market under the trade name 'Taxol' by the pharmaceutical company Bristol Meyers Squibb. The number of paclitaxel manufacturers and those of other taxane-based drugs has expanded in recent years. Taxanes are structurally related to the toxic constituents found in the stem bark, leaves, roots and needles of other Taxus species including *T.wallichiana* (Himalayan yew). Over 100 taxanes have been characterized from Taxus species and taxol is a member of a small group of compounds possessing a four-membered oxetane ring and a complex ester side chain in their structures both of which are essential for anti-tumour activity.

Constituents

Taxol is found predominantly in the bark in relatively low amounts (0.01%–0.02%). Upto 0.033% of taxol has been recorded in some samples of leaves and twigs, but generally it is much lower than in the bark. Significant variation in the taxol content depending on season, geographical location and environmental factors as well as individual population of trees has been noted. The content of some other taxane derivatives in the bark is considerably higher, e.g., upto 0.2% baccatin III. Other taxane derivatives characterized include 10-deacetyl taxol, 10- deacetyl baccatin III (10-DAB), cephalomannine and 10-deacetyl cephalomannine.

Species in Trade and Distribution

Classification of Taxus genus of the Taxaceae family of trees and shrubs is characterized alternately as notoriously difficult or controversial with the species described being discouragingly similar. Depending on the taxonomic authority consulted, the genus contains anywhere from one species with numerous varieties to 24 species with 55 varieties. These are distributed across northern temperate and subtropical regions as far south as El Salvador in Central America and Sumatra in South-East Asia. The species are classified into three groups by differences in leaf epidermal and stomatal features listed below:

1. The wallichiana group with 11 species occurring from central Himalayas to Indonesia and Phillippines, in North America, in the Pacific northwest and from Mexico to Central

America with an isolated occurrence in Florida. There are two subgroups namely wallichiana and chinensis within this group.

2. The baccata group with nine species in temperate Eurasia, Northern Africa and eastern North America. There are two subgroups namely baccata and cuspidata under this group.
3. The sumatrana group with four species overlapping in distribution with the wallichiana subgroup in Asia.

Most species of Taxus are found in the understorey or subdominant canopy of moist temperate or tropical mountain forests. Elevations range from near sea level in northern stations to 3000 m in tropical forests.

T. brevifolia is a slow-growing shrub/tree found in the forests of Northwest Canada (British Columbia) and the United States (Washington, Oregon, Montana, Idaho and North California).

T. wallichiana is wide ranging in Asia occurring in Afghanistan, Bhutan, China, India, Indonesia, Malaysia, Myanmar, Nepal, Pakistan and Vietnam. *T. wallichiana* is said to differ from European *T. baccata* in the longer leaves, which are generally not abruptly cuspidate and may only merit sub-specific rank. The species in the Phillippines and Indonesia is said to be *T. sumatrana* and that in Vietnam T. chinensis var mairei. The population of Taxus in Yunnan is that of *T. wallichiana var. yunnanensis*.

The Asian Taxus species occurs from lowland to montane zones in cool climates with moderate to high evenly distributed rainfall. The North American species (*T. brevifolia* in Western North America, *T. globosa* in Mexico and Central America) are scattered trees of the understorey of conifer and broadleaf forests and along riverbanks and ravines.

In India Taxus species occurs in the northern states of Jammu and Kashmir, Himachal Pradesh, Uttaranchal, Sikkim, Arunachal Pradesh, Assam, Manipur and Meghalaya. Preferred habitats for *T. wallichiana* in Uttaranchal are deeply shaded, moist and sheltered areas such as gorges. This species occurs naturally in Nanda Devi Biosphere Reserve, Garhwal Himalayas, particularly in the north and northwest slopes.

Ongoing research and development in the technology for extracting and synthesizing paclitaxel and other taxanes has widened the range of Taxus species from which these compounds can and are being extracted. These include the European Yew, *T. baccata*, a widely distributed species and also a common ornamental plant, and the North American species, *T. canadensis*, for which commercial propagation trials for taxane production are underway.

Harvest

These are small evergreen trees or shrubs approximately 6–12 m tall. The bark is reddish brown, thin and scaly. Individual trees are either male or female with dioecious flowers. Bark and more recently leaves and twigs of *T. wallichiana* and other Taxus species are harvested for extraction of paclitaxel, 10-DAB and other taxanes. Although not rare Taxus species do not form thick populations and occur only in patches under other species. Also they must be mature (c. 100 years old) to be large enough for exploitation of the bark. At this age, with a trunk diameter of 25 cm, the bark is removed during May through August for *T. brevifolia*, the first identified source of paclitaxel. The harvest method is either pruning or shearing.

Early clinical studies of Taxol created high demand for bark of the species. The harvest approach was destructive and required 52,000–78,000 yew trees annually during the early 1990s. Approximately 10,000 kg of pacific yew bark was required to make 1 kg of taxol with the bark of at least six trees required for a single treatment dose. Concerns regarding the sustainability of

T. brevifolia harvests spurred development of methods to synthesize paclitaxel from 10-DAB also found in other Taxus species including *T. wallichiana*. This new development not only increased the number of species from which to derive paclitaxel, but also expanded the extraction of taxanes to leaves, a more sustainable source of taxanes than bark. Although leaves are needed in large quantities, methods of extraction have become increasingly efficient. By 1993, the amount of Taxus bark required to yield 1 kg paclitaxel was said to have been reduced from approximately 13,500 kg to 6,800 kg, the equivalent bark of some 1000 trees. Three tonnes of leaves are required to make 1 kg paclitaxel.

Slow growing, slow to regenerate and sensitive to canopy disturbance and fire, it appears that this species was declining in some parts of its range countries even before harvest for production of taxanes began. The high demand for bark and leaves for paclitaxel production resulted in a significant increase in the rate of harvest leading to population decline in China, India, Nepal and potentially elsewhere. Cultivation has been promoted in each of these countries, but as yet is not making a major contribution to *T. wallichiana* supplies. It is possible to fully synthesize Taxol. However its molecular structure is complex and its synthesis costly. As a result, harvest of wild or cultivated biomass remains more economically attractive to pharmaceutical companies than full synthesis.

Medicinal and Other Uses

T. wallichiana is a multipurpose tree species valued as a source of timber, fuelwood, fodder, tea, traditional medicine and since the early 1990s, paclitaxel and other taxanes used in anti-cancer medications. For at least several centuries, the young shoots, leaves and bark of *T. wallichiana* have been used for their medicinal properties. In India extracts from bark and leaves are used in Unani medicine as a source of the drug Zarnab, prescribed as a sedative and aphrodisiac and for the treatment of bronchitis, asthma, epilepsy, snake bites and scorpion stings. In Ayurvedic medicine, young shoots are used to prepare a medicinal tincture for the treatment of headache, diarrhea and biliousness. The leaves are also used for the treatment of hysteria, epilepsy and nervousness. Bark and leaves are considered to possess anti-fertility properties. It has been used in steam baths to treat rheumatism. A paste made from the bark is also used to treat fractures and headaches. The inhabitants of the buffer 116 buffer zone villages of Nanda Devi Biosphere Reserve in India collect taxus bark and leaves mainly for traditional teas and for curing colds and coughs, a practice also common in other rural areas.

Herbal formulations using *T. wallichiana* are manufactured in India. Extracts are also used in medicinal hair oils. In Pakistan, decoction of the stem is used against tuberculosis. In North America and Europe, yew was used for making implements, bows, musical instruments, utensils etc. Its wood is valued for strength, durability, decay resistance and decorative characteristics. It is used locally for cabinet making, furniture, veneers, parquet floors, gates and roofs.

Taxol is one of the most promising anti-neoplastic drugs to emerge from the anti-tumour screening of natural products in recent years. It is being used clinically in the treatment of ovarian cancers and is undergoing clinical trials against metastatic breast cancers. It may also have potential value for lung, head and neck cancers. The mode of action is unique in that it enhances the polymerization of tubulin, the protein subunit of the spindle microtubules and induces the formation of stable, non-functional microtubules. As a consequence Taxol disrupts the dynamic equilibrium within the microtubule system and blocks cells in the late G2 and M phase of the cell cycle inhibiting cell replication. Taxol is hydrophobic and therefore the injectable concentrate preparation for intravenous infusion is solubilized in polyoxyethylated castor oil. Before injection, it must be diluted in sodium chloride (NaCl) or dextrose solutions or combinations thereof. Taxotere is a side-chain analogue of Taxol which has also been produced by semi-synthesis from 10-DAB. It has improved water-solubility and is being clinically tested against ovarian and breast cancers. It is considered a faster-growing drug than paclitaxel in US markets. Paclitaxel has also been used in coronary stents.

Trade

Approximately 30,000 kg Taxus biomass (leaves, twigs, bark, needles and roots) is required to produce 1 kg of refined paclitaxel. An estimated 400 kg/year of paclitaxel products are marketed annually in North America and Europe with global amounts estimated at 800–1000 kg. Global demand for paclitaxel in 2004 was estimated at 400 kg/year. However while the US market was described as stagnant the European market was expected to expand with the entry into the market of generic products. Global demand for Taxol is growing and estimated at 800–1000 kg worldwide by 2012. Current market price of Taxus is around US $150–160/kg. World sales of paclitaxel in 2003 were estimated at US $4.2 billion and were expected to grow to US $13 billion by 2008. Bioxel Pharma Inc., a Canadian laboratory producing active pharmaceutical products projected annual sales of US $90 million in 2004. As chemical derivatives rather than plant biomass are the Taxus commodity often traded, the Convention of International Trade in Endangered Species (CITES) Appendix II annotation (Appendix II lists species which though not threatened may become so unless trade is closely controlled) specifically designates all parts and derivatives except seeds, pollen and finished pharmaceutical products.

Taxus biomass in trade is sometimes exported as dried needles and twigs or often in a crude liquid or powdered extracts of varying concentrations. Chemical extracts of Taxus species in trade vary in appearance from a tar-like substance (referred to as 'brown liquor') shipped in drums to a light brown powder. Paclitaxel is a whitish or yellowish crystalline material.

Large paclitaxel production facilities exist worldwide including facilities in India, China, North America and Europe. Taxanes are a global commodity and the distribution of taxus biomass and chemical derivatives for use in pharmaceutical production occurs on a worldwide basis.

The centre of demand for finished products made from paclitaxel and related compounds continues to be in the United States and to an increasing extent in Europe. The US Scientific Authority believes that the bulk of Taxus trade consists of Asian rather than North American species.

Although *T. wallichiana* has been listed in CITES App II since 1995, there remains little information available regarding current rates of harvest and trade due to a combination of factors including

- varying interpretations and confusion regarding the taxonomy of *T. wallichiana* and other Taxus species;
- generally low levels of CITES implementation for medicinal plant species;
- exclusion of chemical derivatives (extracts) from CITES trade controls from 2004–2005 and difficulty in visually identifying the main products in trade (leaves, bark, extract) including with regard to discriminating between parts and derivatives from *T. wallichiana* and other taxus species.

Taxus is processed on an industrial scale within India for the production of Ayurvedic medicines as well as extraction of taxanes such as paclitaxel for re-export. Paclitaxel extraction in India is expanding and India is believed to be one of the world's main producers of paclitaxel, with exports of this and the related taxane docetaxol recorded in India's customs data indicating the scale of processing. Processing involves Taxus species collected within India and from imported *T. baccata.*

Following China's ban on Taxus harvest, Taxus used for extraction of paclitaxel was increasingly imported from other countries. In India, the export of *T. wallichiana* has been prohibited through its listing on the negative list of exports since March 1996 and possibly as early as 1994. India is estimated to have exported 5,500 tonnes of leaves during 1994. Paclitaxel extraction was reported as taking place within India in the 1990s for instance by Indo-Italian companies for export to the United States.

International trade in *T. wallichiana* and other Asian Taxus species involves a combination of leaves, bark and extracts in various stages of processing. Much of the preliminary processing appears to take place within the three range states named above, while the final pharmaceutical products are more likely to be produced and consumed in the United States and increasingly in Europe. There has also been an increasing trade in raw materials from European and North American Taxus species to China in recent years to support processing facilities there.

Paclitaxel is also now being produced via plant cell fermentation technology, although the rights to this technology were apparently initially licensed to a single company. Significant investments in the cultivation of Taxus species suggest that demand for wild-harvested plants will decrease at some stage in the future.

Wild harvest continues to be legal in some states within India, and national export laws allow for the export of formulations made from wild-harvested material. Similarly wild harvest is allowed within Nepal, as is export of value added products (e.g. extracts).

Podophyllum

This consists of the dried rhizomes and roots of *Podophyllum hexandrum* Royle and *Podophyllum peltatum* Linn. of the family Berberidaceae. *P. hexandrum* is found in India, China and the Himalayas and yields Indian Podophyllum, whilst *P. pelatatum* comes from North America and is the source of American Podophyllum.

Commercial Importance

Podophyllum is an endangered but high-value medicinal plant from temperate and cold climatic zones of the globe. It is a source of podophyllotoxin, a natural lignan with cytotoxic, anti-tumour properties. It is the precursor for the semi-synthesis of the widely used anti-cancer drugs etoposide, teniposide and etopophos. It is also a precursor to a new drug that is being tested for rheumatoid arthritis in Europe. Podophyllum resin prepared from the rhizomes has long been used as a purgative, but the discovery of the cytotoxic properties of podophyllotoxin and related compounds has now made Podophyllum a commercially important plant. Preparations of podophyllum resin (the Indian resin is preferred) are effective treatments for warts, and pure podophyllotoxin is available as a paint for soft venereal warts. *P. hexandrum* has an increasing demand in the national and international markets because the percentage of podophyllotoxin is about 20 times more than American Podophyllum.

Habitat and Distribution

Both plants are large-leafed perennial herbs with edible fruits, though other parts of the plant are toxic. The American Podophyllum also called mayapple root, devil's apple, hog apple, wild or American Mandrake is extensively distributed through the Eastern United States growing luxuriantly in moist shady woods and in low marshy grounds from Canada to Minnesota and southwards to Florida and Texas. The drug is collected in Virginia, Kentucky, North Carolina, Tennessee and Indiana.

Indian Podophyllum (Syn: *P. emodi*, *Sinopodophyllum hexandrum*) also called Himalayan Mayapple (Sanskrit: Bakrachimaka, Hindi: Papri) occurs in the forests and open slopes from 2400–4500 m. It is found in India, Afghanistan, Bhutan, China, Nepal and Pakistan. The drug is collected both in India and China. In India, it is distributed in restricted pockets of the Himalayas in Uttarakhand, Garhwal and Himachal Pradesh. Other less common species of Podophyllum (*P. pleianthum*) and related genera (e.g. *Diphylleia*) also contain podophyllotoxin and structurally related lignans.

Harvest

Plants are collected from the wild. American Podophyllum has long-jointed branching rhizomes about 1 m long, which are dug up, cut into pieces about 10 cm long and dried. Indian Podophyllum bears little resemblance to the American one. Rhizomes occur in much contorted pieces of an earthy brown colour about 2–4 cm long, 1–2 cm in diameter. The rhizome is harder and difficult to break. Both plants are propagated by their creeping rhizomes.

Constituents

The roots and rhizomes contain cytotoxic lignans and their glucosides with the Indian Podophyllum containing about 5% and American Podophyllum 1%. The active principles may be obtained in a concentrated form by pouring an ethanolic extract of the root into water. The precipitated podophyllum resin or 'podophyllin' is then dried. While Indian Podophyllum yields about 6% to 12% of resin containing 50% to 60% lignans, American Podophyllum gives 2% to 8% resin containing 14% to 18% lignans.

Both Indian and American Podophyllum have similar lignan constituents, however in different proportions. The Indian drug contains chiefly podophyllotoxin (about 4%) and 4'-demethyl podophyllotoxin (about 0.45%) and the main components in the American root are podophyllotoxin (about 0.25%), β-peltatin (about 0.33%) and α-peltatin (about 0.25%). Deoxypodophyllotoxin, podophyllotoxone, glucosides of podophyllotoxin, 4'-demethyl podophyllotoxin are present in both plants with the Indian root having only traces of peltatins. Fresh rhizomes have more active principles, which are lost on prolonged storage. Also resin preparation results in considerable losses of the water-soluble glucosides.

Uses

American Podophyllum has long been used by native Americans as a vermifuge and emetic and the subsequently obtained resin was employed as a purgative. Its use however declined until 1942 when the resin was recommended for the treatment of veneral warts. Indian Podophyllum has been used in Ayurveda and Unani systems of medicine as purgative, cholagogue, emetic and against warts. Ripe fruits are edible and used against fever. Tibetan medicine uses it for gynecological disorders. Podophyllotoxin and other Podophyllum lignans were found unsuitable for clinical use as anti-cancer agents due to toxic side effects, but the semi-synthetic derivatives etoposide and teniposide made from natural podophyllotoxin have proved excellent anti-tumour agents. They were developed as modified forms (acetals) of the natural 4'-demethyl podophyllotoxin glucoside. Etoposide is a very effective anti-cancer agent and is used in the treatment of small-cell lung cancer, testicular cancer as well as lymphomas and leukemias usually in combination therapy with other anti-cancer drugs. Teniposide has similar anti-cancer properties, and though not as widely used as etoposide has value in paediatric neuroblastoma.

These drugs inhibit the enzyme topoisomerase II, thus preventing DNA synthesis and replication. Topoisomerases are responsible for cleavage and resealing of DNA strands during the replication process. The overall effect of these drugs is the arrest of the cells in late S or early G2 phase of the cell cycle. The anti-mitotic and purgative properties of these compounds depend on a lactone ring in *trans* configuration.

Trade

Mayapple is an important American botanical drug with annual production in several hundred tones supplying both domestic and export demands. The US annual demand for American Podophyllum was more than 130 tonnes in 1970. The commercial interest turned to Indian Podophyllum when it was found to contain more podophyllotoxin than the American root. Indian Podophyllum is considered a rare and threatened species with removal rates exceeding natural regeneration rates. The population of these plants throughout its range was observed to be very sparse, declining and receding towards higher elevations. It has declined considerably to meet the increasing demand of the pharmaceutical industry; 37.3 tonnes of rhizomes were uprooted from 1995 to 2000. Market price of Indian Podophyllum is between Rs.500–660/kg within India. Exploitation of Podophyllum from the wild is prohibited for export from India under CITES. Many Indian research institutes are making great efforts to rescue these species. The annual supply during 1970 was around 50–80 tonnes against a demand of over 100 tonnes. The existing rate per hectare return is estimated at Rs. 141,120 at the rate of Rs. 60/kg.

Liquorice

It consists of the peeled or unpeeled dried rhizomes and roots of various species of *Glycyrrhiza* belonging to the family Leguminosae. A number of different varieties are cultivated commercially:

- *G. glabra var. typica* Reg et Herd is grown in Spain, Italy, England, France, Germany and the United States. Called Spanish liquorice it consists of rhizomes with a few pieces of root and occurs in peeled and unpeeled forms
- *G. glabra var. glandulifera* Weld et Kit is collected in large quantities from the wild in Galicia and Central and Southern Russia along the banks of Volga and other rivers. The dried unpeeled drug from its large root stock with long perennial roots is called Russian liquorice.
- *G. glabra var. violacea* Boiss yields Persian liquorice and is collected in Iran and Iraq in the valleys of Tigris and Euphrates rivers. Usually unpeeled, it occurs in large coarse pieces resembling unpeeled Russian liquorice.
- *G. uralensis* Fischer yields Manchurian liquorice and is an important drug of Chinese commerce. This unpeeled drug, smaller in diameter than the European drug, consists of roots that exfoliate readily and the wood is easier to cut.

Commercial Importance

Most of liquorice produced is used in confectionary and for flavouring including tobacco, beers and stouts. Its pleasant sweet taste and foaming properties are due to saponins. It masks the taste of bitter drugs such as aloe, ammonium chloride and quinine, and increases the foaminess of alcoholic beverages to which it imparts a slightly bitter taste. Following recognition of the anti-inflammatory effects of liquorice extracts and glycyrrhetenic acid present in it, liquorice is being used in the treatment of rheumatoid arthritis, Addison's disease and inflammatory conditions. Anti-ulcerogenic, spasmolytic and anti-ulcer effects of its flavonoids led to its use for sympto-matic relief from peptic ulcer pain. Thus there is a large commercial demand for liquorice.

Harvest

In western Europe liquorice is cultivated, but the Russian and Persian drugs are obtained from wild plants. They are usually propagated by replanting young pieces of stolons but may be grown from the seed. The underground organs are developed to a sufficient extent (ensuring maximum sap sweetness) by the end of the third year when they are dug up after the leaves fall. Some are peeled, and cut up into short pieces before drying, but much of the drug is now used unpeeled. The drug is usually imported in bales. In Southern Italy and to some extent in Spain, Anatolia, etc., a large part of the drug is made into block or stick liquorice. This is prepared by the process of decoction, the liquid being subsequently clarified and evaporated to the consist-ency of a soft extract. This is made into blocks or sticks, dried and exported in boxes lined with laurel leaves.

Constituents

Liquorice contains about 20% water-soluble extracts and much of this is composed of glycyr-rhizin which is typically 3% to 5% of the root, but upto 12% is found in some varieties. Glycyrrhizin is a mixture of the potassium and calcium salts of glycyrrhizinic acid. The bright yellow colour of the liquorice root is provided by the flavonoids (1% to 1.5%) including liquiritin, isoliquiritin and their corresponding aglycones. Considerable amounts of sugars namely glucose and sucrose are also present.

Medicinal Uses

Liquorice has long been used in pharmacy as a flavouring agent, demulcent and mild expecto-rant. Many of the early claims for a broad spectrum of uses of the drugs are borne out by mod-ern pharmacological research. Glycyrrhizin is reported to be 50–150 times sweeter than sucrose. Corticosteroid-like activity has been recognized with liquorice extracts displaying mild anti-inflammatory and mineralocorticoid activities. These have been exploited in the treatment of rheumatoid arthritis, Addison's disease and various inflammatory conditions. Glycyrrhetenic acid is implicated for these activities and it has been found to inhibit enzymes that catalyse the conversion of prostaglandins and glucocorticoids into inactive metabolites. This results in increased levels of prostaglandins, e.g., PGE_2 and $PGF_{2\alpha}$ and hydrocortisone. Flavonoid compo-nent of the root also exerts spasmolytic and anti-ulcerogenic activity. The most significant cur-rent application is to give symptomatic relief from peptic ulcers by promoting healing through increased prostaglandin activity. A semi-synthetic derivative of glycyrrhetenic acid, the hemi-succinate carbenoxolone sodium is now widely prescribed for the treatment of gastric and duodenal ulcers. The mineralocorticoid effects (sodium and water retention) may exacerbate hypertension and cardiac problems.

In Indian medicine, liquorice was one of the prominent drugs of Ayurveda mentioned by Sushruta in his treatise. Called yastimadhu (Sanskrit), mulethi (Hindi) or athimaduram (Tamil), it is a component of several traditional medicinal formulations.

Trade

There exists a large market demand mainly from developed countries for liquorice due to its multiple usages. It is estimated that the global demand for liquorice extracts and roots is around 200–250 thousand tonnnes per year. In 2007 the total value of international trade in liquorice was US $42 million. Bulk of the drug in the international market originates in China, Pakistan and Afghanistan. Turkey, former USSR, Spain, Syria, France, Italy and Iraq are the other major producers. A major portion of the commercial supply comes from wild sources and there is only limited area under cultivation. Total production is between 40–50 thousand tonnes per annum.

China is one of the major suppliers of liquorice roots and extracts in the international trade. Excessive harvesting in this country has reduced its resources from 405 million tonnes in 1950 to 350–450 thousand tonnes in 1983. Even the acreage under liquorice cover declined form 1.53–2 million hectares in 1950s to only 562,400 hectares of land in 2001 with a mere 0.65 million tonnes of reserves remaining. Despite export restrictions imposed for some period, China exported more than 10,000 tonnes each year in the 1980s. Japan, Korea, the United States and China are the dominant importers of liquorice in the world market. Due to unstable global demand and supply, price of liquorice roots in the world market varies from US $1,650/tonne (1988) to US $1200/tonne (2007).

Liquorice does not occur wild in India. Though it grows well in Patiala, Hissar, Jhansi and Lucknow, Indian farmers are hesitant to cultivate it, as profitable returns on the crop come only after three years. The entire Indian requirement for liquorice comes from import.

Cinchona Bark

It consists of the dried bark of the stem and root of various species, races and hybrids of *Cinchona* (Rubiaceae).

Commercial Importance

There are about a dozen different cinchona species in commerce. Cinchona and its alkaloids particularly quinine were of great importance for use in the treatment of malaria before World War II. With the introduction of synthetic drugs, its importance declined but it remains of great economic importance and salts of quinine and quinidine are included in most pharmacoepias. Today it has re-emerged as suitable for the treatment of *Plasmodium falciparum* infections resistant to chloroquine and other synthetic antimalarials. Quinidine, the diastereoisomer of quinine, is employed for the prophylaxis of cardiac arrhythmias and for the treatment of atrial fibrillation. It also has antimalarial properties and like quinine it is effective against chloroquine-resistant organisms.

Species and Distribution

There are over 36 known species and hybrids of cinchona. They are now cultivated in many parts of the world including Bolivia, Gautemala, India, Indonesia, Zaire, Tanzania and Kenya.

Commercially valuable bark is obtained from three main species based on favourable range of alkaloids present. They are

- *C. succirubra* – Cultivated in Belgian Congo and Kenya, it provides what is known as 'red bark' and contains 5% to 7% total alkaloids.
- *C. ledgeriana* – Also cultivated in Belgian Congo and Kenya, it provides 'brown bark' and contains 5% to 14% total alkaloids.
- *C. calisaya* – This and *C. ledgeriana* are natives of Southern Peru and Bilivia. Now also cultivated in India and Indonesia, it yields 4% to 7% total alkaloids.

Selected hybrids can yield upto 17% total alkaloids.

Harvest

The bark was originally obtained by felling wild trees, which led to their destruction. Today production of cinchona bark is a highly specialized section of tropical agriculture employing high-yielding strains, grafting and other techniques. Bark is collected from 6 to 9-year-old trees (with the maximal alkaloid content) during rainy season, sun dried and then dried by artificial heat before being coarsely powdered. It is then processed for the separation of alkaloids.

Constituents

A considerable number of alkaloids have been characterized in the bark, four of which account for 30% to 60% of the alklaoidal content. These are quinine, quinidine, cinchonidine and cinchonine. These are quinoline-containing structures representing two pairs of diastereoisomers. Quinine is usually the major component (one-half to two-thirds of total alkaloids), but the proportions of the four alkaloids vary according to species and hybrids. The alkaloids are often present in the bark in salt combination with quinic acid and cinchotannic acid.

Uses

Galenicals of cinchona have long been used as bitter tonics and stomachics. On account of the astringent effect due to tannins contained, a decoction and acid infusion are sometimes used as gargles. Huge quantities of cinchona bark are consumed in beverages such as vermouth and tonic water.

Quinine was the drug of choice for the treatment of malaria before World War II. However when its source was cut off by Japan during the war, a range of synthetic antimalarials was hastily produced as an alternative to quinine. Many such as chloroquine, primaquine and mefloquine are based on the structure of quinine. These drugs are much more active than quinine but associated with several adverse effects. Due to the ability of *P. falciparum,* the causative oraganism for malaria, to develop resistance to modern drugs, today cinchona alkaloids re-emerge as suitable for the treatment of chloroquine-resistant infections. Mixtures of cinchona alkaloids termed 'totaquine' were used as antimalarials during periods of quinine shortages.

Quinine exerts antimalarial action by intercalation of the quinoline moiety into the parasite's DNA. It also complexes with the toxic breakdown products of haemoglobin formed by the parasite. Quinine finds use in the treatment of nocturnal cramps due to its skeletal muscle relaxant effect. Quinidine is administered in cardiac arrhythmias as it controls fibrillation and uncontrolled contraction of the muscle fibres of the heart.

Trade

Demand for cinchona and quinine products is increasing as they are extensively used not only as antimalarials, but huge quantities are also used in the manufacture of tonic drinks, and soft beverages. Salts of quinine are also added to hair oils, sunburn lotions, moth repellants, insecticides, vulcanization accelerators in rubber industry, polarized lenses and as pickling agent in metal industries.

Indonesia and India, where the Dutch and the British respectively introduced the drug from South America, are important producers of cinchona. A high percentage of the total crop is now grown on plantations in Tanzania, Kenya, Gautemala, Bolivia, Zaire, Rwanda, Sri Lanka, Columbia and Costa Rica. These countries produce approximately 400–500 tonnes of alkaloids, obtained from 8,000–10,000 tonnes of bark produced annually. In 1991 its wholesale price in Hamburg was DM 2.25/kg.

In India cinchona plantations and alkaloid-processing units in Tamil Nadu and West Bengal are of great historical interest. Having originated in the 1860s there was a slump in the cultivation and production from 1955 to 1965 due to various reasons. Due to resurgence of malaria and identification of newer uses of quinine, there has been a revival in the export market for quinine. Today 3,400 hectares in West Bengal and 2,200 hectares in Tamil Nadu are under cinchona cultivation. While *C. officinalis* is cultivated at Nilgiris in Tamil Nadu, *C. ledgeriana* and *C. robusta* (hybrid of *C. officinalis* and *C. succirubra*) are cultivated at Mungpoo on Darjeeling hills in West Bengal.

Ipecac

Ipecacuanha or ipecac consists of the dried rhizomes and roots of *Cephaelis ipecacuanha* (Bortero) or *Cephaelis acuminata* (Karsten) (Rubiaceae).

Commercial Importance

Ipecac in the form of syrup is used in the treatment of drug overdose and poisoning for its emetic effect. Vomiting induced by emetine, a principal alkaloid of ipecac, is used as model to study the therapeutic effect of newer anti-emetics. Emetine is an isoquinoline group alkaloid derived form ipecac and used in the treatment of amoebic dysentery. Emetine and cephaeline, its chief alkaloids, are shown to have anti-tumour and anti-HIV properties, which are being further explored.

Species and Distribution

C. ipecacuanha and *C. acuminata* are low straggling shrubs having horizontal rhizomes with prominently ridged roots. *C. ipecacuanha* yields what is termed Rio, Brazilian or MattoGrasso ipecac and is cultivated mainly in Brazil. It occurs in tortuous pieces. *C. ipecacuanha* is also successfully produced by cultivation in India (Darjeeling hills), Malaysia and in Selangor.

C. acuminata gives Cartagena, Nicaragua, Panama or Costa Rica ipecac and comes principally from Columbia and Nicaragua. The root is of a larger diameter than the Rio root.

Harvest

The plants grow in clumps in the woods and the roots are collected from such wild plants. They are levered from the ground, roots removed and the plant replaced in the ground to produce a further crop of roots and rhizomes. The collected roots are sundried or over fires, freed of adhering soil and packed in bales for export.

Constituents

Ipecac contains 2% to 2.5% alkaloids, the principal ones being emetine and cephaeline typically in the ratio 2:1 in *C. ipeacacuanha* and 1:2 to 1:1 in *C. acuminata*. Minor alkaloids are psychotrine, o-methyl psychotrine, which are dehydro derivatives of cephaeline and emetine respectively. Monoterpenoid isoquinoline glycosides ipecoside, alangoside, iridoid glycosides sweroside, 7-dehydrologanin are also found in the root.

Uses

Ipecac was used as an insect repellant and amoebicide by South American Indians. It was introduced in Europe in the late 16th century and became well known in medicine. Ipecac is used as an expectorant and emetic and in the treatment of amoebic dysentery. Both emetine and synthetic drug 2,3-dehydro emetine are anti-amoebic and act primarily on the intestinal wall and the liver. Emetine hydrochloride has been used extensively as an anti-protozoan in the treatment of amoebiasis, pyorrhea alveolaris and other amoebic diseases. The emetic action of the alkaloids is valuable and the crude drug extract in the form of ipecac emetic mixture is an important preparation used for drug overdose or poisoning. The emetic mixture is often a standard component in poison antidote kits. Ipecac extracts are still components of a number of compound expectorant preparations.

Emetine has more expectorant and less emetic action than cephaeline which is why the Brazilian root is preferred for such mixtures. Emetine may also be prepared by the methylation of cephaeline. Both emetine and cephaeline are potent inhibitors of protein synthesis, inhibiting at the translocation stage. They display anti-tumour, anti-viral and anti-amoebic activity but are too toxic for therapeutic use. In recent studies, o-methyl psychotrine has shown the ability to inhibit viral replication through inhibition of HIV-reverse transcriptase. This gives it a potential in the treatment of AIDS.

Trade

Costa Rica is at present the principal source of the drug. World trade in the root has come down of late due to introduction of highly effective synthetic anti-amoebic drugs. Continuous use of such drugs caused resistant strains of the protozoan, resulting in the revival of demand for ipecac. At present there is a worldwide shortage of the drug. Total production of ipecac in the world is approximately 100 tonnes per year, most of which comes from Nicaragua, Brazil and India. Indian production of ipecac comes exclusively from cultivation at Mungpoo in West Bengal. In India ipecac cultivation is done by the West Bengal Cinchona Department in the Darjeeling district and to a smaller extent in Sikkim and parts of Assam. The annual production ranges between 25–30 tonnes of dry roots and part of the produce, including emetine salts is exported.

Dioscorea

It consists of the tubers or rhizomes of a number of cultivated and wild species of *Dioscorea*, family Dioscoreaceae.

Commercial Importance

A number of species of Dioscorea are cultivated largely for their large starchy tubers, commonly called yams, which are an important food crop in many parts of the world. Apart from several important edible species, a number of species accumulate quite high levels of saponins in their tubers which make them bitter and toxic, but these provide suitable sources of steroidal material for drug manufacture. Such species rich in steroidal sapogenins are of great pharmaceutical importance because of their relationship to compounds such as sex hormones, cortisone, diuretic steroids, vitamin D and cardiac glycosides. Diosgenin, one of the principal sapogenins in several Dioscorea species, is widely used as a precursor in the semi-synthesis of steroid hormones such as progesterone, corticosteroids and anabolic steroids. The cost of progesterone and other important steroids (till then synthesized) fell drastically in the 1940s with their successful semi-synthesis from diosgenin. There was and is thus a great demand for such natural products which will serve as starting materials for the partial synthesis of medicinally important steroids.

Species and Distribution

There are about 15 species of *Dioscorea* genus known to contain diosgenin. Commercially important species are the following:

- *Dioscorea composita*, *Dioscorea mexicana* and *Dioscorea floribunda* found in Mexico, tubers are collected from wild plants.
- *Dioscorea deltoidea* and *Dioscorea prazeri* occurring wild in northwest and northeast Himalayas respectively in India.
- *Dioscorea sylvatica* (Africa).
- *Dioscorea collettii*, *Dioscorea pathaica* and *Dioscorea nipponica* (China).

Disogenin is also sourced from other species such as *Trigonella foenum graecum* (Leguminosae), sisal (*Agave sisalona* –Agavaceae) and *Solanum* species (*S. laciniatum, S. marginatum*).

Constituents

According to species, tubers yield 1% to 8% of total sapogenins, the principal of which is diosgenin with small quantities of the 25β-epimer yamogenin. While *D. composita* may contain 4% to 6% total saponins, *D. floribunda* has 6% to 8% diosgenin. Disogenin is present as a dioscin, the glycosidic form from which it is obtained on hydrolysis.

Harvest

Dioscoreas are herbaceous, climbing, vine-like plants, the tuber being totally buried or sometimes protruding from the ground. Tubers weigh upto 5 kg with 40- to 50-kg tubers being recorded in some species. Drug material is obtained from both wild and cultivated plants with plants collected from the wild having been exploited considerably more than cultivated ones. Commercial cultivation is less economic, requiring a 4- to 5-year growing period and some form of support for the climbing stems. Tubers are collected from 3 to 5-year-old plants (with maximum diosgenin and yamogenin content), when they are dormant by ploughing. They are thoroughly washed of adhering soil and transported appropriately for diosgenin isolation from fresh tubers. In India, the tubers are chopped into smaller units to dry in the sun and then packed.

Exporters grade the material, which is to be ground to prepare powders or processed further to extract diosgenin or 16-dehydro pregnenolone (16-DPA) from it.

Uses

Tubers of many of the dioscoreas have long been used for food, as they are rich in starch. These yams are considered famine foods consumed in times of scarcity. The species is considered a medicinal plant of major importance in higher elevation regions of Nepal, Bhutan, India, Pakistan and southwestern China. The plant is used both as traditional medicine and as a source of steroidal drugs for conventional medicine. Though used traditionally as medicine in Nepal and Pakistan, it is not used in Ayurveda. The rhizomes are traditionally used in western Himalayas to launder raw wool and woollen fabrics owing to their saponin content. Among the hill tribe communities of Jammu and Kashmir, the rhizomes are made into soap used to kill lice. The principal sapogenin diosgenin is an important starting material in the synthesis of steroidal hormones. Diosgenin is converted to 16-DPA, which is then used as a substrate for corticosteroids, pregnenes, androstenes and 19-norsteroids.

Trade

Demand for diosgenin for pharmaceuticals is huge, equivalent to 10,000 tonnes of Dioscorea tuber per annum. Until 1970 Mexican yam was the only source of diosgenin for steroidal contraceptive manufacture. Following nationalization of the Mexican industry, prices increased drastically forcing the search for alternative sources of diosgenin and alternatives to diosgenin. Fenugreek seeds are exploited for their diosgenin content and hecogenin (Agave), sarsasapogenin (Yucca), stigmasterol (soya), solasodine (Solanum) are now being used for the production of 16-DPA. Meanwhile total synthesis of several steroids also became economically feasible and is much used now.

The total turnover of bulk steroids in the world is estimated to be US $500 million and estimated worldwide usage is somewhere between 550 and 650 tonnes of diosgenin. Mexico, Gautemala, Costa Rica, India and China are the major diosgenin-producing countries. Hecogenin is produced in Kenya, Mexico, China and Israel from Agave.

In India *D. deltoidea*, *D. floribunda* and *D. prazeri* are the species cultivated. The cultivation is tedious and expensive. It requires special climatic conditions and protection from virus and other microorganisms. *D. floribunda* commercially released by the Indian Institute of Horticultural Research near Bangalore is introduced for cultivation in Tamil Nadu, Karnataka, Kerala, West Bengal and Assam. *D. deltoidea* is grown at an altitude of 122 m in the Himalayan tracks in Jammu and Kashmir and Himachal Pradesh. Dioscorea species are cultivated by vegetative propagation techniques in about 100 acres of land.

With the introduction of solasodine as a basic analog of diosgenin, the worldwide demand for diosgenin has considerably reduced. Diosgenin is also commercially produced in a low concentration from the tubers of *Costus speciosus*. A number of private units like Cipla, Wyeth, Organon and also CIMAP are engaged in the commercial cultivation of Dioscorea.

Digitalis

It consists of the dried leaves of the 'purple foxglove', *Digitalis purpurea,* belonging to the family Scrophulariaceae

Commercial Importance

Leaves of digitalis species contain medicinally important glycosides of the cardenolide group. Called cardiac glycosides, these C23 steroidal glycosides exert a slowing and strengthening effect on a failing heart. In conventional medicine, glycosides of digitalis are extensively employed in the treatment of congestive heart failure and atrial fibrillation. The worldwide use of the drug amounts to several thousands of kilograms per year. Since these glycosides have so far not been synthesized, digitalis leaves are the only source left to meet the pharmaceutical requirement and hence the commercial importance.

Species and Distribution

D. purpurea and *Digitalis lanata* are the two economically important sources of cardiac glycosides. Both are biennial or perennial herbs growing in semi-shady regions in the wild state. Presently the leaves are collected from cultivated plants. *D. purpurea* is common in UK and most of Europe and naturalized in northern and western USA and Canada. Major centres of cultivation are Suffolk in UK, Wageningen in Holland and Pennsylvania in the United States. It is also grown in Egypt, Japan and India. *D. purpurea* has purple flowers with finger-shaped corolla.

D. lanata is indigenous to central and southeastern Europe and is cultivated in UK, former USSR, Ecuador and the United States. In Holland both the species of *Digitalis* are commercially cultivated. The plants generally resemble purple foxglove but the shape of the corollas is different and the pedicels are covered with woolly trichomes.

Leaves of other Digitalis species namely *D. ferruginea, D. lutea, D. thapsi, D. grandiflora, D. mertonensis, D. nervosa, D. dubia, D. subalpina* also show the presence of cardiac glycosides.

Harvest

D. purpurea is a common ornamental plant of England well known for its medicinal properties. Horticultural varieties grown as garden plants are low in therapeutic glycosides. For pharmaceutical purposes, cultivation is preferable to collection from wild plants because factors such as the climate, soil, age of the plant, season, storage and drying method and genetic makeup of the cultivated strain influence the activity of the drug. The plants are cultivated from the seeds and produce a rosette of leaves in the first year. The first crop of leaves is collected, and the next year the flowering stems which begin to appear are cut off to encourage further leaf growth, which are again collected in the second year. The plants may thus continue to yield a crop of leaves for several years in succession. However total glycoside levels are higher in first-year leaves and medicinally important glycosides are highest in the second-year leaves. Hence the first- and second-year leaves are to be collected as per the pharmacoepias. The leaves have to be collected in dry weather and dried as quickly as possible in the dark at temperatures between 55 and 60° C, since moisture and higher temperatures activate enzymatic degradation of the active glycosides into inactive forms. The dried leaves are to be stored in moisture-free containers and should not contain more than 5% moisture.

Constituents

The cardioactive glycoside content of *D. purpurea* leaves is 0.15% to 0.4% consisting of about 30 different structures. The fresh leaves contain purpurea glycoside A (50% of the glycoside mixture), purpurea glycoside B and glucogitaloxin. These possess at the C-3 position of the aglycone a linear chain of three digitoxose sugar moieties terminated by glucose. On drying, due to enzymatic degradation, the terminal glucose is lost forming digitoxin, gitoxin and gitaloxin respectively. The aglycone gitaloxigenin is less stable and hence digitoxin and gitoxin are the main active components of the drug. Careless storage leads to further hydrolysis resulting in the loss of the three digitoxose sugars leaving the inactive aglycones. Other glycosides present in small quantities involving sugar digitalose and glucose with the same aglycones are present as monoglycosides and diglycosides. Glycosides of gitoxigenin are less active than the corresponding digitoxigenin-derived series. *D. purpurea* leaves also contain anthraquinone derivatives and some saponins. The total cardenolide content of *D. lanata* is upto 1% which is 2–3 times that of *D. purpurea*. The primary glycosides of *D. lanata* resemble those of *D. purpurea*, but are acetylated at the digitoxose moiety next to terminal glucose. This acetyl group makes the compounds easier to isolate from the plant material as they crystallize readily. During drying and storage, deacetylation leads to the same products as of *D. purpurea*. In addition to the three aglycone-based glycosides two additional series of compounds formed on digoxigenin and diginatigenin are found in *D. lanata*. The primary glycosides containing the acetylated tetrasaccharide unit, glucose-(digitoxose)$_3$, are called lanatosides. Lanatosides A and C based on aglycones digitoxigenin and digoxigenin respectively constitute the major components (50%–70%) of the fresh leaf. Some anthraquinone and flavonoid glycosides have also been characterized in *D. lanata*.

Uses

Foxglove leaves are claimed to be used externally by Welsh physicians and its poisonous nature was well known. It has been recorded to be used by a 'witch' healer for the treatment of dropsy. Though introduced into the London pharmacoepia in 1650, it was with William Withering's published clinical findings in 1776 that it came into frequent use. It began to be investigated chemically since 1820. Digitalis was thus used medicinally as leaf, standardized leaf powder and as isolated active constituents. On account of the pronounced cardiac effects of digitalis, the variability in the glycoside content and also differences in the range of structures present due to enzymatic hydrolysis, the crude leaf is assayed biologically. Based on this, the leaf powder was standardized for active glycosides and diluted as required with powdered low-potency digitalis, or with powdered lucerne or grass.

While *D. purpurea* was earlier used as a crude drug, *D. lanata* was never used so. Both are now replaced by pure isolated glycosides. The cardioactive glycosides increase the force of contractions in the heart, thus increasing the cardiac output and allowing more rest between contractions. The improved blood circulation tends to improve kidney function, leading to diuresis and loss of oedema fluid often associated with heart disease. However, the diuretic effect historically important in the treatment of dropsy is now more safely controlled by other diuretic drugs. Digitoxin, digoxin, lanatoside C and desacetyl lanatoside C (deslanide) are the isolated constituents employed in therapy. Acting similar to digitalis leaf, digoxin however has a rapid action. It is more rapidly absorbed from the gastrointestinal tract and is more quickly eliminated than digitoxin and is therefore the more widely used of the cardioactive glycosides. It is also more hydrophilic than digitoxin and binds less strongly to plasma proteins and is mainly eliminated by the kidneys, whereas digitoxin is metabolized more slowly by the liver. Over the past decades, digoxin has become the most widely used drug in the treatment of congestive heart failure. Proprietary preparations of lanatoside A and C are available in various countries but digoxin is more widely used. It is used for rapid digitalization in the treatment of atrial fibrillation and congestive heart failure. Lanatoside C is less absorbed than digitoxin, but it is less cumulative and for rapid digitalization, digoxin is preferred.

Trade

The major digitalis producing countries are the United States, UK, the Netherlands, Switzerland, Germany and the former USSR. In most of these countries *D. lanata* is the source drug. Some 1,000 tonnes of plant material are required annually to meet the world demand. In the long term patients require about 1 mg per day and the worldwide use of the drug now amounts to several thousand kilograms per year.

Though not indigenous to India, digitalis is cultivated chiefly in Himachal Pradesh (Solan), Kashmir, Darjeeling in West Bengal and Nilgiri hills (Kodaikanal) in Tamil Nadu. The total annual demand for the drug in India is estimated at more than 30 quintals. The price of digitoxin in the international market is very high upto Rs.22, 620/kg, while digoxin costs 17,267/kg. The total cost of the raw material imported into India comes to crores of rupees.

Ginseng

It consists of the roots of *panax ginsing* (Araliaceae) and related species such as *P. quinquifolium* and *P. notoginseng*.

Commercial Importance

One of the most ancient drugs of China, ginseng is considered a universal medication in oriental medicine. It has been used for centuries as a tonic, a stimulant to overcome physical and mental fatigue and to counter many conditions arising from the onset of old age. Recently it has become a popular remedy even in the west and is available as a health food in the form of powders, extracts and teas for improvement of stamina, concentration and resistance to stress and disease. It is considered an 'adaptogen' as it helps the body adapt to stress and is popularly promoted as an aphrodisiac, as a performance and endurance enhancer. Modern pharmacological research has reported an array of biological properties for several of its constituents. Many ginseng products are available as OTC products either for oral administration or as cosmetic preparations. Demand for raw material for ginseng-based products has recently increased dramatically.

Species and Distribution

P. ginseng is collected from cultivated plants in China, Korea and Japan. Also called Asian ginseng it is indigenous to the mountainous forests of eastern Asia.

P. quinquifolium called American Ginseng grows in rich woods in eastern USA and Canada. It is collected from cultivated stands and has been exported to China since the early 1700s. It is now an endangered species in the United States.

P. notoginseng also called Sanchi Ginseng is collected from Russia.

P. pseudoginseng ssp. *Himalaicus var augustifolius* (Himalayan Ginseng) found in India (in the mountainous regions of Sikkim and western Himalayas from Pithoragarh district of Uttar Pradesh), Bhutan, Nepal and China.

P. japonicum var major from Japan, *P. vietnamensis* (Vietnamese Ginseng) and *Eleutherococcus senticosus* (Siberian or Russian Ginseng) is an abundant and inexpensive substitute for ginseng and is cultivated in China for the roots which are tonic and sedative.

Harvest

Ginseng plants are perennial herbs growing to a height of 50 cm and having corpulent roots resembling human form. *P. ginseng* is typically a shade-preferring plant exclusively growing under forest shade without the durable impact of direct sunshine. Ginseng was formerly a wild plant growing in the northeastern part of China and northern Korean peninsula. At present it is practically extinct in the forests of China and Korea. The roots are collected from plants culti-vated from seeds, under thatched covers and harvested when 6 years old. The dried and usually peeled root provides white ginseng, whereas red ginseng is obtained by steaming the root, this process generating a reddish-brown caramel-like colour. They are dried first by artificial heat and then sun dried. The roots are graded and packed, with small roots being processed separately to form a separate article of commerce.

Constituents

Ginseng contains a complex mixture of triterpenoid saponin glycosides, which are either tetra-cyclic triterpenes based on steroidal skeleton or pentacyclic triterpenoids structurally related to oleanolic acid. Termed ginsenosides by Japanese workers and panaxosides by the Russian researchers, these are derivatives of two main aglycones, protopanaxadiol and protopanaxatriol. Over 30 ginsenosides have been characterized from different varieties of ginseng. Some of the ginsenosides of *P. quiquifolium* are the same as those of the Chinese and Korean drug; others appear to differ. The roots also contain therapeutically active high molecular weight polysac-charides and acetylenic compounds. The saponin contents of *P. notoginseng* (about 12%) and *P. quinquifolium* (about 6%) are generally higher than that of *P. ginseng* (1.5%–2%).

Uses

For about 2,000 years, the roots of *P. ginseng* have held an honoured place in Chinese medicine. Revered for its strength-giving and rejuvenating powers, the drug was used in the treatment of anae-mia, diabetes, insomnia, neurasthenia, gastritis and sexual impotence. North American Indians used ginseng in many of their herbal formulas. The widespread use of ginseng is accompanied by the availability of abundant literature on the product and its purported activity. Reportedly acting favourably on the metabolism, its CNS-stimulating, CNS-sedative, tranquillizing, anti-fatigue, hypotensive and hypertensive activities have all been demonstrated. Classified as an adaptogen, it helps the body adapt to stress, improving stamina and concentration and providing a normalizing and restorative effect. It is not advisable to take ginseng continuously for three months, as long-term use can lead to symptoms similar to those of corticosteroid poisoning, including hypertension, nerv-ousness and sleeplessness in some people, yet hypotensive and tranquillizing effects in others. Medicinal properties appear to reside in the saponins, ginsenosides and panaxosides.

Trade

Used as medicine since times immemorial, this widely revered drug created international trade by the 3rd century AD, when China's demand for ginseng allowed it to exchange its silk and medicine with Korea for wild ginseng. By the 1900s the demand for ginseng outstripped the available wild supply and Korea began the commercial cultivation of ginseng which continues to this day. American ginseng has been collected from wild plants and from cultivated stands and exported to China since early 1700s. Ginseng trade from Canada and America put an end to Korean monopoly.

One of the earliest marketable herbs to be harvested in America, the ginseng trade continued to flourish until late 1800s. More than 75,000 pounds of wild ginseng roots were exported in 1822 and ginseng sold for 42 cents a pound (2.2 kg). By 1862 ginseng exports exceeded 300 tonnes per year and dried wild ginseng fetched as much as US $300 per pound in today's dollars. Since 1960s trade in American ginseng has grown steadily and today there is a sizeable domestic market for the root.

The market price for ginseng in the world market varies from US $200 to a high of US $1,500 a dried pound for the wild roots. There are several grades in commerce varying from the highly priced, wild roots to smaller roots and root fragments. Korean root is however the most highly prized and expensive. While most of ginseng grown in the United States is exported, ginseng is imported from Korea for sale in the United States. India imports true ginseng mainly from Indonesia and Singapore.

As per ICO 2011 Global Trade Perspective on the World Market for Ginseng Roots, the total world trade in ginseng roots in 2011 was estimated at US $251 million with USA's share at 29% with US $72 million and Canada's share at US $107 million (42%). China ranks third in the world trade of ginseng having exported US $51 million (20%) worth ginseng. India ranks 15 in value out of the 23 countries exporting ginseng. Its export share was US $0.16 million (Rs 1.65 lacs) worth export to France. Hong Kong and the United States are the largest target markets for imported ginseng roots.

Wild ginseng is listed in Appendix II of CITES and in the United States it is monitored by the US Fish and Wildlife Service. Long-term survival of this economically important plant and the future of ginseng trade depend largely on the sustainable cultivation of the roots.

Valerian

It consists of the dried underground parts of *Valeriana officinalis*, Family: Valerianaceae.

Commercial Importance

One of the top selling sedatives in Europe, valerian was a much esteemed root both for its medicinal uses and as a spice and perfume. It is one of the 10 most popular medicinal plants in North America. Valerian preparations are widely used as herbal tranquillizers to relieve nervous tension, anxiety and insomnia. They are used as safe and effective non-addictive alternatives to conventional sleep medications. Various species of valerian are official in the pharmacopeias of many nations such as Belgium, France, Germany, Italy, Switzerland and UK. Considerable quantities of valerian are used by the perfume industry.

Species and Distribution

Native to Europe and parts of Asia, *V. officinalis* is presently obtained from wild and cultivated plants in Britain, Russia, Holland, Netherlands, Belgium, France, Germany, eastern Europe and Japan. It is also cultivated in the United States. Polyploidy is common with *V. officinalis* and there are diploid, tetraploid and octaploid types. British valerian is usually octaploid and central European valerian usually tetraploid.

V. wallichii is the source of Indian valerian and is official in the Indian pharmacopoeia. Consisting of dried rhizomes and roots, it is collected in the temperate zone of western Himalayas. Found near Nagar, Minapin and Bultoria glacier in India, the root is known as 'Tagara' or 'gilgiti valerian' in Hindi.

V. angustifolia yields 'kesso' or Japanese valerian. *V. mexicana, V. sitchensis, V. diocia, V. edulis* are the other species traded as medicinal valerian. Other species such as *Centranthus ruber* root and rhizomes of *Nardostachys jatamansii* (Indian Spikenard) grow in alpine Himalayas of India and show a somewhat similar constituent profile. The latter is used as a sedative in Indian traditional medicine in conditions of hysteria and convulsions.

Harvest

The plant is a hardy perennial growing to a height of 1–2 m. It bears sweet-scented white or pink flowers. Propagated from the seeds and from seedling plantings, valerian is to be harvested in the second year of growth. The vertical rhizomes of the valerian plant with horizontal branches or stolons at about the ground level are collected in autumn. They are washed in running water and the larger rhizomes are sliced and dried along with smaller rhizomes using artificial heat at temperatures not exceeding 40° C. For maximal activity the drug needs to be freshly harvested and carefully dried.

Constituents

The drug yields 0.5% to 1% volatile oil and it should contain NLT 15% of alcohol (60%) extractable matter. The volatile oil consists of esters, alcohols, eugenol, terpenes and sesquiterpenes. It also contains epoxy-iridoid esters called valepotriates, the principal component of which is valtrate (0.4% to 2%). About 0.05% to 1% alkaloids are also present in the dried root. Several other minor valepotriates are also present. During drying and storage, some of them decompose by hydrolysis and oxidation releasing isovalerenic acid that gives the characteristic odour to the roots. GABA (γ-aminobutyric acid) and glutamine have also been identified in the aqueous extract and these have been suspected to contribute to sedative properties.

Uses

Valerian flower extracts were used in perfumery since the 6th century. Employed as an antianxiety agent and sleep aid for more than 1,000 years, valerian is also used an antispasmodic in hysteria and other nervous disorders. Valerian was especially popular during World War I, when it was used to treat shell-shock. It possesses mild sedative and tranquillizing properties and is often prescribed with bromides or other sedatives. It is popularly used as a tea prepared from 2–3 g of the dried herb or equivalent amounts of tincture. Standardized mixtures of valepotriates containing dihydrovaltrate (80%), valtrate (15%) and acevaltrate (5%) are available in some countries. These materials are usually extracted from the roots of other species of valerian which produce higher amounts of valepotriates than *V. officinalis*.

The identity of the sedative components of the root was not ascertained for a long time due to the unstable nature of the active constituents and genetic variability of the plant material. Though valepotriates were thought to be the sedative components, presence of valerenone, a sesquiterpene component of the volatile oil in *N. jatamansii* used as a popular sedative in Ayurveda led to further activity testing. Japanese researchers concluded that the sedative property was due to the sesquitepene components of the volatile oil. Further valepotriates are reported to be toxic *in vitro*.

Trade

There is a large market for valerian for use in pharmaceuticals, food and cosmetic industries. Majority of valerian in trade comes from cultivated material. Most of the drug is now produced in Europe which is also its largest market. Germany is the largest consuming country. Majority of the standardized extracts and crude, cut and sifted material on the domestic market are prepared from European supplies. A variety of valerian root preparations ranging from dried roots, extracts, tinctures, essential oil, etc., are traded. China, France and Hungary are the largest valerian volatile oil producing countries. Recently there is an increase in demand for valerian in Korea. The plant is also being added to flavour tobacco and soft drinks and fruit juices containing valerian are now sold on the market. Japan and the United States are the chief producers of such beverages. While valerian production is increasing, its prices are decreasing. In 2001 there was a surplus of 4,200 tonnes of valerian roots in European countries. Major producing countries of valerian include Belgium, France, former USSR and China. India is the major producer of Indian valerian.

Whole sale price of valerian ranges from US $2.95 to $31.65 per kg.

Papain

It consists of the dried and purified latex obtained form the unripe fruits of *Carica papaya*, Family: Caricaceae.

Commercial Importance

Papain contains several proteolytic enzymes and being similar to pepsin it is referred to as vegetable pepsin. Its protein-cleaving property gives it immense commercial value and it is used for a wide variety of functions such as tenderizing meat, defibrinating wounds in hospitals, clotting milk, digestive aid, shrink-proofing wool and in the treatment of jellyfish and insect stings, corneal skin deformation, edemas and inflammatory processes. A cheap and easily produced enzyme, it has the ability to digest 35 times its own weight of lean meat. It is extensively used as a meat tenderizer and as an ingredient in cleaning solutions for soft contact lenses. It is available in ointment form for removal of dead tissue components from wounds.

Species and Distribution

The papaya tree is indigenous to tropical America and is cultivated throughout the tropical world and warmer parts of the subtropics. On a large scale it is cultivated in India, Sri Lanka, Tanzania, Hawaii, Florida, Phillippines, South Africa and Australia.

Harvest

A large herbaceous tree of 5–6 m height, *Carica papaya* is dieceous but rarely monoecious. The fruit grows to a length of 30 cm and can weigh upto 5 kg. Latex may be collected from incisions made on the full grown unripe green papaya fruit 75–90 days after fruit set. The coagulated latex lumps are collected and incisions continued at weekly intervals till latex no longer exudes. The collected lumps are shredded, dried and purified by dissolving them in water and precipitating with alcohol. Papain when purified is a greyish white hygroscopic powder.

Constituents

Papain contains several proteolytic enzymes and unlike pepsin it can act in acid, neutral and alkaline media. It has peptidase I – which can digest protein into polypeptides – a rennin-like milk-coagulating enzyme, an amylolytic enzyme and a clotting enzyme similar to pectase.

Uses

Because of several proteolytic enzymes it contains, a single sample of papain yields variable results depending on the protein used. Best-grade papain can digest 300 times its own weight of egg albumin. Because of pepsin-like action, it is used as a protein digestant, in combination with other enzymes such as amylases, however over a broader pH range. It is used as an ingredient in cleaner solutions for soft contact lenses to remove protein deposits on them. In the form of a topical application in 10% concentration, it is used to remove dead tissue components from wounds. In the meat packing industry papain is used extensively for tenderizing beef and for freeing food proteins. It is a common ingredient in brewery and meat processing industry. Papain is used as a substitute for rennet in cheese manufacture and is also used for chill-proofing beer. It has been widely employed in the textile industry for degumming silk fabrics and in the tanning industry for dehairing skins and hides. It is also sold in health food outlets as tea and purgative.

Trade

East Africa is currently the world's largest supplier of papain. African nations, especially the Democratic Republic of Congo, are the major exporters of papain. Other suppliers are Zaire, Taiwan, Tanzania, Uganda, Kenya, Israel, Phillippines, India and Sri Lanka. Total market size of papain in Europe is estimated at several 100 tonnes per year. (Exact volume figures are not reported in official government trade statistics.)

Papain-importing countries are the United States, Canada, Japan, England, Belgium, Australia, France, Germany, Denmark, Norway, Sweden, Argentina, Italy, Ireland, Spain, Portugal, Poland and New Zealand.

Papain is purchased and distributed by specialist food ingredient companies mainly in Europe and the United States and redistributed to many other countries. Several plantations that were established during the papain shortage in the early 1990s are just beginning to produce, which has created more available supply for the European and US markets. Demand for papain from breweries is declining as cheaper and more readily available substitutes are being used to emulate papain's function. Papain's use has however continued to expand in the food industry, support-ing the increase in volume. The US market has been estimated at upto double the EU market or roughly 300–400 metric tonnes per year. The Japanese market is relatively small at under 50 metric tonnes per year. Many importing countries particularly Japan, several in Europe and the United States further process their papain imports and re-export the finished product amongst themselves and to others. Direct imports into the United States are mostly sourced from India with smaller supplies coming from China, the Congo and Indonesia.

Papain is sold in both liquid and powdered form. It is commonly imported in a raw form and processed according to the end-user's specifications. The strength of papain is measured in Tyrosine Units (TU); 70–75 TU liquid papain is commonly used by breweries. The price of papain varies with grade and the TU measurement. It varies between US $10/kg and as high as US $80/kg for papain with a high TU measurement.

In India *C. papaya* is cultivated in Maharashtra, Bengal, Bihar and Uttar Pradesh. Papain-producing units are located at Nasik and Bangalore. Several heavy bearing dwarf varieties of *C. papaya* ideal for papain collection are under cultivation in India. There are three major commercial grades each differing in its method of preparation and end use. They are

- Papain BPC (as per British Pharmaceutical Codex, 1954 specifications) used for a variety of applications;
- Papain IP (Indian Pharmacoepia, 1966) used in preparations where a low mineral content is desirable;
- Purified Papain – Highly water soluble and free from colour and odour, it is used in special preparations where an odour-free product of high purity is required.

Total estimated production of papain in India is around 150 tonnes per year. Around 35% is BPC grade papain and the rest is purified papain; 55% of the BPC grade is consumed internally and the rest is exported and 90% purified papain is also exported. A number of industries are coming up to give a boost to the demand of this product.

The current price of BPC Papain is US $40/kg in the international market.

Aloe

Aloe or aloes consists of the solid residue obtained by evaporating the liquid (aloetic juice) which drains from the transversely cut leaves of various species of *Aloe* (Liliaceae).

Commercial Importance

The drug aloes is of historical importance being used as a purgative since 4th century BC by the Greeks. Though it is still of some pharmaceutical significance, the fresh mucilaginous gel (called aloe vera gel) obtained from a group of cells different from those yielding the aloetic juice has in recent years become very big business in the herbal and cosmetic industry. It is advocated for use in numerous conditions and is widely promoted as a moisturizer and wound healing agent for use in the treatment of burns, abrasions and other skin conditions. Aloe is a well-known medicinal plant widely used in modern herbal practice and often available in proprietary herbal preparations.

Species and Distribution

Indigenous to Africa the genus *Aloe* includes herbs, shrubs and trees bearing spikes of white, yellow or red flowers. Many species have been introduced into West Indies and Europe. *Aloe* comprises about 450 species in Africa and Arabia of which about 315 occur in mainland Africa, about 100 are endemic to Indian Ocean islands and 50 occur in Arabia. The taxonomy is complicated by the occurrence of interspecific hybrids both in the wild and in cultivation. The drug aloes is mainly obtained from

- *Aloe barbadensis* Miller (Aloe vera Linne) – known in commerce as Curacao aloes and collected from the West Indian islands of Curacao, Aruba and Bonaire;
- *Aloe ferox* Miller and hybrids with *A. africana* Miller and *A. spicata* Baker – known as Cape aloes cultivated in South Africa and Kenya;

- *A. perryi Baker* – found in east Africa and Arabia and yields Sacotrine and Zanzibar varieties.

Today *Aloe vera* is distributed throughout the tropics and subtropics and is widely grown as a cash crop in dry regions in the Americas, Asia and Australia.

Harvest

Aloe species are grown as ornamentals in gardens and pots. Typical xerophytic plants, *Aloe* species have fleshy leaves which are strongly cuticularized and usually prickly at the margins. Only known as cultivated or naturalized plant, Aloe takes three years to attain harvestable size and can be harvested for seven years. While aloetic juice (for preparations of the purgative aloes) is contained in the large pericyclic cells, it flows out when the leaves are cut. The mucilage of wound healing and cosmetic importance occupying about 3/5th of the diameter of the leaf is present in the large parenchymatous cells. Aloetic juice is collected from leaves transversely cut near the base. About 200 such leaves are arranged round a shallow hole lined with canvas or plastic sheet. The juice draining out of the entire system of pericyclic cells in the leaves gets collected. It is allowed to flow out without applying pressure to prevent contamination with mucilage coming out of the parenchymatous cells. The collected juice is then evaporated suitably and poured into containers for solidification. This is the purgative aloes. The mucilage is collected form the leaves drained of aloetic juice as quickly as possible to avoid degradation of the polysaccharides it contains.

Constituents

Different aloes are associated with different macroscopical features depending on the species and the method of preparation. While cape aloes occurs as dark brown or greenish brown, glassy masses, curacao varies in colour from yellowish brown to chocolate brown. Sacotrine and Zanzibar aloes no longer official are of infrequent occurrence in commerce and they are more opaque and break with porous fracture.

Aloes contain a number of anthraquinone glycosides (10%–30%), principal of which are aloin A and B. They are c-glycosides and the active constituents vary qualitatively and quantitatively according to the species from which they are obtained. Aloesin, aloe resin A and C, aloenin B are resins isolated from aloe species.

The aloe vera gel on the other hand is largely composed of a mucilaginous polysaccharide consisting of glucomannans (acemannans), lectins, sterols, enzymes, pectic substances together with a range of other organic and inorganic compounds.

Uses

Native of northern Africa, *A. barbadensis* was introduced into Barbados islands in the 17th century. Employed as a purgative the drug was known in England in the 10th century. *A. chinensis*, a variety of *A. barbadensis* was introduced into Curacao from China in 1817. The drug was cultivated to a considerable extent in Barbados until the middle of the 19th century.

Though now rarely prescribed alone as a purgative, the activity of aloe is increased when it is administered with small quantities of soap or alkaline salts. Carminatives moderate its tendency to cause griping. Still used as a pharmaceutical aid in Compound Tincture of Benzoin because of its drastic cathartic action, aloe is no longer prescribed as a purgative drug.

Fresh leaf exudate is also taken as laxative or purgative and is externally applied as a refrigerant to treat acne or cuts. Mixed with other ingredients to mask its bitter taste, it is taken to treat asthma and coughs. The exudate is used as a bittering agent for food and beer. Aloe gel, the mucilage from the central cells, has a multitude of medicinal applications. The gel or peeled leaves are generally applied to treat skin afflictions and burns, wounds and abrasions as a poultice on contusions or as a general refrigerant. The gel is also applied externally to cure haemorrhoids. It is further used as hair wash to promote hair growth and against dandruff and as a general cosmetic to improve complexion. As a food supplement, aloe vera gel is used to facilitate digestion and to improve blood and lymphatic circulation, kidney, liver and gall bladder functions.

A stabilized product is prepared from the mucilage by many different proprietary or patented methods, some of which involve expression or solvent extraction under harsh conditions. Scientific studies have substantiated the cell proliferative properties of the fresh mucilaginous gel.

Trade

The International Aloe Science Council (IASC) estimates raw material sales of aloe vera as currently US $70–90 million globally with 35% growth expected in the next five years. The United States is by far the single largest supplier with 60% to 65% of total sales. Latin America constitutes another 20% to 25% and Asia and the Pacific Rim (Australia, China and India) together make up 10% of the market. The total sales value of processed derivatives and ingredients has been estimated by the IASC to be US $1 billion per year in the mid 1990s and has grown continuously since that time. Trade in finished products containing aloe ingredients is estimated to be over $35 billion globally.

High quality aloe vera gel containing 0.5% to 1.3% solid material currently sells for $1.25 and $1.95 per kg (wholesale price) as non-concentrated pure juice. Whole leaf extract (0.95% to 2% solid matter) is available for $2–4. Usually 10x to 40x concentrated gel is supplied. Powder (200 x concentrate) sells for $225–305 per kg.

The major markets for aloe vera and its extracts are Australia, the United States and entire Europe. Cosmetic, food, beverage and dietary supplement industries have a share in the aloe market. Until recently the topical use of aloe gel in cosmetics and skin care products has been emphasized, but the oral use of aloe vera in the form of health juices and liquid supplements has had a market boom in recent years.

Aloetic juice processed either into crystalline or powdered form now called aloe 'bitters' is available for use in the food and beverage industry. Aloe vera was highlighted in 1557 new product launches worldwide by 27,000 global aloe industries with a total turnover of US $33 billion in 2001. The use of the gel has been approved in the United States for the treatment of leukemia in cats, fibrosarcoma in dogs, for wound healing in humans and to dry drysocket (alveolar osteilis) in humans.

In India aloe is grown commercially in almost all parts for its high demand in cosmetic industries as well as in Indian systems of medicine. Aloe, commonly known as 'Musabbar' is a reputed purgative in the indigenous system of medicine. Three varieties of aloes are official in the Indian pharmacopoeia.

- Curacao aloe obtained from *A. barbadensis*;
- Socotrine aloe obtained from *A. perryi*;
- Cape aloe from *A. ferox* and its hybrids.

The leaf juice forms an important constituent of a large number of Ayurvedic preparations. It is also used in veterinary medicine.

About four species have been introduced in India of which *A. barbadensis* has become naturalised in almost all parts of the country, the other species also growing wild in some places. Aloe is known as ghasckumar in the Unani system of medicine and as ghritakumari in the Ayurvedic system. Of the four species introduced and found in India, *A. barbadensis* has established itself in almost all parts of the country. *A. barbadensis, var. chinensis* is common in Maharashtra, Kamataka, Tamil Nadu, Kerala, Andhra Pradesh and Madhya Pradesh. *A. barbadensis'* var. *littoralis* is found on the beach shingle in Tamil Nadu up to Rameswaram. Another variety which thrives on the Saurashtra coast is the source of Jafarabad aloe.

Aloe vera is traded in processed forms such as gel, juice and concentrate.

Tropane Alkaloid-Containing Plants

The term tropane alkaloids refers to a group of more than 200 compounds best known for their occurrence in the family Solanaceae comprising over 100 genera and 3,000 plant species. The most important natural tropane alkaloids are (-)hyoscyamine, its stable racemate, atropine and (-)scopolamine. Important sources of these alkaloids are *Belladonna* sps, *Duboisia* sps, *Datura* sps, *Hysocyamus* sps and *Scopolia* sps.

Commercial Importance

Tropane derivatives are among the economically most important pharmaceuticals. Various pharmaceutical industries are manufacturing over 20 active pharmaceutical ingredients containing tropane moiety in their structures and these are applied as mydriatics, anti-emetics, antispasmodics, anaesthetics and bronchodilators. The natural tropane akaloids are anticholinergic and are themselves of medicinal interest. Atropine has a stimulant action on the CNS and depresses the nerve endings to the secretory glands and plain muscle. Sedative properties of hyoscine enable it to be used in the control of motion sickness and it lacks the central stimulant action of atropine. Hyoscine hydrobromide is employed in pre-operative medication, usually with papaveretum, some 30–60 minutes before the induction of anaesthesia. Atropine and hyoscine are used to a large extent in ophthalmic practice to dilate the pupil of the eye. Homatropine, ipatropium bromide, oxitropium bromide and benztropine are some important drugs related to tropane alakaloids.

The source plants, long known for their poisonous nature, have been used for their medicinal property in traditional herbal medical practice.

Constituents

All the above named solanaceous plants contain the mentioned natural tropane alkaloids together with other minor alkaloids. Table 3.4 lists the important sources of tropane alkaloids.

Species and Distribution

Out of 72 genera of the family Solanaceae, only eight genera namely *Atropa, Hysocyamus, Scopolia, Mandrogora, Physochlaina, Datura, Solandra* and *Duboisia* contain atropine, hyoscyamine and hysocine. The species under these genera can be classified into three categories:

Table 3.4 Important plant sources of tropane alkaloids

S.No	Species/Parts Used	Geographical Source	Total Alkaloid Content	Major	Minor
1.	Atropa belladonna – Deadly nightshade (L & FT)	Europe, USA	0.3–0.6%	Hyoscyamine	Hyoscine
2.	Atropa belladonna (R)	Europe, USA	0.4–0.8%	Hyoscyamine	Hyoscine
3.	Atropa acuminata – Indian belladonna (L & R)	India	0.3–0.8%	Hyoscyamine	Hyoscine
4.	Duboisia myoporoides (L)	Australia	1.5–2%	Hyoscine	Hyoscyamine
5.	Duboisia leichhardtii (L)	Australia	1.5–2%	Hyoscyamine	Hysocine
6.	Scopolia carniolica (R)	Central and eastern Europe	0.5%	Hyoscyamine	Hysocine
7.	Datura stramonium – Thornapple (L)	Germany, France, Hungary, India	0.2–0.45%	Hyoscyamine and hyoscine	Atropine
8.	Datura innoxia (L & FT)	India	0.5%	Hyoscine	Hyoscyamine, atropine
9.	D. metel (L & FT)	India	0.5%	Hyoscine	Hyoscyamine, atropine
10.	Datura metel (S & Sd)	India	0.2%	Hyoscine	hyoscyamine, atropine
12.	Datura ferox (L)	India	0.3%	Hyoscine, meteloidine	Hyoscyamine
13.	Hyoscyamus niger – Henbane (L & FT)	Britain, USA, India	0.045–0.14%	Hyoscyamine	Hyoscine
14.	H. albus – White henbane	India, France	0.04–0.1%	Hyoscyamine	Hyoscine
15.	H. muticus – Egyptian henabane	India, Egypt	0.5–1.7%	Hyoscyamine	Hyoscine
16.	H. reticulatus	India	0.12–0.24%	Hysocine, hyoscyamine	–
17.	H. aureus – Golden henbane	India	0.12-0.24%	Hyoscine	–
18.	H. pusillus	India	0.12-0.24%	Hyoscine	–

L leaves, FT flowering tops, R root, S stem, Sd seeds.

1. Those containing hysocyamine or atropine as the major alkaloid are *Atropa belladonna, A. acuminata, A. boetica, Datura stramonium, D. metel, D. quercifolia, Duboisia leichhardtii, Hysocyamus muticus, Scopolia carniolica, S.anomala, Solandra laevis, Physochlaina praealta;*
2. Those containing hyoscine as the major alkaloid are *D. innoxia, D. metel, Duboisia myoporoides;*
3. Those species containing both hyoscine and hysocyamine, but in low concentration are *Hyoscyamus niger, H. reticulatus, H. albus, Mandrogora officinarum.*

Uses

Several of the solanaceous plants used as sources of tropane alkaloids were well known for their poisonous nature and were also used medicinally. They have been included in the pharmacoepias and have been under cultivation in their source countries.

A. belladonna is a tall perennial herb, commonly referred to as Deadly Nightshade; it was introduced into the London pharmacoepia of 1809. Indigenous to Central and Southern Europe, it is cultivated for drug use in Europe and the United States. The tops of the plant are harvested 2–3 times an year and dried to give belladonna herb. Roots form 3- to 4-year-old plants are less commonly used as a source of alkaloids. While leaves were used internally as sedatives and to check secretions, roots were mainly used externally.

D. stramonium is a bushy annual widely distributed in Europe and North America. Also called thornapple it is now cultivated in Europe and South America. Its leaves and flowering tops have been employed in the Middle Ages by dacoits to drug their victims. It is almost exclusively used in the treatment of spasmodic problems of the respiratory organs.

H. niger or henbane, native to Europe, Persia and India, is now cultivated in Britain, the United States and Central Europe. It was often used to relieve spasms of the urinary tract and with strong purgatives to prevent griping.

Commercially important solanaceous species are sources for the extraction of atropine, hyoscyamine and hyoscine which are anti-cholinergics and stimulants.

Trade

Commercial cultivation of *Duboisia* species in Australia and of *H. muticus* in Egypt constitute the basis for supply of the global demand for tropane alkaloids. Also to a limited extent, *H. niger* is cultivated in the United States, UK and India. Indigenous to Western Europe and temperate forests of India, *A. belladonna* is cultivated in UK, Germany, former USSR, the United States and India. *Duboisia* species are also cultivated in India and Ecuador. *Scopolia* species are cultivated from wild sources and used in commercial isolation of tropane alkaloids in China and Romania. Two of the three species of *Duboisia* are indigenous to Australia and have over 50 years been a major world source of tropane alkaloids. Interest in *Duboisia* was very much stimulated by the demand for hyoscine as a treatment for motion sickness in military personnel during World War II. Even higher levels of alkaloids and higher proportions of hyoscine can be obtained from selected *D. myoporoides* × *D. leichhardtii* hybrids, which are currently cultivated. An important commercial source of medicinal tropane alkaloids, most of the Australian crop (about 1200 tonnes) is exported to Germany, Switzerland and Japan for processing. About 500–600 tonnes of Egyptian henbane are collected from wild sources annually in Egypt and are exported to Germany.

In India *A. belladonna* and *A. acuminata* are cultivated by CIMAP in the Kashmir Valley. The present annual production of belladonna leaves from wild and cultivated sources is around 30 tonnes with yield potential of about 100 kg of total alkaloids per annum.

Out of the 15 species reported from the world, 10 species are found in India. *D. stramonium* is collected from West Himalayas, Nilgiri and Pazhani hills of Tamil Nadu. The present stramonium resources in India are around 40 tonnes per annum.

D. innoxia is by far the commonest species of datura occurring wild in India. Occurring as a weed throughout India, it is more common in the arid regions of Punjab, Rajasthan and the peninsular regions of Andhra Pradesh and Tamil Nadu. The raw material is presently being collected in Andhra Pradesh, Tamil Nadu and Rajasthan with an annual turnover of around 50 tonnes of dry herb.

Plants Containing Laxatives

Of the various plant-based laxative drugs available on the market, Senna (*Cassia angustifolia* and *C. acutifolia,* Family Caesalpinae) and Ispaghula (*P. ovata, P. psyllium,* Family Plantaginaceae) appear to the most widely used plant laxatives others being aloes, cascara, rhubarb along with agar and gums – acacia, tragacanth, sterculia and guar gum.

Commercial Importance

Chronic constipation is one of the most common complaints in clinical medicine. It is estimated that one in five adults worldwide suffers from constipation. Laxatives are drugs that facilitate the passage and elimination of faeces from the colon and rectum thus relieving constipation. Apart from refined diets, several factors are attributed to its increasing incidence and therefore the increasing use and demand for laxatives. The value of laxative sales in the United States for the period 2008–2011 was estimated to be $875 million. Most of the laxative products sold on the market are derived form plant sources. In terms of worldwide usage senna and ispaghula top the list of laxatives sold. Laxative drugs are those products excluding fibre-rich dietary items including fruits, vegetables, functional fibres etc.

Species and Distribution

1. *Cassia angustifolia* (Indian or Tinnevelly Senna) – Indigenous to Arabia, India and Somaliland, it is cultivated in Tamil Nadu, Andhra Pradesh, Gujarat and Rajasthan in India.
2. *Cassia acutifolia* (Alexandrian Senna or Cassia Senna) – Less commonly collected than Indian senna it is cultivated in Sudan, Egypt and northeast African countries.
3. *Plantago ovata* – The genus *Plantago* contains over 200 species with *P. ovata* and *P. psyllium* produced commercially in several European countries, the former USSR, Pakistan and India. About 10 species of Plantago are recorded in India of which *P. ovata* is the most important. Seeds of *P. ovata* (known as Isabgol, blonde psyllium or plantago seeds) are the largest exported plant drug from India cultivated in Gujarat (Sidhpur), Maharashtra, Punjab and Rajasthan.
4. *P. psyllium* seeds are called psyllium or flea seeds and are chiefly produced in Spain, France and Cuba. France was the leading producer of Ispaghula from psyllium seeds until 1890. However now India is the leading producer of Ispaghula products. *P. arenaria* is produced in the Mediterranean Europe and Egypt. Seeds of *P. indica* and *P. afra* (known in commerce as Spanish or French psyllium) along with other species of plantago are produced commercially in several European countries, former USSR, Pakistan and India.

Other purgative drugs of erstwhile importance such as aloes, cascara and rhubarb are no longer prescribed as purgatives because of their drastic mode of action and the severe griping that follows. Gums such as acacia, tragacanth, guar gum and sterculia as also other polysaccharide drugs are used as laxatives to a limited extent due their bulk-forming property. Buckthorn resembles cascara in its cathartic action and is commonly used in Europe in the form of a fluid extract.

Harvest

Senna plants are low-branching erect shrubs. Leaflets and pods are collected from cultivated plants of *C. angustifolia* and from both wild and cultivated plants of *C. acutifolia*. The branches are collected when the fruits are fully formed (but still unripe) and they are rapidly dried in the sun. Leaves are cleaned, sieved to remove leaf fragments and compressed into bales for transportation. Pods are hand picked into various qualities, finer ones being sold in cartons and the inferior ones used for making galenicals. Leaves and pods are important articles of commerce being used in the preparation of extracts, powders and for the isolation of active glycosides.

Indian senna is more carefully collected and has fewer broken leaflets than Alexandrian senna. *P. ovata* is a stemless annual herb from which seeds are collected from fully ripe fruits after drying. Seeds about 3 mm in length are covered with a mucilaginous husk on the concave side. They are very small weighing 1.5 g/1,000 seeds. This mucilaginous husk in the epidermis of the testa being the chief purgative constituent, it is separated from the seeds by crushing in flat stone grinding mills and winnowed to separate it. This forms the 'Ispaghula husk'. Marketed as a separate commodity it fetches more price than the seeds.

Constituents

The active constituents in both senna leaf and pod are dianthrone glycosides, principally sennoside A and B. They are di-O-glucosides of rhein dianthrone (Sennidin A and B) and liberate upon hydrolysis two molecules of glucose and the aglycones sennidin A and B. Minor constituents include sennosides C and D, which are glycosides of heterodianthrones involving rhein and aloe-emodin, palmidin etc. Two naphthalane glycosides have also been isolated from senna.

Senna leaf suitable for medicinal use contains NLT 2.5% dianthrone glycosides, calculated in terms of sennoside B. Sennoside content of Indian senna is 1.2% to 2.5%, while that of Alexandrian senna is 2.5% to 4.5%. Apart from its use in several herbal teas, senna preparations in the form of powdered leaf, powdered pods or extracts are typically standardized to a given sennoside content. Senna glycosides in the form of stabler calcium sennosides are also available.

The chief constituent of Ispaghula is the mucilage contained in the epidermal cells. Two fractions, one soluble in cold water and the other in hot water, have been separated from it.

Uses

Man has been troubled by constipation for more than 7,000 years ever since the switchover from feeding on fruits, roots, vegetables and grains to a wide variety of meat products happened. Constipation is of even greater concern world over today due to the shedding of traditional diets what with the convenience granted by fast foods in today's fast-paced lifestyle. It is also a side effect of drugs such as anticholenergics, anti-psychotics, anti-depressants, antispasmodics and opiates to name a few. The huge trade in purgative drugs, such as aloes, since a long time in history in the west indicates their extensive usage reflecting widespread prevalence of constipation in these societies.

Ayurvedic and Chinese physicians have used many purgative plant drugs including senna and ispaghula to treat various conditions recognized to be linked to constipation. Senna appears to have been used since 9th or 10th century, introduced into medicine by Arabian physicians. Ispaghula is a well-known drug in the Unani system of medicine.

Unlike fibre-rich plant foods such as whole grains that act as bulk laxatives, plants rich in anthraquinone derivatives such as senna, aloes, cascara and rhubarb are stimulant laxatives. The anthraquinone glycosides in the purgative drugs are hydrolysed by the colonic bacteria into active compounds and thus the cathartic action occurs primarily in the colon 8–12 hours after drug administration.

Senna is thus a stimulant laxative acting on the walls of the large intestine, increasing peristaltic movements. After oral administration, the sennosides are transformed by intestinal flora into rhein anthrone which appears to be the ultimate purgative principle. The glycoside residues in the active constituents are necessary for water solubility and subsequent transportation to the site of action. Most of the sennosides are excreted in the faeces as polymers, together with unchanged sennosides, sennidins and rhein anthrone.

Senna is the most widely prescribed laxative, being suitable for both habitual constipation and occasional use. It lacks the astringent after-effect of rhubarb. Despite the availability of a number of synthetics, sennoside preparations remain among the most important pharmaceutical laxatives. Senna products containing total sennosides ranging from 15% to 60% calculated as sennoside B are commercially available.

The laxative action of ispaghula mucilage is purely mechanical and ispaghula seeds are used as an excellent demulcent and bulk laxative in chronic constipation. It is used in irritative conditions of the gastrointestinal tract. The mucilage is not acted upon by digestive enzymes and passes though the small intestine unchanged. It relieves constipation by stimulating intestinal peristalsis by mechanical action.

Though cascara has a similar pharmacological action as senna, in view of its stronger action, its routine usage is not recommended. Aloes and rhubarb on account of their drastic action are largely abandoned from use as purgatives.

Trade

Senna is one of the most traded raw materials in the supplement market. India is the main producer of senna in the world and exports senna leaves and pods worth more then Rs 6 million annually. It is grown on 8,000–10,000 hectares and three-fourths of senna produced in India is exported. Prior to World War II Germany and France used to import large quantities of Indian senna. After the war, the most important markets were the United States and UK. Presently the major importers of Indian senna are Czechoslovakia, France, West Germany, Hong Kong, Hungary, Italy, Japan, Netherlands, Singapore, Spain, Switzerland, UK and the United States. The current world demand is estimated to be 10,000 tonnes of senna leaves and pods per annum. About 700 tonnes are supplied by Sudan, while India exports an average of 450 tonnes per annum. The total yield of senna leaves and pods in India is around 7,150 tonnes.

India is one of the major producers of ispaghula and about 35,000 hectares of land are under ispaghula cultivation with 29,000 tonnes of seeds appearing in the market. Around 90% of seeds and husk worth Rs. 20 crores is exported to the United States, Germany, England and France.

During 1991–1992 India exported 14,393 tonnes of ispaghula husk and 3,151 tonnes of seeds valued at Rs. 620.28 million and 65.2 million respectively. The average price (fob) works out to be Rs.43,100 per tonne for husk and Rs.20,690 per tonne for the seeds. The average import price of ispaghula husk and seed at North European ports was US $1,800–2,000 per tonne and US $600 per tonne respectively during 1992. Seeds of *P. psyllium* grown in France, Spain, Itlay, Belgium and Brazil are similar in appearance to ispaghula, but the former is inferior in quality.

CONCLUSION

Plants have been used for disease treatment and health care since ancient times. Despite a setback in the middle 19th century, medicinal plants still form the basis of traditional or indigenous health systems. Herbs whether being used by a Siddha practitioner in South India, to isolate a new alkaloid in a research lab in Switzerland, as a prescription drug in Germany or as dietary supplement in the United States, the overall demand is on the rise. While medicinal plant materials have been used by a large number of industries both for medicinal and non-medicinal uses, demand for crude plant drugs for medicinal use was largely for the isolation of pure drugs. In fact many of our present drugs are derived directly or indirectly from plants. The past three decades however have seen dramatic changes in the climate for botanical drugs throughout the world. Rapidly rising exports of medicinal plants attests to worldwide interest in these products.

Today medicinal plants are traded in large volumes not only for isolation of single purified drugs, but also as standardized and non-standardized extracts, as also as starting materials for semi-synthesis of ethical drugs. This is in addition to the usage of plants in traditional medical systems such as Ayurveda, traditional Chinese medicine etc. These systems are no longer localized but are adapted and practised by amalgamation into western and other modern herbal therapies.

Global awakening of interest towards safe, effective and natural drugs is one of the factors that has made governments, policy makers, international and national regulatory bodies to streamline their availability. Concerns about the unregulated availability of herbal products, especially in view of the reported toxic effects of some herbal drugs and their interaction with other medications is bringing up issues of ways and means of regulating their availability and usage. Over-exploitation of valuable plant resources, patent issues, protection of indigenous IPR are critical issues to be sorted out. Since the market and regulation of herbal products is diverse throughout the world, time-tested traditional medicines of well-documented systems such as Ayurveda from India are facing several hurdles for their entry into the international market. Improved if not novel quality control procedures are needed to demonstrate the quality of the poly-constituent herbals, since they cannot be evaluated by methods developed for single pure drugs. Such newer methods of standardization will not only help clear the regulatory hurdles for traditional herbal medicines, but will also be the much needed solution to the scientific challenge faced by herbal drugs. The approval of the pending IND for herbal drugs with the US FDA may possibly open the flood gates for the entry of herbal drugs into the ethical drugs market. This hopefully shall be a turning point in the global trade of herbal drugs and related products.

REVIEW QUESTIONS

Essay Questions

1. List the categories of medicinal plant-derived products traded. Describe the significant usage of plant extracts and essential oils.
2. What are functional foods? Discuss the categories, their market safety and regulation.
3. Write an essay on the worldwide trade of tropane alkaloid-containing plants.

Short Notes

1. Challenges in assessment of medicinal plant trade.
2. Sources of plant material in trade.
3. Functional food categories.
4. Taxol – species and trade.
5. Liquorice – uses and trade.
6. Dioscorea – species, uses and trade.
7. Papain – commercial uses and trade.
8. Trade in plant-based laxatives.

4

Herbal Drug Regulatory Affairs

CHAPTER OBJECTIVES

Introduction

Milestones in Herbal Drug Regulation

Specific Objectives of Herbal Drug Regulation

Current Status of Herbal Drug Regulatory Affairs

INTRODUCTION

Use of plants for healing dates back to antiquity in the Indian subcontinent and traditional medical knowledge is very closely knit into the very fabric of Indian culture. In many parts of the world, the practice continues today because of its biomedical benefits and place in cultural beliefs. Increasing global disease burden, disillusionment with synthetic drugs, escalating health care costs are a few of the numerous factors for the rising popularity of plant-derived health care products and traditional medicine world over. The economic reality of the inaccessibility of modern medication for many societies has also played a major role in the broad use of herbal medicines. It has not only continued to be used for primary health care of poor in developing countries, but has also been used in countries where conventional medicine is predominant in the national health care system, with a resulting increase in international trade in herbal medicines and other types of traditional remedies. Recognition of importance of herbal medicines in international trade had led to its growing clinical, pharmaceutical and economic value. Today medicinal plants are important for pharmacological research and drug development, not only when plant constituents are used directly as therapeutic agents, but also as starting materials for the synthesis of drugs or as models for pharmacologically active compounds. This has created the need for greater precision in preparation and evaluation and has stimulated research into the applications and various uses of herbal medicines. Thus herbal medicines have been recognized as a valuable and readily available resource for primary health care, and World Health Organization (WHO) has endorsed their safe and effective use. A few herbal medicines have withstood scientific testing, but others are used simply for traditional reasons to protect, restore or improve health. Most herbal medicines still need to be studied scientifically, although the experience obtained from their traditional use over the years should not be ignored.

The demand for herbal remedies is estimated to grow in the years to come, fuelled by the growth of sales of herbal supplements and remedies. It has been realized that medicinal plants are also a valuable resource for new pharmaceutical products and thus a potential source of new drugs.

The exponentially growing herbal drug trade is consequently shifting global attention to developing nations like India which are treasure troves of medicinal plant wealth. Unsustainable and reckless exploitation of the natural flora of these countries due to vast commercial potential has already resulted in disappearance of germplasm of several plant species, with many of them being endangered, extinct or on the verge of extinction. The United Nations Convention on Biological Diversity states that the conservation and sustainable use of biological diversity is of critical importance for meeting the food, health and other needs of the growing world population, for which purpose access to and sharing of both genetic resources and technologies are essential. Therefore there is an urgent need to bring about legislative control over exploitative harvesting and other unlawful collection practices related to medicinal plant trade in these countries. Regulation of herbal drug trade together with international cooperation and coordination for medicinal plant conservation is essential to ensure their continued availability in the future.

To curb commercial exploitation and to ensure both safety and efficacy of the numerous plant-based remedies that are today available as over-the-counter (OTC) proprietary labelled herbal and other 'natural' medicines, there is a driving need to assess, rationalize and regulate all trade practices related to the manufacture, processing, sale and supply of these herbal drugs, cosmetics and other health enhancers.

MILESTONES IN HERBAL DRUG REGULATION

WHO has recognized the contribution and value of herbal medicines used by a large segment of the world's population. Extensive usage of medicinal plants worldwide has raised concerns of safety, efficacy and quality control of herbal medicines and traditional procedure-based therapies. To enable legislation concerning procedures for registration of herbal medicines, governments need to draft national policies to develop regulatory and legal reforms to ensure good practice and to extend primary health care coverage, while ensuring the authenticity, safety and efficacy of these medicines. Such initiatives shall result in approval of safe and clinically effective drugs by endorsing and encouraging research on herbal medicines for improved utilization by the public.

Some of the significant events that led to the initiation of regulatory changes in herbal drug trade are the following:

The World Health Assembly (WHA) adopted a number of resolutions drawing attention to the fact that a large section of the population in many developing countries still relies on traditional medicine, and that the work force represented by traditional practitioners is a potentially important resource for primary health care. In 1978, the Declaration of Alma-Ata recommended, *inter alia*, the inclusion of proven traditional remedies into national drug policies and regulatory measures.

WHO's policy on traditional medicine was presented in the Director General's report on Traditional Medicine and Modern Health Care to the 44th World Health Assembly 1991. Based on the relevant WHA resolutions, the major objectives of the programme were facilitation of integration of traditional medicine into national health care systems, development of technical guidelines for promotion of rational use of traditional medicine and dissemination of information on various forms of traditional medicine.

The WHA 1989 resolutions urged member states to

- make a comprehensive evaluation of their traditional systems of medicine;
- make a systematic inventory and assessment (preclinical and clinical) of the medicinal plants used by traditional practitioners and by the population;
- introduce measures for the regulation and control of medicinal plant products and for the establishment and maintenance of suitable standards;
- identify those medicinal plants, or remedies derived from them, which have a satisfactory efficacy/side-effect ratio and which should be included in national formularies or pharmacopoeias.

Herbal medicines were included in the International Conference on Drug Regulatory Authorities (ICDRA) since the fourth conference in 1986.

The fourth and fifth ICDRA in 1986 and 1989, respectively, held workshops on the regulation of herbal medicines moving in international commerce and concluded with proposals for WHO to consider preparing model guidelines containing basic elements of legislation and registration for herbal medicines.

A WHO consultation in Munich, Germany, June 1991, drafted guidelines for the assessment of herbal medicines which were adopted for general use by the sixth ICDRA in Ottawa, October 1991. These guidelines define basic criteria for the evaluation of quality, safety and efficacy of herbal medicines to assist national regulatory authorities, scientific organizations and manufacturers to undertake an assessment of the documentation, of submissions and/or dossiers in respect of such products. The WHO guidelines are intended to facilitate the work of regulatory authorities, scientific bodies and industry in the development, assessment and registration of herbal medicines, reflecting scientific results which could be the basis for future classification of herbal medicines and would also accommodate cross-cultural transfer of traditional herbal medicinal knowledge between different parts of the world.

In 1994, the regional office for the Eastern Mediterranean published guidelines for Formulation of National Policy on Herbal Medicines recommending countries to establish a National Expert Committee to identify the steps and plans needed to formulate a national policy on herbal medicine and to develop, direct and monitor the various phases of its implementation.

WHO regional office for the Western Pacific, in 1992, organized a meeting of experts to develop guidelines for research on herbal medicines. Basic scientific principles and special requirements related to their use in traditional practice are incorporated in these guidelines, the main objectives of which are to ensure their safety and efficacy, to promote their rational use, and to provide research criteria for their evaluation. These guidelines provide a basis for member states to develop their own research guidelines, and for exchange of research-related information for generation of data for reliable validation of herbal medicines.

In 1997, with the support of the National Center of Complementary and Alternative Medicine, National Institutes of Health, Bethesda, MD, USA, a WHO informal discussion developed draft guidelines for methodology on research and evaluation of traditional medicine. Since then the draft has been revised four times. The guidelines finalized at a WHO consultation in April 2000, in Hong Kong focus on the current major debates on safety and efficacy of traditional medicine and are intended to raise and answer some challenging questions concerning the evidence base. They clarify certain commonly used but unclear definitions. The guidelines present some national regulations for the evaluation of herbal medicine, and also recommend new approaches for carrying out clinical research.

The summary and recommendations of the sixth ICDRA prompted WHO as part of its Traditional Medicine programme to prepare a technical document entitled 'WHO Monographs on Selected Medicinal Plants' on the basis of the Guidelines for the Assessment of Herbal Medicines. The purpose of this document was to provide scientific information on the safety, efficacy and quality control of widely used medicinal plants and to provide models for member states to develop their own monographs on these and additional herbal medicines.

After discussion and review at the WHO consultation in Munich, Germany in 1996, 28 monographs were adapted and presented at the eighth ICDRA meeting in Bahrain, November, 1996. Another 32 monographs are being prepared. The information in the monographs includes two parts: Part I consists of summaries of the botanical characteristics, major active chemical constituents and quality control of each plant; Part II consists of summaries of clinical applications, pharmacology, posology, possible contraindications and precautions and potential adverse reactions.

Based on national experiences in formulating policies on traditional medicinal products from 52 member states, the WHO has brought out a document reviewing the regulatory situation of herbal medicines in these countries in order to facilitate information exchange on these subjects among the member states and to assist introduction of measures for the registration and regulation of herbal medicines.

SPECIFIC OBJECTIVES OF HERBAL DRUG REGULATION

A significant increase in the use of herbal medicines in the past decade has also seen a resurgence of interest in herbal medicines in developed countries due to a preference for products of natural origin. In addition, manufactured herbal medicines from their countries of origin often follow in the wake of migrants from countries where traditional medicines play an important role.

Herbal drug regulation basically needs to fulfill the following objectives:

- Establish a regulatory pathway for approval of multi-component botanical products such as pharmaceutical drugs.
- Availability of up-to-date and authoritative information on the beneficial properties and possible harmful effects of all herbal medicines to both consumers and health care authorities.
- Draft guidelines at national and international level for the assessment of herbal medicines based on a large corpus of data on how medicinal plant materials and their products should be handled, starting from the collection of materials, through manufacturing, to clinical trials. These shall facilitate the work to be carried out by regulatory authorities, scientific bodies and industry in the development, assessment and registration of herbal products.
- The WHO guidelines so developed should reflect the scientific results gathered in past years in each field of activity related to herbal medicines serving as the basis for future classification of herbal medicines in different parts of the world.
- Identification of categories of medicinal plant-related products in trade as 'traditional medicines' from classical texts, well-known herbal medicines of long-established folklore usage, newer combinations/formulations based on traditional plant drugs etc.

- Taking into account the medical, historical and ethnological background of these products, draft regulatory requirements including the clinical and non-clinical testing and other manufacturing requirements to ensure development of consistent quality herbal products.
- Ensure effective regulation and control of herbal medicines moving in international commerce through close liaison with appropriate national institutions that are able to keep under regular review all aspects of their production and use.
- Address concerns of efficacy, toxicity, safety, acceptability, cost and relative value of herbal drugs by subjecting them to evaluative studies compared with other drugs used in modern medicine.
- Developing system of Good Manufacturing Practices (GMP) covering all aspects of production from starting materials, premises and equipment to the training, personal hygiene of staff, standard operating procedures, work environment, quality assurance, and packaging, storage and waste disposal to ensure reproducibility and establish product consistency.
- Formulate procedures for the registration of herbal drugs after evaluating information on tests conducted, clinical trials, QC methods etc. furnished by the manufacturer.
- Develop standards to ensure control of information supplied as propagation material including labels, product pamphlets or any other type of broadcast statements ruling out misleading information due to misrepresentation of facts.
- Provide assurance of quality and safety through adequate follow-up by appropriate pharmacovigilance to facilitate report of adverse drug reactions occurring either through prolonged use or by inappropriate self-medication.

Despite the fact that the therapeutic benefit and safety of many herbal medicines have been qualitatively established, their potential as drugs has not been fully realized due to lack of economic incentives, absence of strict manufacturing controls, and lack of rigorous proof of efficacy.

CURRENT STATUS OF HERBAL DRUG REGULATORY AFFAIRS

Regulatory mechanism for approval of plant drugs has not been in place in several countries until quite recently. In a WHO question-answer survey of 141 member states, it was found that while 92 countries (65%) have laws and regulations on herbal medicines 48 countries (34%) do not. Information provided by 77 of the member states about the year of issue of the laws/regulations indicates that herbal drug regulation is a recent phenomenon. Over the last 15 years, numbers of member states with laws and regulations on herbal medicines have increased dramatically with the highest number of laws being issued between 1996 and 1999. Herbal medicine practices have been developed in different cultures in different regions without a parallel development of international standards and appropriate methods of evaluation. Legislative controls in respect of medicinal plants have not evolved around a structured control model because of variations between countries with regard to the following:

- Medicinal, pharmaceutical and economic value of medicinal plants;
- Definitions for medicinal plants or herbs or related products;
- Approaches to licensing, dispensing and manufacturing;
- Traditional usage of herbs and trade practices;

- Availability of safety and efficacy data;
- Extent of scientific validation of traditionally used herbal drugs.

According to EU definition herbal medicinal products are 'medicinal products containing as active ingredients exclusively plant material and/or vegetable drug preparations'. Based on their origin, evolution and the forms of current usage, herbal medicines are classified into the following categories:

Category 1: Indigenous Herbal Medicines

Historically used in a local community or region and well known through long usage by the local population in terms of its composition, treatment and dosage.

Detailed information on this category of TM, which also includes folk medicines, may or may not be available. In order to enter market outside the local community or region in the country, such drugs need to meet the safety and efficacy guidelines laid down in the national regulations of that country.

Category 2: Herbal Medicine in Systems

Traditional drugs of long-term usage such as those of Ayurveda, Siddha and Unani and documented along with their therapeutic concepts, accepted by other countries.

Category 3: Modified Herbal Medicines

Drugs of category 1 and 2, modified in form, dose, dosage form, mode of administration, herbal medicinal ingredients, methods of preparation and medicinal indications.

These drugs are to meet the national regulatory requirements of safety and efficacy.

Category 4: Imported Products with a Herbal Medicine Base

All imported herbal medicines including raw materials and products. These need to be registered and marketed in the countries of origin for which the safety and efficacy data has to be submitted to the national authority of the importing country for approval and acceptance.

Important information on the regulatory requirements for some countries is summarized below and Table 4.1 is a brief overview of the current regulatory situation of herbal drugs in a few other countries.

European Union

The market

The herbal medicine tradition in some European countries remains strong, with quoted figures for herbalists being 16,000 for Germany and 4,000 for Denmark. In France as a result of legislation enacted in 1941, the marketing of herbal products passed very much under the control of pharmacists, 65% of total sales being through pharmacies. Many physicians in Europe are now reportedly prescribing an increasing number of medicines based on plant sources, as

Table 4.1 Regulatory situation of herbal drugs in selected countries

Country	Market Size	Regulatory Authority	Current Regulatory Status
Argentina	HPs available through different distribution channels like pharmacies, herboristerias etc. as herbal drugs, mixtures and preparations	Drug law 16.463 under the purview of Instituto Nacional de Pharmacologia y Bromotologia. Herbal drug certification through Laboratorio Central de Salud	Regulation similar to chemical drugs. Approval through grant of certification number at national and provincial level. HD registration as per 1992 regulation published by the Heath Ministry of the Provincia de Buenos Aires
France	US $1.6 billion in 1991. HM sold in pharmacies OTC. Total OTC market US $4 billion in 1994 – HPs formed 29%.	French Medicines Agency (FMA) under the Ministry of Health	Since 1985 HM regulated as OTCs like conventional pharmaceuticals. FMA grants marketing authorization to plant-based drugs not meeting EC pharmacotoxicological criteria, based on abridged dossiers by making reference to traditional use. List of drugs with accepted traditional use first published in 1985 by MOH with several subsequent revisions
Indonesia	TMP being used since 15th century. Current sales for 2007 was US $550 million	Directorate of Traditional Drug Control established under the Directorate General of Drugs and Food Control of Ministry of Health	Imported and locally produced HDs require licence for marketing. The Indonesian Pharmacopoeia and six volumes of 'Materia Medika Indonesia' prescribe formal requirements of crude drugs including GMP and labelling on MOH recommendations
Ireland	HMs sold in pharmacies as prescription and OTC medicines in special outlets without restriction	The Medical Preparations (Licensing, advertisement and sale) regulations 1984 under Irish Medicines Board, Department of Health and Food Safety Advisory Committee under Ministry of Health and Ministry of Agriculture, Food and Forestry	HMs regulated like pharmaceuticals, however HP made up of dried, crushed or comminuted herbs, with indication claims labelled to indicate the herb and the production process excluded from regulation as per information sheet on borderline products issued by the Department of Health in 1988. HP of unestablished composition like extracts, teas and essential oils need marketing authorization if not of GRAS status or not approved by any other regulatory authority or body

(Continued)

Table 4.1 Continued

Country	Market Size	Regulatory Authority	Current Regulatory Status
Italy	US $0.6 billion, 1991 – Plants used traditionally for dietetic and medicinal purpose	Guidelines issued by the Italian Health Authority in accordance with EEC directives	Dietetic products allowed to be sold outside pharmacies in 'erboristeries' using approved labels. Herbs, herb mixtures, teas with therapeutic indications are to be registered as medicinal products and allowed to be sold by pharmacists in pharmacies only
Nicaragua	TM revitalized as alternative to highly priced imported pharmaceuticals during 1985 civil war. Presently QC'd HPs available at low prices through a national network of pharmacies	National Centre for Popular and Traditional Medicine (NCPTM) under the Ministry Of Health, National Autonomous University of Nicaragua	In 1991 TM integrated into local health systems by training nurses and developing courses in basic plant therapy and health anthropology in nursing schools. NCPTM promotes traditional medicine and herbal products included in the basic medicines list of MOH
Norway	HM sold in pharmacies, health food stores, ordinary food stores	Norwegian Medicines Control Authority. Kingdom of Norway issued a National policy on TM/CAM in 2002 as a National Programme	HPs classified as medicines are regulated through marketing authorization process. Others sold as herbal remedies without any medical claims
Singapore	TCM popular with 12% of out-patient attendance being seen by TCM practitioners	Chinese Proprietary Medicines Advisory Committee under the Medicines Act of MOH	Minimal control over Chinese medicinal materials with no registration being required. Present enforcement activities however safeguard public from toxic substances, adulteration and exaggerated claims.
South Africa	HMs in use through self-care and on advice of 200,000 strong traditional healers	Medicines Central Council (MCC)	Unregulated; a few regulated herbal medicines are according to USP standards. Governments' Reconstruction and Development Programme has Drug Policy section which includes HMs
Turkey	Though used traditionally, HPs are of limited use at present. Prior to 1984 crude drugs available in 'Akthar shops'	Herbal Committee under the Ministry of Health issues HD authorizations	V Symposium on crude drugs at Ankara undertook a resolution to regulate HPs. All 'Akthar shops' require licensing and herbal products listed into three categories for registration purposes

HM: herbal medicines; HP: herbal products; HD: herbal drugs; TCM: traditional Chinese medicine.

distinct from synthetic ones. The European market for herbal remedies in 1998 is estimated to be $5.5 billion.

Legal status

The European market has harmonized regulations for the marketing of herbal medicinal products and issued the Traditional Herbal Medicinal Products Directive (THMPD). It came into force on 30 October 2005 and requires traditional, over-the-counter herbal remedies to be made to assured standards of safety and quality and in conformity with regulations so that these are standardized across Europe. According to the directive no herbal medicinal product shall be allowed in the European Union (EU) market without a licence since its implementation and it intended a simplified registration procedure with a seven-year transition period for traditional herbal medicinal products to obtain a medicine licence.

The EU directive thus allows the licensing and over-the-counter sale of herbal products that have a history of use anywhere in the world for at least 30 years, 15 of which must be in an EU member state. The European Medicines Evaluation Agency (EMEA) issued Guidelines on Specifications, Test Procedures and Acceptance, Criteria for Herbal Substances, Herbal Preparations and Herbal Medicinal Products in 2005 to ensure the quality of the starting plant material, development, in-process controls, GMP controls and process controls, and by specifications applicable to them throughout development and manufacture.

According to the THMP Regulations 2005, no traditional herbal medicinal products shall be placed on the market or distributed wholesale, unless a traditional herbal registration has been obtained in accordance with the relevant community provisions by the licensing authority.

Registration of herbal products

Herbal product manufacturers having available the services of a Qualified Person, a resident of an EU member state, need to apply to the Medicines and Healthcare Products Regulatory Agency (MHRA) for the grant of a traditional herbal registration for every product and each must comply with the official published standards. The application should include

1. Statement indicating whether the herbal medicinal product is one that should be available only from a pharmacy or should be on general sale.
2. Product medicinal indications must be as per the listing in the annexures to the EMEA Guidelines.
3. Safety data put together as a bibliographic review along with an expert report on both non-clinical and clinical aspects of safety. As per EMEA the expert can be a registered doctor, registered pharmacist or other scientifically qualified individual with relevant competence, for example, a toxicologist or an herbal practitioner who is a member of a professional body that is working towards the statutory regulation of the herbal medicine profession, or a registered herbal practitioner.
4. As covered in the 'Key Requirements' section, the application will need to be accompanied by bibliographic or expert evidence that the medicinal product or a corresponding product has been in medicinal use throughout a period of 30 years. The new European Committee, the Committee on Herbal Medicinal Products (HMPC) will establish the 'European positive list' provided for in Directive 2004/24/EC.

5. Product quality should be supported with a technical dossier covering quality of herbal ingredients and the finished product including details of all necessary physicochemical, biological and microbiological tests, covering residual solvents, pesticide residues, microbial limits and heavy metal residues.

6. Finished product specifications should include summary of stability studies undertaken (conditions, batches, analytical procedures) results and conclusions, the proposed storage condition and shelf life.

7. The labelling and patient information as per requirements of MHRA Guidance Note 25 should include name of the product, strength, pharmaceutical form, quantity of active ingredients posology, method of administration, indications, contraindications, excipients, shelf life and any special warnings and precautions for use and a summary of product characteristics.

An independent body concerned with the advancement of the status of phytomedicine in Europe is the European Scientific Cooperative of Phytotherapy (ESCOP). It is an umbrella organization representing national herbal medicine phytotherapy associations across Europe. Among its other activities ESCOP endeavours to assist with the harmonization of the regulatory status of phytomedicines at the European level. In particular it provides state-of the-art reviews of the therapeutic use of leading herbal medicinal products based on leading expertise across Europe. From 1997 to 2010, it has published 108 monographs and has coordinated and completed EU BIOMED research programme determining European standards for the safe and effective use of phytomedicines.

United Kingdom

The market

In Britain alone, an estimated 6,000–7,000 tonnes of herbs are extracted annually for use as ingredients of herbal remedies and for the health food market in 1983 it was estimated that the sale of herbal, homeopathic and other remedies amounted to £15M. The market for licensed herbal medicines in the UK was estimated to be worth £38M in 1996, representing over one half of the total market for complementary remedies.

Legal status

The manufacture of these products is carried out by relatively few companies and, as distinct from the sale of an unprocessed herb, these preparations require a product licence for their manufacture and sale. This EC requirement was introduced in 1972 for new products and was subsequently extended to review all products irrespective of how long they have been marketed. The demonstration that a particular remedy complied with the imposed standards of quality, safety and efficacy as applied to medicines in general was, by nature of the mixed herbal preparation, difficult or impossible to show without extremely costly research. Some limited cognizance of this fact was taken by the national regulatory bodies of member EC countries but interpretation of the EEC directive varied considerably with different states.

Large amounts of traditional medicines are imported into Britain, legally and illegally. Herbal remedies in Britain can be obtained through a medical herbalist or medical practitioner on prescription and as OTC products from pharmacies and other retail outlets.

In practice, medical herbalists of the European herbal tradition, who constitute a relatively small professional body (about 300 in UK), are not consulted by the majority of the public who purchase herbal preparations. General practitioners rarely prescribe herbal remedies although, with complementary treatment – especially traditional Chinese and Indian herbal medicine – now being available through the NHS, referral to an herbal practitioner is becoming more common. Presently there is a marked increase in pharmacies stocking herbal medicines and it is estimated that this sector represents 45% of the total sales for UK. Health food stores and similar sources are still the principal outlets for OTC products.

The supply of medicines in UK is controlled by the Medicines Act 1968 and by the Retail Sale or Supply of Herbal Remedies Order .The General Sales List of the Medicines Order contains about 341 herbal medicines which, with reasonable safety, can be sold or supplied other than under the supervision of a pharmacist. A further stricture on the supply of herbal and other medicines relates to the very limited claims which may legally be made for a preparation, these being restricted to relatively minor ailments.

Part I of the Schedule on herbal drugs in the Medicines Act 1968 lists plants that may be sold or supplied only from a registered pharmacy. Those listed in Part II and III may be used by practitioners who sell or supply herbal remedies where they are for administration to a particular person following a personal consultation, but are not for retail in circumstances other than through pharmacy.

Herbal medicine licensing

The requirements of the licensing system in the United Kingdom are set out in Part II of the above act. Without the appropriate licence it is an offence to manufacture, sell, supply, export or import a medicine into UK, unless some exemption is provided in the act or regulations. However unprocessed plant material, without any written therapeutic recommendation, sold or supplied by its botanical name with reference to the process of manufacture are exempt from licensing requirements.

Herbal medicines indicated for conditions capable of self-diagnosis were granted a licence when sufficient evidence of efficacy was established, and the authority required the product label to mention traditional use. Combination products containing a large number of herbal ingredients or mixtures of herbal and non-herbal ingredients were not accepted and licence holders were asked to consider retaining ingredients attributed with therapeutic activity . In December 1995, 'A guide to what is a medicinal product' was published by the Medicines Control Agency. In accordance with Directive 65/65/EEC it tries to give examples for clarification where the borderline lies between medicinal products such as cosmetics and foodstuffs, taking into consideration claims for the product, the properties of its ingredients, the labelling, promotional literature, product form and whether there are similar licensed products on the market. The new guideline does not intend to affect the status of products legally sold without a licence or the current exemptions for herbal remedies.

Australia

The market

Australia is one of the leading countries in the world with regard to practice and teaching of alternative and complementary medicine. The alternative and complementary medicine industry in Australia is growing rapidly and the current estimated market worth is over one billion dollars, with more than 20% of that market being herbal medicine and related products. This market appears to be growing at about 30% per year. The rapid growth is largely due to a growing demand from the public, with reportedly more than 50% of Australians using herbal or complementary medicines.

Western herbal medicine is one of the most popular forms of alternative medicine and the National Herbalists Association of Australia is the national body for practising herbalists. Traditional Chinese medicine (TCM) has existed in Australia since the influx of Chinese migrants to the gold fields over 100 years ago and many herbal practitioners even incorporate some Ayurvedic principles and herbs into their practice though there are very few purely Ayurvedic practitioners in Australia. Herbs used in these systems are all imported from overseas.

Legal status

Therapeutic goods for human use including traditional medicines which are imported or manufactured in Australia must be included in the Australian Register of Therapeutic Goods (ARTG) in accordance with the Therapeutic Goods Act 1989. Instituted by the Common wealth Department of Health and Aged Care, the overall objective of the act is to ensure the quality, safety, efficacy and timely availability of therapeutic goods. The act controls the standard of all ingredients used in manufacture, advertising and label claims for products, registration of products on the ARTG, manufacturing and packaging conditions and controls (GMP). The Therapeutic Goods Administration (TGA) of the government has established a Traditional Medicines Evaluation Committee (TMEC) to make recommendations on safety, quality and efficacy of herbal substances which are required to be listed or registered with ARTG. Appointed by the Minister, TMEC provides expertise for the evaluation of non-prescription traditional medicines and consists of six to nine members who are experts in clinical practice or teaching of alternative medicine: pharmacy professionals with expertise in pharmacognosy or plant toxicology, manufacture of alternative medicine, traditional medicine practitioners and clinical pharmacologists.

Australian register of therapeutic goods

Registered medicines are classified as high risk and low risk. The high-risk ones are assessed individually for quality, safety and efficacy and should be manufactured under GMP. The low-risk ones are listed medicines and contain ingredients permitted by the TGA for use in low-risk medicines restricted to indication and claims relating to health maintenance, health enhancement or non-serious, self-limiting conditions. These are not assessed individually for efficacy, but must certify to the TGA that they hold evidence to support all indications and claims made for their products. These too should be manufactured under GMP and require post-market regulatory activities, including reporting of adverse reactions, audit of manufacturers and laboratory testing.

Listed drugs

Australian herbal remedies being considered by the TGA to be 'reasonably safe with less adverse reactions than conventional pharmaceutical treatments' are allowed to enter the register at a lower level than other pharmaceuticals. Herbal products made from starting materials of pharmacopoeial standards, approved by the TGA, with claims within Advertising Code guidelines containing active ingredients prescribed in the regulations receive a LISTING and an AUSTL number. Though a LISTING does not specifically require submission of efficacy or stability data, TGA reserves the right to call for this data.

Listed medicines may only contain ingredients that have been evaluated by the TGA to be low risk. TGA has a list of substances that may be used as active ingredients in listed medicines. The safety of ingredients for use and quality standards for ingredients acceptable to the TGA are given in Therapeutic Goods Order (TGO). The Australian Regulatory Guidelines for Complementary Medicines (ARGCM) contains guidance on the criteria for compositional guidelines which is a summary of descriptions, tests and limits that define the composition and relevant characteristics of the substance. These guidelines have been developed to assist sponsors in determining the appropriate evidence to support indications and claims made in relation to listable medicines. Where the claims/indications do not appear to be consistent with the evidence guidelines, the TGA may request the sponsors to submit full text copies of all relevant reference materials for evaluation. The guidelines offer advice on the levels and kinds of evidence to support claims on therapeutic goods.

According to general requirements for labels of medicines, herbs are included in the list of Australian approved names for pharmaceutical substances which is published by the TGA in its edition 'TGA Approved Terminology for Drugs' dated January 1993, with amendments. There are also special regulations in the expression of quantity or proportion of active ingredients in drug products, with special requirements for herbal ingredients. Post-market regulatory activities include targeted and random desk-based audits of listed products, monitoring of adverse reactions to complementary medicines, targeted and random laboratory testing of products and ingredients, targeted and random surveillance in the market place, an effective, responsive and timely recall procedure, audit of GMP, effective controls for the advertising of therapeutic goods, adverse drug reaction reporting and monitoring adverse reactions to complementary medicines. Traditional medicines such as Ayurvedic and Chinese medicines are classified as 'complementary medicines' and are generally required to meet the same standards of quality and safety as other modern medicines to meet their legislative obligations. Once a therapeutic claim is made or implied, then the goods become therapeutic and subject to the requirements of the Australian Therapeutic Goods Act 1989.

Canada

The market

Over the last decade there is a reported increase in the sale and use of herbs in Canada. In North America herbal remedies constitute a $2-billion-a-year industry that is growing at a pace of 15% annually.

Legal status

Herbal products were generally regulated as foods or drugs under the Food and Drugs Act coming under the supervision of the Directorates of both Food Safety and Drug Safety. Since some of the products sold as food with medicinal claims were considered harmful the Canadian Government has entrusted Health Canada to control the registration of herbal products through a body called the Natural Health Products Directorate (NHPD). Its objective is to provide safe, effective and high quality natural health products and prevent adverse effects to consumers. NHPD has established the Food and Drugs Act to regulate herbal remedies, homeopathic medicines, vitamins, traditional medicines, probiotics, amino acids and essential fatty acids. The regulations include provisions on product licensing, site licensing, GMP, adverse reaction reporting, clinical trials and labelling.

In order to address the issue of regulation of herbs, Health Canada has constituted Expert Advisory Committees on herbs and botanical preparations and has been issuing information letters, guidelines and policy statements to develop an appropriate framework for regulating herbal remedies. Today herbal remedies are regulated as drugs in Canada and must therefore conform to labelling and other requirements as set out in the Food and Drugs Act and Regulations. Thus in contrast to the United States, large numbers of herbal medicines with indication claims are legally sold on the Canadian market.

Herbs and botanicals are acceptable as drugs on the basis of acknowledged claims and quantitative statements of the active ingredient. Under the Food and Drugs Act herbal products are generally regulated either as foods or as drugs depending on the pharmacological activity of the ingredients, the intended purpose of the product and the representations made regarding its use including medicinal claims.

Amendments to the Food and Drugs Act in the form of Schedule 705 outlines substances not permitted for use in or as food and those substances acceptable as foods under specified conditions. In response to certain concerns raised, an Expert Advisory Committee reconstituted in 1993 recommended removal of seven herbs and botanical preparations from the 'unacceptable as food' list. Of these seven, five – namely wormwood, feverfew, Levant wormseed, mugwort, St. John's wort – are now acceptable as food, with the other two – goldenseal root and Oregon grape root – now acceptable as food under specified conditions. According to legislations in the form of Bills C-85/C-7/C-8 to the Controlled Drugs and Substances Act (CSDA), some products such as cannabis and khat are controlled substances with different regulations and restrictions applicable to their sale and supply. Further an information letter issued by the Canadian Health Protection Branch contains a list of herbs considered hazardous.

The regulations of the Food and Drugs Act require a marketed herbal product claiming to have medicinal properties to carry a drug identification (DIN) or general public (GP) number. These numbers indicate that there has been a review of the product's formulation, labelling and instructions for use, and are intended to provide assurance that any content and health claims are accurate. All natural health products require a licence and information on the product, including medicinal ingredients, source, potency, non-medicinal ingredients and recommended use. If a product number is preceded by the distinct letters NPN, then the product has been reviewed and approved by Health Canada for safety and efficacy. As a general practice, herbal remedies used for minor self-limiting conditions are allocated DINs based on logical pharmacological rationale and bibliographic references which include verified traditional uses that have not been superceded by more recent research and study.

An information letter issued on 5 January 1990 outlines the regulatory requirements of herbal medicines and provides advice on the mechanisms for applications for DIN for these products. Herbal medicinal products in this letter are classified into two major groups:

1. Herbs listed in pharmacopoeias and major pharmacological reference works: they generally have their properties, dosage, indications and contraindications for a well-established use. Products containing such herbal ingredients are reviewed in the same manner as other drug products and are widely available on the market either on prescription or as non-prescription drugs.

2. Herbs which have received relatively little attention in scientific literature and therefore may not be well known in Canada. Nonetheless, there is literature available on their traditional

use on an empirical basis, and these references are considered to be useful in supporting acceptability of herbal drug products. It was expected that herbal drugs from this group would be used for minor self-limiting conditions. These products which are based on traditional or folkloric use should be designated as traditional medicines, and some details for application for DIN have been announced.

Registration of herbs and botanical preparations

Furthermore in order to provide a specific framework for the registration of herbs and botanical preparations, a concept of review involving 'Standardized Drug Monographs' (SDM) has been proposed to facilitate registration of those drugs containing herbs that meet requirements of the monographs. Products making reference to such an SDM would require less individual premarket scrutiny on a product-by-product basis and would result in more rapid issuance of DIN, but would be balanced with additional post-market compliance monitoring and activity. Combinations of herbs outlined in such monographs would be accepted if justified on sound therapeutic principles. Claims in respect of prevention or treatment of serious diseases and those which are inappropriate for self-diagnosis and treatment are prohibited within this procedure. The review of DIN applications involving SDMs should enable a manufacturer to certify that products meet the conditions outlined in the SDM.

In October 1990, guidelines on 'Traditional Herbal Medicines' were published by the Health Protection Branch, by authority of the Minister of National Health and Welfare, to assist manufacturers in completing applications for DIN and in labelling products that fall within the category of Traditional Herbal Medicine (THM) as outlined in the information letter on 5 January 1990.

A site licence is required to manufacture, package, label and import for sale any natural health product. The manufacturing has to be done in conformity with GMP to ensure product safety and quality, including appropriate standards and practices regarding product manufacture, storage, handling and distribution. GMP covers specifications on premises and equipment, personnel, sanitation programme, operational procedures, quality assurance, stability studies, record keeping, lot or batch sampling and recall reporting. Adverse drug reaction reporting is statutory based on risk assessment and the corresponding management of risks so that advisories, where appropriate, to the public could be issued. The Natural Health Products regulations require that product licence holders monitor all adverse reactions and report serious adverse reactions to Health Canada.

In case of non-traditional products, clinical trials are required to establish the product's clinical, pharmacological or pharmacodynamic effects to identify any adverse events related to its use, to study its absorption, distribution, metabolism and excretion and to determine its safety and efficacy.

Labelling requirements are very stringent to enable consumers to make informed choices. A label should include the product name, ingredients and composition, quantity of product in the bottle, recommended conditions of use, health claim, dosage form, dose, route of administration, any cautionary statements, contraindications, ADR and storage conditions.

Applications for traditional medicine manufacture must include a draft version of the label with a clear claim or indication for the use of the traditional herbal medicine. The claim should be supported by references. If an SDM is available for an herb, and if the proposed claims are within the scope of the monograph, a statement to this effect is an acceptable replacement for other references. Terms such as tonic, supplement, purifier, depurative, and similar wordings are not accepted. Some combinations of herbs that seem illogical, e.g., diuretics combined with laxatives and those with contradictory effects are regarded as questionable.

The assessment is primarily based on traditional references for efficacy and dosage. The claims are restricted to those that are acceptable for self-monitoring. If there are safety concerns, modern research will be taken into account instead of traditional references.

Germany

The market

Herbal medicine sales is growing in Germany and herbal remedies represent an important share of the German pharmaceutical market. According to an Institut fur Medizinische Statistik (IMS) report, presented during an ESCOP Symposium in Brussels in October 1990, the German herbal medicines market was worth US $1.7 billion in 1989, which was equal to 10% of the total pharmaceutical market in Germany. A representative study carried out by the Allensbach Institute among the German population in June 1989 confirmed usage of natural medicines by a large number of people in Germany. The study showed that 58% of the population has taken such remedies, 44% of them within the previous year. It could also be shown that over the years the number of younger people using natural remedies has increased significantly. According to the study report, natural medicines were generally considered more harmless than chemical drugs. A majority among the German population (85%) believed that the experience of physicians, practitioners and patients should be accepted as proof for the efficacy of natural medicines. The rising popularity is driven by German patients, who began demanding herbal alternatives to synthetic drugs. Medical schools responded by reintroducing lessons on a topic that had been phased out of medical curriculum.

Herbal medicines are distributed through OTC sales in pharmacies and other distribution channels and on medical prescription through pharmacies. They are, in principle, reimbursable by the health insurance system unless special criteria for their exclusion apply, for example, specified indications such as common cold or laxatives or substances with a negative assessment by Commission E. Except for a few preparations, herbal medicines are not prescription-bound but can be prescribed by physicians or practitioners for reimbursement.

The total turnover of non-prescription-bound herbal medicines in pharmacies was DM 4.5 billion in 1995, which was equal to almost 30% of the total turnover of non-prescription-bound medicines (DM 15.2 billion). Preparations sold on prescription amounted to DM 2.4 billion and those purchased through self-medication to DM 2.1 billion of the total turnover of non-prescription-bound phytomedicines. Herbal medicines can be found among the 2,000 most important drugs prescribed by medical doctors and reimbursed by health insurances.

Legal status

In Germany, issues surrounding quality control and standardization of herbal products are less of a concern than elsewhere because ethical botanical manufacturers use the same high-quality production standards found in the synthetic drug industry. However in terms of legal status, herbal medicines are fully considered as medicines according to the Second Medicines Act of

1978 which determines the standards for the granting of marketing authorization in accordance with the European framework for the handling of medicines. Under this new regulation, proof of quality, safety and efficacy became an essential precondition for the registration of medicines. All products on market at the time of issuance of the directive were allowed to continue being marketed with a so-called fiction marketing authorization for a 12-year transition period until 31 December 1989. To meet the requirements of the new Medicines Act, the authorities were obliged to carry out a review of active principals, which resulted in monographs and product-specific verification of pharmaceutical quality and conformity with published monographs. The review largely focused on active ingredients and established an *a priori* criterion for the same. The review of herbal remedies was done by a pluridisciplinary commission of experts – the Commission E – with pharmacists, pharmacologists, toxicologists, clinical pharmacologists, biostatisticians, medical doctors from hospitals and general medical practitioners. Established in 1978, Commission E is an independent division of the German Federal Health Agency that collects information on herbal medicines and evaluates them for safety and efficacy.

This commission responsible for the evaluation of more than 300 medicinal plants received pharmaceutical, pharmacological and clinical data along with data from international side-effect monitoring system and publications from the Health Authority. The work also supported by the 'Kooperation Phytopharmaka' resulted in the compilation of a prepublished draft monograph that was open for remarks from companies and other interested parties. Later the monographs covering most of the ingredients of industrially prepared herbal medicines were published officially in the Federal Gazette, Bundesanzeiger, and this scientific evaluation formed the basis for marketing authorizations and review decisions of the Federal Institute for Drugs and Medical Devices, Bundesinstitut fur Arzneimittel und Medizinprodukte (BfArM), responsible for the assessment of medicines and the verification of submitted dossiers with respect to quality, safety and efficacy. The monographs include analytical test requirements and also texts for labels and package leaflets with 279 monographs of standardized marketing authorizations for herbal teas. While 'positive monographs' pertain to those that cover all relevant indications including package leaflet or consumer information such as drug composition, form of applications, indications, contraindications, warnings, dosage etc. a substantial number of 'negative monographs' is for those that involved risks from active ingredients or had no reasonable proof of efficacy. The work of all review commissions including the Commission E regarding the evaluation of bibliographic data and preparation of monographs was finalized in the Fifth Amendment of the Medicines Act. The commissions are now advisory boards to the health authorities in making decisions on the registration of new drugs, and in the individual assessment of old medicinal products already on the market.

Registration criteria

Criteria for registration and requirements for marketing authorizations for herbal remedies are as set out by European Directives and guidelines, such as the Note for Guidance on Quality of Herbal Remedies, the European Pharmacopoeia, and national guidelines and directives such as the guidelines for testing of drugs following section 26 of the Medicines Act. While bibliographic data on well-established use of herbal medicines is accepted, the criteria developed by Commission E and positive monographs are widely used to document safety and efficacy of herbal remedies. Monographs can to a large extent replace pharmacological, toxicological and clinical documentation as can bibliographic data. Medicines or groups of medicines which do not pose a direct or indirect risk to the health of man or animal can be exempted from the requirement of individual marketing authorization according to section 6 of Medicines Act. To ensure their quality, safety and efficacy, each such medicinal product referring to this procedure must comply exactly with a monograph of a standardized marketing authorization published by the Ministry of Health.

The fifth amendment of the German Medicines Act, which became effective in August 1994, widened the scope of existing legislation for herbal medicinal and other products already on the market. Traditional medicine usage instead of reasonable proof of efficacy is accepted for a certain category of products, mostly sold outside pharmacies. These products have to be labelled as 'traditionally used' and in accordance to section 109a of the Medicines Act, the BfArM has compiled lists stating which preparations are allowed to refer to this regulation and which traditional indications can be claimed. This new system offers a legal possibility for a large number of preparations without sufficient documentation as proof of efficacy to be re-registered under such a simplified procedure.

On a 'higher level', 'non-traditional' are admissible, provided that these are based on monographs or on individual clinical studies with defined preparations. In contrast to herbal medicines, the quality dossiers of 'traditional' products are not checked by the health authority. The regulation contrasts with EU requirements for the marketing of medicinal products. Hence the new regulation offers a legal possibility for herbal and non-herbal preparations to stay on a strictly national market without sufficient documentation as proof of efficacy and safety and without thorough control of pharmaceutical quality. In Germany three possibilities for marketing herbal drugs exist:

1. Temporary marketing authorization for old herbal drugs until they are evaluated for safety and efficacy;
2. Monographs of standardized marketing authorization;
3. Individual marketing authorization.

United States of America

The market

The use of herbal medicines in the United States is less widespread than in the majority of developed nations as wider distribution through pharmacies is difficult because no medical claims may be made and consumers are dependent on advice from pharmacists who, in majority of cases, have little knowledge about medicinal herbs. Also distribution of herbal products is limited to health food stores frequented by only a small proportion of the population.

Legal status

Ever since the passing of the Food, Drug and Cosmetic Act in the late 1930s the Food and Drug Administration (FDA) has regulated as drugs any products which claim to treat, cure, mitigate or prevent a disease. Thus for any herbal medicine claims to be allowed, the same procedures must be followed as for a chemical drug. Thus most natural products in the United States are regulated as foods or food additives even though many are used by consumers as folk medicines. Even for herbs 'generally recognized as safe' (GRAS) and related products that are not misbranded or adulterated, no claims are allowed. Natural products theoretically have GRAS status, as long as qualified experts confirm this and are not contradicted by other experts. Also the requirement of 'common use in food' is not only restricted to use in the United States, but applied also to herbs without a history of use in the United States. Though some better-known medicinal herbs were initially listed by the FDA for OTC status, they were dropped as the US herbal drug industry failed to submit evidence to support their use as such.

Following the 'Proxmire Bill' of 1976, according to a civil regulation for the Health Food Market, foods including dietary supplements are not categorized as drugs. This law kept the FDA from making monographs on dietary supplements, vitamins, minerals and herbs as has been done for several kinds of drugs.

Nutrition Labelling and Education Act (NLEA) passed by the Congress in 1990 required all food products to have nutritional labelling and the FDA was required to establish criteria for approving such health benefit labelling. Vitamins, minerals, herbs and similar nutritional substances that are consumed differently from conventional food were considered for exemption and leniency with respect to standards of evidence for their health benefits. The Dietary Supplement Health and Education Act (DSHEA) of 1994 recognized the usefulness of dietary supplements in preventing chronic diseases and helping limit long-term health care costs. Herbs and other botanicals, vitamins and minerals too now fall under the definition of a dietary supplement which is presented in a dosage form such as capsules, tablets, liquids etc. Dietary supplements do not include substances first sold as drugs and later as dietary supplements, nor do they include substances undergoing clinical studies which were not first sold as dietary supplements.

Regulation

According to the law dietary supplement is considered to be food which does not need pre-market approval by the FDA, and not as a food additive which needs a pre-market approval by the authority. A statement on the label of a dietary supplement is allowed if a benefit is claimed related to a classical nutrient deficiency, if the role of the ingredient is described, or if the documented mechanism of action to maintain a function is characterized. Also it must be clearly stated that this statement has not been evaluated by the FDA, and that this product is not intended to diagnose, treat, cure or prevent any disease. The ingredients, the plant and/or its parts and their quantities must be clearly listed. If the supplement claims to conform to an official compendia standard (USP) for which there is an official specification and fails to meet that standard, the product is regarded as misbranded. Products not covered by official compendia failing to meet the claimed identity, strength, quality and purity are also considered misbranded. The signing into law of the DSHAE has accelerated the recognition and importance of herbal products in the US market, with the law giving an opportunity to market these products as dietary supplements, provided there is data to support claims with reasonable substantiation and to show that the products are safe.

However since the FDA does not accept bibliographic evidence of effectiveness and prefers randomized controlled trials as evidence of efficacy, at present it is not possible to market a herbal product as a drug in the United States. Otherwise the guidelines for the manufacture of herbal products, quality of evidence to the claims made etc. like elsewhere are in accordance with GMPs established by the FDA.

China

The market

TCM has a long history of use of more than 4,000 years. Discovery of medicinal materials in ancient times was closely related to the life and the labour of people and their natural conditions of living. People found that many natural materials could be used to treat diseases, and great experience in this field has gradually been accumulated. The Chinese Materia Medica is one of the best documented and most extensive sources, as well as one that enjoys the most continued use, containing references to more than 7,000 species of medicinal plants.

The constitution of the People's Republic of China stipulates that modern and traditional medicines should be developed simultaneously. Therefore since the founding of the People's Republic of China, TCM has developed steadily. By the end of 1995, there were 2511 TCM hospitals with a total of 276,000 beds. Most of the general hospitals have a TCM department. There are 940 factories and plants for the manufacture of herbal medicines. The total sales volume of traditional herbal medicines in 1995 was 15 billion Yuan, an increase of 123% compared to 1990. From 1978 to 1993, sales of patent herbal medicines and raw plant materials increased by 10.8% and 2.3%, respectively.

The 1998 edition of The Chinese Pharmacopoeia included 784 articles on TCM and 509 articles on Chinese patent medicines. The monographs describe the source or the substances used, prescriptions, methods of preparation, identification, examination, extraction, effects and main indications as well as methods of use, dosage and precautions.

Legal status

Herbal medicines in China are normally considered as medicinal products with special requirements for marketing that include quality dossiers, safety and efficacy evaluation, special labelling etc. The Drug Administration Law of the People's Republic of China enacted in 1984 encourages the state to develop both modern and traditional drugs and the state protects the resources of wild herbal drugs and encourages domestic cultivation of herbal drugs. While traditional experiences with regard to therapeutic efficacy are held in esteem, modern scientific and technical knowledge is used in appraising the therapeutic effects and quality of modified traditional medicines, thus contributing administratively to the exploitation of TCM. According to article 5 of the Drug Administration Law of China an herbal drug manufacturing enterprise should be staffed with an adequate number of technical personnel and skilled workers capable of handling large-scale drug production. Units engaged in handling plant material need to be staffed with pharmaceutical professionals familiar with the property of raw materials and registered with the health bureau above the county level. Article 6 requires medicinal plant material processing to be carried out in compliance with the pharmacopoeia of the People's Republic of China or the processing norms stipulated by the health bureau of the province, autonomous region or municipality. The Drug Administration Law also stipulates the places of disbursement and sale of medicinal pant materials and has under its purview norms for the export, import, patenting and clinical trial requirements of such products.

Even new drugs are examined and approved according to the Drug Administration Law. Upon approval, a New Drug Certificate is granted an approval number and the factory is permitted to put the product on the market. 'New Drugs' are referred to as drugs which have not been produced previously in China, or drugs for which a new indication, a change in the route of administration or a change of dosage form is to be adopted.

Traditional Chinese medicines are often composed of multiple herbs, which have been selected by a TCM practitioner to treat specific diseases in individual patients. Since these are 'individualized' converting a TCM into a pharmaceutical product is challenging as the latter requires a specific composition. Defining a specific composition can be tricky because the efficacy of a TCM preparation may be used over a range of compositions. Overall, developing TCM as pharmaceutical drugs presents unique challenges, including coping with multiple herbs, controlling the cultivation of the biomass and steps for processing it adhering to GMP. Applicants engaged in the development, production, distribution, prescription, inspection and surveillance of new drugs must adhere to the provisions of articles 21 and 22. The regulation includes general principles concerning new drugs, their classification, research, clinical trials, approval and manufacture. Appendices to the document provide detailed information on the application form, list of documents required and technical requirements of toxicological and clinical studies on new modern drugs and new TCM drugs.

Regulation of medicinal material and pharmaceutical forms

Based on the amendment and Supplemental Regulation of Approval of New TCM Drugs implemented in 1992 [The approval of new pharmaceuticals (concerning the revision and the additional regulations on the sections on Chinese Traditional Medicine) implemented on 1 September 1992. Ministry of Health of the People's Republic of China], new TCM drugs are classified under five categories:

Category 1

1. Artificial imitations of TCM herbs
2. Newly discovered medicinal plants and their preparations
3. Single active principal extracted from TCM plant materials and their preparations

Category 2

1. Chinese medicinal herbal injections
2. Parts of TCM medicinal plants newly employed as a remedy and their preparations
3. Non-single components extracted from TCM and natural plants and their preparations
4. TCM materials obtained by artificial techniques *in vivo* and their preparations

Category 3

1. New TCM preparations
2. Combined preparations of TCM and modern medicine in which TCM medicine is the main component
3. Cultivated material which traditionally is imported

Category 4

1. New dosage forms or new routes of administration of TCM drug
2. Materials introduced from other parts of the country and those for cultivation instead of harvesting in the wild

Category 5

1. TCM products with new and additional indications.

For these categories, different requirements have to be fulfilled for medicinal materials and the pharmaceutical form. All research on new medicines should provide data on toxicity, pharmacological properties and clinical research, as well as detailed documentation on the quality of the medicinal material and the pharmaceutical preparation. Proprietary medicines included in the national pharmacopoeia and new medicines approved by the Ministry of Public Health are exempted from clinical testing when only the dosage form is changed, such as from powder to capsules, or from tablets to granular form infused with boiling water, without changes in the indications for cardinal symptoms or dosage. As per the technical requirements for pharmacological studies, tests on major drug effects are to be designed in such a way that the special characteristics of TCM are taken into consideration. Two or more methods shall be selected for research on the major drug actions, based on the effects of the new medicines on the complex of symptoms or the illness. For new medicines in categories 1, 2 and 3 this research shall be sufficient to verify the major therapeutic functions and effects. For new medicines in category 4, two tests on the major effects are required or well-documented material has to be submitted. For new medicines in category 5, only tests on the major effects of the medicine on 'new' cardinal symptoms are required. Research on general pharmacology shall be performed on the nervous system, on the cardiovascular system and on the respiratory system. Technical requirements for studies on toxicity are as required by the document. While clinical trials are divided into three phases, clinical verifications do not have phases. Clinical trials shall be conducted for new medicines of categories 1, 2 and 3 and clinical verifications are required for new medicines of categories 4 and 5.

Medicines in categories 1 and 2 which have either toxic or incompatible compounds need to go through Phase 1 clinical trial to study the reaction and tolerance of the human body to the new medicine and to assess the safe dosage.

Phase 2 clinical trials are undertaken to obtain an accurate evaluation of the curative effects of the new medicine and its safety and consists of two stages. While the first applies when treatment is performed, the second is applicable when it is to be expanded. Selection of cases, methods used are all as per standard norms and when curative effects are determined, four ratings are applicable, namely – clinical recovery, significantly effective, effective and non-effective. The evaluation of the curative effects shall be based on the clinical symptoms, objective standards for curative effects and the ultimate results on the patient. The objective of the Phase 3 clinical trial is the further investigation of the safe use or effectiveness of the new medicine on the basis of the findings of Phase 2.

Clinical verification applicable to new medicines of categories 4 and 5 is to observe their curative effects, contraindications and precautions.

Summary of the clinical trial shall be objective and comprehensive and shall be an accurate reflection of the whole process. The discussion in the final report shall include the conclusion which is based on the outcome of the tests, the functions and effects on cardinal symptoms, the scope of application of the new medicine, its administration, the course of treatment, curative effects, safety, adverse reactions, contraindications and precautions.

The Amendment and Supplemental Regulation of Approval of new TCM drugs has a special chapter on the technical requirements for studies on quality standards for Chinese medicinal material and medicines. These include the prescription, the way of processing, the properties, the identification, the examination and the assay in accordance with the general guidelines laid down in the pharmacopoeia. It also describes the requirements for studies on stability.

Japan

The market

Traditional medicine in Japan may be divided into folk medicine and Kampo medicine, i.e., Chinese medicine from ancient China. Herbal medicines have been used effectively in Japan for the past 1,400 years and similar to the situation in China, today raw medicinal herbs used as folk medicine are combined with modern preparations in many cases. The per-capita consumption of herbal medicine in Japan is the highest in the world with among the top 100 items of OTC drugs sold, 45 correspond to the raw herb combined preparations representing 34% of sales with considerable economic importance. Kampo drugs are extremely popular in Japan and each Kampo drug is a formula consisting of 5–10 different herbs. Since 1957, several original formulae of Kampo drugs are being produced in modern ready-to-use industrialized granular, powdered forms based on the classic decoction. Today more than 95% of Kampo drugs used in Japan are taken in such ready-to-use forms as ethical drugs.

Legal status

Since 1961, 100% of the Japanese population has been covered by the National Health Insurance (NHI) and in 1972 Ministry of Health Labour and Welfare (MHLW) designated 210 formulas as OTC drugs based on the experience of doctors practising Chinese galenical medicine. In 1976, 43 Kampo drugs were included in the NHI Drug Price Tariff as prescription drugs and today 147 Kampo drug preparations available as ethical drugs are already registered by the MHLW without the need for clinical validation studies.

Regulation

For new drugs to be included as prescription drugs, applications with specified data on safety, stability, clinical test results etc. are required. New Kampo drugs are regulated in essentially the same way as Western drugs in Japan. They are regarded as a form of combined drug, and the same data required for new western drugs are required for new Kampo drugs in the Pharmaceuticals and Medical Devices Agency (PMDA). All the mandatory toxicity study results including special toxicity tests such as for mutagenicity, carcinogenicity and teratogenicity are required as also are the results of three-phase clinical trials.

The high value of Chinese medicines in modern medical practice is indicated by its remarkable growth as prescription drugs in the Japanese market. While 19% physicians recorded having prescribed Chinese medicines in 1979, the percentage increased to 79% in 1989. According to another survey, at least 65% physicians administered both Chinese and modern medicine. Physicians generally recognize Chinese medicine as a complement to modern medicine and it is common knowledge in Japanese society that traditional drugs are safe. As per an in-hospital side-effect monitoring report in 1989, Chinese medicines accounted for a low 1.3% of all cases.

Quality standards of folk and Kampo medicines are based on different evaluation methods, with the effect of the former being assessed on the sum of pharmacological actions of the effective ingredients contained in the raw herb similar to chemical substances. With respect to evaluation and safety, those raw herbs, components of an industrial product with long-established use as folk medicine, are listed in the corresponding monograph and are freely usable within the range of the monograph.

For the evaluation of Chinese medicines on the other hand, importance is given to the 'empirical facts or experience' such as reference data, clinical test reports etc. Safety and efficacy is estimated based on general methods employed by modern medical science.

Since the policy of requiring scientific evidence for safety and efficacy was instituted by the Japanese Government in the year 1967, the MHLW has been running a programme for the re-evaluation of all drugs marketed before this. Results of the first re-evaluation of ethical drugs approved prior to 1967 have been made public since 1973 and those of second re-evaluation of ethical drugs approved from October 1967 to March 1980 since 1988. These two re-evaluations completed 99% and 58% respectively of the total number of products. In addition a new system to re-evaluate the efficacy and safety of all ethical drugs every five years was launched in 1988. The methods of re-evaluation of Chinese medicines not being clearly established, an official notification has been issued on 1 February 1991 and a first selection was made of eight prescriptions, with the manufacturers being requested to furnish necessary data to prove their effectiveness and safety.

All these measures resulted in the improvement of the quality control of Kampo drugs in the mid-1980s. An Advisory Committee for Kampo Drugs was established in 1982 in close association with the Pharmaceuticals Affairs Bureau of the MHLW. A working group on the quality of Kampo drugs was established and three years later, a new regulation was issued by the Pharmaceutical Affairs Bureau setting standards for the manufacture and quality control of Kampo drugs. The regulation calls for quality monitoring of specific ingredients, using at least two different chemical or physical methods to test them. Also since 1986, GMP, a standard required of pharmaceutical drugs issued by MHLW in 1976 applies to Kampo drugs too. In addition, in 1988, the Japan Kampo Medicine Manufacturers' Association drew up self-imposed guidelines that take into consideration the unique nature of Kampo drugs. In 1985 guidelines for extract-based ethical drugs in oriental medicine formulations were developed, according to which data from a comparative study of the extract and a standard decoction have to be provided by the manufacturer of an ethical extract product. Besides data on the crude drug and on the standard decoction prepared in accordance with the TCM prescription, a comparative study has to describe the content of an indicator ingredient in the finished product, which is required to be more than 70% of the content of the indicator ingredient in the standard decoction. For collection of data on adverse drug reactions in Japan there are three major systems of the MHLW:

1. The Adverse Drug Reaction Monitoring System monitors 2,915 designated monitoring hospitals, which have been requested to report cases of adverse reactions to MHLW. This is a voluntary monitoring system, and 1,158 cases of adverse reaction were reported in 1990, of which 15 cases pertained to Kampo drugs.
2. The Pharmacy Monitoring System formed by 2,733 pharmacies mainly collects data on cases of adverse reactions to OTC drugs; 400 cases have been reported annually in the recent years, among which common adverse reactions caused by Kampo drugs are minor, involving symptoms such as gastric discomfort and skin problems.

3. Manufacturers' Adverse Reaction Reporting involves reporting by the concerned companies, wherein recently several severe cases of 'Shosikoto', including drug-induced hepatitis and pneumonitis documented at medical conferences and journals have been reported to MHLW.

In addition, since 1988 the newly drafted Good Post-Marketing Surveillance Practice (GPMSP) has been used on a pilot scale for western drugs dispensed in Japan. When new Kampo drugs are approved and appear on the market, these guidelines will also apply to them.

India

The market

Traditional medical knowledge in India dates back to antiquity and use of herbs for curative properties have been recorded in the Vedas, some of the oldest written records in the world. Ayurveda, the oldest written medical system, is richly supplemented with ancient medical compilations and current scientific research is validating the traditional medicine claims of herbs and several healing practices. Such medical wisdom was so assimilated in the cultural ethos of the nation that despite years of foreign rule and suppression of native medicine, a great deal of folk knowledge exists even today among ordinary people about traditional use of herbal medicines.

Medicinal herbs have been in use in one form or another under indigenous systems of medicine like Ayurveda, Siddha and Unani. Today with about 6,000 plants representing about 75% of the medicinal needs of the third world countries, India is a major worldwide exporter of raw medicinal and aromatic plants and processed plant-based drugs.

Ayurveda is recognized by WHO and is widely practiced world over. While it is difficult to quantify the market size of traditional Indian systems since most practitioners formulate and dispense their own recipes, the present annual turnover of products manufactured by large companies is estimated at approximately US $300 million, compared to a turnover of approximately US $2.5 billion for modern drugs.

Legal status

General physicians educated and trained in modern medicine are relatively unfamiliar with Ayurvedic products and prescribe these drugs only when no other treatment option is available, though the efficacy of several Ayurvedic products is scientifically proven. However patent and proprietary Ayurvedic medicines are sold OTC in pharmacies and these products appear to represent a major share of branded traditional products in India. There is a huge market for these Fast Moving Consumer Goods (FMCG) because of self-medication by the populace for minor ailments such as cold, cough, diarrhoea and stomach problems adding to the large quantum of drugs being prescribed by traditional medical practitioners of Ayurveda, Siddha, Unani and Homeopathy.

Modernization and scientific validation of traditional remedies though initiated on a large scale is yet to catch up with the rapid advances and competition from China, Japan and Korea. Multi-herb composition of traditional drug formulations, individualization and subjectivity of drug dispensing, holistic treatment approach and dearth of standardization methodologies for these preparations as per WHO requirements, reckless exploitation of medicinal plant wealth are some of the contributing factors to the lack of empirical support of modern medical science to traditional drugs from India.

In India there are currently about 250,000 registered medical practitioners of the Ayurvedic system with approximately 291,000 for all systems combined, compared to 700,000 modern medicine practitioners. In every Indian state, about one-third government medical posts are occupied by physicians who belong to the traditional systems.

Regulatory activity

In India, national policy on TM/Complementary and Alternative Medicine (CAM) was introduced in the form of Drugs and Cosmetics Act of 1940 and the Drugs and Cosmetics Rules of 1945. This has been updated in 1964, 1970 and 1982. These govern and regulate the import, manufacture, distribution and sale of drugs and cosmetics. In 1959, the Government of India recognized the traditional Indian systems of medicine and amended the Drugs and Cosmetics Act to include drugs derived from traditional Indian medicine.

A number of expert committees have been appointed for different forms of TM/CAM, the earliest was established in 1962. There are also a number of national research institutes; the first was the Central Council of Indian Medicine established in 1970.

According to the Drugs and Cosmetics Act, herbal medicines are regulated as prescription and OTC medicines and dietary supplements. Herbal medicines may be sold with medical, health and nutrient content claims. No products derived from traditional Indian medicines may be manufactured without a licence from the State Drug Control Authorities. Patent and proprietary medicines derived from traditional systems must contain ingredients which are mentioned in the recognized books of the above systems, as specified in the Drugs and Cosmetics Act. The government is advised by a special committee and an advisory board for Ayurvedic, Siddha and Unani (ASU) drugs. Criteria for all ASU drugs whether misbranded, adulterated or spurious are laid down under specific sections of the act as also the regulations for the manufacture, licensing and sale of these drugs. Categories of offences and penalties are also stipulated under this act. The Department of AYUSH further drafted certain rules to amend the Drugs and Cosmetics Rules, 1945 in the Gazette of India. The draft claims that the certificate of GMP to manufacturers of ASU drugs shall be issued to licensees who comply with the requirements of GMP of ASU drugs as laid down in Schedule T of the act. According to rules 157, 158 and 159 of the Drugs and Cosmetics Act, failure to comply with GMP's notified Schedule T of the Drugs and Cosmetics Act and Rules leads to revocation of the manufacturers' licence by the State Drug Licensing Authorities.

India has two multi-volume national pharmacopoeias – the Ayurvedic Pharmacopoeia of India and the Unani Pharmacopoeia of India. Both are considered to be legally binding. Several sources are used for national monographs, including a national database on medicinal plants used in Ayurvedic medicine and monographs contained in the national pharmacopoeias. Manufacturing regulatory requirements include adherence to information contained in pharmacopoeias and monographs and the same GMP rules required for conventional pharmaceuticals. Drug licensing, inspection and testing are employed to ensure compliance with these requirements. Safety requirements include those required for conventional pharmaceuticals, as well as special requirements of traditional use without demonstrated harmful effects and reference to documented scientific research on similar products. No control mechanism is used for these requirements, as the long-standing use of herbal medicines in the Ayurveda, Unani and Siddha systems demonstrates their safety for human use.

In 1993 an expert committee appointed by the Indian Government developed guidelines for the safety and efficacy of herbal medicines which were intended to be incorporated into the

Drugs and Cosmetics Act and Rules. It was proposed that no new herbal medicines other than those authorized by the licensing authorities be allowed to be manufactured or marketed, except for those mentioned in and manufactured in compliance with the formulae given in the 'authoritative' books for ASU herbal medicines. A manufacturer of a new herbal medicine must include safety data and appropriate efficacy data in the marketing authorization application. Herbal preparations are defined as natural products in which the predominant active constituents are of plant origin. A classification for herbal medicines was proposed depending on their market availability, and the nature of herbs.

- Category 1: already in use for more than 5 years
- Category 2: in use for less than 5 years
- Category 3: new medicines.

The classification depends on whether the herbal medicines contain processed or unprocessed parts of plants and whether they contain potentially poisonous plants. Requirements for safety and efficacy vary according to the classification and market availability of the product. Depending on the nature of herbs and market availability, different requirements exist for submission of clinical trial data and toxicity data.

There are 4,246 registered herbal medicines and essential drug lists exist separately for the three systems of traditional medicine in India; the Ayurveda has 315 herbal medicines on its essential drug list, the Unani list has 244 herbal medicines and the Siddha list has 98. These lists were issued in 1999, 2000 and 2001, respectively. In India, herbal medicines are sold in pharmacies as prescription and OTC medicines, in traditional medicine outlets by licensed practitioners without much restriction. Annual herb sales figures, based on sales of 162 medicinal plants between 1999 and 2000, were estimated at Rs. 6,705 million (US $149 million). Recognizing the global demand, the Government of India mandates GMPs for pharmacies manufacturing ASU medicines to improve the quality and standard of drugs in the June 2000 amendment to the Drugs and Cosmetics Act, 1940. Department of Indian Systems of Medicine and Homeopathy (ISM&H) has framed safety and efficacy regulations for licensing new patent and proprietary botanical medicines. Indian pharmacopoeia covers a few Ayurvedic medicines and monographs have been given for some Ayurvedic drugs like clove, guggul, opium, mentha and senna. The Ayurvedic Pharmacopoeia of India gives monographs for 258 different Ayurvedic drugs and The Indian Drug Manufacturers Association (IDMA) has published Indian Herbal Pharmacopoeia with 52 monographs of widely used medicinal plants found in India. The latest available scientific data has been incorporated in these monographs.

Traditional Knowledge Digital Library (TKDL) is an original proprietary database fully protected under national and international laws of Intellectual Property Rights containing information on names of traditionally used medicinal plants, traditional description of diseases under their modern names and therapeutic formulations. Enabled by decoding software it facilitates automatic conversion of information from Sanskrit to various European languages. Also the Indian Medicines Development Corporation Bill, 2005 established a corporation exclusively to promote and develop Indian systems of medicine. The Traditional Herbal Medicines Act, 2006 was introduced in the Indian Parliament to regulate the sale of traditional herbal medicines which are being marketed without any licence and control under the cover of being manufactured as traditional formulations.

For herbal remedies and medicinal plants that are to be clinically evaluated for use in the allopathic system and which may be used in allopathic hospitals, the procedure laid down by the office of the Drugs Controller General of India for allopathic drugs should be followed. When an extract of a plant or a compound isolated from the plant has to be clinically evaluated for a therapeutic effect not originally described in the texts of traditional systems or if the method of preparation is different, it has to be treated as a new substance or new chemical entity (NCE) and the same type of acute, sub-acute and chronic toxicity data will have to be generated as required by the regulatory authority before it is cleared for clinical evaluation.

An extract or a compound isolated from a plant which has never before been mentioned in ancient literature should be treated as a new drug, and therefore, should undergo all regulatory requirements before being evaluated clinically.

The June 2000 amendment to the Drugs and Cosmetics Act provides general guidelines on clinical trials of herbals, toxicity studies, need for standardization and compliance with GCP in all clinical trials. Some of its recommendations include adherence to GMP guidelines for manufacture and standardization. For herbal remedies, it is not necessary to undertake Phase I studies and for those requiring usage for more than three months, 4–6 weeks' toxicity studies in two species of animals are needed for Phase II and Phase III trials. Clinical trials should be carried out with herbal preparations only after standardization and identification of markers to ensure that the substances being evaluated are always the same. Also ethical guidelines for biomedical research like patient information, informed consent, protection of vulnerable populations etc. should be followed. Clinical trials should be approved by the appropriate scientific and ethical committees of the concerned institutes. Clinical trials should be carried out when a competent ASU physician is a co-investigator.

Saudi Arabia

The market

In Saudi Arabia, herbal medicines are sold in pharmacies as prescription and over the counter medicines and in special outlets without restriction. A national research institute on herbal medicines is part of King Saud University.

Legal status

The Kingdom of Saudi Arabia is currently developing a national policy, laws and regulations on TM/CAM.

Herbal products come under the purview of The Practice of the Pharmacy Profession and Trade in Pharmaceuticals and Medical Products Act. According to articles 44 and 50 issued by the Royal Decree, registration of medicinal products by the Ministry of Health is obligatory. As per paragraphs 13A of the special provision of regulation for registration amended through ministerial resolution, apart from drugs all products with medical claims or containing active ingredients with medicinal effects such as herbal preparations, health and supplementary food, medicated cosmetics, antiseptics and medical devices need to be registered.

Regulation

Herbal medicine regulation in Saudi Arabia was established in 1996 is the issue of a separate law specifically for herbal medicines. The regulatory categories for herbal medicines include over the counter medicines, dietary supplements, health foods and functional foods. By law, medical, health, nutrient content and structural function claims may be made. An herbal preparation is defined as a product prepared for therapeutic and/or prophylactic use, the active ingredients of which are of plant origin. The definition is limited to preparations to be administered locally, orally, rectally or by inhalation. In accordance with 'Regulations for Registration of Herbal preparations, Health and Supplementary Food, Cosmetics and Antiseptics that have medicinal claims' issued by the Ministry of Health of the Kingdom of Saudi Arabia, the formal application for registration which is submitted to the General Directorate of Medicinal and Phamaceutical Licences at the Ministry of Health is based on registration of the products in the country of origin. Therefore documents such as manufacturing licences, free sales certificates and GMP certificates have to be submitted with information on composition, therapeutic category, certificate of analysis, percentage of alcohol and in case of ingredients of animal origin, the kind of animal. Furthermore full specifications and methods of analysis of the finished product, data on stability studies and storage conditions, six samples of the product and of the outer package and label together with abstracts of scientific references testifying to the efficacy and safety of the product have to be submitted. Handling of locally produced or imported products is prohibited before registration by the Ministry of Health. After registration it is not allowed to make any change in the composition, specification, method of manufacturing, indications, container or package unless it has been approved by the authority. A registration may be cancelled by the authorities under certain preconditions. The registration committee reviews registered products after three years from the date of registration, or as deemed necessary, to consider for re-registration.

CONCLUSION

The last few decades have witnessed pandemic herbal drug usage against the setting of rising global disease burden outweighing the technological advancements and introduction of newer synthetics and biologicals in the growing pharmaceutical industry. Explosive population growth in the developing world, increasing interest in industrialized nations and ensuing huge international market for herbal products is driving health authorities across nations to regulate herbal drug trade. The need of the hour is more productive assessment and greater availability of safe and effective herbal medicines through operative regulation of long-used traditional remedies. In exploring specific analytical solutions tailored to evaluate the unique/holistic pharmacology of these traditional remedies lies the key to realizing these goals. Work of the WHO combined with the regulatory efforts of its member states supplemented with future research solutions will hopefully resolve herbal drug quality control issues resulting in enhanced health care on a worldwide basis.

(**REVIEW QUESTIONS**)

Essay Questions

1. Outline the milestones that resulted in the need for herbal drug regulation.
2. Compare the regulatory status of herbal drugs in the Canada and European Union.
3. Write an essay on the current regulatory status of TCM in China.

Short Notes

1. Kampo drugs.
2. US regulatory bodies for Herbal drugs.
3. Herbal drug status is Germany.
4. Indian Herbal drug regulation.
5. Objectives of herbal drug regulation.

Herbal Institutes and Industries Working on Medicinal Plants in India

5

CHAPTER OBJECTIVES

Introduction

Global Volume of Trade in Herbal Drugs

India's Advantage

India's Initiatives

Central Governmental Establishments

State Level Governmental and Non-governmental Organizations

Commercial Herbal Drug Industry

INTRODUCTION

Global resurgence of interest in medicinal plants has resulted in explosive growth of the herbal drug industry. Today modern medicine uses 7,000 compounds that may be sourced to plants. Natural products have until recently been the primary source of commercial medicines and drug leads. A recent survey revealed that 61% of the 877 drugs introduced worldwide can be traced to or were inspired by natural products. Lukewarm results for the search for new compounds from synthetic chemistry and/or combinatorial chemistry has led only recently to a newfound respect for the privileged structures inherent within natural products. The World Health Organization (WHO) estimates that 80% of the population of developing countries relies on traditional medicines, mostly plant drugs for its primary heath care needs. Even the modern pharmacopoeia contains at least 25% drugs derived from plants and many others, which are semi-synthetic, are built on prototype compounds isolated from plants. Medicinal plants are the major components of all indigenous or alternative systems of medicine. Use of indigenous drugs from plant origin forms a major part of complementary and alternative medicine.

GLOBAL VOLUME OF HERBAL DRUG TRADE – INDIA'S CONCERN

Medicinal plants are essentially consumed either as traditional medicines administered by traditional practitioners to the local population or as plant-derived commercial medicines dispensed as patented/licensed products on prescription or as over-the-counter (OTC) drugs. The latter mostly are products of allopathy with even products of traditional systems of medicine such as herbal nutritional supplements, cosmetics and essential oil formulations coming under this category. The economic value of both these categories of products depends on several factors:

- Multiple medicinal applications and usage in a number of formulations because of higher therapeutic effect as in the case of 'elite species' like neem and sandalwood.
- Single plant species of great market value on account of being the only known curative, for e.g., *Catharanthus roseus* yields vincristine that is specifically used to treat leukemia.
- Overexploited, high-in-demand medicinal plants like Rauwolfia that are difficult to cultivate and occur in localized areas in specific environmental conditions, on account of their low availability fetch high prices.
- High processing costs due to poor yield e.g. 1 tonne of vinca leaves are to be processed to isolate 1 g of vincristine.
- Structural complexity, novelty and powerful biological activity of plant-derived biomolecules that are either difficult to synthesize and/or are less efficacious.
- Urgent need for processed, consumer usable, value enhanced product rather than direct-harvested plant material.

In addition, costs of cultivation, transportation, packaging, further screening, processing, compound isolation, standardization, clinical testing etc. determine the overall cost of plant-based products.

The global trade in medicinal plants being secretive and unregulated, a large part of it is neither documented nor do trade statistics distinguish the therapeutic value of a plant from its other uses. However the current world market for herbal medicine including herbal products and raw materials has been estimated at US $62 billion with an annual growth rate of 5% to 15%, and it is expected to grow to US $5 trillion by the year 2050. The herbal food supplement market is estimated to have an even higher growth rate of 25%. A similar trend is envisaged for the herbal cosmetics market. The importance accredited to herbal drugs is reflected in the resent upsurge in the demand for herbal remedies in the international market. This is partly fuelled by the recognition of plant-based drugs in the policies of the United States and United Kingdom. These countries have set up national institutes and departments of complementary and alternative medicines that are investigating the scientific basis of the efficacy of traditional medicines. In the global herbal market European Union (EU) has the biggest share of 45% while North America accounts for 11%, Japan 16%, Asian countries 19% and rest of EU 4.1%. The rising demand for herbal drugs has put pressure on the ecosystems of the developing countries from where the bulk of the raw material is derived from the wild. This growing market demand is to be taken as an opportunity by these countries to explore the potential of medicinal plants for their sustainable socio-economic development.

The global market for medicinal plant-based raw drugs alone is estimated to be worth more than US $5 billion per annum. India's export share in this is about 8% with China (24%) and the United States (11%) being the leaders. However India's global market share becomes negligible

(0.3%) if the annual global herbal market including medicines, cosmaceuticals and food supplements valued at US $62 billion is taken into consideration. Thus India's contribution to the global herbal market however is a meager US $1 billion annually. Countries like Japan, China and South Korea have successfully marketed their traditional medicines abroad. Their alternative therapies are well accepted in Europe and the United States. Products like ginseng – the famed aphrodisiac similar in property to ashwagandha, an Ayurvedic medicine, – accounts for over US $800 million of international market as compared to all our herbs put together. Thus in the level of penetration of the global market, India does not figure anywhere near China or Japan.

The global herbal trade is estimated to be growing at an annual rate of about 7%. While the likelihood of a proportional increase in India's share in the raw drug component is fairly high, a similar increase in its share in the finished product component is a highly doubtful. It is especially so in view of the stringent and unfavourable drug control legislations in the developed countries towards Indian Systems of Medicine (ISM) formulations.

India is unable to benefit from the escalating growth trend of the herbal drug trade due to the following constraints:

1. Need for evaluation of therapeutic potential of traditional drugs of age old usage as per WHO guidelines.
2. Ensuring availability of these drugs in standardized form as products of uniform quality.
3. Lack of information on the full potential of traditional drugs in the international community due in part to the lack of complete comprehension of Ayurvedic therapeutics in current scientific understanding.
4. Lack of awareness of the needs of the international market by traditional drug manufacturers along with dearth of technology to upgrade their produce to global needs.
5. Need for extensive documentation of traditional usage of medicinal herbs since centuries to protect them from exploitation and biopiracy as well as for patent protection.
6. Need for the development of sustainable cultivation methods and processing technologies to harness traditional medical knowledge for socio-economic development without threat to our biodiversity.
7. Ruling out adulteration, substitution, heavy metal and microbial contamination in every plant-based product that has been documented properly with regard to the identification of species and specific plant part utilized.
8. Lack of well-organized management of medicinal plant trade with adequate promotional strategies concurrent to orientation of indigenous population towards increasing global demand for medicinal plants to ensure employment and equitable profits to the grass-root level people.

INDIA'S ADVANTAGE

India however has the richest medical tradition in the world. It is a gold mine of well-recorded and traditionally well-practised knowledge of herbal medicine. It is the largest producer of medicinal herbs and is rightly called the botanical garden of the world. There are very few medicinal herbs of commercial importance which are not found in this country. India officially recognizes over 3,000 plants for their medicinal value. It is generally estimated that over 6,000 plants in India are in use in traditional, folk and herbal medicine, representing about 75% of the medicinal needs of the third world countries. Three of the 10 most widely selling herbal medicines in the developed countries namely preparations of *Allium sativum*, *Aloe barbadensis* and *Panax* species are available in India. It covers only 7% of the earth's land surface, yet harbours more than 70% of the total plant species. It has a vast variety of flora and fauna commanding 7% of the world biodiversity and supports 16 major forest areas.

A land of immense biodiversity in which 2 out of the 18 hot spots of the world are located, India is also one of the 12 mega-biodiversity countries in the world. The total number of plant species of all groups explored so far is 45,000. Of these seed-bearing plants account for nearly 15,000–18,000. India enjoys the benefits of varied climate, from alpine in Himalaya to tropical wet in the south and arid in Rajasthan. Such climatic conditions have given rise to rich and varied flora in the Indian subcontinent.

With the large growth forecast figures for the herbal drug market by the year 2050, it is evident that herbal remedies would become increasingly important especially in developing countries. Low cost of man power, rich accumulated traditional knowledge on medicinal plants, large biodiversity and lowering international trade barriers give India a tremendous potential and advantage in this emerging area, which need to be capitalized on.

INDIA'S INITIATIVES

The National Health Policy, 1983 has reiterated the efficacy and cost effectiveness of Indian traditional medicine and recognized the need for ending the long neglect of these systems in our health care strategy. The policy emphasized the need for a meaningful phased integration of ISM with modern medicines and has called for augmentation of budgetary support and extension of fiscal incentives and concessions available to the modern pharmaceutical industry to be made available to the ISM sector. Recognizing the urgency to explore India's potential advantage and expand India's share in the world herbal drug market, the Indian government initiated the establishment of several premier organizations (Figure 5.1) all over the country to engage in a plethora of medicinal plant-related promotional activities ranging from fundamental research to identification, cultivation, documentation, training, standardization etc. To this effect it has restructured and expanded existing bodies, instituted newer programmes to enable planned, integrated progress in all areas of health care and human development particularly agriculture and food products, rural development, education, social welfare, tourism, housing, water supply, sanitation etc.

The Planning Commission of India in its 'Task force on Conservation and Sustainable Use of Medicinal Plants' had recommended the following action plan among others for the comprehensive development of the medicinal plant sector:

1. Establishment of 200 Medicinal Plant Conservation Areas.
2. Establishment of 200 'Vanaspati Van' in forest areas for commercial supply of crude drugs to pharmacies and exports to be managed by a registered society.
3. About 100 endangered, rare and threatened medicinal plants should be grown in botanical gardens.
4. Direction to the three gene banks at Central Institute of Medicinal and Aromatic Plants, Lucknow, National Bureau of Plant Genetic Resources, New Delhi and Tropical Botanical Garden and Research Institute at Trivandrum to store germplasm of all medicinal plants.

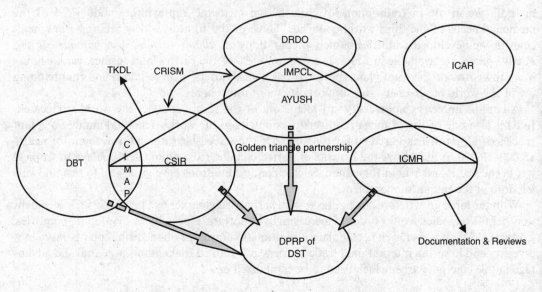

Figure 5.1. Governmental agencies promoting herbal drug sector

5. Forest Departments to effectively identify and map areas rich in medicinal plants, manage the harvesting, extraction and transport of medicinal plants from the wild and maintain list of traders, private agents, wholesale dealers and final consumers of medicinal plants to streamline trade activities.

6. Identifying non-governmental organizations (NGOs) to aid the government in promoting awareness and availability of seeds and planting material to farmers, encouraging medicinal plant cultivation through organic farming.

7. Initiate efforts to ensure quality of herbal drugs through standardization, active molecule identification and overall quality improvement utilizing tools and techniques of biotechnology and genetic engineering.

8. Accelerate search for new molecules and their development as new drugs concurrent to their standardization and patenting.

9. Formalizing and organizing medicinal plant trade through the establishment of a National Medicinal Plants Board with adequate representation being given to all stakeholders.

10. Ensuring appropriate policy, legislation and financial support to the sector towards greening the country, generating employment and enhancing health care standards.

11. Cataloguing ancient medical manuscripts to retrieve the wealth of knowledge that is lying scattered in oriental libraries and in private collections. Creation of such a database shall rightfully establish our claim on this knowledge thus protecting our medical wisdom from overseas patenting.

As part of efforts towards meeting these goals, the Government of India launched several schemes:

(i) Extra Mural Research project of AYUSH to enable accreditation of organizations for research and development (R&D) in traditional medical systems;

(ii) Golden triangle partnership (GTP) scheme between AYUSH, CSIR and ICMR;

(iii) National Medicinal Plants Board was set up for coordinating all matters relating to medicinal plants, including drawing up policies and strategies for conservation, proper harvesting, cost effective cultivation, R&D, processing, marketing of raw material in order to protect, sustain and develop this sector;

(iv) AYUSH identified as nodal agency to enable Traditional Knowledge Digital Library for the documentation and digitalization of indigenous knowledge for availability to patent examiners to prevent grant of patents to indigenous knowledge;

(v) New Millennium Indian Technology Leadership Initiative (NMITLI) launched by CSIR to attain a global leadership position in a 'team India spirit' for Indian industry by synergizing the best competencies of publicly funded R&D institutions, academia and private industry;

(vi) Technology Development Board (TDB) provides financial assistance to industrial concerns and other agencies attempting development and commercialization of indigenous technology to wider domestic applications;

(vii) Scheme on home-grown technology of TIFAC of DST basically promotes Indian capabilities for the development of novel products and processes in different areas including the pharma sector and herbal sector;

(viii) Drugs and Pharmaceuticals Research Programme of DST is implemented to synergize the strength of R&D institutions and Indian pharmaceutical industry for discovery and introduction of new drugs;

(ix) National Panel on Bhasmas for identification of thrust areas of R&D in the areas of Bhasmas and Kushtas – much more economical drug delivery systems – and setting up of national facilities for the said purpose.

In addition to the government initiatives, several national and international organizations are actively involved in different parts of India to promote awareness, documentation and conservation strategies for medicinal plants. Several NGOs are working in the areas of conservation and developing cultivation strategies. A brief overview of the agenda and achievements of prime governmental and non-governmental agencies involved in promoting research and utilization of Indian medicinal plants follows.

CENTRAL GOVERNMENTAL ESTABLISHMENTS

1. AYUSH

Department of Ayurveda, Yoga and Naturopathy, Unani, Siddha and Homeopathy was formerly called the Departments of Indian Systems of Medicine and Homeopathy (ISM&H). AYUSH is the latest statutory effort in the series of attempts at reviving traditional medicine in India.

Ayurveda and Siddha, ancient medical systems in vogue in this country since earliest times, are fully developed medical traditions that have been serving the needs of our people. Complete by themselves they developed gradually and systematically over the centuries under the aegis of legendary scholars and physicians on the basis of a unique philosophy guided by time-tested methodologies and practices prevalent in that era. Foreign invasions, cross-cultural interaction and lack of support from the ruling British were the reasons for the stagnation of these ancient medical systems. The wealth of medical knowledge of these systems, which is presently receiving worldwide recognition is what was current and updated centuries ago. This reflects the potential of the therapeutic knowledge, which is answering several unaddressed medical needs of today, despite lying mostly untapped since then.

The beginning of the 20th century saw efforts to revive these systems. The members of the Imperial Legislative Council passed a resolution to investigate and recognize these systems and it was accepted in the year 1916. This led to the establishment of a number of colleges of Ayurveda. In the post-independence era, the efforts to develop research gained momentum. As per the recommendations of the various committees, grant-in-aid projects were sanctioned to selected colleges. The Central Council for Ayurvedic Research as an advisory body was established in 1962 and finally the Central Council for Research in Indian Medicine and Homeopathy (CCRIM&H) was established in 1969. This council initiated research programmes in ISM and homeopathy in different parts of the country and started coordination at the national level for the first time. Upon its reorganization the Central Councils for Research in Ayurveda and Siddha (CCRAS) and Homeopathy (CCRH) were established in 1978 for the formulation, coordination and development of research in these systems on scientific lines. An independent identity under the Ministry of Health and Family Welfare was created for The Indian Systems of Medicine and Homeopathy (ISM&H) in 1995. It was renamed Department of AYUSH, Ayurveda, Yoga and Naturopathy, Unani, Siddha and Homeopathy, in November 2003.

Agenda of AYUSH

Developing and propagating these officially recognized traditional medical systems by

1. Encouraging scientific research and regulating education standards;
2. Promoting cultivation and regeneration of medicinal plants;
3. Laying down pharmacopoeial standards to ensure quality drugs by following good manufacturing practices (GMP) and evolving good laboratory practices;
4. Supplementing state governments' efforts in setting up speciality clinics of AYUSH in allopathic hospitals and AYUSH wing in district allopathic hospitals;
5. Creating and spreading awareness by effective communication strategies to reach all sections of people.

While the Central Acts empower implementation of the set objectives, Ayurveda, Siddha, Unani and Homeopathy drugs are covered under the purview of Drugs and Cosmetics Act, 1940. AYUSH medicines being predominantly plant derived, the National Medicinal Plants Board was set up to promote cultivation of medicinal plants and to ensure sustained availability of quality raw material. A separate National Policy on ISM is in place since 2002.

The infrastructure under AYUSH sector consists of 1,355 hospitals with 53,296 bed capacity; 22,635 dispensaries; 450 undergraduate colleges; 99 colleges having post-graduate departments; 9,493 licensed manufacturing units; and 7.8 lakh registered practitioners of ISM and homeopathy in the country. An outlay of Rs. 4,000 crores has been allocated for the department during the 11th five year plan with Rs. 440 crores for medicinal plants alone. The administrative units under AYUSH umbrella is given in Figure 5.2. The department has three subordinate offices, one public sector undertaking, two statutory organizations, four research councils, 11 educational

---

Subordinate Offices
Pharmacopoeial Laboratory for Indian Medicine
Homeopathic Pharmacopoeial Laboratory
Ayurved Hospital, New Delhi

Public Sector Undertaking
Indian Medicines Pharmacopoeial Corporation

Statutory Regulatory Councils
Central Council of Indian Medicine
Central Council of Homeopathy

Research Councils
Central Council of Research in Ayurveda and Siddha
Central Council of Research in Unani Medicine
Central Council of Research in Homeopathy
Central Council of Research in Yoga and Naturopathy

National Institutes
National Institute of Ayurveda, Jaipur
National Institute of Siddha, Chennai
National Institute of Unani Medicine, Bangalore
Morarji Desai National Institute of Yoga, New Delhi
National Institute of Naturopathy, Pune
National Institute of Homeopathy, Kolkata
The Rashtriya Ayurveda Vidyapeeth, Delhi
The All India Institute of Ayurveda, New Delhi
North Eastern Institute of Folk Medicine, Pasighat
Institute of Post-Graduate Teaching and Research in Ayurveda, Jamnagar
North Eastern Institute of Ayurveda and Homeopathy, Shillong

National Medicinal Plant Board
35 State and UT level Medicinal Plant Boards

Figure 5.2. Administrative units under AYUSH

institutions and a national medicinal plant board (with 35 state/UT level boards) under its administrative fold.

Subordinate offices

The pharmacopoeial laboratories situated at Ghaziabad have been set up as national drug testing laboratories to lay down the standards and undertake testing for identity, purity and quality of drugs under the respective medical systems. The worked out standards are published as monographs under the respective pharmacopoeias. The Ayurved Hospital at New Delhi, established in 1978, provides general and specialized therapies in Ayurveda.

Central public sector undertaking

Established at Mohan (Almora Dist.), Uttarakhand, Indian Medicines Pharmaceutical Corporation (IMPCL) manufactures over 300 authentic Ayurvedic and Unani medicines according to classic texts for catering to the needs of dispensaries of Central Government Health Scheme (CGHS), units of Central Research Councils of Ayurveda and Unani and state government institutions. A cGMP certified lab, it attained a record sale of Rs. 8.42 crores in the year 2005–2006.

Statutory regulatory councils

The statutory regulatory councils are the Central Council of Indian Medicine (CCIM) and the Central Council for Homeopathy (CCH). Set up under the Acts of Parliament, these councils are primarily concerned with regulating education and practice of the respective systems of medicine. They advise the government regarding education, prescribe course curricula, evolve and maintain standards of education and maintain Central Registers of Practitioners in these medical systems.

Research councils

The four apex councils, namely CCRAS, Central Council for Research in Unani Medicine (CCRUM), CCRH and Central Council of Research in Yoga and Naturopathy (CCRYN), implement research and development activities related to AYUSH under their various intra- and extra-mural research programmes.

CCRAS is an autonomous body under the Department of AYUSH, Ministry of Health and Family Welfare, Government of India. Its activities are carried out through its 38 institutes/units located all over India and through a number of units located in universities/institutes/hospitals of Ayurveda and Siddha. The practice, education and research in the Amchi System of Medicine is also under the supervision of CCRAS. The council funds research studies in all these disciplines with emphasis on finding effective, low-cost remedies for selected diseases through systematic research. Research activities of the council include clinical research, health care and drug research, nutraceutical and cosmaceutical research, literary research and family welfare research.

CCRUM, also an autonomous organization, was established in 1979 to initiate, develop and coordinate scientific research in Unani system of medicine. The council's research programme comprises clinical research, drug standardization, i.e., development of standard operating procedures for compound formulations, survey, development of agro techniques for domestication and cultivation of medicinal plants and literary research. Its activities are carried out through a network of 22 institutes/units functioning in different parts of the country.

CCRH, fully funded by the government, functions through a network of 40 institutes/units throughout the country and is engaged in fundamental and basic research on mechanism of action of homeopathic medicines, clinical trials for predetermined protocols, drug-proving research, drug standardization, survey, collection and cultivation of medicinal plants.

CCRYN is a society registered under the Societies Registration Act as an autonomous body under AYUSH. Its basic objective is to conduct scientific research in the field of yoga and naturopathy and also to regulate education, training and propagation of these disciplines. Currently it is identifying NGOs to engage in clinical verification, literature research/translation/publication-related activities, establishment of treatment-cum-propagation centres and patient care centres.

National institutes

The following are the 11 national institutes under AYUSH established to promote excellence in ISM and Homeopathy education:

1. National Institute of Ayurveda, Jaipur
2. National Institute of Siddha, Chennai
3. National Institute of Unani Medicine, Bengaluru
4. Morarji Desai National Institute of Yoga, New Delhi
5. National Institute of Naturopathy, Pune
6. National Institute of Homeopathy, Kolkata
7. The Rashtriya Ayurveda Vidyapeeth, Delhi
8. The All India Institute of Ayurveda, New Delhi
9. North Eastern Institute of Folk Medicine, Pasighat.

10. Institute of Post Graduate Teaching and Research in Ayurveda, Jamnagar
11. North Eastern Institute of Ayurveda and Homeopathy, Shillong.

National Medicinal Plant Board (NMPB)

Medicinal plants are a living resource, exhaustible if overused and sustainable if used with care and wisdom. They are not only a resource base for the traditional medicine and herbal industry but also provide livelihood and health security to a large segment of the Indian population. About 960 species of medicinal plants are estimated to be in trade of which 178 species have annual consumption levels in excess of 100 metric tonnes. Domestic trade of the AYUSH industry is of the order of Rs. 80–90 billion. India at present exports herbal materials and medicines to the tune of Rs.1,000 crores only while it has been estimated that this can be raised to Rs. 12,000 crores by 2012. World trade in herbal products being US $120 billion, it is expected to reach US $7 trillion by 2050. The Chinese export based on plants including raw drugs, therapeutics and other is estimated to be around Rs. 18,000–Rs. 22,000 crores. In view of the innate Indian strengths which inter alia include diverse ecosystems, technical and farming capacity and a strong manufacturing sector, the medicinal plants area can become a huge export opportunity after fulfilling domestic needs.

Apart from requirement of medicinal plants for internal consumption, India exports crude drugs mainly to developed countries, namely the United States, Germany, France, Switzerland, UK and Japan, who share between them 75% to 80% of the total export of crude drugs from India. Medicinal plants market in the country is today unorganized due to several problems that affect it directly and indirectly.

1. At present 95% collection of medicinal plants is from the wild. Current practices of harvesting are unsustainable and many studies have highlighted depletion of resource base.
2. Pharmaceutical companies are partly responsible for inefficient, imperfect, informal and opportunistic marketing of medicinal plants.
3. There is a vast, secretive and largely unregulated trade in medicinal plants, mainly from the wild, which continues to grow dramatically in the absence of serious policy attention with environmental planning.
4. Confusion also exists in the identification of plant material where the origin of a particular drug is assigned to more than one plant, leading to adulteration in such cases.
5. Marketing is a daunting problem, since marketability of products is a crucial factor in determining the success of a product.

A clear understanding of both supply-related issues and the factors driving the demand and size of the medicinal plants market is vital. This will ensure both the conservation and sustainable use of the habitats of these plants as well as ensure continued availability of the basic ingredients.

The medicinal plant board was set up under a government resolution to establish an agency which would be responsible for coordination of all matters relating to medicinal plants, including drawing up policies and strategies for conservation, proper harvesting, cost-effective cultivation, research and development, processing, marketing of raw material in order to protect, sustain and develop this sector.

Agenda of NMPB

- The board will address all issues connected with the conservation and sustainable use of medicinal plants leading to remunerative farming, regulation of medicinal farms and conservation of biodiversity.
- The work would continue to be carried out by the respective departments and organizations, but the board would provide a focus and a direction to the activities. In pursuance of the guidelines of the National Board, all the 35 Indian states and union territories have constituted State Medicinal Plant Boards to implement the schemes of NMPB and to explore the medicinal plant wealth of their states.
- The National Board will coordinate the efforts at the central and state levels to facilitate inter- ministry, interstate and institutional collaboration to avoid duplication of efforts.

Functions of the board

Coordination with ministries/departments/organizations/state/UT governments for development of medicinal plants in general and specifically in the following fields:

1. Assessment of demand/supply position relating to medicinal plants both within the country and abroad;
2. Advise concerned ministries/departments/organization/state/UT governments on policy matters relating to schemes and projects for development of medicinal plants;
3. Identification of market and market segmentation to address issues relating to import/export and establishment of an export authority;
4. Provide guidance in the formulation of proposals, schemes and projects by agencies with cultivable land and infrastructure for collection, storage and transportation of medicinal plants;
5. Identification, inventorying and quantification of medicinal plants;
6. Promotion of *ex situ* and *in situ* cultivation and conservation of medicinal plants;
7. Promotion of cooperative effort among collectors and growers and assisting them to store, transport and market their produce effectively;
8. Through its statutory status, the board will regulate registration of farmers, cooperative societies and transporters towards effective marketing of medicinal plants, their proper procurement and supply to the pharmaceutical industry;
9. Encouraging the protection of patent rights and IPR and facilitating the prevention of patents being obtained for medicinal use of plants which are in the public domain;
10. Matters relating to import/export of raw material, as well as value-added products either as medicine, food supplements or as herbal cosmetics including adoption of better techniques for marketing of products to increase their reputation for quality and reliability in the country and abroad;
11. Undertaking and awarding scientific, technological research and cost-effectiveness studies;
12. Development of protocols for cultivation and quality control.

The board offers various promotional and commercial schemes for the overall development of the designated 32 medicinal plants and even other plants of well-assured market to government organizations, registered growers, association/federations of growers, traders, manufacturers, societies, pharmaceutical companies, NGOs and recognized private research institutes or any group of people who have three years' experience in the medicinal plants sector.

The board considers promotional and commercial schemes relating to survey and inventorying, *in situ* conservation and *ex situ* cultivation, creating region-specific or species-specific herbal gardens, improved agro techniques including germplasm generation, awareness generating communication-related activities, demand-based marketing strategies, value addition or semi-processing products of medicinal plants and other research and development activities of medicinal plants for financial assistance.

Overseas Establishment of AYUSH – Centre for Research in Indian Systems of Medicine (CRISM)

Centre for Research in Indian Systems of Medicine (CRISM) is an Indo–US joint venture whose aim is to facilitate scientific validation and acceptance of ISM through collaborative research between India and the United States. It was jointly initiated under Memorandum of Understanding (MoU) for scientific cooperation in the field of botanicals between CSIR through its constituent Indian Institute of Integrative Medicine, Jammu with University of Mississippi through NCNPR in 2005. Department of AYUSH, CSIR, NCNPR and other external agencies including industry both in India and the United States are the partners of CRISM.

Department of AYUSH, having provided the financial support to this venture, also provides the necessary skill, expertise, knowledge and resources through its constituent councils, departments and other associated institutes engaged in R&D and teaching in areas of ISM and natural products for the development of ISM/herbal and botanical pharmaceuticals.

Agenda of CRISM

1. It encourages and facilitates cooperation for research activities between Indian and US academic and industrial institutions.

2. It facilitates dialogue between scientific community and regulatory bodies of the two countries to evolve a platform for such regular exchange.

3. This centre aims to provide and promote authentic information about the strengths of Indian system of medicine and to help demystify the misconceptions about these systems of medicine in the United States.

4. CRISM endeavours to get global recognition for our health care systems in order to position our products in the world market by enabling standardization of classical formulations, ensuring GMP and strengthening regulatory mechanism within India.

Achievements of Ayush

1. Collaboration with Russia – Three MoUs have been signed between the Government Institute of Ayurvedic Medicine, St.Petersburg and Indian Institutes namely National Institute of Ayurveda, Jaipur, CCRAS and Morarji Desai National Institute of Yoga, New Delhi.

2. On the request of an NGO based at Hungary a team of Ayurveda experts were deputed to this country in 2008 to give authentic training of Ayurvedic health care, massage and panchkarma methods to health personnel and masseurs of wellness units and spas.

3. The second meeting of the inter-ministerial task force was constituted by Department of AYUSH for promotion of traditional Indian medicine with the objective of identifying focus countries, creation of a database of NGOs working for AYUSH in foreign countries and AYUSH experts for international cooperation activities.

4. An MoU between AYUSH and The State Administration of Traditional Chinese Medicine, China was signed to envisage cooperation in policies relating to regulation and administration of traditional medicine in India and China.

5. A framework of cooperation was signed between Department of AYUSH and International Trade Center, Geneva with regard to international market development of Ayurveda, Siddha and Unani products.

6. An Ayurveda conference-cum-exhibition was organized by the Indian Embassy in Budapest, Hungary to showcase the strengths of Ayurveda and to explore the opportunities of possible collaborations with educational institutions and universities in the field of education and research.

7. AYUSH participated in WIPO's Intergovernmental Committee on Intellectual Property and Genetic Resources, Traditional Knowledge and Folklore at Geneva and highlighted India's concerns regarding misappropriation of its traditional knowledge and the need for an internationally binding legal instrument for protection of traditional knowledge and genetic resources.

8. Department of AYUSH deputed experts in Ayurveda for a period of one month in 2007 to the United States to deliver lectures to medical students under CME modular teaching at the medical schools of University of Connecticut and University of Washington.

9. As a part of an ongoing Indo-EU dialogue under the aegis of India-EU strategic partnership for economic cooperation, a three-member expert team from European Union Commission visited India in 2007 on a fact-finding mission to understand the regulatory, educational and other related aspects of Ayurveda. They suggested a simplified registration system for traditional medicinal products based on bibliographic evidence of safe use in the form of textual references of authentic classic texts and pharmacopoeias and formularies, absence of microbial impurities, pesticides, heavy metals etc.

10. India is represented by AYUSH in the International Regulatory Cooperation on Herbal Medicines, a network setup under the aegis of WHO. The forum provides a platform for electronic exchange of regulatory information of herbal/traditional medicines through a collaborative web space provided to individual focal points of each member country.

2. Council of Scientific and Industrial Research

The Council of Scientific & Industrial Research (CSIR), a premier industrial R &D organization in India was constituted in 1942 by a resolution of the then Central Legislative Assembly. It is an autonomous body registered under the Registration of Societies Act of 1860. CSIR aims to provide industrial competitiveness, social welfare, a strong science and technology base for strategic sectors and advancement of fundamental knowledge. Today CSIR is recognized as one of the world's largest publicly funded R&D organizations having linkages to academia, R&D organizations and industry. CSIR's 37 laboratories not only knit India into a giant network that impacts and adds quality to the life of each and every Indian, but is also party to the prestigious Global Research Alliance that seeks to apply global knowledge pool for global good through global funding. CSIR's R&D portfolio embraces areas as diverse as aerospace, biotechnology, chemicals etc. covering the entire spectrum of scientific activity in Indian science.

Health care, drugs and pharmaceuticals is a prominent sector under CSIR's mandate. CSIR has geared itself to face the challenges in this sector through measures to prioritize research programmes, creation of state-of-the-art facilities, induction of new talent and networking research within CSIR with other national agencies/industry to capitalize on their combined strength.

CSIR projects in this sector focus on new drugs based on our traditional knowledge, biodiversity, marine resources, new molecular targets for selected pathogens, *in silico* biology, predictive medicine, new animal models and animal substitute technologies.

Recent advances in biology such as genome sequencing have opened up unlimited opportunities in medicine. Technologies of combinatorial synthesis and high-throughput screening offer the potential to speed up drug discovery. CSIR has made valuable contributions to the industry and society by the development of several novel drugs.

Products developed under CSIR's composite mandate in the sector of health care, drugs and pharmaceuticals include herbal medicines, nutraceuticals, new drugs, diagnostics, vaccines, inventions, devices and gadgets for monitoring air, water, food contaminants/adulterants all of which comply with international regulatory requirements, quality and standards. Some of the CSIR laboratories at the forefront of herbal drug-related research are listed below (Figure 5.3).

a) Central Institute of Medicinal and Aromatic Plants, Lucknow

Popularly known as CIMAP, it is a frontier plant research laboratory, originally established as Central Medicinal Plants Organization (CMPO) in 1959. CIMAP is steering multidisciplinary

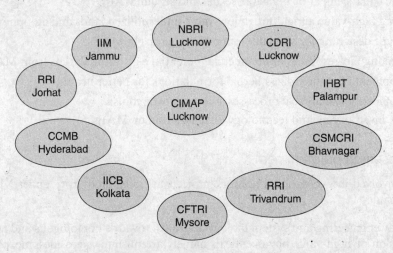

Figure 5.3 CSIR laboratories in herbal drug research

high-quality research in biological and chemical sciences and extending technologies and services to farmers and entrepreneurs of medicinal and aromatic plants (MAPs) with its research headquarters at Lucknow and research centres at Bangalore, Hyderabad, Pantnagar and Purara. CIMAP research centres are aptly located in different agroclimatic zones of the country to facilitate multilocation field trials and research. Fifty years since its inception CSIR today has extended its wings to Malaysia with CSIR-CIMAP having signed two bilateral cooperation agreements between India and Malaysia in research, development and commercialization of MAP-related technologies.

CIMAP's contribution to the Indian economy through its MAP research is well known. Mint varieties released and agro-packages developed and popularized by CIMAP have made India the global leader in mints and related industrial products. It has released several varieties of MAPs, their complete agro-technology and post-harvesting packages which have revolutionized MAP cultivation and business scenario in the country.

Facilities

CIMAP is equipped with state-of-the-art multidisciplinary laboratories, ultra-modern instrumentation facilities and scientific expertise in agriculture, genetics and plant breeding, molecular taxonomy, molecular and structural biology, plant biotechnology, biochemistry, microbiology, bioenergy and chemical sciences, apart from development of herbal products. CIMAP houses the National Gene Bank of MAPs, in addition to seed gene bank, tissue and DNA bank. Further Field Gene Bank of different varieties of MAPs is maintained at CIMAP and its four research centres situated across the country.

Major research areas

1. Gene bank utilization strategies, conservation and bio-prospecting genes/molecules/products;
2. Genetic enhancement of obligate asexual and sexual MAPs;
3. Enabling high-value agriculture in low-value underutilized lands and cropping systems;
4. Genotype designing for speciality/opportunity crops in MAPs;
5. Prospecting bio-resources of commercial potential e.g., antimalarials from MAPs;
6. Development of standardized herbal formulations for better health;
7. Development of analytical processes and diagnostic tools;
8. Survey, inventorying and technology dissemination of MAPs.

Flagship research programmes

CIMAP is involved in two national network projects as nodal laboratory under XII Five Year Plan that include

a. Pathway engineering and system biology approach towards homologous and heterologous expression of high-value phytoceuticals namely artemisinin, picrosides, morphine, withanolides, podophyllotoxin etc.

b. Biological and chemical transformations of plant compounds for production of value-added products of therapeutic/aroma value.

CIMAP is a participating laboratory in seven national network projects on
   a. Exploitation of India's microbial diversity;
   b. Remediation/eco-restoration and clean-up of contaminated ground water and water resources;
   c. Discovery, development and commercialization of new bioactive and traditional preparations;
   d. Comprehensive traditional knowledge digital documentation and library;
   e. Neem and artemisia.

Publications

To facilitate laboratories to market journey of medicinal and aromatic crops, CIMAP documents and creates scientific knowledge base relevant to MAPs for their effective utilization through its various publications namely

   i. Farm bulletins in Hindi, English and regional languages on various economically important MAPs, e.g., mint, lemongrass, palmarosa, geranium, withania, artemisia etc.
   ii. Training manuals – 'Aus Saathi' MAPs Companion
   iii. Crop calendars
   iv. Composite research journal – Journal of Medicinal and Aromatic Plant Sciences.

Patents

CIMAP has an IP portfolio of more than 135 foreign and Indian patents granted in

- major medicinal and aromatic plants including molecules and bioactives – 17
- improved new processes – 52
- new methods and techniques – 13
- Formulations and compositions – 36
- Plant varieties – 23
- Cell cultures/enzymes/strains – 06

Major impact-making patents that resulted in major marketable technologies from CIMAP are

- Artemisia cultivation method (US 6,39,376)
- CIM-Arogya herb processing for artemisinin (IN 176679)
- Development of arteether (IN 173947)
- Artemisinin extraction process (US 5,955,08)
- CIM-Arogya, genetically tagged high-yielding variety of Artemisia annua and its cultivation technology (US 6,393,763)
- Cultivar Himalaya and Kosi of menthol mint (PP 10935, PP 12426)
- Method of producing mint plant kushal (US 6,420,174).

Recognition

CIMAP Gene Bank established in 1993 as a follow-up action taken in the summit of G-15 countries held at Caracas is one of the three national gene banks of the country that focuses on the conservation of MAPs of India in the form of seed, field, tissue and DNA banks.

CIMAP has been designated by Protection of Plant Varieties and Farmers' Rights Authority (PPV&FRA) as the nodal laboratory for developing National Test Guidelines for plant varieties' protection and distinctiveness, uniformity and stability (DUS) testing of MAPs and seed species.

National Biodiversity Authority of India has recognized CIMAP as a Designated National Repository (DNR) under the Biological Diversity Act, 2002, to keep in safe custody specimens of different categories of biological material.

CIMAP has been recognized as the focal point for South East Asia by International Centre for Science and High Technology, United Nations Industrial Development Organization (ICS-UNIDO).

National and international linkages

1. CIMAP has established alliances with Indian Institute of Agricultural Research (IIAR), Gandhinagar (Gujarat) and North East Institute of Science and Technology (NIEST), Jorhat (Assam) for multiplier effect for its endeavour in western and northeast region respectively.
2. Scientific collaboration with Bulgarian Academy of Science for rose oil technology.
3. CIMAP has entered into a scientific agreement with Special Innovation Unit (UNIK) Office of the Prime Minister of Malaysia and Monash University, Sunaway Campus, Malaysia, envisaging establishment of a Joint Innovation Accelerator Centre to carry out research on areas of mutual interest such as green technologies, MAPs and other innovative technologies using CIMAP expertise in Malaysia. CIMAP and UNIK will explore and develop the use of herbs, plants, flowers and fruits for medicinal and aromatic purposes in Malaysia by way of improving extraction techniques, modern processes and herbal products.

Academic alliances

In order to strengthen functional relationship between the universities and laboratories of CSIR, CIMAP has signed MoUs with several universities including Jawaharlal Nehru University (JNU), GB Pant University of Agriculture & Technology (GBPUAT), Pantnagar, Chandra Shekhar Azad University of Agriculture and Technology (CSAUAT), Kanpur, Banaras Hindu University (BHU), Universities of Allahabad and Lucknow among others.

Towards the mission of bringing scientific excellence through university-research institution joint efforts, CIMAP has been recognized by JNU, New Delhi as its centre for research and academic activities in the field of Life Sciences.

b) Indian Institute of Integrative Medicine, Jammu

Formerly Regional Research Laboratory, Jammu, it is one of the premier institutes engaged in two areas of research namely, drug design and development and microbial biotechnology.

Established in 1941 as a low-key research and production centre known as Drug Research Laboratory of J&K State, it was later taken over by the CSIR in 1957. Sri Ramnath Chopra, an outstanding luminary in the field of medical education and research and widely acclaimed as the Father of Indian Pharmacology, was its founder director. The track record of achievements of RRL, Jammu, which has widened its scope of prospecting biodiversity of various geographical niches of the country, has been recently recognized and renamed Indian Institute of Integrative Medicine (IIIM).

Facilities

A multidisciplinary organization, it has all the infrastructural facilities and Science & Technology (S&T) manpower on all aspects ranging from development of agro-technologies to the production of finished value-added products from medicinal plants.

Major areas of research

1. Standardizing the agro-technology of MAPs and their propagation techniques;
2. Isolation of active fraction/s and single molecules from such plants;
3. Bioactivity screening of plant fractions and molecules;
4. Exploring microbes for useful reactions;
5. Identification and standardization of chemotypes and genotypes of plants by molecular fingerprinting;
6. Screening microbial wealth of North West Himalayas for isolation of enzymes for industrial processes;
7. *In silico* screening studies of a huge repository of natural and synthetic compounds.

Knowledge network on medicinal plants

An extension of Government of India-UNDP Umbrella Programme on Herbal Drugs that helped in fostering and promoting cooperation amongst participating developing countries, this knowledge network on medicinal plants and National Centre for Training and Technology Transfer has been established at IIIM to accelerate the development of herbal drugs through mediation of a comprehensive knowledge base on herbal drugs. The centre will endeavour to serve as a national clearing house of information on herbal drugs. It also holds national and international workshops for human resource development in this area in the developing world.

c) National Botanical Research Institute, Lucknow

The National Botanical Research Institute (NBRI) is a premier plant-based multidisciplinary, state-of-the-art national R&D centre of CSIR undertaking research from classical taxonomy to cutting edge areas of modern biology, including both, applied and basic research in multifarious fields ranging from biochemistry to bioinformatics, for the conservation and sustainable utilization of the non-crop plant genetic resources of the country.

To keep pace with the upsurge in the demand for plant-derived products, to accelerate R&D output, NBRI has instituted the Central Instrumentation Facility (CIF) with high-tech sophisticated instruments to cater to the analytical needs of its research projects.

This NABL-accredited lab is equipped with complete instrumentation required to carry out the entire spectrum of testing of plant-based products. It has been recognized by AYUSH as a centre for standardization and quality control of herbal drugs and is also involved in the preparation of monographs for Ayurvedic Pharmacopoeia of India.

Other CSIR laboratories engaged in research on plant drugs are

1. Central Drug Research Institute (CDRI, Lucknow)
2. Indian Institute of Chemical Biology (IICB, Kolkata)
3. Indian Institute of Chemical Technology (IICT, Hyderabad)
4. Centre for Cellular and Molecular Biology (CCMB, Hyderabad)
5. Institute of Himalayan Bio resource Technology (IIHBT, Palampur)
6. Central Salt & Marine Chemicals Research Institute (CSMCRI, Bhavnagar)
7. Regional Research Laboratory (RRI, Jorhat)
8. Regional Research Laboratory (RRL, Thiruvananthapuram)
9. Central Food Technological Research Institute (CFTRI, Mysore)

Accomplishments of CSIR

CSIR has earned the distinction of developing 11 out of the 16 new drugs developed in India. It has developed cost-effective and innovative processes for around 25 generic drugs, standardization of over 50 herbal drugs and devised new diagnostic tools. The production of over 25 drugs/ drug intermediates, technologies for which have been developed and successfully commercialized, is valued at around Rs. 600 million annually. Several of these drugs are exported and save net foreign exchange through export substitution. Some noteworthy accomplishments in the area of herbal drug research are listed below:

I. Products commercialized

1. *Bacopa monniera* standardized extract developed, manufactured and marketed under trade name 'Promind' by Lumen Marketing Company, Chennai.
2. A polyherbal standardized drug for asthma 'Asmon' commercialized by Herbochem Remedies India Limited, Kolkata.
3. Spermicidal saponins of *Sapindus mulkrossi* developed as 'Consap' is to be marketed by Hindustan Latex Ltd.
4. 'Shallaki', an anti-inflammatory drug for the treatment of rheumatoid arthritis and osteo-arthritis produced from *Boswellia serrata,* is marketed by Gufic (P) Ltd., Mumbai.
5. 'Livzon', a multi-herbal formulation with hepatoprotective property, marketed by M/s Hind Chemicals Ltd., Kanpur.
6. 'Imminex', a multi-herbal formulation with immunomodulatory property, marketed by M/s Hind Chemicals Ltd., Kanpur.
7. Technology for the development of an eco-friendly cosmetic from multiple natural colours fortified with natural aromas has been transferred to M/s Ayur Herbal (Pvt) Ltd.

II. Products available for commercialization

1. A saccharifying amylase in pure form is identified in the aqueous extract of *Tinospora cordifolia* stem. With a huge potential for use in the pharmaceutical industry it has been patented by IICB.
2. NMITLI-HA-002, a multi-herbal formulation as hepatoprotective against alcoholic cirrhosis and viral cirrhosis is under multi-centric trials.
3. VIJAYASAR, a single plant based anti-diabetic drug under multi-centric clinical trials sponsored by ICMR.
4. End-to-end technology on *Hypericum perforatum*, a mild anti-depressant, passed on to M/s Nicolas Piramal Ltd., Mumbai.

III. Diagnostic kits/probes

1. RJ-NE-299E a plant-based adjuvant for use in anti-hepatitis vaccine replacing the usual $Al(OH)_3$ is in advanced stage of development with DST, Bharat Biotech having extended financial support for this.

IV. Products under development

1. A unique plant-based therapeutic agent that specifically targets cancer cells, ignoring normal cells, for chronic myelogenous leukemia, which constitutes 80% of blood cancers, has been developed by IICB.
2. Two strong candidate anti-cancer drugs being developed out of more than 20 short-listed plant extracts/fractions by RRL Jammu.
3. 97 M, an iridoid glycoside mixture from *Vitex* species being developed as a hepatoprotective for alcoholic cirrhosis.

V. Technology available for commercialization

1. Production of phytopharmaceuticals – colchicine, colchiside, silymarin, boswellic acid, diosgenin, 16-DPA, berberis hydrochloride and rutin.
2. End-to-end technology of standardized extract of *Tinospora cordifolia*.

VI. Traditional Knowledge Digital Library

The rich traditional knowledge of India lying in common knowledge of our people, having been passed on from generation to generation by word of mouth was largely not documented. Though part of this knowledge is available in ancient classic medical and other literature, it is inaccessible to the common man and rarely understood in the context of its original notion. Documentation of such knowledge, available in public domain, on various traditional systems of medicine has become imperative to safeguard the sovereignty of this knowledge and to protect it from being misappropriated in the form of patents on non-original innovations, which has been a matter of national concern.

India fought successfully for the revocation of turmeric and basmati patents granted by United States Patent and Trademark Office (USPTO) and neem patent granted by European Patent Office (EPO). As a sequel to this, in 1999, the Department of AYUSH constituted an inter-disciplinary task force, for creating a traditional knowledge digital library (TKDL). The project TKDL was initiated in the year 2001.

TKDL provides information on traditional knowledge existing in our country, in languages and format understandable by patent examiners at International Patent Offices (IPOs), so as to prevent the grant of wrong patents. TKDL thus acts as a bridge between the traditional knowledge information existing in local languages and the patent examiners at IPOs.

TKDL is a collaborative project between CSIR and Department of AYUSH, Ministry of Health and Family Welfare, and is being implemented by CSIR. An inter-disciplinary team of traditional medicine experts, patent examiners, IT experts, scientists and technical officers are involved in the creation of TKDL for ISM.

Project TKDL involves documentation of the traditional knowledge available in public domain in the form of existing literature related to Ayurveda, Unani, Siddha and Yoga, in digitalized format in five international languages, namely English, German, French, Japanese and Spanish. Traditional knowledge resource classification (TKRC) is an innovative structured classification system for the purpose of systematic arrangement, dissemination and retrieval, evolved for about 25,000 subgroups in relation to medicinal plants, minerals, animal resources, effects and diseases, method of preparations and mode of administration. This was an improvement over the few subgroups that were available in the earlier version of the International Patent Classification (IPC). Thus, TKRC developed by TKDL led to the creation of World Intellectual Property Organization-Traditional Knowledge (WIPO-TK) task force constituting participation of patent offices from the United States, EU, Japan, China and India to consider linking TKRC with IPC. This resulted in the inclusion of a new group with 207 subgroups covering different categories of plants in the IPC.

Thus TKDL gives legitimacy to the existing traditional knowledge and enables protection of such information from getting patented by the fly-by-night inventors acquiring patents on India's traditional knowledge. It also breaks the format and language barrier making it accessible to patent examiners at International Patent offices for the purpose of carrying out search and examination.

3. Department of Science and Technology

The Department of Science and Technology (DST) is a department within the Ministry of Science and Technology in India established in 1971 with the objective of promoting new areas of science and technology and to play the role of a nodal department for organizing, coordinating and promoting scientific and technological activities in the country.

The DST in collaboration with NBRI has initiated an All India Coordinated Project on Plant Based Health System involving women. Under this, women are trained on different improved techniques relating to the cultivation of medicinal plants, preparation of herbal products and their marketing. Several NGOs have also been involved in this project and they have been instrumental in implementing it in different states of India.

In 1994–1995, DST initiated the Drugs and Pharmaceuticals Research Programme (DPRP), a scheme for promoting R&D in the drugs and pharmaceuticals sector. It aims at synergizing the strength of R&D institutions and the Indian pharmaceutical industry for the discovery and introduction of new drugs. Managed by Drug Development Promotion Board it covers all systems of medicine and supports the following national facilities:

1. IICB, Calcutta – Immunomodulatory Potential of Natural Products
2. IICT, Hyderabad – National Facility for Analysis of Herbo-Metallic Products

3. CARISM, SASTRA, Thanjavur – Central Facility for Pre-Clinical Studies for Research in ISM

4. IICT, Hyderabad – National Facility for Combinatorial Natural Products.

Among the 22 projects granted to the pharma sector, 3 are related to ISM; 6 product patents and 13 process patents were filed in India and abroad out of various projects financially supported under the above programme. One product patent and four process patents filed are related to AYUSH systems.

Accomplishments

- In a project related to traditional herbal drugs, plant extracts of *Asparagus racemosus* and *Terminalia chebula* showed significant immunopotentiating effect while plant extract of *Centella asiatica* possessed significant memory-enhancing activity.
- A novel process with a marked reduction in the time for the preparation of 'Asavas' and 'Aristas' using yeast strains instead of the traditionally used flower buds was developed.

The vision of DPRP is to create more industry-institutional alliances with respect to both traditional and conventional medicine, set up more national facilities on pharma informatics, standardization and quality control and evaluation of safety and efficacy of traditional medicines for disorders like atherosclerosis, arthritis, reproductive problems, diabetes, cancer and communicable diseases like hepatitis, tuberculosis, malaria, leishmaniasis, filariasis, leprosy etc.

4. Department of Biotechnology

The setting up of a separate Department of Biotechnology (DBT) under the Ministry of Science and Technology in 1986 gave a new impetus to the development of modern biology and biotechnology in India. The department's efforts at promoting and accelerating the pace of development of biotechnology in the fields of agriculture, health care, environment and industry are now culminating into products and processes.

Biotechnology of MAPs and plants is a major area under the R&D programmes of DBT. Major Scientific achievements of DBT in this sector are listed below:

I. Conservation and characterization

- A national network of four gene banks on MAPs at TBGRI, Thiruvananthapuram, CIMAP, Lucknow, NBPGR, New Delhi and IIIM, Jammu were further strengthened and now have a total of about 8,500 accessions of prioritized species conserved in different forms.
- A germplasm bank for medicinal plants used in Ayurveda has been set up at Arya Vaidya Sala, Kotakkal, Kerala.

II. Micropropagation

- *In vitro* propagation protocols for selected MAPs such as *Garcinia indica, Holarrhena anti-dysenterica, Lavandula officinalis, Pterocarpus marsupiam, Chlorophytum borivilianum*

- Successful multi-locational field trials on performance of tissue culture-derived crop of *Pogostemon cablin* carried out on a total of 32 acres involving five centres.
- Field evaluation of the performance of tissue culture-raised elite varieties of large cardamom (*Cardamomum subulatum*) over a total area of 50 acres in Uttaranchal initiated in association with the spices board.

III. Cell culture production of therapeutic agents

- Generation of podophyllotoxin from *Podophyllum hexandrum*, hyoscyamine from *Hyoscyamus niger*, guggulsterones from *Commiphora wightii* and camptothecin from *Ophiorrhyza* species.
- Four fast-growing cell cines of *P. hexandrum* capable of synthesizing podophyllotoxins devoid of α-peltatins were developed.
- A 15 l bioreactor set up for upscaling cell culture production of podophyllotoxin, anthraquinones and other therapeutic agents.
- Cell suspension cultures raised from leaf and hairy root derived callus of *Hyoscyamus muticus* have been scaled up in bioreactor towards production of hyoscyamine.

IV. Process upscaling for lead compound extraction

- Processes for the generation of 10-Deacetyl-abeo-baccatin from *Taxus wallichiana* needles, camptothecin from *Nothapodytes foetida* and silymarin from *Silybum marianum* have been upscaled for commercial production

V. Cell-based screening systems

- *In vitro* bioscreen to identify anti-diabetic, anti-cancer and immunomodulatory agents from plants developed and a multi-institutional project implemented on using it along with cell signal targets.
- Using a cell-based screen developed for evaluating anti-amoebic activity of plant extracts, an active extract has been identified for further standardization and product development.

VI. Isolation and characterization of new bioactives/therapeutic agents

- Based on *in-vitro* screening of 60 traditional medicinal plants a total of 35 lead molecules have so far been identified – anti-cancer-15, anti-diabetic-5, immunomodulatory-15.
- Two anti-cancer lead molecules (from *Aegle marmelos* and *Phyllanthus urinaria*) have been patented.
- A patent filed for a plant extract demonstrating osteogenic activity *in vitro* and *in vivo*.
- An anti-mycobacterial lead fraction from *Piper longum* effective against both sensitive and resistant strains of *Mycobacterium tuberculosis* has been identified.

VII. Development of standardized herbal formulation

- A collaborative project to develop a standardized and safe herbal product for left ventricular dysfunction from *Terminalia arjuna* based on leads already available is underway.

VIII. Genomic resources and metabolic pathways

- Patent filed for capsaicin synthase enzyme – key enzyme involved in the biogenesis of capsaicin – characterized from the placental tissues of *Capsicum* species.
- Five lines of *Catharanthus roseus* hyperproducing serpentine and its product ajmalicine developed through DNA marker assisted pyramidation of the concerned gene loci.

5. Indian Council of Medical Research

The Indian Council of Medical Research (ICMR), New Delhi, the apex body in India for the formulation, coordination and promotion of biomedical research, is one of the oldest research bodies in the world. The ICMR is funded by the Government of India through the Department of Health Research, Ministry of Family and Health Welfare. The council's research priorities coincide with the national health priorities and its charter of activities is aimed at reducing the total disease burden and at promoting health and well-being of our people.

Accomplishments

I. Reviews on Indian medicinal plants

The past several decades have seen the accumulation of enormous scientific research/information on multidisciplinary aspects of medicinal plant research owing to the global resurgence of interest in herbal medicine. This enormous literature lies widely scattered not only in ancient manuscripts, but also in the form of recent results of the work of various laboratories/institutions in various scientific journals. The focus of the medicinal plant unit of ICMR is to consolidate this multidisciplinary published research work in the form of review monographs. As part of this programme, nine volumes (10th in print) have been brought out in a series of publications, entitled Reviews on Indian Medicinal Plants on about 2,206 medicinal plant species. The publication includes 40,814 citations. Each monograph includes

- Regional names of each medicinal plant
- Sanskrit synonyms as well as the Ayurvedic description
- Habitat and parts used
- Ethnobotanical, botanical, pharmacognostical, chemical, pharmacological and clinical data
- Complete references and bibliography on each aspect of the information cited
- Colour photographs of important medicinal plants.

II. Quality standards of Indian medicinal plants

To ensure laying down quality parameters of crude drugs, the ICMR has initiated a programme which has resulted in the compilation of eight volumes (ninth in print) on Quality Standards of Indian Medicinal Plants. It contains data on 274 medicinal plants commonly used in India. These volumes cover

- Authentic botanical names, synonyms, parts used
- Detailed macroscopic and microscopic description of the part used as drug

- Diagnostic characters and colour photographs
- Limits of foreign matter
- Total ash, acid-insoluble ash, water and ethanol soluble extractive values
- Chromatographic finger print profile
- Pharmacological, clinical and toxicity study results.

III. Phytochemical reference standards of selected Indian medicinal plants

Monographs on the spectral and analytical data on 30 marker compounds generated by Agharkar Research Institute, Pune through a project sanctioned to it by the ICMR is being brought out by the council similar to its earlier publications.

IV. Medicinal plants monographs on diseases of public health importance

Monographs on select diseases of public health importance in line with national health priorities shall incorporate a unique collection of data namely

- Disease etiopathogenesis and other medical information
- Drugs of choice in allopathic system of medicine
- Plant drugs indicated in ancient traditional medical texts
- Up-to-date research data on these plants and its constituents
- Scientific basis of use of ISM drugs
- Strengthen claims in respect of IPR/patents for global acceptability.

The first volume in this series has been brought out on the 'Prospective of Indian medicinal plants in the management of liver disorders'. Other thrust areas for which similar review monographs are initiated are immunomodulators, Kala-azar, malaria, filariasis, diabetes mellitus, liver disorders and anti-inflammatory drugs.

6. Defence Research and Development Organisation

The Defense Research and Development Organisation (DRDO) is an agency of the Republic of India, responsible for the development of technology for use by the military. It was formed in 1958 by the merger of technical development establishment and the Directorate of Technical Development and Production with the Defence Science Organisation. The DRDO has a network of 52 laboratories engaged in developing defence technologies covering various fields, such as aeronautics, armaments, combat vehicles and naval research and development. The organization includes more then 5,000 scientists and about 25,000 other scientific, technical and support personnel.

Thrust areas of DRDO in life sciences research are

1. Development of life support technologies to improve combat efficiency
2. Enhancement of soldiers' health even in extreme environmental and operational conditions
3. Building the human capital for armed forces
4. Development of novel food technologies to ensure appropriate military nutrition

5. Strengthening man-machine interface through human factor engineering
6. Enhancing the morale and motivation of the troops.

DRDO's achievements in the field of MAPs research are as follows:

1. To counter high-altitude health challenges, the Defence Institute High Altitude Research (DIHAR) has developed, mostly using high-altitude MAPs

   (a) Herbal tea technology for its commercial production being transferred and introduced in high altitude ration of army;
   (b) A herbal antioxidant supplement to counter high-altitude maladies, formulated and technology transferred with IMPCL, Ministry of Health;
   (c) A non-toxic herbal appetizer which is undergoing clinical studies;
   (d) Herbal UV protective oil against high-altitude UV radiation;

2. Standardized bulk extraction process of sea buckthorn seed oil using supercritical fluid CO_2. Its biochemical profiling being undertaken, its soft gel capsules have been formulated. Toxicological studies for the same are in progress.

3. Floristic wealth of Ladakh and Lahaul-Spiti with emphasis on MAPs have been surveyed, identified and documented.

4. Rare, endangered and threatened medicinal plants such as *Aconitum* species, *Dactylorhiza* species, *Ephedra* species, *Inula* species, *Podophyllum* species have been enlisted and conserved *ex situ.*

5. Technology for the propagation and commercial cultivation of 30 high-altitude MAPs has been developed.

6. Established an alpine herbal garden of 50 MAPs for R&D activities at Pithogarh, Uttarakhand.

7. Under its Transfer of Technology programme, technology for the formulation of the following polyherbal formulations developed by DRDO has been transferred to M/s AIMIL Pharmaceuticals Pvt Ltd., New Delhi:

   (a) Leuskin for leucoderma developed in the form of ointment and liquid oral dosage has been evaluated on 100 patients with leucoderma.
   (b) Eczit, a polyherbal for eczema, as an ointment evaluated in 50 patients with different clinical features and extent of disease.
   (c) Amtooth, a polyherbal solution to check and treat toothache due to dental nerve inflammation has been evaluated for clinical efficacy.

8. Patents obtained for

   (a) Multivitamin herbal beverage – process of preparation from sea buckthorn fruits
   (b) Process of preparation of herbal jam from fruits of sea buckthorn
   (c) Formulation of DRDO herbal tea from trans-Himalayan herbs
   (d) Process for preparation of a radio-protective herbal extract
   (e) Formulation of herbal antioxidant supplement
   (f) Formulation of herbal UV-protective oil.

7. Indian Council of Agricultural Research

The Indian Council of Agricultural Research (ICAR) is an autonomous organization under the Department of Agricultural Research and Education (DARE), Ministry of Agriculture, Government of India. Formerly known as Imperial Council of Agricultural Research, it was established in 1929 as a registered society under the Societies Registration Act, 1860 in pursuance of the report of the Royal Commission on Agriculture. The council is the apex body for coordinating, guiding and managing research and education in agriculture including horticulture, fisheries and animal sciences in the entire country. With 97 ICAR institutes and 47 agricultural universities spread across the country, this is one of the largest national agricultural systems of the world.

The Directorate of Medicinal and Aromatic Plants Research (DMARP) – formerly National Research Centre for Medicinal and Aromatic Plants – at Boriavi in Anand district of Gujarat is a national institute of ICAR. It is mandated to develop appropriate production, protection and processing technologies for important MAPs through basic, strategic and applied research and thus contribute to the growth and development of medicinal and aromatic sectors in India.

The Food and Agriculture Organization (FAO) of the United Nations, India and DMARP of ICAR have together developed an interactive training toolkit to facilitate better application of the WHO guidelines for good agriculture and collection practices (GACP) for medicinal plants. The adoption of GACP in medicinal plant sector will improve livelihood by adding premium price to the produce and also generating additional employment in rural sector for educated youth. This training toolkit is based on the guidelines of GACP for medicinal plants that were developed by the WHO in 2003 to ensure safety, efficacy and quality of raw materials used in herbal medicine. In 2009, the NMPB, in collaboration with the WHO country office for India, developed a set of country-specific guidelines and standards for GACP.

STATE LEVEL GOVERNMENTAL AND NON-GOVERNMENTAL ORGANIZATIONS

In addition to government initiatives, several national and international organizations are actively involved in different parts of India to promote awareness, documentation and conservation strategies for medicinal plants. Several NGOs are working in the areas of conservation and developing cultivation strategies. The international development and research centre has initiated a Medicinal and Aromatic Plants Programme in Asia (MAPPA) which promotes collaboration through national and international networks. It also promotes research on approaches to sustainable production and processing of medicinal plants.

The volume of developmental activity as a result of governmental initiatives is complemented by the pioneering work being carried out in individual states towards promotion and enhancement of the medicinal plant sector in their regions. Apart from the state medicinal plant boards that are implementing the board's directives, efforts to conserve, sustain and effectively utilize the medicinal plant wealth within each state are being undertaken by several governmental and non-governmental agencies that include

- Forest research institutes
- Research programmes of agriculture and medical – governmental, autonomous and deemed – universities
- Government departments of agroforestry

- Traditional medicine practitioners' forums
- Private charitable trusts
- Registered societies
- Educational institutes with departments in Botany, Medicinal Chemistry, Biotechnology and Phytochemistry
- Departments of selected Indian Institutes of Technology
- Government-run traditional medicine manufacturing units
- 7,000-unit strong Herbal Drug Industry in India manufacturing traditional medicines with or without standardization.

Selected establishments, both governmental and NGOs, making significant contributions in this sector are listed below statewise.

1. Andaman & Nicobar Islands

The atypical forest coverage of these groups of islands made up of 12 different types of forests constitutes 86.2% of its total land area. From these reserve and protected tropical rain forests so far 2,200 varieties of plants have been recorded out of which 200 are endemic and 1,300 do not occur in mainland India. About 170 medicinal plants have been identified on these islands of which 150 species are endemic to the islands. A digital database on plant resources of the islands indicates the medicinal value of over 400 plant species.

(1) Andaman & Nicobar Medicinal Plants Board was constituted with objective of developing conservation strategies for the cultivation of 14 selected prioritized medicinal plants in the islands.
(2) ICMR's Regional Medical Research Centre is documenting traditional healing practices of the indigenous population of these islands.

2. Andhra Pradesh

Andhra Pradesh's (AP) varied topography from hilly ranges to the shores of Bay of Bengal support varied vegetation types enriched by a variety of flora and fauna. The variations are accentuated by the various types of ecosystems such as hilly, wetland, manmade systems, mangroves, estuaries and forests that are largely dry deciduous to scrub. Out of a total number of 2,586 species, around 1,800 species are estimated to be medicinal plants. The AP government in an effort to conserve the gene pool of medicinal plants occurring in the forests has taken up *ex situ* cultivation to effectively harness the state's medicinal plant wealth. Ethnobotanical gardens of about 400 species are established in the four regional research centres in the state located at Rajamundry, Tirupati, Mulugu (near Hyderabad) and Achuthapuram in Khammam District.

(1) AP Forest Development Corporation
(2) Acharya N.G. Ranga Agricultural University
(3) CIMAP Resource Centre at Hyderabad
(4) Herbal Folk Research Centres, Hyderabad, Warangal, Tirupati (BIO-TRIM) and Rajamundry
(5) Chaitanya Bharathi Seva Sangam, Guntur

    (6) Santhagiri Ayurveda and Siddha Vaidya Sala – 371 units spread across the state

    (7) Venkateshwara Ayurveda Nilayam, Chintaluru

    (8) Siris Impex, Vijayawada

3. Arunachal Pradesh

Situated in the Eastern Himalayan Range with the largest forest cover next to Madhya Pradesh, Arunachal Pradesh has over 20 forest types ranging from tropical to alpine. Possessing a phenomenal range of biological diversity in flora and fauna, it has been recognized as the 25th biodiversity hot spot in the world and is among the 200 globally important eco-regions.

    (1) Arunachal Pradesh Forest Development Corporation, Deemali (Tirpa Dist.)

    (2) State Forest Research Institute, Itanagar

    (3) Ayurveda Regional Research Institute, Itanagar

    (4) Division of Plant Sciences & Ecology, RRL, Jorhat

    (5) Van Vigyan Kendra, Chessa

    (6) High Altitude Botanic Garden, Bondila

    (7) Germplasm Bank and Experimental Station, Namsai

4. Assam

One of the richest repositories of medicinal and aromatic plants in the world, the state is rich in bioresources and ethnocultural diversity. It is a forerunner in the production of MAPs with more than 300 species of commercially important medicinal plants produced in the state. To promote scientific approach for the exploration, conservation and value addition in the field of medicinal and aromatic plants several research centres have been created.

    (1) Assam Bioresource Centre under the Science, Technology & Environment Council (ASTEC), Madan Kamdev (Kamrup Dist.)

    (2) Regional Research Laboratory (CSIR), Jorhat

    (3) The Energy & Resource Institute (TERI), Guwahati

    (4) Prahar Gusthi, Nagoan District

    (5) Agro Development and Social Welfare Organization, Berpeta (Bhawanipur Dist.)

    (6) International Centre for Integrated Mountain Development, Ministry of Environment and Forests, Dimapur.

5. Bihar

With 61.18% of land under cultivation, Bihar is endowed with three agroclimatic zones where 200 species of medicinal plants are found and several of them are cultivated in a total of 2,600 hectares. Mentha and lemongrass are largely grown in the state.

    (1) Rajendra Agricultural University, Pusa, Samastipura

    (2) Anne Marg, Patna

    (3) State Medicinal Plant Board, Patna

    (4) Baidyanath Ayurved Bhawan, Patna

6. Chattisgarh

Situated in the Deccan biogeographical area, Chattisgarh has forests under two major types, tropical moist deciduous forest and tropical dry deciduous forest. The 22 varied forest sub-types existing in the state contributing to its rich biocultural diversity and dependence of the large forest-dwelling population on medicinal plants are the reasons for the government declaring it the 'Herbal State' in 2001. Thus Chattisgarh forest policy is specially provided to facilitate conservation of the medicinal plants which are in the category 'Nationalized Non-Wood Forest Produce'.

(1) State Medicinal Plant Board, Raipur

(2) Chattisgarh High Tech Herbal Farm, Raipur

(3) Golden Roots Organic Herbal Farm, Mohranga, Raipur

(4) Jai Maa Bamleshwar Herbal Hi-Tech Farm, Rajnandgaon

(5) Research and Extension, Social Forestry Division, Bilaspur

(6) Vanoshadhalaya Sankra, Dhamtari

7. Chandigarh

The first planned city of India, Chandigarh is located near the foothills of the Shivalik range of Himalayas in northwest India. Most of the city being covered by dense banyan and eucalyptus plantations, Asoka, cassia and mulberry trees flourish in the forested ecosystem that surround the city.

8. Delhi

(1) DEEKSHA, Sarvodaya Kanya Vidyalaya, Madanpur Khader,

(2) Directorate of ISM&H, Government of NCT of Delhi

(3) College of Forestry, Dr. Balasaheb Savant Konkan Krushi Vidyapith, Dapoli (Ratnagiri Dist.)

(4) Technology Development Mission – IIT, Delhi

(5) The Energy and Resources Institute (TERI), Lodhi Road, New Delhi

(6) NBPGR, Issapur Farm Station

(7) Jamia Hamdard, Hamdard Nagar

(8) Mother Herbs (P) Ltd., Delhi

(9) Jeevan Herbs and Agro Farms, Delhi

(10) Knight Queen group of Industries, New Delhi

(11) Essential Oil Association of India, New Delhi

9. Dadra and Nagar Haveli

Located at the foothills of the Sahayadri mountain range, this UT is landlocked between Maharashtra and Gujarat. Tropical moist deciduous forests with 201 sq. km of protected reserve forests and wildlife sanctuary in this UT constitute 42% of total geographic area as against the national average of 23%.

(1) Dadra and Nagar Haveli State Medicinal Plants Board, Forest Department, Silvassa

10. Daman and Diu

The second smallest UT, it is located in Gujarat and agriculture is an important economy. It is situated on an alluvial coastal plain, though headlands and low plateaus are created in the area due to outcrop of basalt.

(1) Daman and Diu Department of Medical and Health Services, Moti

11. Goa

Goa has more than 33% of its geographic area under government forests owing to its location on the Western Ghats range classified as a biodiversity hotspot of the world. This equatorial forest cover and the grasslands of Goa have more than 1,512 documented species of plants with 57 species of medicinal plants.

(1) Goa State Medicinal Plant Board, Forest Development Corporation, Panaji
(2) Western Regional Centre (TERI), Goa

12. Gujarat

A highly industrialized state, its forest cover is less than 10% of the total geographical area: 1,315 medicinal plants are identified out of which 270 are widely utilized; 201 of them are found in Gujarat with 148 collected from wild and 53 cultivated. The total demand for medicinal plant raw material is 3,755 metric tonnes annually out of the utilized 270 species of medicinal plants.

(1) State Medicinal Plant Board, Gandhinagar
(2) State Forest Development Corporation
(3) DMARP, Boriavi, Anand
(4) Medicinal and Aromatic Plants Division, Anand Agricultural University
(5) National Research Centre for Medicinal and Aromatic Plants, Anand
(6) Gujarat Ayurved University, Jamnagar
(7) Center for Environment Education, Ministry of Environment and Forests, Ahmedabad
(8) Gujarat Institute of Desert Ecology, Bhuj
(9) Aditya Ayurvedics, Vapi, Valsad
(10) Ajay Pharmacy, Kalapinagar, Amreli
(11) National Research Centre for Medicinal and Aromatic Plants (NRCMAP), Anand
(12) Akhandanand Ayurvedic Aushadhi Nirman, Lambha, Ahmedabad
(13) Alicon Pharmaceuticals (P) Ltd., Sarigam, Valsad
(14) Amlani Ayur Pharmacy, Ram Tekara, Porbandar
(15) Amruitumbh Ayurvedic Pharmacy, Banaskantha
(16) Ayurlab Herbal (P) Ltd., Panchamahal
(17) Atul Pharmacy, Banaskantha
(18) Bharat Chemical Laboratories, Panchamahal
(19) Bharatbhai Jivandas Bhatiya Ayurvedic Pharmacy, Kutch
(20) Bhavsar Chemicals (P) Ltd., Surat

(21) Bright Pharma, Sabarkantha

(22) Cadila Health Care (P) Ltd., Sabarkantha

(23) Dang Jila Ayurvedic Pharmacy Cooperative Society Ltd., Dang

(24) Gayatri Pharmacy, Narmada Girnar Ayurvedic Products, Junagadh

(25) Government Ayurvedic Pharmacy, Narmada

(26) Government Ayurvedic Vikas Mandal Pharmacy, Junagadh

(27) Gurukrupa Pharmacy, Bhavnagar

(28) Helios Phamaceuticals, Mehsana

(29) IPCA Health Products Ltd., Bharuch

(30) Indigenous Drug Pharmaceuticals, Sabarkantha

(31) Intercare Ltd., Mehsana

(32) JB Chemicals and Pharmaceuticals Ltd., Bharuch

(33) Janak Ayurvedic Pharmacy, Amreli

(34) Kalyan Kanpani Ayurvedic Pharmacy, Rajkot

(35) Madhu Medicine manufacturers, Junagadh

(36) Mars Pharmaceuticals, Vadodara

(37) Medical Labs, Ahmedabad

(38) Megh Pharmaceuticals, Sabarkantha

(39) Moon Drugs Ltd., Sabarkantha

(40) Nagarjuna Pharmaceuticals (P) Ltd., Ahmedabad

(41) Nar Narayan Ayurvedic Pharmacy, Ahmedabad

(42) Navjivan Herbal Remedies, Anand

(43) Nimbark Ayurvedic Pharmacy, Mehsana

(44) Norissa Medicines Ltd., Ankleshwar, Bharuch

(45) Ojas Pharma, Suman, Desaiwada, Surat

(46) Orient Ayurvedic Pharmacy, Banaskantha

(47) Paras Pharmaceuticals, Mehsana

(48) Prasanth Pharmaceuticals, GIDC, Narmada

(49) Priya Pharmacy, Navsari

(50) Rajkumar Sevashram, Kutch

(51) Rakesh Pharmaceuticals, Mehsana

(52) Rashmi Aushadhi Nirman Industries, Gandhigram, Kutch

(53) Research Drugs and Pharmaceuticals Ltd., Ahmedabad

(54) Saga Laboratories, Ahmedabad

(55) Sanskar Pharma, Pachmahals

(56) Sehat Pharma (P) Ltd., Sabarkantha

(57) Selus Pharmaceuticals, Sabarkantha

(58) Shelter Pharmacy, Sabarkantha

(59) Shivam Pharmaceuticals, Rajkot

(60) Shri Shankar Ayurvedic Pharmacy, Ahmedabad

(61) Shri Akshar Pharma (P) Ltd., Sabarkantha

(62) Shri Brahmani Van Bij Bhandar, Gandhinagar

(63) Shri Sarveshwar Ayurvedic Pharmacy, Banaskantha

(64) Shriji Herbal Products, Sabarkantha

(65) Surya Ayurvedic Pharmacy, Dahod

(66) Trio Pharma, Ahmedabad

(67) Unjha Ayurvedic Pharmacy, Mehsana

(68) Unjha Formulations Ltd., Mehsana

(69) Vasu Pharmaceuticals (P) Ltd., Vadodara

(70) Vihosi Pharma, GIDC, Vapi, Valsad

(71) Vilco Laboratories (P) Ltd., Bhavnagar

(72) Y.E. Hadavaid, Rajkot

(73) Zandu Pharmaceuticals, Vapi, Valsad

13. Haryana

Primarily an agricultural state with almost 80% of its land under cultivation, 3.52% of its geographic area is under notified forest. Thorny dry deciduous forest and thorny shrubs can be found all over the state. Shiwaliks of Haryana are a large source of a number of valuable medicinal plants and about 40 species are collected from the forests legally and illegally.

(1) State Medicinal Plant Board, Panchkula

(2) Choudury Devi Lal Herbal Nature Park, Chuharpur, Yamunanagar District

(3) Haryana Agro Industries Corporation, Panchkula

(4) Yamuna Pharmacy, Yamunanagar

(5) Yugal Pharmacy and Chemical Works, Yamunanagar

(6) Maharishi Ayurveda Products (P) Ltd., Faridabad

(7) Bhrigu Pharma, Jagadhari

(8) Ayulabs (P) Ltd., Rajkot

(9) Jackson Herbocare, Yamunanagar

14. Himachal Pradesh

Known for its varied agroclimatic conditions, Himachal Pradesh (HP) is most suitable for cultivation, conservation, propagation and development of medicinal plants. About two-thirds of the geographical area of this hill state being a designated forest, around 2,500 tonnes of medicinal plant-related material from 165 species is officially harvested from the state's forests and exported every year. The legal annual trade in medicinal plants in the state is worth about Rs.10 crores over and above the parallel illicit trade suspected. Due to various anthropogenic pressures, the state's forests are getting degraded and fragmented posing serious risk of extinction to many high-value medicinal plant species. The trade in medicinal plants is thus largely unregulated, secretive and exploitative with cultivation being restricted to only a few species with 60 medicinal plants being red-listed.

Centrally coordinated, participative nature of management of the medicinal plant trade is needed to regulate and effectively utilize/conserve the natural wealth bestowed upon the state.

(1) State Medicinal Plant Board, Shimla
(2) Advanced Centre for Hill Bioresources and Biotechnology, Palampur
(3) Himalayan Forest Research Institute, Shimla
(4) Department of Ayurveda, Research Institute in Indian System of Medicine, Joginder Nagar, Mandi
(5) Department of Silviculture and Agroforestry – Dr. Y.S. Parmar University of Horticulture and Forestry, Nauni-Solan
(6) Himalayan Research Group, DST, Chotta Shimla
(7) Himachal Pradesh Medicinal Plants Society, HP Forest Department
(8) Himachal Pradesh Krishi Vishwa Vidyalaya, Palampur, HP
(9) Herbal Garden, Herbarium and Research Institute, Government of HP, Joginder Nagar, Shimla
(10) National Board of Plant Genetic Resources, Regional Station, Shimla
(11) Ayush Herbs, Nagrota Bagwan
(12) Baijnath Pharma, Baijnath
(13) Chadda Traders, Nagrota Bagwan
(14) Dhanwantri Herbals, Solan
(15) Bioveda Action Research (P) Ltd., Dharamkot
(16) Government Ayurvedic Pharmacy, Jogendar Nagar, Majra, Paprola
(17) Hemma Herbs (P) Ltd., Solan
(18) Himachal Ayurveda Pharmacy, Kangra
(19) Kangra Hill Care and Cure Products, Kangra
(20) Vets Farma Ltd., Una
(21) Yogmaya Pharmacy, Kangra

15. Jammu and Kashmir

Phytogeographically the most complex and diverse, Jammu and Kashmir (J&K) has a fairly rich diversity of plant life. Floristically it is divisible into three ranges, namely alpine desert vegetation of Ladakh, temperate vegetation of Kashmir and sub-tropical vegetation of Jammu. The flora of Himalayan Kashmir comprises about 3,054 species, with 880 species in Ladakh and 506 species in Jammu. While the whole Himalayan belt is one hotspot megacentre having eight critical areas which include Ladakh and Kashmir, the latter is one of the 26 hotspots in India where there are high rates of deforestation and endemicity. This area is a storehouse of MAPs used in pharmaceutical and perfume industries. The list includes 55 species of important medicinal plants, several of which grow wild in temperate and alpine habitats. Some native medicinal plants like *Dioscorea deltoidea* have been taken up for cultivation.

(1) State Medicinal Plant Board, Directorate of Indian Systems of Medicine, Srinagar and Jammu
(2) PCCF, Forest Department

(3) Field Research Laboratory (DRDO), Leh Forest Division, Ladakh

(4) Indian Institute of Integrative Medicine, Jammu, Srinagar

(5) Traditional Medical-Cultural Association, Leh, Ladakh

(6) S.K. University of Agricultural Sciences and Technology, Shalimar

(7) J&K Medicinal Plants Introduction Centre, Pulwama

16. Jharkhand

The state of Jharkhand is a part of biodiversity-rich regions of India because of its diverse physiographic and climatic conditions. It forms part of the Chotanagpur plateau province of the Deccan peninsula biographic zone. Nearly 50% of the country's minerals are located in the state; 30% of its geographic area is covered with tropical dry deciduous forest, moist deciduous forest, dry peninsular forest and dry mixed deciduous forest types. They form catchments of three main rivers namely Koel, Damodar and Subernekha. The landscape of the state has a mix of wild, semi-wild and cultivated habitats. Though 29.6% of its total area is a notified forest, the biodiversity of the state is under threat due to unsustainable harvest of natural resources that has resulted in the loss of regeneration capacity of medicinal plants like *Rauwolfia serpentina*, *Adathoda vasica*, *Gloriosa superba* and *Achyranthes aspera*.

(1) State Medicinal Plant Board, Ranchi

(2) Institute of Forest Productivity, Ranchi

17. Karnataka

The state is one of the highly biodiverse regions of India as it is endowed with great diversity of climate, topography and soils. It spans the seacoast with rich aquatic bed and mangrove swamps at the mouth of estuaries. It harbours verdant tropical evergreen forests, paddy fields, coconut and arecanut plantations on the narrow coast flanked by the Western Ghats. The latter is known to have more diversity of wild relatives of cultivated plants than any other region of comparable size in the world. The aquatic biodiversity is also very rich with many endemic species. The state has around 4,500 species of flowering plants and the Karnataka State Medicinal Plant Board is concerned with medicinal plant cultivation under the aegis of the state forest department.

(1) Karnataka Forest Department, Bellur, Dharwad, Madikeri

(2) CIMAP Resource Centre, Allasandra, Bangalore

(3) University of Agricultural Sciences, G.K.V.K. Campus, Bangalore

(4) Indian Institute of Horticultural Research, Bangalore

(5) Karnataka Medicinal Plant Authority, Bangalore

(6) Bayir Groups, Bangalore

(7) Hill Green (Extracts), Bangalore

(8) Sami Labs Ltd., Bangalore

(9) Natural Remedies (P) Ltd., Bangalore

(10) Southern Regional Center (TERI), Bangalore

18. Kerala

One of the most land-hungry states in India with lowest per capita land holding, much of Kerala's notable biodiversity is concentrated and protected in the Western Ghats. Almost a fourth of India's 10,000 plant species are found in the state. Amongst the almost 4,000 flowering plant species – 1,272 of which are endemic to Kerala and 159 threatened – 900 species are medicinal plants. Its 9,400 square kilometers of forests include tropical wet evergreen and semi-evergreen forests, tropical moist and dry deciduous forests and montane subtropical and temperate forests. Altogether 24% of Kerala is forested. Two of the world's Ramsar Convention listed wetlands – Lake Sasthamkotta and the Vembanad-Kol wetlands – as well as the 1,455.4 square kilometer vast Nilgiri Biosphere are in Kerala. The state of Kerala is well known for its rich tradition of Ayurvedic medicine. Apart from the world renowned Kottakkal, it has 20 governmental and 6 non-governmental research organizations engaged in medicinal plant research and production. Overall the State Medicinal Plant Board at Thrissur supervises the medicinal plant cultivation activities in the state.

(1) Forest Head Quarters, Trivandrum, Peechi, Thrissur
(2) All India Coordinated Research Project on Medicinal and Aromatic Plants, Kerala Agricultural University Campus, Thrissur
(3) Rehabilitation Plantation, Kollam
(4) Tropical Botanical Garden and Research Institute, Thiruvananthapuram
(5) NBPGR, The Pharmaceuticals Corporation, 'Oushadhi' Thrissur
(6) Floriculture and Medicinal Plants Cooperative Society, Kozhikode
(7) Kottakkal Arya Vaidya Sala, Kottakkal, Malappuram
(8) State Medicinal Plant Board, Thrissur
(9) Amala Pharmaceuticals, Ernakulam
(10) Amruth Ayur Pharma, Malappuram
(11) Aranya Ayurved Vaidyasala, Kozhikode
(12) Aravind Ayurvedic Pharmaceuticals, Ernakulam
(13) Arya Vaidya Pharmacy Ltd., Kanjikode
(14) Ashoka Pharmaceuticals, Kannur
(15) Ashwini Ayurvedic Pharmacy, Wayanad
(16) ATV Pharmacy, Malappuram
(17) Chaitanya Herbals, Thiruvananthapuram
(18) Chandra Ayurvedic Medical Store, Kochi
(19) Changampally Ayurveda Vaidya Sala, Valanchery
(20) Cochin Arya Vaidya Sala, Ernakulam
(21) Enpees, Chombala
(22) Everest Pharma, Thrissur
(23) Falcon Pharma, Alleppey
(24) Focus Drug Research Lab (P) Ltd., Thiruvananthapuram
(25) Greenlife Pharmaceuticals, Ernakulam
(26) Eastern Herbals (P) Ltd., Malappuram

(27) Hareethaki Pharma, Kollam

(28) Himalaya Pharmaceuticals, Kozhikode

(29) Ilaj Ayurveda Pharmacy, Malappuram

(30) K.P. Namboothri's Dhanta Davana, Ernakulam

(31) Kakkanat Ayurveda Ashramam, Shoranur

(32) Kalan Arya Vaidya Sala, Thrissur

(33) Kalan Nellai, Thrissur

(34) Kas Pharma, Alappuzha

(35) Kerala Ayurveda Pharmacy Ltd., Aluvai

(36) Kozhikode Ayurveda Pharmacy, Wayanad

(37) Kurunhikattil Pharmacy, Malappuram

(38) MVS Ayurvedic Research Centre, Malappuram

(39) Madhava Pharmaceutical Laboratories, Ernakulam

(40) Mangalodayam Pharmaceuticals, Malappuram

(41) Marmachikitsalayam Herbal Products, Malappuram

(42) Mykeel Pharmaceuticals, Kannur

(43) Nagarjuna Herbal Concentrates Ltd., Idukki

(44) Nalanda Ayurvedic Pharmacy, Ernakulam

(45) Nangelil Pharmacy, Ernakulam

(46) Oushadha Kala Pharmaceuticals, Thrissur

(47) Oushadhi (The Pharmaceutical Corporation (I.M) Kerala Ltd.) Thrissur

(48) PVS Vaidya Sala, Calicut

(49) Pattarumadom Dispensary, Ernakulam

(50) Peringattuthodiyil Herbals, Malappuram

(51) RMN Vaidya Sala, Thrissur

(52) Rani Drug House, Thrissur

(53) Reliance Herbal Products, Thrissur

(54) Rishi Valley Herbaceous Pharmaceuticals (P) Ltd., Kochi

(55) Santhosh Pharmacy, Kadalundi

(56) Santiniketan, Kozhikode

(57) SDV Manufacturing Co., Kollam

(58) Sen and Sen's Ayurvedic Pharmaceuticals, Kollam

(59) Select Drugs and Pharmaceuticals, Ernakulam

(60) Siddhashrama Sivananda Vijayam Oushadhasala, Kannur

(61) SMV Herbal Products, Kollam

(62) SNA Oushadhalaya (P) Ltd., Thrissur

(63) Sree Santhosh Ayurveda Pharmacy, Kottarakkara

(64) Surya Ayur Products, Calicut

(65) TK Ayurvedic Pharmacy, Koyilandy

(66) Udaya Ayurvedic Pharmacy, Kodakara

(67) Vaidyaratnam Oushadha Sala, Thrissur

(68) Varma's Ayurveda Pharmacy, Alappuzha

(69) Vederpacha Pharmaceuticals, Kollam

(70) Vijaya Pharmacy, Punalur

19. Lakshadweep

This group of islands off the coast of Kerala in the Arabian Sea contains diverse reef formations, hosting several endangered plant and animal species. Endowed with an unparalleled natural scenic beauty, Lakshadweep has a rich biodiversity and is home to more than 400 species of terrestrial plants.

(1) State Medicinal Plant Board, Directorate of Medical & Health Service, Kavaratti

20. Madhya Pradesh

With 9.38% geographical area of the country Madhya Pradesh accounts for 12.44% of the country's forests; 34.8% of the geographical area of the state amounting to 9.5 million hectares is under forests. Dry and moist deciduous forests abundant in the state are extremely rich in terms of both floral and faunal biodiversity. The tribal areas of Sidhi, Shahdol and Mandla are rich in MAPs. Ashwagandha, safed musli and turmeric are under cultivation.

(1) Centre for Forestry Research and Human Resource Development, Chindwara

(2) Social Forestry Division, Jabalpur

(3) Research and Extension Circle, Forest Department, Sagar

(4) Shilpa Chem, Indore

(5) MP Gramin Vikash Mandal, Khadi

(6) Gramodyog Bhandar, Balaghar

(7) Mahila Utkarsh Sansthan, Indore

(8) Mahila Jagriti Manch, Indore

(9) Jawaharlal Nehru Krishi Vishwa Vidyalaya, Jabalpur

(10) Tropical Forest Research Institute, PORFRC, Jabalpur

(11) State Forest Research Institute, Polipather, Jabalpur

(12) Madhya Pradesh State MFP Cooperative Federation, Bhopal

(13) Amsar (P) Ltd., Indore

(14) Ammi Pharma, Sehore

(15) Pushpak Pharmaceuticals, Indore

(16) Ajmera Pharmaceuticals, Indore

(17) Asrani Essential Oils, Jabalpore

21. Maharashtra

Maharashtra is known for dissimilar climatic conditions and dynamic topography. Its rich flora and fauna perfectly reflect the diversity of climate and geography as the topography of the region varies from arid desert and tropical rain forest to mountain ranges over 4,000 feet in altitude.

However with changing circumstances, the diverse ecosystem of Maharashtra's Western Ghats faces a threat from growing population and unabated development measures. Resultant dense forest degradation is perpetually affecting forests leading to a large increase in open forests. Today, recorded forests cover approximately one-fifth of Maharashtra's geographical area which is 61,939 square kilometers of which 79.47% constitute reserved forests and 13.23% protected forests. Unclassified forests comprise 7.3% of the total forest area.

(1) Social Forestry Division, Kolhapur

(2) Maharashtra State Horticulture and Medicinal Plants Board, Pune, Mumbai

(3) Directorate of Social Forestry, Pune

(4) Applied Environmental Research Foundation, Pune

(5) Bharti Vidyapeeth University, Pune

(6) Chaitanya Pharmaceuticals (P) Ltd., Nashik

(7) Charak Pharma (P) Ltd., Mumbai

(8) Jambhule Farms, Dhule

(9) Central Research Station, Dr. Punjab Rao Deshmukh Krishi Vidyapeeth, Akola

(10) Mahatma Phule Krishi Vidyapeeth, Rahuri

(11) Shree Dhootapapeshwar Ltd., Mumbai

(12) Zandu Pharmaceutical Works Ltd., Mumbai

22. Manipur

The state of Manipur in northeastern India is known for its ecologically distinctive and rich biodiversity, having many endemic flora and fauna. Traditional conservation practices of the indigenous population protecting small forest patches by dedicating them to the local deity have contributed to their conservation. Such forest patches called 'sacred groves' are tracts of virgin forest harbouring rich biodiversity and are repositories of rare and endemic species – remnants of the primary forest left untouched by the local inhabitants due to religious belief. As a result these groves possess a great heritage of diverse gene pool of many forest species having socio-religious attachment and possessing medicinal values. A total of 166 sacred groves distributed in different locations are inventoried from Manipur Valley. Among these only a few (11%) are well preserved, while most are threatened (58%) and others threatened (3%) due to anthropogenic pressures such as developmental activities, urbanization and population explosion.

(1) Manipur State ISM&H Development Society, Imphal

(2) Silviculture and Training Division, Forest Department. Government of Manipur, Imphal

(3) Manipur Tribal's Pioneer Association, Imphal

(4) State Medicinal Plant Board, Imphal

(5) International Centre for Integrated Mountain Development, Ministry of Environment and Forests, Imphal

23. Meghalaya

A hilly strip in eastern India, one-third of the state is forested. Its mountain forests are distinct from the lowland tropical forests to the north and south. The wettest state in India, the

Meghalaya subtropical forest ecoregion encompasses the state and it supports a vast floral and faunal biodiversity. The flora has a large variety of phanerophytes which include a variety of trees and shrubs, parasites, epiphytes and succulent plants. The state is rich in timber such as teak and sal woods and medicinal plants such as *Cinchona* and *Taxus baccata*. The most significant floras of Meghalaya are 325 different species of orchids. In addition small pockets of forest groves protected for religious purpose similar to Manipur are rich in rare plant and animal species.

(1) NBPGR, Regional Station, Shillong
(2) Forest Division – Khasi Hills, Lower Lacumiere – Shillong, Jaintia Hills Territorial Division, Jowai
(3) State Medicinal Plant Board, Shillong
(4) International Centre for Integrated Mountain Development, Ministry of Environment and Forests, Shillong

24. Mizoram

A land of rolling hills, rivers and lakes, as many as 21 major hill ranges run through the length and breadth of Mizoram. Its forests are tropical wet evergreen, tropical semi-evergreen and montane sub-tropical pine type. Of these the tropical wet evergreen forests are rich in valuable timber. More than 400 ethnomedicinal plants have been recorded in the state of which about 230 species have medicinal value. Out of this, 65 species are categorized as threatened at the state level and 64 species are recorded as new ethnomedicinal plants.

(1) State Medicinal Plant Board, Directorate of Health Sciences and Department of Health & Family Welfare, Aizawal
(2) International Centre for Integrated Mountain Development, Ministry of Environment and Forests, Aizwal

25. Nagaland

Though geographically a small state, Nagaland has several types of forests on account of its varying physiographic and geoclimatic conditions. Forests occupy an area of approximately 8,62,930 hectares of which government forests account for 11.7%. The state is located in one of the 25 biodiversity hotspots of the world. It supports 2,431 species belonging to 963 genera and 186 families under angiosperms. Gymnosperms also register their presence with 90 species under 6 genera from 5 families. A few areas of the state are pristine, covered with gigantic trees, where sunrays cannot penetrate, harbouring a wide variety of endemic plants, animals and microorganisms. However in recent times, the biodiversity of the state is facing serious threats due to increasing population, pressure on agriculture to bring more areas under cultivation and other developmental activities.

(1) State Medicinal Plant Board, Directorate of Health Sciences, Kohima
(2) Nagaland University School of Engineering and Technology, Dimapur
(3) International Centre for Integrated Mountain Development, Ministry of Environment and Forests, Dimapur

26. Orissa

The state of Orissa located in the eastern coast of Indian peninsula is quite rich in natural resources and is one of the richest biodiverse regions in southeast Asia. It has varied and wide-spread forests harbouring dry deciduous forests as well as mangroves with several unique, endemic, rare and endangered floral and faunal species. There are seven major river deltas formed by the rivers Subernekha, Budha balanga, Baitarani, Brahmani, Mahanadi, Rushikulya and Bahuda. This region has five morphological zones namely the coastal plains, the middle moun-tainous and highland regions, the central plateaus, the western rolling uplands and major flood plains. The dominant vegetation type being mangrove, there are 94 species of orchids and 1,076 species of other plants including 2 species of orchids which are endemic, 8 endangered, 8 vulner-able and 34 rare species of plants.

(1) Orissa Forest Research Institute, Bhubaneshwar

(2) Natural Products Department, RRI (CSIR), Bhubaneshwar

(3) Orissa Forest Development Corporation Ltd., Bhubaneshwar

(4) Jaydev Foundation Trust, Bhubaneshwar

(5) Gurukul Mahavidyalaya, Amsena

(6) Tapobhoomi Trust, Narayanipada, District Khurda

(7) State Medicinal Plant Board, Forest and Environment Department, Bhubaneshwar

27. Punjab

A fertile alluvial land area, the state has abundant water supply owing to large rivers and an extensive irrigation canal system. A belt of undulating hills extends along the northeastern part of the state at the foot of the Himalayas. While there are no natural forests in the plains, extensive tracts occur covered only with grass, shrubs and bushes. Agriculture is the largest industry in Punjab. The Shiwalik area is richest in terms of floral and faunal diversity and has been identified as one of the micro-endemic zones of India. Among angiosperms, about 355 species of herbs, 70 tree species, 70 species of shrubs or undershrubs, 19 climbers and 21 species of twiners have been recorded from the area. Three species of pteridophytes, 27 of bryophytes and 1 of gymnosperms have also been recorded. Hanke, Kanjli and Ropar wetlands of Punjab are inhabited by diversity of flora and fauna that include some rare plants and animals.

(1) Shyam Nikunj Educational and Social Welfare Society, Patiala

(2) Vir Sawarkar Social Welfare Society, Kapurthala

(3) National Institute of Pharmaceutical Educational and Research, Mohali

(4) State Medicinal Plant Board, Chandigarh

28. Puducherry

A quiet little town on the southern peninsular coast, Puducherry is not rich in flora and fauna.

(a) State Medicinal Plant Board, ISM & H, UT of Puducherry

29. Rajasthan

The main geographic features of Rajasthan are the Thar desert and the Aravalli range which runs through the state from southwest to northeast. Despite little forest cover, the state has rich and varied flora and fauna. Forests mostly confined to the east of the Aravalli range constitute just about 9% of the total area of the state. Natural vegetation in Rajasthan is mostly ephemeral occurring only during the monsoon season. The shallow wetlands of eastern Rajasthan are dotted with shrubs, creepers, bushes and herbs. The Ranthambore National Park has 75 tree species, 30 species of grasses, 13 types of shrubs and over 100 medicinal plants

(1) Central State Farm, Sriganganagar, Suratgarh District

(2) Jagadguru Ramanandacharya Rajasthan Sanskrit University, Jaipur

(3) Paryavaran Chetana and Sodhan Sansthan, Jaipur

(4) Department of Botany, Jai Narayan Vyas University, Jodhpur

(5) State Medicinal Plant Board, Jaipur

(6) Government Ayurvedic Pharmacy, Unit I, II, III and IV

30. Sikkim

One of the 26 biodiversity hotspots, Sikkim is a veritable treasure house of some of the world's most beautiful streams, lakes and waterfalls. The state has rich flora and fauna despite having only 0.5% of the land of the country. It is a land of vast variation in altitude within very short distances. Elevation plays a prime role in fashioning the ecoregions of the state. Based on altitude, tropical, sub-tropical, temperate-alpine and trans-Himalayan are the four vegetation zones of the state of which the alpine is rich in medicinal plants. Sikkim has 4,500 species of flowering plants with more than 450 species of orchids.

(1) Department of Horticulture and Cash Crops, Government of Sikkim, East Sikkim

(2) State Medicinal Plant Board, Department of Forest, Environment and Wild Life Management, Gangtok

(3) Eshwaramma Social Welfare Association, Gangtok

(4) International Centre for Integrated Mountain Development, Ministry of Environment and Forests, Gangtok

31. Tamil Nadu

Tamil Nadu (TN) is endowed with rich biodiversity and has the unique distinction of having two biosphere reserves, The Nilgiri Biosphere Reserve (NBR) and Gulf of Mannar Biosphere Reserve (GOMBR). The main natural habitat types are forests, mountains, rivers, wetlands, mangroves and beaches. One-sixth of its land mass is covered with forests. The total forest cover of the state is 22,643 square kilometers constituting 4.75% of the geographic area and 20.03% of the recorded forest area. Forests in TN are rich repositories of a number of valuable medicinal plants. With 5,640 species, nearly one-third of the total flora of India, it ranks first among all the states. This includes 533 endemic species, 230 red-listed species, 1,559 species of medicinal plants and 260 species of wild relatives of cultivated plants. TN has 4 indigenous and 60 introduced species of

Gymnosperms. An area of 307.85 square kilometers of forest area has been brought under national parks. The NBR is the first biosphere reserve to be established in India in 1986. Also the first internationally designated biosphere reserve, it is located in the Western Ghats and encompasses two of the 10 biogeographic zones of India. Rich in plant diversity, NBR has about 3,200 species of flowering plants of which 132 are endemic.

The GOMBR between Rameswaram and Kanyakumari is among the world's richest marine biodiversity regions. Extending over 1,500 square kilometers, it includes 21 islands and has about 3,600 species of flora and fauna. However habitat destruction, overexploitation, pollution and species introduction are the major causes of biodiversity loss in TN.

(1) Forest Productivity and Agroforestry Division, Institute of Forest Genetics and Tree Breeding, Forest Campus, Coimbatore

(2) Agricultural College and Research Institute, Tamil Nadu Agricultural University, Madurai

(3) Departments of Botany, Horticulture – Annamalai University, Annamalai Nagar

(4) Tamil Nadu Aromatic and Medicinal Plant Cooperative Limited (TAMPCOL), Chennai

(5) Indian Medicine Practitioners Cooperative Pharmacy and Stores Ltd (IMPCOPS), Chennai

(6) Arya Vaidya Nilayam, Madurai

(7) Cavin Care (P) Ltd., Chennai

(8) Centre for Advanced Study in Botany, University of Madras, Guindy Campus, Chennai

(9) Department of Botany, St. Joseph College, Tiruchirapalli

(10) Amrita Vishwa Vidyapeetham, Coimbatore

(11) Child Jesus Educational and Charitable Trust

(12) Community Action Trust, Tiruchirapalli

(13) Trust for Socioeconomic Development, Tiruchirapalli

(14) Technology, Information, Forecasting and Assessment Council's Centre of Relevance & Excellence in Herbal Drugs (TIFAC CORE), JSS College of Pharmacy, Ooty

(16) State Medicinal Plant Board, Commissioner of Horticulture and Development, Commissioner of ISM&H, Chennai

(17) Indfrag, Chennai

(18) Kothari Phytochemicals International, Madurai

32. Tripura

Endowed with vast natural resources, the state has 603.65 square kilometers of forests within four sanctuaries at Sipahjala, Gumti, Trishna and Roa. Geographically, it lies in a strategic zone as it falls in between the Indo-Malayan and Indo-Chinese biological realms. Thus Tripura stands at the gateway of floral and faunal confluence. Its forests are classified as evergreen and deciduous occupying 0.32% area of India that accounts for 12.78% of the plant resources of the country. Its forest density is 17.35% as against the national average of 11.73%. Listed as one of the 26 endemic centers in India, it possesses 1,545 plant species, 379 trees species, 320 shrubs, 581 herbs, 165 climbers, 34 ferns, 45 epiphytes out of which 7 are endangered, 7 endemic and 18 rare species. The state also has 24 species of orchids and 266 species of medicinal plants. It has the maximum

Plant Diversity Index of 5.23, one of the highest in India. Over the years, habitat destruction mainly by rampant felling of forests and shifting cultivation, the forest cover dwindled from 76% to 33%. The state government is setting up 30 biological hotspots and the forest department has undertaken the task of enacting the three-tier Panchayati Raj System to increase awareness through people's participation.

    (1) Medicinal Plant Board of Tripura, Agartala.

33. Uttarakhand

Declared one of the five UNESCO's World Heritage Biodiversity states, Uttarakhand in India occupies an area of 53,483 square kilometers of which 93% is mountainous and 64% is covered by forests. Perched within diverse geographical features ranging from an array of snow-capped mountain peaks and tropical forests, it is a state of natural beauty with some of the untouched and well-preserved natural habitats. Its biodiversity includes sacred groves that exhibit a rich wealth of flora and fauna and several rare and threatened species of plants and animals.

    (1) Kedarnath Vanya Jeev Prabhag, Gopeshwar

    (2) GB Pant University of Agriculture and Technology, Pantnagar

    (3) Soil Conservation Forest Division (Narendra Nagar, Didihet, Tons), Uttarkashi

    (4) Herbal Research and Development Institute, Chamoli (Gopeshwar Dist.)

    (5) Divya Yog Mandir Trust, Kankhal

    (6) High Altitude Plant Physiology Research Centre, HNB Garhwal University, Srinagar-Garhwal

    (7) Uttaranchal Cooperative Marketing Federation, Dehradun

    (8) Jula Besaj and Sahakari Vikas Sangh, Sumari, Tilwara District

    (9) CIMAP Resource Centre, Pantnagar

  (10) Alakananda Soil Conservation, Forest Division, Chamoli

  (11) Jila Besaj Sahkari Vikas and Kriya Vikriya Sangh Ltd., Chamoli

  (12) Department of Ayurvedic and Unani Services, Dehradun

  (13) Uttaranchal Youth and Rural Development Centre, Chamoli

  (14) Society for Himalayan Environment Research (SHER), Dehradun

  (15) Society for Rural Research and Development (SRRD), Garhwal

  (16) Dhauli Krishi Utpadan Evam Vignana Sahkari Samiti, Chamoli

  (17) M/s India Glycols Ltd., Dehradun

  (18) National Bureau of Plant Genetic Resources (NBPGR), Regional Station, Bowali

  (19) G.B. Pant Institute of Himalayan Environment and Development, Almora

  (20) Indian Council for Forestry Research and Education (ICFRE), Dehradun

  (21) Divya Pharmacy, Haridwar

  (22) The Himalaya Drug Company, Dehradun

  (23) Gramin Krishi Evam Paryavaran Vikas Samiti, Pithoragarh

  (24) Himalayan Centre (TERI), Mukhteshwar

34. Uttar Pradesh

Being situated on the uplands, it accommodates the upper catchments of major river systems. The Gangetic plain in the centre with highly fertile alluvial soil and the Vindhya Hills and the plateau in the south are the distinct geographical features of Uttar Pradesh. Forests constitute about 12.8% of its total geographic area, which are the tropical moist deciduous, tropical dry deciduous and tropical thorny. The Himalayan region and the Terai and Bhahar area in the Gangetic plain have the most forests. The state is rich in flora and fauna with an amazing variety of some 1,000 woody plants including 3,000 trees, 400 shrubs and 100 woody climbers.

   (1) Social Forestry Division, Etawah
   (2) CIMAP, Lucknow
   (3) Department of Forestry, C.S.A. University of Agriculture and Technology, Kanpur
   (4) Shanmol Gramodyog Sansthan, Lucknow
   (5) Jeevaniya Society, Lucknow
   (6) National Botanical Research Institute, Lucknow
   (7) Narendra Dev University of Kumarganj, Faizabad
   (8) Central Institute of Medicinal and Aromatic Plants, Lucknow
   (9) I.C.F.R.E. Forest Research Institute, Dehradun
 (10) NVS Bioresearch Pvt. Ltd., Moradabad
 (11) Dabur India Ltd., Sahidabad.

35. West Bengal

On the eastern bottleneck of India, stretching from the Himalayas in the north to the Bay of Bengal in the south, West Bengal has diverse flora and fauna due to the varying altitude through the state. Forests however make up 14% of the geographical area which is less than the national average of 23%. Phytogeographically, the southern part of the state is divided into two regions namely the Gangetic plain and the Littoral mangrove forests. In the latter are located part of the world's largest mangrove forest, The Sunderbans. Protected forests cover 4% of the state area.

   (1) Indian Institute of Technology, Kharagpur
   (2) North Bengal University, Siliguri
   (3) University of Calcutta, Kolkata
   (4) Institute of Alternative Medicine and Research Institute, Kolkata
   (5) Y.S. Parmar University of Horticulture & Forestry, Nauni-Solan
   (6) West Bengal State Medicinal Plants Board, Kolkata
   (7) Baidyanath Ayurved Bhavan, Kolkata
   (8) Chemi Homeo Laboratory Private Limited
   (9) RHB Trades, Kolkata
 (10) Cal-Trade, Kolkata
 (11) Dey's Medical Stores, Kolkata
 (12) TCG Life Sciences, Kolkata

COMMERCIAL HERBAL DRUG INDUSTRY

In India about 880 species of medicinal plants in active trade estimated at 1,28,000 tonnes of medicinal plant-based raw material is consumed by around 8,300 licensed units manufacturing herbal medicines and products across the country. Of these 80% is sourced from the wild. Plant-based crude drugs exported are estimated worth Rs.463 crores, the major export destinations being the United States, Germany, Japan, UK, France, Taiwan, Italy, Pakistan and Hong Kong. Taking into account the volume of domestic trade and export of plant-based raw material, the annual medicinal plant based trade was worth Rs.850 crores during 2001 with the national herbal sector growing at 30%.

While herbal medicines are produced by several thousand companies in India, most of them are quite small, including numerous neighbourhood pharmacies that compound ingredients to make their own remedies. The industry is however dominated by less than a dozen major companies for decades, joined recently by a few others, so that today there are 30 companies doing more than Rs.5 crore business per year. The products of these companies are included within the broad category of 'Fast Moving Consumer Goods'(FMCG) which include herbal medicines for internal consumption, health foods, toiletries etc.

Dabur, Baidyanath and Zandu together have about 85% of India's domestic market. Some of the major units engaged in herbal drug manufacture are listed below.

Dabur India Ltd

India's largest herbal medicine supplier and the fourth largest producer of FMCG, it was established in 1884 and has grown to Rs.65 crores annual turnover in 2003. With 15% sales volume being herbal drugs and the rest mostly food and cosmetics, Dabur's Ayurvedic Specialities Division has over 260 medicines for treating a range of conditions from common cold to chronic paralysis. These constitute only 7% of Dabur's total revenue with Dabur Chyawanaprash having a market share of 70% and Chewable Hajmola digestive tablets 88%. Other major products are Dabur Amla Hair Oil, Vatika (shampoo) and Lal Dant Manjan (tooth powder).

Sri Baidyanath Ayurvedic Bhawan Ltd was founded in 1917 in Kolkata and specializes in Ayurvedic medicines. It has expanded into FMCG with cosmetic and hair-care products. With a total sales volume of Rs.35 crores, it has over 700 Ayurvedic products made at 10 manufacturing centres with 1,600 employees. One of its international products is Shikakai Shampoo with other items being herbal teas, patent medicines, massage oils and chyawanaprash.

Zandu Pharmaceutical Works incorporated in Bombay in 1919 was named after an 18th century Ayurvedic physician. Its primary business being herbal drugs, today it also has chemicals and cosmetics divisions. With total sales volume at Rs.4.5 crores one of its current projects is to develop a plant-derived dopamine drug for Parkinsonism for which an NDA has been filed with the US FDA.

Himalaya Drug Company was established in 1934 in Bangalore. With Rs.50 crores annual turnover it has a US Distribution Division (Himalaya USA). It is well known in the United States for Liv-52 a liver protective for the treatment of viral hepatitis.

Charak Pharmaceuticals founded in 1947 has three distribution centres across India. 'Evanove' its product for menopause contains herbal estrogen receptor modulators in addition to soya and asparagus.

Vicco Laboratories established in 1958 mainly produces topical therapies based on Ayurveda. It is best known internationally for its tooth paste Vajradanti, which has been in the market in the United States for more than 25 years.

The Emami Group founded in 1974 provides a diverse range of products, with an annual turnover of Rs. 11 crores. Its Himani line generates a small revenue out of chyawanaprash and other health care goods; however toiletries and cosmetics are its major products.

Aimil Pharmaceuticals Ltd. incorporated in 1984 and engaged in manufacture and sales of both generic and proprietary Ayurvedic medicines has an annual business turnover of Rs.2 crores. Its wide range of Ayurvedic herbal formulations, covering most therapeutic segments, is well known for products meant for hepatitis, diabetes, menstrual disorders, digestive and urinary diseases.

Universal Medicaments Pvt. Ltd. a unit of Universal Pharmaceuticals Group, is best recognized for its formulations Karnim (anti-diabetic supplement), Herbokam (anti-Stress formula), Chetak (stimulant) and Tonabolin (iron supplement). With 15 main proprietary products that are a gradual move away from traditional formulas like teas, ghee preparations etc. Universal is engaged in manufacture and export of both pharmaceutical formulations and research-based herbal medicines. The herbal products in general are for lipid regulation, blood sugar lowering, cardiovascular health, menopause, liver protection and detoxifying regimens. It has joint ventures for research and manufacture of herbal products with Cipla and Lupin.

Surya Herbal, New Delhi is involved in manufacture and export of wide range of Ayurvedic generic, branded specialities and other OTC herbal health care products. It is one of the few facilities that blend modern production technology and advanced quality measures into the area of herbal personal care products and medicines. Established in the year 1999, it was promoted by Surya Roshini Group having interests in lighting and steel pipes businesses which later diversified to herbal commerce. The company produces 15 formulations, which match, for the most part, the categories of natural therapeutics in demand worldwide.

Sami Labs is the Research and Development group of Sabinsa Corporation, a US company with affiliates in India. It produces herbal extracts and special powders in standardized forms sought after by herbal product manufacturers.

Maharishi Ayurveda Products International Inc. Established in 1985 it was first set up as a 100% export-oriented unit. With an annual sales turnover of nearly Rs. 5 crores, ISO 9001 certified Maharishi Ayurveda produces over 900 medicinal formulations and presently it exports to over four countries with the United States alone consuming 50% of its turnover.

Kottakkal Aryavaidya Sala is a century-old charitable institution engaged in the practice and propagation of Ayurveda. Established at Kottakkal in Kerala in 1902 by the visionary physician and philanthropist the Late Vaidyarathnam P.S.Varier, today the trust manages Ayurvedic hospitals at Kottakkal, Delhi and Kochi. It has two Ayurvedic medicine manufacturing units established with current infrastructure and instrumentation. With branches at 15 major cities all over India, it has over 900 authorized dealers for the sale of its products.

Cholayil is amongst Kerala's most famous and respected Ayurvedic families practising Ayurveda for generations and also presently manufacturers of the world's largest selling Ayurvedic soap 'Medimix'. A Chennai-based Rs.100-crore FMCG, Cholayil Pharmaceuticals is the flagship company of the Cholayil group and produces products focussed on the toiletries, personal care and health care segments. Cholayil creates products blending native elements into the most contemporary forms. It has 15% market share in talc and 17% in bath soap in Kerala. Its products include both traditional formulations and herbal contemporary dosage forms.

Emami, Johnson & Johnson, Dechane and Amrutanjan are some of the other reputed industry giants leading in the herbal drug manufacture and research.

With the growing demand for safe, effective remedies from time-tested knowledge, several allopathic drug manufacturers like Ranbaxy, Novartis, as also personal care product leaders like Cavin Care and other reputed business groups like HCL are all venturing into the herbal drug market.

CONCLUSION

India is home to an amazing diversity of plants, with over 46,000 plant species recorded and approximately 760 known to be harvested from the wild for use by India's large herbal medicine industry. An immensely vast repository of traditional knowledge in therapeutically used plants adds to its rich biodiversity, giving India a clear leeway to become a major player in the growing herbal drug market. Awareness of this potential, largely through both governmental and non-governmental initiatives together with technological advancement has brought about phenomenal growth of the Indian herbal drug sector. Despite stringent regulation against exploitative hoarding of the nation's plant wealth, illicit collection of rare and endangered plants still continues unchecked. Enforcement of enacted laws requires people's awareness of the hazards faced by our valued ecosystems. The need of the hour is to minimize destructive utilization of medicinal plant resources by replacing conservative cultivation methods with newer agro-technological breeding techniques. In order to step up India's share in the global herbal market, there is an urgent need to showcase the worthiness of our traditional herbal products in the international market by developing newer approaches to their standardization to meet WHO requirements. A well-established herbal drug market complemented with adequately modernized and regulated traditional medical systems akin to China shall go a long way in tackling the nation's growing disease burden.

REVIEW QUESTIONS

Essay Questions

1. Write an essay on the agenda, achievements: Research councils under AYUSH.
2. Discuss the contributions of any two CSIR labs in herbal-drug research.
3. Outline the accomplishments of ICMR and DRDO in herbal drug development

Short Notes

1. India's initiatives to promote herbal industry.
2. NMPB.
3. Herbal.
4. Major players in Indian Herbal drug Industry.
5. TKDL.

6

Quality Control and Standardization of Herbal Drugs

CHAPTER OBJECTIVES

Introduction

Standardization of Herbal Drugs

Important Parameters for the Quality Control of Herbal Drugs

INTRODUCTION

Using herbs as medicine is the oldest form of health care known to humanity and to this day over 80% of the world population depends on herbal medicines and products for healthy living. There is increasing awareness and general acceptability of the use of herbal drugs in today's medical practice. Medicinal plants constitute a source of raw materials for both traditional systems of medicine and modern medicine. As such they represent a substantial portion of the drug market.

Commercialization of the manufacture of these medicines to meet the increasing demand has resulted in a decline in their quality, primarily due to lack of adequate regulations pertaining to this sector of medicine. Often herbal raw materials are procured and processed without any scientific evaluation and launched onto the market without any mandatory safety and toxicology studies because there is no effective machinery to regulate manufacturing practices and quality standards. Rise in the use of herbal products has also given rise to various forms of abuse and adulteration of herbal products resulting in some instances in fatal consequences.

All drugs whether single pure drugs or multi-constituent herbal products should fulfill the basic requirements of being safe and effective. Herbal drugs are plants or plant parts that have been converted into phytopharmaceuticals by means of certain simple processes involving harvesting, drying and storage. Hence they are capable of variation caused by differences in growth, geographical location and time of harvesting. Variability of constituents in herbs or herbal preparations due to genetic, cultural and environmental factors has made the use of herbal medicines more challenging.

The quality of herbal drugs is influenced by factors not applicable to single pure drugs, such as the following:

1. Herbal drugs range from parts of plants to isolated purified constituents.
2. They consist of complex mixtures of compounds of several chemical groups.
3. The active principals in most cases are unknown.
4. Selective methods of analysis or reference compounds may not be commercially available.
5. Plant materials are chemically and naturally variable.
6. Varieties and cultivars of plants differing in chemical composition exist.
7. There is a great deal of variation in the source and quality of the raw material.
8. Methods of harvesting, drying, storage, transportation and processing (mode of extraction, extracting solvent, constituent instability etc.) have an effect.

STANDARDIZATION OF HERBAL DRUGS

Standardization is the process of prescribing a set of standards or inherent characteristics, constant parameters, definitive qualitative and quantitative values that carry an assurance of quality, efficacy, safety and reproducibility. It is the process of developing and agreeing upon technical standards. Specific standards are worked out by experimentation and observations, which would lead to the process of prescribing a set of characteristics exhibited by a particular herbal medicine. Hence standardization is an important tool in the quality control process.

Though herbal products have become increasingly popular throughout the world, one of the impediments to their acceptance is the lack of standard quality control. The herb or herbal drug preparation in its entirety is regarded as the active substance and the constituents are either of known therapeutic activity or are chemically defined substances or group of substances generally accepted to contribute substantially to the therapeutic activity of the drug.

The profile of constituents in the final product, however, has implications on its efficacy and safety. But due to the complex nature and inherent variability of constituents of plant-based drugs, and the limited availability of simple analytical techniques to identify and characterize the active constituents solely by chemical or biological means, it is difficult to establish quality control parameters.

Herbal drug manufacturers undertake quality control testing of their products based on certain preliminary parameters. This is because it is not possible to identify/quantify the presence of all/active ingredients claimed in a formulation. Assay methods so far developed are for single pure drugs at the best quantifiable in a formulation containing a limited number of other similar or non-similar constituents. Plants being constituted of innumerable complexes of closely related and unrelated groups of compounds, it is not an easy task to standardize plant drug formulations, which may even be polyherbal in composition.

A vast array of modern chemical analytical methods involving Ultraviolet/Visible (UV/VIS) spectrophotometry, thin layer chromatography (TLC), high performance liquid chromatography (HPLC), gas chromatography-mass spectroscopy (GC-MS) and a combination of these are employed for herbal drug standardization when the active constituents are known. The task of standardization is all the more perplexing where the active constituents are not known.

Currently there is a need to develop internationally recognized guidelines for quality assurance. Ensuring the purity, safety, potency and efficacy of herbal drugs being of cardinal importance, various standards of quality are being developed for herbal drug raw material and finished products. Such standards prescribed in pharmacopoeias, formularies, WHO and ESCOP monographs and herbal drug PDRs are rigidly being followed by regulatory authorities world over.

IMPORTANT PARAMETERS FOR THE QUALITY CONTROL OF HERBAL DRUGS

The last two decades has seen a significant increase in the use of herbal medicines. Plant materials are employed throughout the industrialized and developing world as home remedies, over-the-counter (OTC) drugs and ingredients for the pharmaceutical industry. As a result of WHO's promotion of traditional medicine, countries have been seeking the assistance of the organization in identifying safe and effective herbal medicines for use in National Health Care systems. The World Health Assembly in its resolutions of 1978, 1987 and 1989 has emphasized the need to ensure the quality of medicinal plant products by using modern control techniques and applying suitable standards. Deliberations on the regulation of herbal medicines that were part of the Fourth and Fifth International Conferences of Drug Regulatory Authorities in 1986 and 1989 were concerned with the commercial exploitation of traditional medicines through OTC products. This was followed by model guidelines prepared by WHO to define basic criteria for the evaluation, safety and efficacy of herbal medicines.

Quality control and standardization of herbal drugs involves several steps. These take into consideration all aspects that contribute to their quality right from the source and quality of raw material, subsequent manufacturing operations, analytical methods of evaluating the potency up to clinical evaluations where needed. WHO guidelines for the quality control of herbal drugs encompasses various physicochemical, biological and analytical evaluation techniques. These processes and procedures include the following quality indication parameters:

Good Agricultural Practices and Good Manufacturing Practices

Source and quality of the raw material is an important determinant in the quality control and standardization of herbal drugs. Such variations multiply during storage and further processing. Due to the inherent variability of plant material, batch-to-batch variation starts from the collection of raw material. Using cultivated plants under controlled conditions instead of those collected from the wild can minimize most of these factors. Following accepted good agricultural practices (GAP) and good manufacturing practices (GMP) can play a pivotal role in ensuring quality of herbal drug products. GAP involves right seed selection, growth conditions, use of fertilizers, harvesting, age and part of the plant collected, time and method of collection, drying and storage. Active principals may be destroyed by enzymatic processes that continue for long periods from collection to marketing resulting in variation of composition. Thus using uncontaminated plant material, right temperature of processing, exposure to light, method of extraction and other GMPs largely influences the quality of herbal drugs. Thus GAP and GMP are an integral part of herbal drug quality control.

Botanical Identity of Plant Material

Herbal ingredients must be authenticated by correct identification of their botanical source referred by their Latin binomial. Different batches of herbal materials may still be subject to inter-and intra-species variation. Other related information required are synonyms, vernacular names, parts of the plant used for each preparation and detailed instructions for agricultural production and collection conditions as per the country's GAP.

Sampling

Accurate identification of herbal material by macroscopic and microscopic examination by comparison with authentic material or descriptions of authentic herbs is the first important step. Prior to such an evaluation, a sample is to be drawn for analysis. Reliability of any conclusions drawn from the analysis will depend upon how well the sample represents the whole batch. For sampling material in bulk 10% of the packaging units need to be sampled if they are more than 50 in number. For 6–50 units, sample from 5 and for less than 5 units, all units need to be sampled. All damaged units are to be individually sampled. From each container three samples from the top, middle and bottom respectively are to be taken. Seed samples are to be taken with a grain probe. The pooled samples are to be adequately mixed and one-fourth of them are taken. The process is repeated as necessary till the required quantity prescribed for the particular plant part is reached, for example 100–200 g for flowers and up to 10 kg for certain roots.

For material in retail packages from boxes and cartons selected for sampling, randomly selected two consumer packages are to be taken. For small batches of wholesale containers, 10 consumer packages are to be taken. The samples are then pooled and sorted by the same quartering procedure described above to get the final sample. The selected samples are then subjected to further testing.

Macroscopic Evaluation

For whole drugs, macroscopic/sensory evaluation is usually enough for the drugs to be identified. Visual inspection in terms of shape, size, surface characteristics, colour, consistency, odour, taste, fracture and appearance of the cut surface of the drug provide the simplest and quickest means to establish its identity, purity and even quality. Comparison with the authentic drug will often reveal features not described in the requirements. Where needed measurements such as diameter of seeds and fruit samples are taken. General appearance of the sample itself will indicate whether it is likely to comply with standards. For example, percentage of clove stalks in cloves, ash in valerian, brittle broken leaves in leaf samples, horny fracture of starch-containing drugs, colour of the fractured surface (gentian) indicate improper processing during drug preparation.

Drug prices in the case of important drugs such as senna leaflets, senna pods, nutmeg, ginger and chamomile flowers are largely dependent on their macroscopic characters. Since these are judged subjectively and substitutes and adulterants may closely resemble the genuine material, it is often necessary to substantiate the findings by microscopy and physicochemical analysis.

Presence of Foreign Matter

Herbal materials should be entirely free from visible signs of contamination by moulds or insects and other contaminants including animal excreta. No abnormal odour, discolouration, slime or signs of deterioration should be detected. Since it is difficult to obtain plant materials in an entirely pure condition, pharmacopoeias contain statements as to the percentage of other parts of the plant or other organic matter which may be permitted. However, no poisonous, dangerous or otherwise harmful foreign matter or residue should be allowed. During storage products should be kept in a clean and hygienic place to avoid contamination. Special care should be taken to avoid formation of moulds, since they may produce aflatoxins. Any soil, stones, sand, dust and other foreign inorganic matter must be removed before herbal materials are cut or ground for testing.

Foreign matter is material consisting of parts of herbal material or those other materials not named within the limits specified for the concerned herbal material in the respective monographs. For examination of presence of foreign matter, weighed quantity ranging from 50–500 g based on the type of drug (roots, rhizomes, bark –500 g, leaves, flowers, seeds and fruit –250 g, cut herbal material – 50 g) is carefully spread in a thin layer. It is then examined using a magnifying lens (6x or10x) for sorting the foreign matter into groups which are then separated for weighing. The remaining sample is sifted through #250 sieve, dust being regarded as mineral admixture. The separated foreign matter is weighed and percent content calculated. Drugs containing appreciable quantities of potent foreign matter, animal excreta, insects or mould should be rejected even though the percentage of such substances are insufficient to cause rejection of the drug on the basis of percent foreign matter (as given in herbal pharmacopoeias). Detection of foreign matter in powdered drugs requires microscopic examination. When foreign matter consists of a chemical residue, TLC is often needed to detect the contaminant.

Microscopic Evaluation

Establishment of identity of powdered drugs depends on the microscopic recognition of characteristic cell types and cell contents. Microscopic analysis is indispensable for the identification of the correct species and/or the right plant part that is to be present. For example, pollen morphology may be used in the case of flowers to identify the species and presence of leaf stomata to identify the plant part used. Stinging nettle (*Urtica urens*) is a classic example where the aerial parts are used to treat rheumatism, while the roots are applied for benign prostate hyperplasia. The basic aim of microscopic examination is to determine the size, shape and relative positions of different cells and tissues, chemical nature of cell walls and form and chemical nature of cell contents.

Powdered drugs or adulterants which contain a constant number, area or length of characteristic particle/mg such as starch grains, epidermis, trichome ribs, fibres etc. can even be determined quantitatively using lycopodium spores as indicator diluent. Other microscopic determinations are percent foreign organic matter in powdered drugs, calculation of vein-islet number, palisade ratio, stomatal numbers and stomatal indices for leafy drugs. Average fibre length (Ceylon and cassia cinnamon), length of epidermal cells (Indian and European squill) number of characteristic sclereids/mg (clove stalks and coconut shells) may be estimated for comparison with known standard for genuine drugs to identify the adulterant or the variety present in the powdered drug.

Prior to microscopic examination the sample has to be treated with chemical reagents. Dried material requires softening before preparation for microscopy preferably by being placed in a moist atmosphere (for leaves) or by soaking in water. Bark, wood and other dense and hard materials need to be soaked in water or equal parts of water, ethanol and glycerol overnight. Botanical sections of the plant material may need to be made and sections of the drug material are necessary for the examination of mucilage or water-soluble cell components. Disintegration serves isolation of specific tissues and bleaching and defatting techniques for observing deeply coloured materials and fatty seeds respectively. Clearing agents and suitable stains are required to highlight cell walls and cell contents. Powdered material is to be mounted in a few drops of water, glycerol/ethanol TS or chloral hydrate before microscopic examination.

Examination of microscopic morphology of both powdered and unground drugs is valuable to establish the identity of many adulterants. For instance, varieties of senna may be identified by vein-islet numbers and palisade ratios, adulterants of belladonna herb by stomatal index and stomatal number or by trichomes.

Knowledge of the microscopic features of genuine materials and of frequently encountered adulterants is essential for their detection in powdered drugs. For example, ginger is character-ized by non-lignified vessels, varieties of aloes by the presence or absence of aloin crystals and cinchona bark by the absence of sclereids.

Determination of Moisture Content

An excess of water in herbal materials encourages microbial growth, presence of fungi or insects and deterioration following hydrolysis. At suitable temperatures, enzymes are activated leading to hydrolytic degradation of active constituents (e.g. digitalis). As most vegetable drugs contain all the food requirements for the growth of moulds, insects and mites, deterioration is very rapid once infestation takes place. Limits for water content should therefore be set for every herbal material. This is especially important for drugs that absorb moisture easily or deteriorate quickly in the presence of moisture. Many methods are now available for moisture content determination.

The test for loss on drying employed in British Pharmacopolia (BP), Extra Pharmacopolia (EP), United States Pharmacopolia (USP) and Indian Pharmacopolia (IP) determines both water and volatile matter. Drying can be carried out either by heating to 100–105° C or in a desic-cator (spreading thin layers of weighed drugs over glass plates) over phosphorous pentoxide R under atmospheric or reduced pressure at room temperature for a specified period of time. The desiccator method is especially useful for materials that contain considerable proportion of vola-tile matter and/or those that melt to a sticky mass at elevated temperatures (balsams and resins). For materials such as digitalis, aloes, starch and fibres which contain little volatile matter, direct drying to constant weight can be employed. Use of moisture balance that combines both drying process and weight recording is suitable where large numbers of samples are handled and where a continuous record of loss in weight with time is required.

The azeotropic method of moisture determination gives a direct measurement of the water present in the material being examined. When the sample is distilled together with an immiscible solvent such as toluene, xylene or carbon tetrachloride, the water present in the sample is absorbed by the solvent. The water and solvent are distilled together and separated in the receiv-ing tube on cooling. To avoid water remaining absorbed in the solvent even after distillation, the solvent is saturated with water before use.

Chemical method of moisture content determination using Karl Fischer reagent is employed for expensive drugs and those which contain small quantities of moisture. Dry extracts of alka-loid-containing drugs, alginic acid and fixed oils such as arachis, castor oil and sesame oil for parenteral use are usually evaluated by this method. Other chemical methods for water determi-nation include treating the sample with various carbides, nitrides and hydrides and measuring and analysing the gas evolved using GC.

Determination of Volatile Oils

Crude drugs containing volatile oils are mostly characterized by typical odoriferous nature. Because they are considered the 'essence' of herbal material and are often biologically active, they are also known as essential oils. Chemically usually composed of mixtures of monoterpenes, sesquiterpenes and their oxygenated derivatives, they are volatile at room temperature. For volatile oil-bearing crude drugs, minimum standards for the percentage of volatile oil present in a number of drugs are prescribed by many pharmacopoeias.

To determine the volatile oil content of a crude drug, the plant material is distilled with water and the distillate is collected in a graduated tube. The aqueous portion separates automatically and is returned to the distillation flask. For oils with relative densities equal to or greater than water, separation from water is assisted by placing a known volume of xylene in the receiver and reading off the combined oil and xylene. Time taken to complete the distillation of the oil varies with the nature of the drug and its state of size reduction, but about four hours is usually sufficient. Solution of the volatile oil in a fixed oil such as in powdered drugs of umbelliferae may retard distillation. Pharmacopoeial standards for volatile oil contents of powdered drugs are lower than those for corresponding whole drugs.

Extractable Matter

The determination of matter extractable into solvents such as water, alcohol and ether is generally used for evaluating plant drugs, the constituents of which are not readily estimated by chemical or biological methods. Extractive values thus provide assay for drugs such as linseed, which contain fixed oil as an important constituent. Here ether-soluble extractive is required to fall within the prescribed range. Similarly water-soluble extractive values for drugs like liquorice, valerian and gentian provide an assay process. Yield of drugs to solvent which normally do not have much action upon the drug itself may be used to detect and approximately determine the amount of an adulterant which dissolves in the solvent. For example, when colocynth seeds are used with the pulp in powdered colocynth, its petroleum ether-soluble extractive is higher than normal. On the other hand the amount of insoluble matter will also indicate the presence of an unreasonable amount of woody matter or pieces of bark or vegetable debris in drugs such as myrrh, balsam of tolu, catechu, benzoin etc. However when assay methods are developed, e.g., assay for anthraquinone drugs, the extractive tests are no longer required as pharmacopoeial standards.

Extraction of drugs is by maceration or by percolation. Water, ethanol, ether and petroleum ether are the usual solvents used. Concentration of ethanol specified in the test procedure for the herbal material is used for extraction (90% ethanol for ginger and jalap, 60% ethanol for valerian and 45% ethanol for quillaia).

Ash Values

The ash remaining following ignition of herbal materials is a measure of the total amount of the inorganic material left after burning. For some drugs this value gives an indication of the care taken in the preparation of the drug. Adulteration with mineral matter will give higher ash values than for pure unadulterated drug. Determination of ash is useful for detecting low-grade products, exhausted drugs and excess of sandy or earthy matter, especially in powdered drugs. Different types of ash values such as total ash, acid-insoluble ash, sulphated ash and water-soluble ash are measured.

The total ash is determined by incinerating 2–4 g of air-dried drug by gradually increasing heat up to 450° C. The objective is to remove the carbon at as low a temperature as possible. This is because volatile alkali chlorides may be lost at high temperatures without leaving an ash. EP and BP use sulphated ash which involves treatment of the drug with dilute sulphuric acid before ignition. All oxides and carbonates are thus converted to sulphates and the ignition is carried out at 600° C.

For water-soluble ash, the total ash is boiled with water and filtered. The insoluble matter is further ignited in an ashless filter paper. The weight of the formed ash subtracted from the total ash value gives the water-soluble ash.

Total ash is treated with dilute hydrochloric acid, filtered and the insolubles on ignition give acid-insoluble ash. This measures the amount of silica present, especially as sand and silicious earth.

Total ash consists mainly of carbonates, phosphates, silicates and silica. It includes both 'physiological' ash which is derived from the plant itself and 'non-physiological' ash, which is the residue of extraneous matter such as sand, soil, chalk or lime (used for coating drugs such as nutmeg, ginger etc.) that may be present.

Total ash is not useful in detecting adulteration with earthy matter when it varies within a wide range as it does for rhubarb (8% to 40%), because of the variable calcium oxalate content. In such cases acid-insoluble ash which removes the variable calcium oxides or carbonates formed will indicate the presence of earthy matter likely to be present in roots, rhizomes and pubescent leaves such as digitalis and henbane.

Water-soluble ash detects material exhausted by water. E.g., tea and ginger, if admixed with exhausted drugs will show much greater reduction in water-soluble ash than total ash. It is therefore an important indicator when exhausted material is substituted for the genuine drug.

Crude Fibre

Crude drugs may be processed to separate crude fibre, which is a means of concentrating the more resistant cellular material of drugs for microscopic examination. This is especially applicable when the amount of foreign matter in a powder is small. Preparing a crude fibre concentrates the resistant parts of adulterants in a small amount of tissue thus facilitating better microscopic examination. It is particularly useful for starchy drugs such as ginger, which are rich in oleoresin and starch. The technique involves defatting the powder and boiling in turn with standard acid and alkali with suitable washing of the insoluble residue obtained in different stages. The procedure disintegrates the tissues readily such that the resistant material is suitable for microscopic study. The crude fibre so obtained is employed quantitatively to assay the fibre content of foods and animal feedstuff and also to detect crude drug adulteration, such as clove stalks in cloves. For detection of insect infestation, it is possible to further treat the crude fibre with acetic anhydride and sulphuric acid to destroy all lignified matter in the fibre. What is left will be only insect particles that may be easily visualized. Crude fibre values vary widely for many drugs making it difficult to apply as the only evidence of adulteration.

Detection of Hazardous Chemical Contaminants and Residues

Herbs and herbal products ideally need to be free of pesticides, fumigants and other hazardous contaminants. At best they may be controlled for the absence of unsafe levels. Herbal drugs are prone to pesticide residues, which accumulate from agricultural practices, such as spraying, treatment of soils during cultivation and administration of fumigants during storage.

Presence of contaminants or residues in herbal drugs can either be accidental or intentional. They may be classified into physicochemical contaminants and biological contaminants. A variety of agrochemical agents and some organic solvents may be important residues in herbal medicines. Contamination should be avoided and controlled through quality assurance measures such as GAP for medicinal plants and GMP for herbal medicines. Chemical and microbiological contaminants can result from the use of human excreta, animal manures and sewage as fertilizers. As per WHO guidelines on GAP for medicinal plants, human excreta must not be used as a fertilizer and animal manures should be thoroughly composted. The level of some contaminants and residues present at the stage of harvesting may change as a result of post-harvest processing (e.g. drying) in herbal preparations such as extracts and in finished herbal products during the manufacturing process.

Hazardous contaminants/residues likely to be present in herbal drugs are discussed below.

(i) *Toxic metals and non-metals*: Presence of lead, cadmium, mercury, chromium, copper, arsenic or nitrite in herbal drugs is attributed to many causes including environmental pollution (contaminated emissions from factories, leaded petrol, contaminated water from rivers, lakes and sea, pesticides etc.). They can pose clinically relevant dangers for the health of the user. The potential intake of the toxic metal can be estimated by the level of its presence in the product and the recommended or estimated dosage of the product. This potential exposure can then be put into a toxicological perspective by comparison with the Provisional Tolerable Weekly Intake values (PTWI) for toxic metals which have been established by the Food and Agriculture Organization of the WHO.

A simple, straightforward determination of heavy metals can be found in many pharmacopoeias and is based on colour reactions with special reagents such as thioacetamide or diethyl dithiocarbamate. The amount present is estimated by comparison with a standard. Instrumental analyses have to be employed when the metals are present in trace quantities, in admixture or when the analyses have to be quantitative. The main methods commonly used are atomic absorption spectrometry (AAS), inductively coupled plasma analysis (ICPA) and neutron activation analysis (NAA). The use of herbal medicines is not generally expected to contribute significantly to the exposure of the population to heavy metal contaminants. Still it is recommended that their levels be minimized.

(ii) *Pesticides, agrochemical residues and other persistent organic pollutants*: Organic chemicals such as synthetic aromatic chlorinated hydrocarbons generated inadvertently as by-products of combustion or industrial processes and persistent pesticides such as dioxin aldrin, chlordane, DDT, dieldrin, endrin, heptachlor, mirex are likely to remain in herbal medicines.

Insecticides, fungicides, nematocides, herbicides, ascaricides, molluscicides, rodenticides and fumigants such as ethylene oxide, ethylene chlorhydrin, methyl bromide and sulfur dioxide are classes of pesticide residues that may accumulate in herbal drugs. Agricultural practices like soil treatment, spraying, fumigation during storage are the sources of such contamination. Of these, only chlorinated hydrocarbons and related pesticides and a few organophosphorous pesticides (e.g. carbophenothion) have a long residual action. Though use of these pesticides is widely discontinued, residues like DDT may still remain in the environment. Copper-based pesticides, though essential in terms of plant nutrition, at higher levels of ingestion (70 mg/day) can have serious adverse effects on health. Also copper is strongly bio-accumulated in nature and therefore is likely to persist in herbal materials. Though most pesticides have very short residual action, herbal materials need to be tested for the presence of organically bound chlorine and phosphorous as a preliminary screening method. Even though there are no serious reports of toxicity due to the presence of pesticides and fumigants, herbal products have to be controlled for their presence to safe levels.

TLC and GC methods are available for the determination of organochlorine and urea derivatives, enzymatic methods for organophosphorous compounds, colorimetric methods for urea derivatives and spectroscopic techniques for paraquat triazines and heavy metals. Toxic residues in herbal drugs may be substantially reduced or eliminated by the use of infusions of the dried plant material by the extraction of the useful plant constituents. Storage at 30°C has been shown to reduce rapidly the ethylene oxide residues in senna pods to tolerable levels.

HPLC and GC are the principal methods for the determination of pesticide residues when coupled with MS. Samples are extracted by a standard procedure, impurities are removed by partition and/or adsorption and the presence of a moderately broad spectrum of pesticides is measured in a single determination. However these techniques are not universally applicable. Some pesticides are satisfactorily carried through the extraction and clean-up procedures, others are recovered with a poor yield and some are lost entirely. Following chromatography, the separations may not always be complete. Pesticides may decompose or metabolize and many of the metabolic products are still unknown. As a result of the limitations in the analytical technique and incomplete knowledge of pesticide interactions with the environment, it is not yet possible to apply an integrated set of methods that is satisfactory in all situations.

Generally the methodology should be adapted to the type of herbal material being tested, and modifications may be necessary for different samples – including seeds, leaves, oils, extracts and finished products – and for samples containing different quantities of moisture. Also, the spectrum of pesticides to be tested for is dependent on the specific pesticides used on the herbal material and the history of use of persistent pesticides in the region.

It is therefore desirable to test herbal materials of unknown history for broad groups of compounds rather than for individual pesticides. Various methods are suitable for this purpose. Pesticides containing chlorine in the molecule, for example, can be detected by the measurement of total organic chlorine; insecticides containing phosphate can be measured by analysis for total organic phosphorous, whereas pesticides containing arsenic and lead can be detected by measurement of total arsenic or total lead, respectively. Similarly, the measurement of total bound carbon disulphide in a sample will provide information on whether residues of the dithiocarbamate family of fungicides are present.

Importantly, where such general methods are employed, care must be taken to ensure that results are not adversely affected by contributions from certain plant constituents containing the targeted elements. If the pesticide to which the herbal material has been exposed is known or can be identified by suitable means, an established method for the determination of that particular pesticide residue should be employed. General aspects of analytical methodology and commonly recommended procedures for the qualitative and quantitative determination of important pesticide groups are as per WHO guidelines and pharmacopoeias.

(iii) *Solvents:* Solvents used in herbal drug processing can be detected as residues in herbal preparations and finished products. Depending upon their potential risk (benzene: class I, methanol, hexane: class II, ethanol: class III), they have to be controlled through GMP and QC.

(iv) *Radioactive contamination*: A certain amount of ionizing radiation including nuclides occurring naturally in the earth and atmosphere is unavoidable. WHO in collaboration with several other international organizations has developed guidelines to prevent widespread contamination by radionuclides in the dangerous consequence of a nuclear accident such as in Chernobyl and Fukushima. Taking into consideration the quantity of herbal medicine normally consumed, this is an unlikely health risk. Thus at present no limits are proposed for radioactive contamination.

Biological Contaminants

Parasites, microbial contaminants, mycotoxins and endotoxins are the classes of biological contaminants likely to be found in herbal materials.

(i) *Parasites*: Protozoa, nematodes and their ova may be introduced during cultivation or during processing and manufacturing if personal hygiene measures have not been taken by handling personnel. As a result zoonosis may occur especially if uncomposted animal excreta are used during cultivation.

(ii) *Microbiological contaminants*: Medicinal plants may be associated with a broad variety of microbial contaminants represented by bacteria, fungi and viruses. This microbiological background depends on several environmental factors and affects the overall quality of herbal products and preparations.

A large number of bacteria and moulds often originating in soil or derived from manure are found in herbal materials. Some of them form the naturally occurring microflora of medicinal plants of which aerobic spore-forming bacteria frequently predominate. Improper methods of harvesting, cleaning, drying, handling and storage may cause additional contamination and microbial growth.

Microbial contamination may also occur during processing of herbal materials. Failure to control moisture levels during transportation and storage as well as failure to control the temperature of liquid formulations and finished products could be the reason. Presence of *Escherichia coli* and *Salmonella* species and moulds may indicate poor quality of production and harvesting practices. GAP and GMP are thus critical for effective control of microbial contamination. Laboratory procedures investigating microbial contamination limit their levels as indicated by values laid down in pharmacopoeias as well as in WHO guidelines. Generally a complete procedure consists of determining the total aerobic microbial count, the total fungal count and the total *Enterobacteriaceae* count, together with tests for the presence of *E. coli*, *Staphylococcus aureus*, *Shigella*, *Pseudomonas aeruginosa* and *Salmonella* species. As per WHO guidelines, *Salmonella* and *Shigella* species must not be present at any stage in herbal medicines intended for internal use. Different pharmacopoeias have different testing requirements.

Vegetable drugs tend to show much higher levels of microbial contamination than synthetic products. European pharmacopoeias hence allow higher levels of microbial contamination in herbal drugs than in synthetic pharmaceuticals. The allowed contamination level may also depend on the method of processing of the drug. For example, higher levels are permitted if the final herbal preparation involves boiling with water. Presence of fungi should be carefully monitored since common species produce toxins which can pose acute and chronic risks to health.

These fungal toxins called mycotoxins are usually secondary metabolic products which are non-volatile, have a relatively low molecular weight and may be secreted onto or into the medicinal plant material. They may help parasitic fungi invade host tissues. Mycotoxins are of four main groups namely aflatoxins, ochratoxins, fumonisins and trichothecenes, all of which have toxic effects.

Aflatoxins have been extensively studied and are classified as group I human carcinogens by the international agency for research on cancer. Aflatoxin-producing fungi sometimes build up during storage. Procedures for their determination in herbal drugs are published by the WHO. After a thorough clean-up procedure, TLC is used for confirmation. Mycotoxins produced by the species of fungi including *Aspergillus*, *Fusarium* and *Penicillium* are the most commonly reported. In addition to the risk of bacterial and viral contamination, herbal materials may also carry bacterial endotoxins. Found mainly in the outer membranes of certain Gram-negative bacteria and released during cell disruption, they are complex lipopolysaccharide molecules that elicit an antigenic response, cause altered resistance to bacterial infections and have other serious effects. Certain plant constituents are susceptible to chemical transformation by contaminating microorganisms. Withering leads to enhanced enzymatic activity, transforming some of the constituents to other metabolites not initially found in the herb. These newly formed constituents may cause adverse effects along with formed moulds such as *Penicillium nigricans* and *P. jensi*.

Tests for the presence of microbial contamination on herbal drugs should be performed in dosage forms in compliance with the requirements of national, regional or international pharmacopoeias. BP for example requires drugs such as acacia, agar and powdered digitalis to be free of *E. coli* in the quantity of the material stated. Others like alginic acid, cochineal and tragacanth are also tested for the absence of Salmonella. Drugs such as agar and guar gum galactomannan should not have total viable count of 10 microorganisms/gm. Generally manufacturers will ensure that for crude drugs to be taken internally, the limits for bacterial and mould contamination as applicable to food stuffs are adhered to. Considerable quantities of drugs are sterilized in special equipment by treatment with ethylene oxide.

Phytochemical Standardization

To ensure quality of herbal drugs, it is necessary not only to establish the identity, but also to ensure batch-to-batch reproducibility. Apart from macroscopic and microscopic evaluation, tests to identify principal chemical groups are the next priority. These cover identification and characterization of the crude drug with respect to phytochemical constituents. Several analytical techniques are to be employed for this.

a. Physicochemical standards: applicable to groups of specific constituents

(i) Fixed oils, volatile oils and related substances

Physical constants such as specific gravity, optical rotation, viscosity and refractive index are especially valuable for oils and fats, oleoresins, balsams, gums and similar substances. A number of quantitative chemical tests such as acid value, iodine value, saponification value, ester value, unsaponifiable matter, acetyl value, volatile acidity (Reichert Meissl value) are mainly applicable to fixed oils. Hence some of these tests are also useful in the evaluation of resins (acid value, sulphated ash) volatile oils (acid value, acetyl value, ester value) and gums (methoxyl determination, volatile acidity). The pharmacopoeias prescribe range of values of these physical and chemical parameters for different fixed oils, oleoresins, volatile oils, balsams etc. as appropriate for each of them. Experimental determination of these indices for the crude drug/derived product to evaluate if the values are within the pharmacopoeial limits will thus indicate their standard.

(ii) Swelling index/swelling factor

Crude drugs especially gums and those containing an appreciable amount of mucilage, pectin or hemicellulose are of specific therapeutic or pharmaceutical utility because of their swelling properties. The swelling index is the volume (in ml) taken up by the swelling of 1g of herbal material under specified conditions. Its determination is based on the addition of water or a swelling agent as specified in the test procedure for each individual herbal drug (either whole, cut or powdered). Using a glass-stoppered measuring cylinder, the material is shaken repeatedly for one hour and then allowed to stand for a required period of time. The volume of the mixture (in ml) is then read. The mixing of whole herbal material with the swelling agent is easy to achieve, but cut or pulverized material requires vigorous shaking at specified intervals to ensure even distribution of the material in the swelling agent. BP prescribes standard for agar as ≤10, linseed ≥4 for whole drug, ≥ 4.5 for powdered drug, Ispaghula husk ≥10, powder ≥90.

(iii) Foaming index

Saponin-rich plant drugs can cause persistent foam when an aqueous decoction is shaken. The foaming ability of an aqueous decoction of herbal materials and their extracts is measured in terms of foaming index; 1 g of the herbal material (powdered and passed through #1250 sieve) is transferred to a 500 ml conical flask containing 100 ml of boiling water. After 30 minutes of moderate boiling, cool, filter into a 100 ml standard flask and make up the volume with sufficient water. Transfer successive portions of 1 ml, 2 ml, 3 ml up to 10 ml of the decoction respectively into 10 stoppered test tubes and make up to 10 ml volumes with water. Stopper and shake them for 15 seconds and set aside for 15 minutes. Measure the height of the foam. If it is less than 1 cm in all tubes, the foaming index is taken as less than 100. If it is more than 1 cm in all tubes, the foam index is over 1,000 and the test is to be repeated by dilution, such that foam height of about 1 cm is got in at least one of the tubes. The volume (in ml) (a) of the decoction used for preparing the dilution in the tube where foaming of 1 cm height is observed is used to determine the foaming index using the formula 1000/a.

(iv) Determination of haemolytic activity

Ability to cause haemolysis is a characteristic property of saponins. Many herbal drugs, especially those derived from families Caryophyllaceae, Araliaceae, Sapindaceae, Primulaceae and Dioscoreaceae, contain saponins. Saponins when added to a suspension of blood produce changes in erythrocyte membranes, causing haemoglobin to diffuse into the surrounding medium.

The haemolytic activity of herbal materials, or a preparation containing saponins, is determined by comparison with that of reference saponin drug R, which has a haemolytic activity of 1,000 units/g. A suspension of erythrocytes is mixed with equal volumes of a serial dilution of the herbal material extract. The lowest concentration to effect complete haemolysis is determined after allowing the mixtures to stand for a given period of time. A similar test is carried out simultaneously with the reference drug R. Procedures proposed for the determination of the haemolytic activity of saponin-containing drugs are all based on the same principle, although the details with respect to the source of erythrocyte suspension, preparation or experimental method may change. In order to obtain reliable results, it is essential to standardize the experimental conditions and especially determine the haemolytic activity by comparison with that of the reference saponin drug R.

(v) Determination of bitterness value

Herbal drugs such as gentian that have a strong bitter taste called 'bitters' are employed therapeutically mostly as appetizing agents. Their bitterness is said to stimulate gastric secretions. Bitters can be determined chemically. However since they are composed of two or more constituents with various degrees of bitterness, it is to be measured by taste.

The bitter properties of herbal material are determined by comparing the threshold bitter concentration of an extract of the materials with that of a dilute solution of quinine hydrochloride R. The bitterness value is expressed in units equivalent to the bitterness of a solution containing 1g of quinine hydrochloride R in 2,000 ml. Safe drinking water should be used as a vehicle for the extraction of herbal materials and for mouth wash after each testing. Taste buds dull quickly if distilled water is used. The hardness of water rarely has any significant influence on bitterness. Sensitivity of bitterness varies from person to person, and even for the same person it may be different at different times. Therefore the same person should taste both the material to be tested and the quinine hydrochloride solution within a short space of time. The bitter sensation is not felt by the whole surface of the tongue, but is limited to the middle section of the upper surface of the tongue. A certain amount of training is required to perform this test. A person who does not appreciate a bitter sensation when tasting a solution of 0.058 mg of quinine hydrochloride R in 10 ml water is not suitable to undertake this determination.

The preparation of the stock solution of each individual herbal material should be specified in the test procedure. In each test series, unless otherwise indicated, the determination should start with the lowest concentration in order to retain sufficient sensitivity of the taste buds. Bitterness value of herbal drugs is to be done only after their identity has been confirmed.

b. **Phytochemical screening**

It is essentially a first step in a series of procedures such as extraction, purification and characterization of the active constituents of pharmaceutical importance. These constituents are either of known therapeutic activity or are chemically defined substances or a group of substances generally accepted to contribute substantially to the therapeutic activity of herbal drugs.

Phytochemical screening involves a preliminary extraction of the crude drug with a suitable solvent such as alcohol by any of the general methods of extraction such as maceration, percolation etc. The concentration extracted is subjected to a battery of qualitative chemical tests to identify various classes of phytoconstituents such as alkaloids, lipids, anthraquinones, terpenoids, flavonoids, tannins, coumarins, saponins, volatile oils, resins etc. Alternatively the drug is subjected to successive extraction with solvents of increasing polarity to isolate constituents of corresponding polarity in the respective solvents. These upon concentration yield extracts that are qualitatively evaluated for the presence of groups of phytoconstituents. Qualitative chemical tests may identify specific constituent groups like alkaloids, sugars, lipids etc. A combination of techniques, especially chromatography, is now employed for the positive identification of phytoconstituents.

c. **Quantitative chemical evaluation**

Assaying herbal drugs with known active principals is another method of ensuring product identity and purity. An assay is established to set criterion for the minimum accepted percentage of active substances. A crude drug may be assayed for a particular group of constituents, for example, total alkaloids in cinchona or total sennosides in senna. Alternatively it may be necessary to evaluate specific components like reserpine content in Rauwolfia species. A plethora of analytical methods based on chemical and physical assays are available for routine standardization.

- Gravimetric assays are used for drugs such as colchicines in colchicum corm, podophyllum resin, total balsamic esters, caffeine in tea etc.
- Simple physical separation assay based on complex formation with cresol is used for determining cineole content in eucalyptus oil.
- Acid-base titration based assays are routinely employed to determine the total alkaloid content of tobacco, opium or cinchona as also are strychnine in nux vomica, cinnamaldehyde in cinnamon, free alcohols in peppermint oil, carvone in oil of caraway, citral in lemon oil.
- Spectrophotometric methods including colorimetric and flourimetric assays are developed for most active ingredients of herbal drugs.
- Several newer assay techniques based on HPLC, GC, radioimmunoassay, enzyme-immunoassay are being developed for assaying phytoconstituents.

Chromatographic Techniques

Chromatography is the science which studies the separation of molecules based on differences in their structure and/or composition. In general it involves moving (in a mobile phase) preparation of materials to be separated over a stationary support. Based on their differential affinity between the mobile and stationary phase, molecules in the preparation get separated between the phases. Chromatographic separations can be achieved on a variety of supports. Immobilized silica on glass plates in TLC, highly subdivided silica on aluminium sheets in HPTLC, volatile gases in GC, paper in PC and liquids with incorporated hydrophilic, insoluble molecules in HPLC are some of the supports effecting separations.

Chromatographic techniques are invaluable in the analysis of herbal drugs as they offer very powerful separation ability such that even complex chemical components in herbal drugs can be separated into relatively simple sub-fractions. Despite advances in chromatography with sophisticated instrumentation, basic techniques like column chromatography and TLC are still invaluable aids for the separation of phytoconstituents in quantity and identification of phytoconstituent profiles respectively.

a. Thin layer chromatography

TLC was the common method of choice for herbal drug analysis long before instrumental chromatographic methods like GC and HPLC were established and in use even now. Its ease of usage, versatility, sensitivity, simplicity of sample preparation and simultaneous applicability to multiple samples make it a convenient tool for the detection of quality and adulteration in herbal drugs. TLC is a powerful and relatively rapid technique to distinguish between chemical classes, where macroscopy and microscopy may fail. Chromatograms of essential oils are widely published in scientific literature and can be of invaluable help in herbal drug identification.

b. High performance thin layer chromatography

It is a sophisticated, advanced and an automated version of TLC, which combines the simplicity and precision of TLC with the speed and efficient quantitation which modern instrumentation provides. It employs high performance precoated silica gel plates which give more efficient and reproducible separation than conventional grades of silica. Very small accurately measured volumes may be applied at predetermined rate on exact locations at measured distances from neighbouring spots if any. Development time is much smaller and the developed chromatogram may be evaluated by comparison with reference standards. It may also be quantified with greater sensitivity and precision than is possible with conventional TLC.

Forced-flow planar chromatography (FFPC), rotation planar chromatography (RPC) and over pressured layer chromatography (OPLC) are some of the updated techniques in TLC being employed in herbal drug analysis.

c. Gas chromatography

Separation and analysis of volatile oil components such as essential oils and fatty oils are best undertaken on GC. A GC chromatogram gives a reasonable fingerprint of the volatile oil that is used to identify the plant. The composition and relative concentration of the organic compound in the volatile oil are characteristic of the particular plant and presence of impurities may be readily detected. GC enables straightforward extraction of volatile oil and it can be standardized by component identification using GC-MS analysis. GC-MS is the first online combination of chromatography and spectroscopy and is widely used in the analysis of essential oils. Monitoring relative quantities of components will assess changes in volatile oil composition, indicating oxidative and other changes. GC with flame ionization detector (FID) gives sensitivity of detection of all volatile compounds in a mixture. However GC is not convenient for polar compounds and non-volatile compounds.

d. High performance liquid chromatography

HPLC is the most preferred method for quantitative analysis of more complex mixtures. It is easy to learn and use and is not limited by the volatility or stability of the compound. HPLC in general can be used to analyse almost all compounds in herbal drugs. Extensively applied for herbal drug analysis, reversed phase columns are most used for analytical separation of phytocompounds. It is simplest to use once conditions are optimized that require skill, expertise and experience.

Micellar electrokinetic capillary chromatography (MECC), high-speed counter current chromatography (HSCCC), low-pressure size exclusion chromatography (SEC), reversed phase ion-pairing HPLC (RP-IPC-HPLC), strong anion-exchange HPLC (SAX-HPLC) are some of the newer methods that provide better opportunities for good separation of specific extracts of some herbal drugs. Their versatility is an advantage since most phytoconstituents are non-chromophoric. HPLC coupled with evaporative light scattering detector (ELSD) is an excellent detector of non-chromophoric compounds. It provides direct analysis of many pharmacologically active components in herbal drugs. The response of ELSD depends on size, shape and number of eluate particles rather than on the structure and/or chromatophore of analytes as does a UV detector.

HPLC-MS is useful for direct structure elucidation of phytoconstituents in herbal drugs. It provides the advantage of both chromatography as separation method and MS as identification method.

e. Chromatographic fingerprint analysis

Herbal drugs, singularly and in combinations, contain a myriad of compounds in complex matrices in which no single active constituent is responsible for the overall efficacy. This creates a challenge in establishing quality control standards for raw materials and standardization of finished herbal drugs. Botanical extracts made directly from crude plant material show substantial variation in composition, quality and therapeutic effects. Standardization involves adjusting it to a defined constituent or group of constituents with known therapeutic activity. When active principals are unknown, marker constituents are to be established among the known constituents of the extract for standardization purposes.

Markers are chemically defined constituents of an herbal drug that are important for the quality of the finished product. Ideally, the chosen marker should also be responsible for the therapeutic effect of the herbal drug. When the marker is a definite constituent or group of constituents associated with therapeutic activity, it is true standardization.

Ginkgo with its 26% ginkgo flavones and 6% terpenes is a classic example. Such extracts are highly standardized and no longer represent the whole herb and are now considered as phytopharmaceuticals.

Markers are basically of the following three types:

- Active principals – One or a few constituents specific to the particular herbal drug responsible for the claimed activity. E.g. curcumin for turmeric, E- and Z- guggulsterones for guggulipid, ginsenosides for ginseng, andrographolide for kalmegh, silymarin for milk thistle, sennosides for senna, piperine for pepper.

- Chemical markers – Compounds reported from the respective drugs but not specific to them. Activity specific to the marker may or may not be proven. E.g. Vasicine from *Adhatoda vasaca* is its major alkaloid, active principal and an important biomarker. However it cannot be considered as marker specific for Vasaka because it is also present in other species of *Adhatoda*, *Sida* sps, *Paganum harmala* etc. Likewise hyoscyamine is present in several Solanaceous species. On the other hand constituents such as rutin, quercetin or lapachol are found in a number of related plants and therapeutic activity of the drugs may not be attributed to these compounds.

- General markers – Compounds widely present in many plants such as gallic acid, lupeol, stigmasterol, β-sitosterol for which activity may or may not be reported.

Thus traditionally only a few markers of pharmacologically active constituents were employed to assess the quality and authenticity of complex herbal medicines. However, the therapeutic effects of herbal medicines are based on the complex interaction of numerous ingredients in combinations which are totally different from those of chemical drugs. Thus many kinds of chemical fingerprint analysis methods to control the quality of herbal drugs have gradually come into being. Development of fingerprint profiles of plant extracts is one of the most salient requirements in herbal drug standardization.

Chromatographic fingerprint of a plant extract is its chromatographic pattern developed under a standard, repeatable set of experimental conditions.

Developing such reproducible and highly specific chromatographic patterns for herbal drug extracts has been a significant milestone in herbal drug standardization. Thus these extract-specific chromatographic patterns are considered the 'fingerprint' of the analysed extract.

TLC fingerprinting is of key importance for herbal drugs made up of essential oils, resins and gums. In TLC fingerprinting, the data that can be recorded using a HPTLC scanner includes the chromatogram, retardation factor (R_f) values, the colour of the separated bands, their absorption spectra, λ_{max}, and shoulder inflections of all the resolved bands. Information generated from a HPTLC chromatogram has potential application in the identification of an authentic drug by excluding adulterants and also in maintaining the quality and consistency of the drug. HPLC fingerprinting includes recording of the chromatograms, retention time of individual peaks and the absorption spectra with different mobile phases. GC is used for generating the fingerprint profiles of volatile oils and fixed oils.

Such fingerprint profiles are usually distinctive and form a benchmark for the drug when either the active principals are not known or when chemical markers are not available. Also markers, either active principals or chemical markers, can be quantified by HPLC, GC and HPTLC methods from the developed chromatograms. E.g. phyllanthin, hypophyllanthin, gallic acid, ellagic acid content in *Phyllanthus amarus* whole plant; eugenol, gallic acid, ursolic acid, oleanolic acid content in *Ocimum sanctum* leaf. Several methods for quantification of phytochemicals using HPLC are widely reported in literature.

Fingerprint analysis of herbal drugs therefore represents a comprehensive qualitative approach for the purpose of species authentication, evaluation of quality and ensuring the consistency and stability of herbal drugs and their related products. The entire pattern of compounds can then be evaluated to determine not only the presence or absence of desired markers or active constituents but the complete set of ratios of all detectable analytes.

According to the concept of photoequivalence the chromatographic fingerprint of an herbal product is to be identical or similar to a similar profile of a clinically proven reference product.

Apart from serving the purpose of standardization and quality control, the fingerprint profiles, especially of TLC, aid in the experiments for bioassay-guided fractionation leading to the isolation of active compounds.

The chemical fingerprints obtained by chromatographic and electrophoretic techniques, especially by hyphenated chromatographies, are strongly recommended for the purpose of quality control of herbal medicines, since they might represent appropriately the 'chemical integrities' of herbal medicines and therefore be used for authentication and identification of the herbal products.

To summarize, TLC, HPLC and GC, quantitative TLC (QTLC) and HPTLC can determine the homogeneity of a plant extract. OPLC, infrared and UV-visible spectrometry, MS, GC, liquid chromatography (LC) used alone, or in combinations such as GC-MS, LC-MS and nuclear magnetic resonance (NMR) spectroscopy and electrophoretic techniques especially by hyphenated chromatographic techniques are powerful tools, often used for standardization and in quality control of both the raw material and finished herbal drugs including polyherbals. The results from these sophisticated techniques provide a chemical fingerprint as to the nature of chemicals or impurities present in the plant or extract. Methods based on information theory, similarity estimation, chemical pattern recognition, spectral correlative chromatograms (SCC), multivariate resolution, the combination of chromatographic fingerprints and chemometric evaluation for evaluating fingerprints are all powerful tools for quality control of herbal products.

CONCLUSION

Global market for medicinal plants is growing exponentially as plant materials are being increasingly used both in developing countries and in the industrialized world. Today there is a substantial market for herbal drugs both as traditional medicines and in modern medicine. Their widespread availability and lack of effective machinery to regulate manufacturing practices and quality standards have raised concerns over the safety and efficacy of such unregulated availability and usage. Urgent need to develop uniform standards to ensure quality of herbal drugs has resulted in the drafting of model guidelines by WHO to define basic criteria for the evaluation, safety and efficacy of herbal medicines. Several standards prescribed in pharmacopoeias, formularies, WHO and ESCOP monographs and herbal drug PDRs are rigidly being followed by regulatory authorities world over. Such standards include various physicochemical, biological and analytical evaluation techniques. Modern instrumental analytical methods on HPTLC, HPLC, GC and other hyphenated techniques are being developed to standardize multi-constituent complexes of herbal drugs. Formulating uniform standards applicable to herbal drugs in general still seems an arduous task. Meanwhile indiscriminate use of herbs, unlike the closely monitored traditional medicine usage of yesteryears, is clearly an unsafe and questionable practice. Reported adverse and toxic effects of several commonly used herbs and their potential interaction with modern medicines and even some dietary articles have raised alarm over their unsupervised sale and usage. Hence quality control and standardization of botanicals must be the topmost priority if the global demand for safe and effective herbal drugs is to be rightly capitalized upon.

REVIEW QUESTIONS

Essay Questions

1. What are the factors influencing the quality of herbal drugs? Outline the significance and methods for macroscopic and microscopic evaluation of herbal drugs.
2. Discuss the role of chromatographic techniques in herbal drug standardization. Add a note on marker compounds.
3. Describe the phytochemical parameters to be analysed for herbal drug standardization.

Short Notes

1. Quality indication parameters for herbal drug standardization.
2. Crude fibre content.
3. Extractable matter and ash values.
4. Hazardous chemical contaminants and residues in herbal drugs.
5. Evaluation for detection of biological contaminants.

7 Phytochemical Analysis— An Introduction

CHAPTER OBJECTIVES

Introduction

Some General Principles of
Phytochemical Analysis

Extraction, Isolation, and Identification of
Some Phytochemical Classes

Applications of Chromatography to
Phytochemical Analysis

INTRODUCTION

Recent global acceptance and renewed interest toward plant-derived drugs, nutraceuticals, and other natural products, has generated a lot of commercial as well as research activity in phytochemistry. Earliest drug discoveries made possible by random sampling of higher plants, used simpler operations for the separation, purification, and identification of phytoconstituents. Further, research developments with the introduction of chromatographic, spectroscopic, and high throughput screening techniques have enabled beneficial amalgamation of organic chemistry, phytochemistry, pharmacology, and analytical instrumentation. Today phytochemical analysis has advanced to the level of making compound characterizations possible with even tiny fractions of phytoisolates. Direct identification of phytoconstituents from fresh plant parts, extracts, essential oils, and formulations is a straightforward task. However, phytochemical analysis for the isolation and purification of plant active constituents is still a challenging issue because plant drugs are constituted of an enormous variety of organic substances of complex chemical nature. The range and number of discrete molecular structures produced by plants is vast. While molecules of plant primary metabolism are of universal distribution, plant secondary metabolites are of more limited distribution within restricted taxonomic groups, and are of greater therapeutic interest due to their unique physiological effects.

One of the greatest challenges facing phytopharmacological research is the identification of exact active constituents of therapeutically effective polyconstituent plant drugs of alternative or traditional medicine streams. Attempts at isolations have often resulted in frustration due to the loss of activity resulting in compounds of lesser or no activity in comparison to that of multi-constituent plant drugs. Extraction and isolation procedures need to be carefully monitored at each stage to follow the active constituent being isolated. It is found that, with many time-tested and therapeutically efficacious traditional drugs, the activity is not attributable to a single chemical constituent. The observed biological effect could be a synergistic phenomenon resulting from the multipharmacological effects of the complex chemical profile of the drug.

Once active metabolites are successfully identified, a wide range of extraction techniques are available for the isolation of different classes of phytoconstituents.

Equipped with sophisticated separation techniques, current phytochemical analysis is concerned with the development of:

- Techniques to identify classes of bioactive compounds in plant tissues/extracts/herbal recipes prior to their isolation
- Methods and tools for the isolation of such active constituents without much loss of activity
- Analytical techniques to standardize polyconstituent herbals
- Procedures for estimation of heavy metals, pesticides, and other contaminants in plant drugs.

SOME GENERAL PRINCIPLES OF PHYTOCHEMICAL ANALYSIS

Most of the underlying principles of phytochemical operations are traceable to the early nineteenth-century methods of plant drug isolations. Comprehensive knowledge of the physicochemical nature of targeted constituent is an essential prerequisite before its isolation may be attempted. Extraction refers to the physical separation of soluble active metabolite from the insoluble, inactive/inert plant cellular matrix. Depending on the nature of the active constituent, an appropriate method of extraction may be adopted from the innumerable extraction techniques that are available today.

Following is a brief listing of some basic principles of phytochemical isolations:

- Authenticated plant material of established botanical identity free from adulteration and other contaminants shall be the source material.
- Fresh plant parts are used for the direct isolation of active constituents as in the case of essential oil components.
- In general, however, the plant parts are appropriately dried and size reduced before further processing.
- To avoid unwanted chemical changes and enable long-term storage, an extract representative of the chemical constituents of the plant material is prepared.
- Maceration, percolation, hot continuous percolation, digestion, decoction, aqueous-alcoholic extraction by fermentation, and enfleurage are some of the conventional methods of extraction.
- Super critical fluid extraction, microwave-assisted extraction, ultrasonication-assisted extraction, accelerated pressure–assisted solvent extraction, pressurized counter–current liquid extraction, thermal desorption, and phytonic desorption with hydrocarbon solvents are some of the newer methods of extraction.
- Hydrodistillation, sublimation, solvent extraction, enfleurage, and expression are some of the methods applicable to volatile constituent isolations.

- Head space trapping, solid-phase micro-extraction, protoplast extraction, microdistillation, thermodistillation, and molecular distillation are the newer extraction techniques applicable to essential oil components.

- Selection of solvent and method of extraction are dependent on the nature of the plant material, purpose of extraction, and the properties of constituents targeted for isolation.

- When the classes of active constituents are unknown, a preliminary phytochemical screening using qualitative chemical tests will reveal the classes of compounds of relatively high yield.

- The prepared extract may be further fractionated with solvents of varying polarity to segregate the phytoconstituents.

- Further processing of the prepared extract or its fractions is the general approach to the isolation of individual active constituents.

- All extraction and isolation processes need careful monitoring at every stage since processing conditions are likely to bring about chemical degradation due to enzymatic or nonenzymatic hydrolysis, loss of volatile matter, molecular rearrangements, racemization of optically active compounds, proteolytic degradation, artifact formation, etc. These changes may lead to loss of activity.

- Chromatographic separation on a column is a conventional and still the only widely used method for the isolation of constituent compounds in large-scale extractions.

- GC and GLC are ideally suited for the detection and analysis of volatile compounds and volatile derivatives of nonvolatile compounds.

- Volatile mixtures of compounds and single constituents are isolated using simple or fractional distillation.

- Preparative separations of mixture of compounds from fractionated extracts may be undertaken by preparative TLC using adsorbents laid thicker on the supporting medium.

- Paper chromatography and thin-layer chromatography are indispensable tools guiding chromatographic processing as they enable preliminary identification of phytoconstituents in plant extracts by means of co-chromatography with authentic sample of the compound.

- High-speed counter-current chromatography and droplet counter-current chromatography are some of the advanced liquid–liquid chromatographic processing techniques used for the detection and isolation of a range of phytoconstituents.

- High-performance liquid chromatography is one of the most preferred automated separation techniques that gives much rapid and improved separations over conventional column chromatography. From a range of stationary phase columns available, it is possible to effectively use it for the efficient separation and analysis of a number of phytoconstituents of different polarities.

- The versatility of HPLC for the isolation of many classes of phytoconstituents (however, in smaller quantities relative to column chromatography) using preparative columns has made it a convenient separation technique in phytochemistry.

- Characterization of newly isolated constituents is now undertaken with relative ease on milligram quantities of samples using a combination of UV, IR, Mass, NMR, X-ray crystallography and optical dispersion methods.

- Quantitative determination of phytoconstituents is a significant aspect of phytochemical analysis. Newer analytical techniques available today enable accurate estimation of secondary metabolites in multicomponent plant extracts, galenicals, body fluids, and formulations.

EXTRACTION, ISOLATION, AND IDENTIFICATION OF SOME PHYTOCHEMICAL CLASSES

Alkaloids

Alkaloids constitute the single largest class of plant secondary metabolites. Around 10,000 of them are reported and many more newer ones are being identified. They are generally referred to as organic nitrogenous bases of plant origin that are pharmacologically active. All alkaloids cannot be described by a clear-cut definition because not all are basic, and though most commonly encountered in the plant kingdom, to a lesser extent they are also found in bacteria, fungi and animals.

Structurally alkaloids are extremely diverse ranging in complexity from relatively simple molecules to very complex structural forms. Typically alkaloids contain one or more nitrogen atoms present as primary, secondary, or tertiary amines usually as part of a cyclic system. They are extremely variable with respect to their botanical, biochemical origin, chemical structure, and pharmacological action. Though several forms of classification is possible, alkaloids may be conveniently classified based on their biogenetic origin or on the nature of the nitrogen-containing ring system. They usually occur either free or as salts bound to a typical organic acid or occur as N-oxides. Protoalkaloids are those that do not have nitrogen in a ring system, and steroidal terpene alkaloids and purines not derived from amino acids are referred to as pseudo alkaloids. The degree of basicity of alkaloids is variable, depending on the structure and presence and location of other functional groups within the molecule.

Distribution of alkaloids in the plant kingdom is restricted to specific groups of families and genera. In angiosperms they are well represented in many dicotyledonous families. To a very limited extent, they are also distributed in monocots as also in gymnosperms and pteridophytes. Toxic alkaloids of more than 24 classes are reported from skins of amphibians. Many alkaloid-containing plants have been used since early times as drugs, poisons, stimulants, and as psychedelics. Many of our present drugs include alkaloids or their synthetic substitutes and they are of great medicinal significance on account of their powerful pharmacological/toxicological properties.

Properties

Despite their great diversity, alkaloids have many common physical and chemical properties. In general, alkaloids are colourless, crystalline (a few are amorphous) with an intensely bitter taste, and have sharp melting points. Alkaloids like nicotine and coniine are liquids and berberine and sanguinarine are coloured. Presence of nitrogen in their structure confers basic properties and they unite with acids to form salts. This facilitates their isolation as water-soluble salts in the presence of mineral acids. Alkaloids are mostly optically active substances.

They are insoluble or sparingly soluble in water. They are soluble in ether, chloroform, and other nonpolar immiscible solvents. Salts of alkaloids formed on reaction of the bases with acids are water soluble, but insoluble in nonpolar solvents. Solubilities of different alkaloids and their salts show considerable variation. N-oxide alkaloids, protoalkaloids, and pseudoalkaloids are water soluble.

Extraction and isolation of alkaloids

There are several methods reported for the extraction of alkaloids and the choice of method is dependent on the purpose of isolation and scale of operation. For small-scale isolations column chromatography will effectively separate the alkaloids from the initially prepared plant extracts. However, on a commercial scale, large volumes of aqueous extracts of plant materials are pumped through huge metallic columns packed with cationic resins, which in turn collect all basic components (cations). Subsequently, the basic alkaloids are conveniently washed off by flushing the column with a moderately strong acid. Such cationic resins may be reused.

It is rare to find alkaloids occurring single and they are found in plant parts as a mixture of closely related compounds. Hence, the total alkaloids are to be initially extracted prior to attempting separation of individual alkaloids.

Being basic, they occur either free or as salts and can be normally extracted from the plant material into a weakly acidic alcoholic solvent. Most alkaloids may be extracted into an organic solvent after basification. Volatile alkaloids may be isolated by steam distillation and all alkaloids have to be subsequently purified wither by chromatography or by recrystallization using a combination of solvents.

Following is one general method for the isolation of total alkaloids from plant material.

1. Plant material is dried at a temperature not exceeding 60°C and finely powdered.
2. Macerate the powdered material with sufficient quantity of ethanol and set aside overnight. Most alkaloids and their salts being alcohol soluble will get dissolved in the solution.
3. Filter and concentrate the extract to 1/4th the initial volume. Complete the evaporation of the remaining solvent at a temperature not exceeding 50°C.
4. Treat the residue with dilute sulphuric acid and filter to remove resins, fatty matter, and other unwanted substances.
5. Basify the solution by the addition of alkali such as ammonia as it effectively precipitates most alkaloids and because of its volatility, it can be conveniently removed by heating in subsequent processing steps.
6. Extract this solution with successive portions of chloroform or till complete extraction of all the alkaloids is effected.
7. Concentrate the pooled organic layer to yield a crude mixture of total alkaloids of the plant material.
8. Dissolve the above residue in dilute sulphuric acid and filter if necessary.
9. Basify the solution with ammonia and successively extract with chloroform.
10. Run the pooled chloroform layers through a bed of anhydrous sodium sulphate and evaporate to dryness. Note the weight of the mixture of total alkaloids.

Fractionation of the mixture thus obtained into individual alkaloids may be done using a number of techniques such as column chromatography, ion exchange chromatography, counter current liquid–liquid partitioning, HPLC, and preparative TLC.

However, they may also be separated by fractional crystallization or by salt formation.

Alkaloids may be separated from one another based on their relative differential solubilities either in a single solvent or in a mixture of miscible solvents. Most alkaloids are more soluble in chloroform than in other solvents such as acetone, ethanol, methanol, ethyl acetate, ether, benzene, and hexane. Thus the mixture of alkaloids may be dissolved in minimum quantity of chloroform by warming and another solvent such as ethanol may be added in drops. The alkaloid which is less soluble in ethanol than chloroform will crystallize out of the solution. On cooling, crystals of this alkaloid, less soluble in ethanol, can be separated. In this way, the other alkaloids of the mixture could be fractionally crystallized using any of the other solvents in which they may be less soluble compared to chloroform.

For separation of alkaloid by salt formation, the mixture of alkaloids is dissolved in minimum quantity of a warm solution of 10% acetic acid or hydrochloric acid in methanol. Cool the solution and add ether drop by drop for the precipitation of the salt of the alkaloid. Separate the precipitated material by suction filtration and carefully transfer the precipitate into a very small quantity of hot acetone. Addition of drops of methanol will precipitate the salt of the alkaloid. Volatile alkaloids such as nicotine may be isolated by simple distillation of the plant material.

Identification

Alkaloids are precipitated from a neutral or slightly acid solution by a number of metallic salts. These precipitation reactions may be used for the detection of the presence of alkaloids in solution. Some of the metallic salts also give colour reactions with proteins and hence results need to be interpreted with caution. Following are some of the common chemical tests used to detect alkaloids.

1. A solution of the alkaloid treated with dragendroff's reagent (solution of potassium bismuth iodide) gives an orange red precipitate.
2. A solution of the alkaloid when treated with Mayer's reagent (potassiomercuric iodide solution) gives a cream-coloured precipitate.
3. A solution of the alkaloid when treated with Wagner's reagent (solution of iodine in potassium iodide) gives a reddish-brown precipitate.
4. A solution of the alkaloid when treated with Hager's reagent (a saturated solution of picric acid) gives an yellow precipitate.
5. A solution of the alkaloid with solution of tannic acid gives a buff-coloured precipitate.
6. Murexide test: A solution of the alkaloid is mixed with a very small quantity of potassium chlorate and a drop of hydrochloric acid. It is evaporated to dryness and a drop of ammonia is added. A purple colour is formed with purine alkaloids like caffeine, which do not precipitate most other alkaloidal reagents.

Alkaloid form precipitating complexes with phosphomolybdic acid, phosphotungstic acid, and chlorauric acid and chlorplatinic acids and these may be used for their identification.

TLC identification

Alkaloids being chemically heterogeneous, cannot be identified in plant extracts using a single chromatographic test. However, the following general procedure may be used for the preliminary detection of alkaloids in plant tissues.

1. Macerate the dried plant material in 10% acetic acid in methanol for about 4 hours, filter and concentrate to 1/4th the original volume.

2. Add ammonia drop by drop for the precipitation of the alkaloid. Centrifuge the solution and carefully collect the precipitate.

3. Dissolve the precipitate in a few drops of ethanol and spot it on a Silica gel TLC plate.

4. Develop in methanol: ammonia (200:3) and spray with dragendroff's reagent. Presence of alkaloids is indicated by the development of an orange red–coloured spot.

The presence of alkaloids may be confirmed by measuring the UV absorbance of a sample of the alkaloid dissolved in 0.1 M sulphuric acid. Typical maxima values range from 250–303 nm. Alkaloids with aromatic rings in their structures may absorb at longer wavelengths.

Lipids

Lipids are a heterogenous group of compounds widely distributed throughout the plant kingdom. In plants they occur in the seeds, nuts, and fruits; in animals they are stored in adipose tissues, bone marrows, and nervous tissues. They are found in all organisms as structural components of the cell membrane.

Based on the chemical composition, lipids may be classified into three subgroups. Simple lipids are those that upon hydrolysis yield an alcohol and one or more fatty acids. Oils, fats, and waxes are simple lipids. Compound lipids have elements such as Phosphorous, Sulphur, and Nitrogen in their composition. Derived lipids include hydrolytic products of lipids as well as other lipid-like compounds like sterols, carotenoids, essential oils, aldehydes, ketones, alcohols, hydrocarbons, etc.

Plants store excess energy as carbohydrates, which later are converted to energy-rich triglycerides. These are converted back to carbohydrates during germination. Triglycerides are found in seeds, which are the source of most vegetable oils. Plants contain storage lipids mainly in the seeds. Some plants store it in the pericarp (olive, palm, avocado) and rarely in tubers (tiger nut tubers—*Cyperus esculentus*). In seeds storage lipids may be accumulated in one or both of the main types of seed tissue, that is, embryo or endosperm. For example, in sunflower, linseed or rapeseed, lipids are stored in the cotyledons of the embryo and in castor bean, coriander, or carrot, the endosperm is the main site of lipid accumulation. Tobacco, however, stores lipids in both embryo and endosperm tissues.

Hydrocarbons and waxes are found on the cuticle of fruits and leaves and these serve as protective coatings and as aids of water retention. Carnauba wax, Japan wax, and Ouricury wax are some examples of plant waxes.

Lipids comprise 7% of the dry weight in leaves in higher plants and they are important as membrane constituents in the chloroplasts and mitochondria. The amount of lipids in plant parts vary from 0.1–70%.

Polar lipids—phospholipids and glycolipids are structural components of plant cell membranes. Galactolipid are unique plant lipids enriched in plant membranes, particularly chloroplasts. As plants have no mechanism for controlling their temperature, they must possess membrane lipids that remain mobile at relatively low temperatures.

In addition to serving the function of food or energy storage, fats and oils are important products pharmaceutically, industrially, and as food. They are of tremendous importance in nutrition as they rank the highest among food in calorific value. In addition, they find use for cooking, soap making, glycerol manufacture, and for medicinal purposes.

Composition

Oils and fats, the principal plant lipids, are esters of long-chain fatty acids and alcohol or of closely related derivatives. Chemically fixed oils and fats are composed predominantly of triacyl glycerols having identical or different fatty acids esterified to the three hydroxyl positions on the glycerol molecule. Numerous fatty acids are now known in plants, common ones being saturated or simple unsaturated compounds of C16- C18 –chain length. Palmitic acid (C16 acid), is the major saturated acid in leaf lipids and it also occurs in quantity in seed oils such as groundnut oil. Stearic acid (C18) is less prominent in leaf lipids, but is a major saturated acid in seed fats in a number of plant families. Unsaturated acids are widespread in both leaf and seed oils. Oleic acid comprises 80% of the fatty acid content of olive oil, 59% in groundnut oil and is often accompanied by the di-unsaturated linoleic acid. The tri-unsaturated linoleic acid is common, occurring in linseed oil along with linoleic and oleic acids. Rarer fatty acids such as petroselinic acid, erucic acid, and sterculic acids are found as lipid components occurring characteristically in seed oils of a few related plants.

Waxes are esters of high molecular weight fatty acids and monohydric alcohols and the chain length varies from 24–36 carbon atoms. They vary with nature of the monohydric alcohol which could be a sterol such as cholesterol, stigmasterol, ergosterol, or others such as acetyl alcohol, myricyl alcohol, etc. In addition, many plant waxes contain varying quantities of higher saturated hydrocarbons, long-chain ketones, and secondary alcohols. Higher fatty esters of carotenols, free and combined sterols in combination with higher acids are also found. A number of glycerol containing fatty substances with physical properties similar to that of waxes are also referred to as true waxes. Japan wax is one such wax and it has a high melting point and is nongreasy to touch because of the presence of high molecular weight dibasic acids.

In addition to triacylglycerols, mono and di-acylglycerols and free fatty acids may be present in oils and fats depending on the maturity and physical condition of the natural source at the time of lipid extraction.

Phospholipids are characterized by a phosphate ester joined to either choline, ethanolamine, inositol, or serine attached to the C-1 position of glycerol and fatty acids are esterified to the C-2 and C-3 positions. Diacylgalactoglycerol and diacylgalabiosylglycerol are glycolipids playing an important role in chloroplast metabolism.

Leaf cutin acids, though not fat components, are formed from fatty acids by chain elongation and they have a longer chain length ranging from C24-C32. These acids have hydroxyl groups in their structures.

Properties

The properties associated with lipids are dependent on the nature and extent of its fatty acid composition. Lipids are in general defined by their solubility properties. They are soluble in organic solvents (ether, petroleum ether, benzene, chloroform, alcohol, etc.) and sparingly soluble in water. Greasy in nature, they yield a permanent translucent stain when applied on paper. They are colourless liquids or solids, lighter than water and immiscible with it. More or less they are viscous and possess a characteristic odor (waxes are odorless). They are nonvolatile, cannot be distilled, and decompose on heating giving an irritating odor of acrolein. Oils and fats readily form emulsions when agitated with water in the presence of soap, gelatin, or other emulsifiers. On prolonged exposure to air, moisture, and light, they develop a rancid odor, which is due to the oxidation of esters partly due to microorganisms. Glycerides may be readily sapinified into glycerol and salts of fatty acids.

Oils such as linseed having a high degree of unsaturation absorb oxygen on exposure to air and undergo oxidation and polymerization forming a tough protective film on the surface. This property makes it a drying oil of much use in the paint industry. Some fixed oils like cotton seed oil, dry very slowly and are called semi-drying oils. The economic value of several oils of commercial importance is dependent upon their composition and purity.

Waxes are more resistant to saponification than fats and oils.

Extraction and isolation

Due to their special solubility properties, lipids may be extracted from plant tissues with alcohol or ether. Such an extraction removes other classes of lipids like leaf alkanes and steroids. The actual method of isolation of lipids from natural sources is largely dependent on the nature of the lipid and its source.

Conventional vegetable oils are separated from the plant tissue by expression. In this, the seeds are crushed by rollers and pressed in hydraulic press or continuous expellers, when the oil separates leaving behind the "oil cake," which was earlier used as fodder. Such oil is called virgin or cold-pressed oil. When heat assists expression, it is hot-pressed oil. Solvent extraction is used to extract the remaining oil from the pressed cake. The crude oil or fat is treated with a little alkali to neutralize free acid and also to coagulate any colloidal impurities present. It is then bleached by warming at 70–80°C with animal charcoal, fuller's earth, or plaster of paris. After about half an hour, the decolorized oil is filtered through filter press and then deodorized by passing superheated steam through it. The oil is then quickly cooled and withdrawn, so that its odor may not be impaired. Seeds being rich sources of oils may be conveniently processed by expression.

For small-scale laboratory isolation of simple lipids, the fresh plant material may be coarsely injured and then subjected to hot continuous percolation with hexane or petroleum ether for complete extraction of all the fatty matter. The percolate may then be evaporated to yield the lipids present in it.

When plant tissue is being processed for the separation of lipids, the following general procedure may be used:

1. The freshly collected plant material is homogenized in 100 parts of isopropyl alcohol (to inhibit lipases that rapidly hydrolyze the plant lipids releasing free fatty acids). For tissues such as cereals in which the lipids are very tightly bound, extraction with chloroform: ethanol: water (200:95:5) is preferred.

2. It is filtered and the marc is re-extracted with 1:1 v/v chloroform, isopropanol by sufficient mixing.

3. It is filtered and the combined filtrates are vacuum evaporated. The residue is dissolved in minimum volume of 2:1 v/v chloroform, methanol.

4. This solution is then washed with 1/5th volume of 0.9% sodium chloride solution. After gentle vortexing, the mixture is centrifuged at 2000 rpm to separate the two phases.

5. The upper phase containing the polar lipids is taken for appropriate analysis and the lower phase containing the neutral lipids is vacuum evaporated to yield the pure lipid.

6. Alternatively the residue in step 3 can be column chromatographed on silica gel in ethereal solution. The neutral lipids such as oils and fats will pass through, leaving the phospholipids and glycolipids adsorbed.

7. These can be recovered by eluting the column with chloroform–methanol mixture.

Plant lipids are being extracted using a number of techniques such as super critical fluid extraction, pressurized fluid extraction, ultrasound-assisted extraction, and even automated robotic extraction.

Identification

- Small quantities of lipid material extracted from plant tissues may be tested by simple tests such as checking the greasy spot left on paper when stained with it, or by checking its insoluble nature in water.
- When obtained in quantity specific gravity of lipids is usually in the range 0.87–0.97.
- Fixed oils, fats and waxes in general are defined by their solubility, consistency, hardness, colour, specific gravity, viscosity, melting point, solidifying point, optical rotation, and refractive index.
- Some well-known chemical tests may be used to identify fixed oils like Halphen test for cottonseed oil, Baudouin test for sesame oil, and Fitelson test for tea seed oil.
- On account of the complexity of mixture of fatty acids normally present in fixed oils, no single method is available for their separation or analysis. Chemical parameters like acid value, iodine value, saponification value, acetyl value, Reichert-meissl value, and peroxide value are used as indicators for the quality of fixed oils.

Plant lipids may be conveniently identified by chromatographic techniques. For a preliminary analysis and to identify lipid fractions or products of saponification, TLC is best suited. Isolated lipid components or products of hydrolysis can be derivatized into methyl esters and analyzed directly by GLC.

1. Preliminary identification of the total lipids of plant tissue may be undertaken by TLC using appropriate marker lipids. Neutral lipids such as oils and fats may be analyzed by development on silica gel using isopropyl ether-acetic acid (24:1) and petroleum ether-ethyl ether-acetic acid (90:10:1) as successive solvents systems on the same TLC. For detection the plate is sprayed with 25% sulphuric acid, followed by heating the plate to 230°C. Glycerides and hydrocarbons are seen as pale brown-coloured spots. Hydrocarbons are seen near the solvent front and phospholipids remain near the origin. Triglycerides move ahead of diglycerides, which are ahead of monoglycerides.

2. Phospholipids and glycolipids may be identified on TLC in silica gel plates developed in chloroform-methanol-acetic acid-water (170:30:20:7). The plate is sprayed with a solution of 0.2% ethanolic 2′,7′-dichlorofluorescein. Presence of fluorescent green spots in UV light, against a purplish violet background indicates the presence of phospholipids and glycolipids.

3. To identify the lipid composition, the total lipids isolated-neutral or polar lipids are subjected to alkaline or acid saponification. Acid hydrolysis is carried out with 2M sulphuric acid under nitrogen at 100°C for 6 hours. Upon dilution with water, the fatty components are extracted into chloroform.

- The aqueous portion is neutralized and further analyzed by TLC for the presence of glycerol, galactose, phosphates, etc. Paper chromatography in n-butanol-pyridine-water (7:3:1) for about 40 hours along with the authentic sample of glycerol or sugars will reveal their presence when activated with alkaline silver nitrate reagent. For phosphate detection, TLC of the neutralized aqueous portion on silica gel in methanol-1M ammonia-10% trichloroacetic acid-water (10:3:1:6) is done and activated by spraying with 1% aqueous ammonium molybdate followed by 1% stannous chloride in 10% hydrochloric acid. Presence of blue spots indicates the presence of phosphate and hence phospholipids.

- The chloroform portion is analyzed for the presence of amines and fatty acids. Alternatively, the lipid may be saponified by heating under reflux with 5% ethanolic potassium hydroxide on a water bath for 1 hour. It is then filtered and acidified. This or the chloroform layer obtained in the acid hydrolysis may be analyzed by GLC for the determination of its fatty acid composition.

4. Fatty acids may also be isolated from the saponification mixture by fractional crystallization, fractional distillation, preparation and debromination of polybromides, column chromatography, or by the formation of urea-fatty acid complexes.

5. Plant waxes on the other hand may be directly extracted by quickly dipping the unbroken leaves or stems in hexane or ether. In so doing, the surface waxes are extracted into the solvent without disturbing the cellular contents.

- On concentration the extracted wax may be further fractionated by passage through an alumina column to separate into alkanes or related hydrocarbons.

- Direct TLC of the wax dissolved in chloroform on silica gel in chloroform-benzene (1:1) and development by spraying with 0.5% ethanolic Rhodamine B fluorescein will indicate the presence of hydrocarbons and other fractions as yellowish spots against a pink background.

- Constitution of waxes is deduced by studying the products of hydrolysis. Saponification of waxes is generally more difficult than that of saponification of fats.

Glycosides

Glycosides are a large and varied group of plant metabolites found universally distributed in higher plants and also in some lower plants. They are defined by the common property of yielding sugars among the products of their hydrolysis. Chemically they are considered sugar ethers as they are formed by the condensation of the –OH group of the sugar with the –OH group of a nonsugar component referred to as aglycone. The aglycone or the sugar component is most frequently glucose with rhamnose, fucose, cymarose, and digitoxose being among the other sugars. Based on the α or β configuration of the sugars, both forms of glycosides are possible. However, only β forms do occur in plant glycosides, with α-linkages being common among carbohydrates.

Some glycosides contain more than one sugar being linked to each other as a disaccharide or trisaccharide. In many glycosides, the sugar could be a sugar derivative such as glucuronic acid, galacturonic acid, etc.

When the glycosidic linkage between the sugar and nonsugar takes place through oxygen, they are O-glycosides. Such glycosides are easily hydrolyzed to the parent sugar and the aglycone by either enzymes or acids. When the linkage is between the –OH of the sugar and the –CH group of the aglycone they are C-glycosides. These glycosides resist normal acid hydrolysis and can be successfully hydrolyzed only by oxidative hydrolysis with ferric chloride. N-glycosides are those in which the linkage is formed between the amine group of the aglycone and the OH group of the sugar and S-glycosides are formed through linkage of the –OH group of sugar with –SH group of the aglycone.

Aglycone of a glycoside includes representatives of many numerous groups of hydroxyl compounds occurring in plants ranging from small molecules to tetracyclic and pentacyclic triterpenoid moieties, hydroxyanthraquinones, naphthaquinones, anthocyanins, thiocyanates, cyanogenetic, phenylpropanoid, flavones-related compounds, coumarin, furanocoumarin, etc.

Classification of glycosides may be done under different criteria such as the nature of the aglycone, nature of the sugar, nature of the glycone–aglycone linkage, or on therapeutic property.

Some biologically important groups of glycosides based on the aglycone are as follows:

1. *Anthraquinone glycosides*: Sennosides from Senna leaves and pods, Cascarosides from Cascara bark, Aloin from Aloe sps, rhein, aloe-emodin from Rhubarb rhizome.

2. *Cardiac glycosides*: These are based on C23 or C24 steroids called cardenolides and bufadienolides respectively. For example, Digitalis glycosides from digitalis leaves, strophanthus glycosides from strophanthus seeds are cardenolides. Toxic glycosides of red and white squill are bufadienolides.

3. *Saponin glycosides*: are based on either tetracyclic or pentacylcic triterpenoid moiety. For example, dioscin from Dioscorea tubers, ginsenosides form Ginseng roots, Glycyrrhizin from liquorice stolons, Quillaia saponins from soap bark, senegin from Senega roots, etc.

4. *Cyanogenetic glycosides*: yield HCN on hydrolysis. For example, Amygdalin from bitter almonds, manihotoxin from poisonous manihot root, linamarin from linseed, Prunasin from wild cherry bark.

5. *Thiocyanate glycosides*: Based on algycones with thiocyanate (SCN) grouping, for example, sinigrin from black mustard.

6. *Flavonol glycosides*: based on flavone and its derivatives, these occur both in the free state and as glycosides. They form the largest group of naturally occurring phenols. These coloured compounds are widely distributed in nature. For example, rutin from buck wheat, hesperidin from citrus fruits, silymarin from silybum sps, etc.

7. *Coumarin and furanocoumarin glycosides*: For example, visnagin from dried ripe fruits of Visnaga, psoralen from dried ripe fruits of Psoralea, etc.

8. *Naphthaquinone glycosides*: For example, lawsone from Henna leaves.

9. *Phenol glycosides*: Aglycones are based on phenolic groups. For example, salicin from Populus sps, vanillin from vanilla sps, tannin glycosides, etc.

Glycosides accumulate in plant organs at definite stages of growth and characteristic glycosides are found in maximum proportion in young organs in the cell elongation stage. Physiologically glycosides have an important role to play in the metabolism, self defense, and excretory functions of the plant. Because of the large variety of compounds involved, glycosides vary widely physically, chemically, and pharmacologically. They include many therapeutic compounds with an array of biological activities, such as cardiac glycosides, purgative anthraquinone glycosides, flavonoid glycosides, saponin glycosides, etc.

Properties

The basic physical and chemical properties of glycosides are dependent on the nature of the aglycone and sugar–nonsugar linkage. Some general properties are:

1. Glycosides are crystalline or amorphous nonvolatile substances that are soluble in water and dilute alcohol. They are insoluble in organic solvents like chloroform and ether.
2. The aglycone moiety is soluble in nonpolar solvents like benzene, ether, etc.
3. They are easily hydrolyzed by water, mineral acids, and enzymes.
4. They are optically active and normally laevorotatory.
5. Glycosides do not reduce Fehling's solution until they are hydrolyzed.
6. Some glycosides occur in one part of the plant while a hydrolytic enzyme occurs in another. Tissue injury, germination, or other physiological activity of the plant brings them in contact with each other, resulting in hydrolysis of the glycoside. A large number of such enzymes are found in plants.
7. Therapeutic property of a glycoside is dictated by the aglycone part. The sugar facilitates absorption of glycoside and helps in transportation of the aglycone portion to the site of action.

Extraction and isolation

Inactivation of enzymes that may be present in plant tissues is an important first step before isolation of glycosides is attempted. This is especially so when fresh plant material is being processed. Dried material does not require such precaution as these enzymes are active only in fresh tissues.

Due to the wide range of physical and chemical properties of glycosides, it is not possible to follow a single general method for the isolation of all glycosides. Different methods of isolation, based on the nature of the aglycone and the type of sugar–nonsugar linkage of the glycoside are followed for the isolation of specific glycosides.

Following is a general method suited for the isolation of glycosides from plant tissues:

1. The plant part containing the glycoside is carefully and quickly dried and powdered. It is exhaustively extracted with 95% ethanol using hot continuous percolation. Heating deactivates the enzymes. For thermolabile glycosides, the temperature should not exceed 45°C.
2. Alternatively, the fresh plant part is boiled under reflux with 95% ethanol for 30 min for the inactivation of hydrolytic enzymes. The residue of the plant material is then size reduced and further extracted with the same solvent.
3. The combined ethanol extracts or the extract of step 1 is evaporated to dryness in the presence of a little $CaCO_3$ under reduced pressure at a temperature not exceeding 50°C.
4. The dry residue is dissolved in minimum quantity of water (equivalent to 1g/ml of fresh tissue) and 10% basic lead acetate solution is added until there is no further precipitation (of tannins).
5. A further $1/10^{th}$ of the earlier added volume of lead acetate solution is added to the solution taken in a mortar.

6. To this mass, add anhydrous sodium sulphate in small portions (1g/ml of lead acetate solution is added first). This is to render the non-glycosidal components insoluble.

7. The above mass thoroughly mixed is allowed to air-dry to become a semi-solid mass.

8. This is then spread out on glass or porcelain tiles and allowed to air dry to a powdery state.

9. The fully dried product is broken up and treated with successive portions of ethyl acetate, ether, chloroform, ethanol, or ethyl acetate-ethanol (4:1). Different solvents are used depending on the solubility of the glycoside.

10. The mixture is filtered and concentrated with ether being added in final stages. The glycoside crystallizes out.

11. Further if the glycosides occur as mixtures, they may be separated using column chromatography, preparative TLC, or fractional crystallization.

Identification

Glycosides on account of their varied nature are first analyzed for the nature of the sugar and then tested according to the characteristic of the aglycone. Many glycosides are coloured, fluorescent, or chromogenic and are therefore tested accordingly. Different chemical tests specific for the aglycone are used to detect them after hydrolysis.

I. Some of the general tests for glycosides are:

1. A solution of glycoside gives a deep red colour with concentrated sulphuric acid.

2. To a pinch of the substance dissolved in glacial acetic acid, add a few drops of ferric chloride solution followed by concentrated sulphuric acid. Appearance of a red ring at the junction of two layers indicates the presence of glycosides.

II. Tests specific for sugars in glycosides

1. Molisch' test: To a pinch of the drug dissolved in water add 1 ml hydrochloric acid and heat to boiling. Cool and treat with α-naphthol and a few drops of concentrated sulphuric acid. Formation of a purple colour indicates the presence of a glucoside, a glucose containing glycoside.

2. Treat about 0.2 g of the crude drug with 5 ml dilute sulphuric acid and warm on a water bath for 2 minutes. To the supernatant add equal volumes of Fehling's solution A and Fehling's solution B and heat for 2 minutes. A brick-red precipitate indicates the presence of glycosides.

3. Keller-Kiliani test: Dissolve a pinch of the glycoside in 3 ml glacial acetic acid containing 2 drops of 5% ferric chloride. Carefully transfer this to the surface of 2 ml concentrated sulphuric acid. A reddish-brown layer forms at the junction of the two layers and the upper layer slowly becomes bluish-green and darkens on standing. This test is specific for glycosides containing desoxy sugars

4. Paper chromatography for the identification of sugars

A solution of the hydrolyzed mixture of the glycoside is spotted on a paper along with marker sugars. It is developed in the upper layer of butanol-acetic acid-water (4:1:5) system. After a run of about 24 hours, air dry the paper, and spray with aniline hydrogen phthalate solution. Sugars are seen as visible brown-coloured spots. Comparable R_f of the sugar with that of the authentic samples will indicate the sugar present in the glycoside.

III. Tests specific for aglycones

1. Cardiac glycosides answer keller-kiliani test. In addition they answer tests for the presence of the unsaturated lactone ring and tests for steroids. (See under "Identification of digoxin" (Chap 8, p. 284).) Strophanthus glycosides reduce tollen's reagent and they also give a precipitate with tannic acid.

2. Tests for anthraquinones

    i. *Born Trager's test*: Boil 0.1 g of the drug with 2 ml dilute sulphuric acid and centrifuge. Pipette off the supernatant, cool and shake with an equal volume of carbon tetrachloride and separate it. Treat 1 ml of it with half its volume of dilute ammonia. A rose-red colour is formed in the ammoniacal layer indicating the presence of anthraquinones. To another 1 ml of the organic layer add methanolic magnesium acetate solution; an orange colour is formed.

    ii. *Modified Born Trager's test*: Boil 0.1 g of the drug with 1 ml dilute hydrochloric acid and 2 ml of 5% aqueous ferric chloride solution. Filter while hot, cool, and shake the filtrate with carbon tetrachloride. Separate the organic layer and shake it with 2 ml dilute ammonia. A rose-red colour is formed in the ammoniacal layer. C-glycosides such as carcarosides may be identified by this modified test as they are resistant to normal acid hydrolysis and require oxidative hydrolysis with ferric chloride for the cleavage of the sugar–nonsugar bond.

3. Tests for triterpenes and flavonoids discussed under saponin and flavonoid glycosides.

4. *Tests for cyanogenetic glycosides*: Moisten a pinch of the drug with water and add a small amount of dilute sulphuric acid. Heat the flask gently and as heating progresses suspend a strip of filter paper previously moistened and dried with sodium picrate solution into the test tube clamped between the test tube cork closure. Hydrocyanic gas is released as a result of hydrolysis and this turns the picrate paper to a red colour.

Flavonoids

Flavonoids are a large group of naturally occurring plant polyphenolic compounds based on the C_6-C_3-C_6 carbon skeleton. These non-nitrogen plant pigments are responsible for flower coloration and are involved in UV filtration, symbiotic nitrogen fixation, metabolic oxidation-reduction processes and play an important role in reproductive physiological processes in higher plants. These ubiquitous compounds of large variety and relatively low toxicity are extensively investigated for their possible physiological action and the beneficial effects of fruits, vegetables, tea, and red wine is attributed to their flavonoid composition. Recent research is demonstrating their role as dietary anti-oxidants—their polyphenolic nature enabling them to scavenge free radicals. *In vitro* studies have shown them to be biological response modifiers with anti-inflammatory, anti-allergic, anti-thrombotic, vaso protective, tumor inhibitory, and gastroprotective properties. Several traditional herbal remedies of use in cardiovascular disease and certain forms of cancer are increasingly being reported to be rich in flavonoids and derived tannins. Several flavonoid containing plants are used as anti-spasmodics, diuretics, anti-bacterial, and antifungal agents.

Some ten classes of flavonoids are known—all are structural variants based on flavone and occur in all vascular plants both in the free state and as glycosides. More commonly found as glycosides—both as O- and C-glycosides—they are found in plants as mixtures of different classes and even a single flavonoid aglycone may occur in a single plant in several glycosidic combinations. As of now some 2500 flavonoids are known with nearly 500 occurring in the free state.

Basic skeleton of flavonoid compounds

Flavonoids have been extensively used as chemotaxonomic markers and they are found abundantly in Polygonaceae, Rutaceae, Leguminoseae, Umbelliferae, and Compositae. Dimeric compounds such as colourless biflavonyls are found in Gymnosperms.

Properties

Most flavonoids are coloured in crystalline masses and faintly coloured or colourless in microgram quantities. Anthocyanins, chalcones, and aurones possess deep colours even in trace amounts. In general, flavonoids are coloured, water-soluble compounds insoluble in organic solvents, while non glycosidic flavonoids are sparingly soluble in water and soluble in ether. They range in complexity from being non-glycosidic to highly methylated/glycosidic forms having up to three sugar residues. The various structural types of favonoids differ in the degree of oxidation of the C ring and in the substitution pattern in the A and B rings. Most of them are present as mono or diglycosides.

Thus in terms of solubility characteristics, they could be ether soluble-water insoluble non-methylated substances to ether insoluble-water soluble glycosides with up to three attached sugars.

Flavonoids are crystalline substances with sharp melting points. Flavones, isoflavanes, flavanones, flavanonols are colourless crystals; flavones, flavonoles, chalcones and aurones are yellow or vividly yellow. Anthocyanines are sap pigments and the actual colour of the plant organ is determined by the pH of the sap. Flavanols (cathechins) are optically active.

Flavanones and flavononones are unstable compounds. Treated with oxidants, they turn into chalcones and leucocyanidins accordingly.

Being phenolic, they dissolve in alkalis, giving yellow solutions, which on addition of acid become colourless. They contain conjugated aromatic systems and thus show intense absorption bands in the UV and visible regions of the spectrum.

Different classes of flavonoids are anthocyanins (e.g., delphinidin, pelargonidin), proanthocyanidins (e.g., resveratrol, catechin), flavones (e.g., luteolin, apigenin), flavonols (e.g., quercetin, kaempferol), glycoflavones (e.g., vitexin, isovitexin), flavanones (e.g., hesperitin, naringenin), flavanonol (e.g., taxifolin), chalcones (butein, isoliquiritigenin), aurones (e.g., aureusidin, sulphuretin), and isoflavones (e.g., genistein, daidzein). A high proportion of these occur as water-soluble glycosides and classification of flavone type in a plant tissue is based on a study of solubility properties and colour reactions.

Extraction and isolation

No single extraction procedure is ideally suited for all flavonoids due to the differences in their solubility characteristics. Also when the class of flavonoid present in the plant material is not known, a preliminary TLC examination of the hydrolyzed plant extract is essential in order to determine this. Chromatographic separation of the flavonoid rich fraction and its subsequent TLC analysis using known markers shall reveal the class of flavonoid contained. According to Harborne, a routine screening of plant tissues for the presence of flavonoids may be undertaken by two-dimensional paper chromatography of concentrated alcoholic extracts using butanol: acetic acid: water (4:1:5-top layer) and 5% acetic acid. Flavonoids having characteristic colours may be distinguished depending on their relative positions on the chromatogram. Some flavonoids are seen in visible light and majority may be visualized under UV light. Fuming the chromatogram with ammonia yields further information on the compounds from the colour changes observed. Use of standard markers such as rutin, quercetin, kaempferol, delphinidin, luteolin, and orientin will cover most classes of flavonoids.

Flavonoids of flower, fruit, leaves, bark, roots, rhizomes, and resinous exudates occur only as glycosides, while flavonoid aglycones are most typically found in wood tissues. Since most flavonoid glycosides are readily hydrolyzed by acid, care is to be taken where the fresh material is used. Hydrolyzed plant extracts on shaking with ethyl acetate segregate most flavonoids (except anthocyanins) into the organic layer.

Flavonoids may be extracted from fresh or dried plant material by extraction with methanol or ethanol. Preliminary extraction with petroleum ether removes waxy material.

1. Fresh plant material (flowers) is extracted with hot aqueous ethanol and filtered
2. The filtrate is concentrated in vacuo, and the residue washed with ether.
3. Dissolve it in dilute hydrochloric acid and extract with equal volume of ethyl acetate. Wash the ethyl acetate extract first with dilute hydrochloric acid and then with water.
4. Pass the ethyl acetate layer through anhydrous sodium sulphate, concentrate *in vacuo* to a syrupy mass, cover with toluene, and store in a refrigerator.
5. Collect the formed precipitate by centrifugation, dissolve in hot water, wash with ether, and set aside the aqueous layer.
6. Separate the crystallized flavonoid glycosides and purify by recrystallization from 50% aqueous ethanol.

Identification

Typically coloured anthocyanins are detected in aqueous alcoholic solutions by red to blue colour pigmentation. Flavones and flavonols are readily detected in white or pale yellow tissues by the appearance of yellow or red colours when the tissue is exposed to ammonia. In general, solutions containing flavonoids change colour when treated with alkali. Following are some common colour tests for flavonoids:

1. *Shinoda's test*: A few milligrams of the flavonoid dissolved in alcohol is treated with magnesium turnings. Concentrated hydrochloric acid is then added in drops. Flavonoids especially flavones, flavonols, and flavanones produce crimson red colours. Chalcones and aurones do not show such colour changes.

2. Treat an aqueous alcoholic solution of the flavonoid with aqueous sodium hydroxide solution. Anthocyanins give blue to violet colours. Flavones and flavonols deepen in colour. Chalcones and aurones show red to purple colours. Flavonones give nearly colourless to yellow solutions, which turn deep red on heating (due to isomerization to corresponding chalcones). Isoflavones give brown solutions in visible light or exhibit brilliant blue colours in UV light.

3. An aqueous alcoholic solution of the flavonoid when treated with dilute sulphuric acid gives intensely yellow or orange solutions in the case of anthocuanins, flavones, and flavonols. Flavonones give orange to crimson colours. Chalcones and aurones give deeply red, crimson or magenta colours.

4. All flavonoids in solution when treated with aqueous solutions of ferric chloride give colours ranging from green, purple, to brown.

5. To an aqueous alcoholic solution of the flavonoid, add a few ml of lead acetate solution. Flavones give yellow to deep red-coloured precipitate and chalcones and aurones show deep orange red colours.

6. Solutions of flavonoids either in water or alcoholic solvents, post acid hydrolysis, show typical absorption maxima. Anthocyanins exhibit visible maxima between 515–545 nm. Flavones show spectral maxima at 330–350 nm, flavonols at 350–386 nm, chalcones and aurones at 370–410 nm, flavonones exhibit different spectral properties with peaks at 225, 288, and 300 nms.

Saponins

Saponins are high molecular weight, foam-forming glycosides based on the tetracyclic (steroidal) and pentacyclic tritepene groups and are characterized by their property of producing frothing aqueous solutions even at very low concentrations.

Detected in over 70 plant families, saponins occur as complex mixtures of glycosides, differing from one another in nature of sugar attachment or in the structures of the aglycone. The sugar may be glucose, galactose, glucoronic acid, xylose, rhamnose, or methyl pentose. The great complexity of saponin structure arises from the variability of the aglycone structure, the nature of the side chains, and the position of attachment of these moieties on the aglycone. Their glycosidic pattern is complex with as many as five sugar units attached and glucuronic acid is a common component. Saponins cause hemolysis when injected into the blood stream due to lysis of RBCs and increase in permeability of the plasma membrane. On account of their toxic nature, extracts of several saponin containing plants have been used as arrow poisons. However, they are harmless when taken orally due to low absorption and hydrolysis and plant foods such as lentils, beans, soyabeans, spinach, and oats are rich in saponins.

Steroidal alkaloids are nitrogen analogues of steroidal saponins and share their foaming and hemolytic property. However, they are toxic when ingested. Examples include solasodine and tomatidine from Solanum species.

On account of their surfactant properties and biological activities, saponins are in commercial demand with applications in the food, cosmetic, and pharmaceutical industries.

Plants rich in saponins have long been used in different parts of the world for their detergent properties and they are of great economic interest. Sarasaparilla rich in steroidal saponins is widely used in the manufacture of non-alcoholic drinks. Steroidal saponins are of great pharmaceutical importance as they can be easily transformed into medicinally important steroids such as cortisone, diuretic steroids, vitamin D, sex hormones, and cardiac glycosides. Though total synthesis of therapeutic steroids is today commercially feasible, there is a large demand for plant-derived steroidal sapogenins to be used as starting materials for partial synthesis of these steroids. Diosgenin (Dioscorea sps), hecogenin (Agave sps), sarsasapogenin (Yucca and Smilax sps), and sarmentogenin (Strophanthus sps) are some of the steroidal sapogenins—aglycones of saponins, commercially exploited for semi synthesis of such steroids. Steroidal alkaloids are also commercially employed for steroid manufacture as the semi synthesis involves removal of the ring systems containing the side chain and hence presence of O or N in the side chain is inconsequential.

Because of their surfactant properties, saponins such as quillaic acid (Quillaia bark) are used pharmaceutically for emulsifying fats. Pentacyclic triterpenes are of medicinal importance especially those of the β-amyrin type. Examples include Glycyrhhizin from liquorice, Ginsenosides from Ginseng, Aesculin from Horse chestnut.

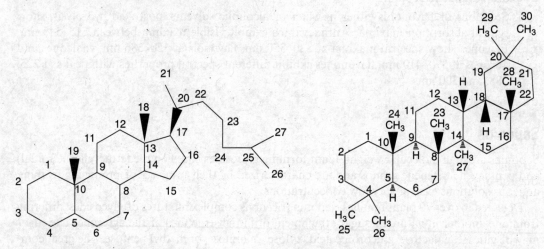

Ring structure of steroidal saponins   Ring structure of pentacyclic triterpenoid saponins

Properties

Saponins are high molecular weight, high polarity compounds which on hydrolysis yield, sugars, uronic acids, and steroidal or pentacyclic triterpenoid aglycones. Both have C-3 sugar linkage and have a common biogenetic origin. Many saponins have an additional sugar at C26 or C28 position. Natural sapogenins differ in their configuration at C-3, C-5, and C-25 positions and in the orientation at C-22 position. Steroidal saponins are C_{27} sterols in which the side chain of cholesterol has undergone modification to produce a spiroketal as in dioscin. All steroidal saponins have the same configuration at the C-22 spirocenter. Additional stereoisomers at C-25 co occur as mixtures in the plant. They occur in Monocot families such as Dioscoreaceae (Dioscorea sps), Amaryllidaceae (Agave sps), Liliaceae (Yucca and Trillium sps).

Pentacyclic triterpenes (C_{30}) are more widely distributed in nature and occur abundantly in dicots and are based on α-amyrin, β-amyrin, and lupeol. More than 360 different sapogenins representing 750 different glycosides are known. Plant materials contain these saponins in considerable amounts, for example, Liquorice (2–12%), Quillaia (10%), Primula root (5–10%) and Horse chestnut (13%). Oleanolic acid is a common saponin occurring in beet root, thyme, guaiacum sps, and in the free state in olive leaves and clove buds.

Saponins form colloidal solutions in water having a bitter, acrid taste. They occur as milky white amorphous powders and are soluble in water, ethanol, and methanol. They are insoluble in chloroform and benzene. Drugs having saponins are characterized by their sternutatory property and they cause irritation of the mucous membrane. On hydrolysis saponins yield sapogenins, which are readily crystallizable compounds. A large number of carbon atoms in their structure makes them lipophilic and the presence of water soluble sugars gives them a hydrophilic/lipophilic asymmetry resulting in the lowering of surface tension in aqueous solution. This causes foaming in aqueous solutions. Saponins are much more polar than sapogenins because of their glycosidic attachment.

Extraction and isolation

As saponins occur as complex mixtures their isolation in a state of purity is somewhat tedious. In general, various chromatographic techniques are employed for their isolation and acetylation renders them crystallizable. Different extraction procedures are followed depending on the nature of saponin, amount present, and nature of the plant tissue. For the isolation of steroidal sapogenins, fresh plant material is usually used, though it is not uncommon to extract them from dried-size reduced plant material.

Ideally, fresh plant tissues are homogenized in aqueous solution and set aside for the autolysis of the glycosides through the action of endogenous glyosidase enzymes present in plant tissues. This also achieves cyclization of open-chain saponins in addition to cleaving off the sugar attached, yielding the sapogenin. This is a standard approach employed in the commercial production of steroidal sapogenins. Several newer methods of separation such as high speed counter current chromatography coupled with evaporative light scattering detector are being employed for the isolation of spaonins.

Following is a general method that may be adapted for the isolation of steroidal sapogenins:

1. 1 kg of the fresh plant material sufficiently size reduced is extracted with 95% ethanol at 100°C for 12 hours.
2. Filter hot and evaporate the filtrate under vacuum to a pasty residue.
3. Add 300 ml 1M Ethanolic hydrochloric acid and heat under reflux for 2 hours.
4. Filter, cool, and add 400 ml ether. Treat the solution with equal volume of water and discard the aqueous layer. Some methods adapt chromatographic separation of the saponin on a column of silica gel at this stage.
5. Wash the solution with 5% sodium hydroxide solution and again with water. Reject the aqueous layers and evaporate the solution to dryness.
6. Hydrolyze the dried residue with 10% alcoholic potassium hydroxide solution for 30 minutes and cool the solution.
7. Extract with 4 × 25 ml ether and evaporate the ether layers.
8. The product may be purified by recrystallization from acetone.

Identification

Formation of persistent foams during plant extraction and concentration is a good indicator for the presence of saponins in the plant tissue.

1. Shake an aqueous alcoholic extract of the plant material in a test tube. Formation of persistent foam above the liquid surface indicates the presence of saponins. Stable foam in alkaline medium indicates the presence of steroid saponins. Pentacyclic triterpenoid saponins form foam that is stable both in alkaline and acidic media.

2. TLC test: To 10 g of the dried powdered plant material, add 100 ml of 1M hydrochloric acid and heat under reflux for 2 hours. Cool, neutralize with alkali, and evaporate to dryness. Extract with 3 × 30 ml chloroform and concentrate to about 15 ml. Spot it on a TLC plate and develop in acetone:hexane (4:1). Air dry and activate the plates by spraying with antimony trichloride in concentrated HCl. Sapogenins may be detected as pink or purple-coloured spots.

3. *Liebermann–Burchard reaction*: To a small quantity of the drug dissolved in alcohol, add a few drops of acetic anhydride followed by concentrated sulphuric acid. Formation of a bluish-green ring at the junction of two layers indicates the presence of steroids.

4. *Sange's test*: To a solution of the saponin, add a solution of vanillin in sulphuric acid. [0.5 g in sulphuric acid-ethanol (4:1)]. Development of a yellow colour indicates the presence of steroidal saponins.

5. *Lafon's reaction*: To a solution of the saponin in methanol, add a few drops of concentrated sulphuric acid and 1 ml of ferric sulphate solution. Formation of a bluish green colour indicates the presence of saponins.

6. To a solution of the saponin in water add 3 ml of 25% lead acetate solution. Formation of a dense precipitate indicates the presence of saponins.

Volatile Oils

Volatile oils are defined as oily liquids, which are entirely or almost entirely volatile without decomposition. They are also called essential oils as they are said to represent the essence of the odor constituents of the plants from which they are obtained. Volatile oils have been used in medicine, perfumery, and for flavoring since ancient times. Today they are used industrially as flavors in food, confectionary, and in the spice, perfume, and cosmetic trade. They are of considerable importance to the pharmaceutical industry as flavors and perfumes, and also due to their antiseptic, anesthetic, carminative, stimulant, insect repellant properties. Volatile oil components are also used as starting materials for the synthesis of other compounds (eugenol for vanillin).

Recent interest in aromatherapy has revived interest in essential oils due to their claimed curative effects.

Depending on the plant family, volatile oils are secreted in oil cells, in secretion ducts, or in glandular hairs of plants. They may be formed directly by the protoplasm, by decomposition of the resinogenous layer of the cell wall, or by the hydrolysis of certain glycosides. Volatile oils are present in every plant part, namely flowers, seeds, leaves, roots, bark, etc. In plants, they may act as insect repellants or insect attractants and are frequently associated with gums and resins.

The constituents of volatile oils are called terpenes referring to their biogenetic origin as they are formed from the head to tail condensation of isoprene units. The chemical nature of the volatile oil is dependent on the nature of the terpene constituents it contains. Terpenes are diverse as a chemical class and volatile oils in general are rich in mono and sesquiterpenes. These occur as mixtures of hydrocarbons and oxygenated compounds derived from these hydrocarbons. In some oils like turpentine oil, the hydrocarbons predominate and oils such as that of clove abound in oxygenated derivatives. In the case of many oils, the oxygenated terpenes determine the odor, taste, and even therapeutic properties of the oil and the hydrocarbons merely act as diluents in the oil.

Monoterpenes are biogenetically formed from 2 isoprene units and are categorized as acyclic, monocyclic, and bicyclic terpenes.

- Acyclic monoterpenes are considered the most important isolates in perfumery and occur as optical or geometrical isomers, which may be found together in the same oil or in different oils. For example, citral, geraniol, linalol, citronellol, and nerol are oxygenated; myrcene and ocimene are hydrocarbons.
- Monocyclic monoterpenes also occur as optical and structural isomers. For example, limonene is a widely distributed monocyclic hydrocarbon and terpineol, cineole, menthol, and carvone are oxygenated.
- In bicyclic monoterpenes, the first ring has six members and common to all, while the size of the second ring varies. These also occur as isomers with both forms occurring in the same or different plant sources. For example, pinene is a hydrocarbon, and camphor, borneol, and eugenol are oxygenated.

Sesquiterpenes are formed from three isoprene units and they constitute the higher boiling fraction of essential oils. On the basis of the number of rings in the structure, they are divided into four groups:

- *Acyclic*: For example, farnesene is a hydrocarbon; farnesol and nerolidol are oxygenated.
- *Monocyclic*: For example, zingiberene and bisabolene are hydrocarbons; gingerol is oxygenated.
- *Bicyclic*: For example, cadinene and caryophyllene are hydrocarbons; santalol is oxygenated.
- Tricyclic: For example, longifolene and copaene are hydrocarbons; patchoulol is oxygenated.

Properties

1. Volatile oils are light, mobile, highly odorous liquids, which can be distilled without decomposition.
2. They are volatile in steam and differ entirely in physical and chemical properties from fixed oils.
3. They are optically active and their specific gravity varies from 0.8–1.15 with most of them below 1.00. (Oil of clove and oil of cinnamon have specific gravity more than 1.00.)
4. They have a characteristic odor and taste and are freely soluble in ether and chloroform and fairly soluble in alcohol. They are slightly soluble in water.
5. When stained on paper they give a translucent stain (unlike fixed oils, which leave a permanent stain), which is temporary as it disappears when the oil volatilizes.

6. They undergo oxidation when exposed to moisture, light, or air, forming compound of altered/objectionable odor characteristics.

7. Oxygenated terpenes are odoriferous and much more soluble in water and alcohol than hydrocarbon terpenes.

8. When oils are specifically enriched with respect to oxygenated terpenes by the removal of hydrocarbons, such oils are called "terpene less" oils.

9. Extraction and isolation

Volatile oils are traditionally obtained by distillation of the plant parts containing the oil. Some volatile oils which undergo undesirable changes in the oil composition and organoleptic features due to distillation are separated by methods not involving heat application. In addition to these several newer methods such as super critical fluid extraction may now be conveniently applied for their isolation. Following are some of the usual methods of isolation of volatile oils.

1. *Water or hydrodistillation*: This method is applied to plant material that is dried and not subject to injury by boiling. The plant material is boiled along with water in a distillation chamber over naked flame until all the volatile oil distills over along with water. In some cases the plant material is allowed to macerate in water before being subjected to distillation. Turpentine oil, predominantly being constituted of hydrocarbons is unaffected by heat. It may be distilled from the fresh, un dried plant material by this method.

2. *Steam distillation*: This method is applicable to fresh plant material that may be subject to damage and loss of constituents by direct heat. Fresh plant material is directly taken to the distillation still in which it is charged on the perforated bottom. Steam generated in another boiler is passed through the still having the fresh material with sufficient moisture content. Droplets of the essential oil along with water vapor are carried through the condenser, whereby it condenses and collects in the receiver as a biphasic liquid of water and the immiscible essential oil. Ideally steam distillation enables maximal and rapid diffusion of steam through the plant cell membranes keeping hydrolysis and decomposition of constituents minimal. For example, peppermint and spearmint oils are isolated by steam distillation.

3. *Water and steam distillation*: This method is employed for the separation of volatile oils from plant material either dried or fresh, which tend to be injured by direct heat or steam. The plant material is charged under a layer of water over a perforated grid in the distillation chamber. Steam is passed through the macerated mixture, which is also heated underneath. The volatile oil vapor and water vapor arising from the charge, pass through the condenser to eventually get collected in the receiver. Because of different specific gravities, water and the oil get separated and the oil is drained or siphoned. For example, cinnamon and clove oil are isolated by water and steam distillation.

4. *Expression and distillation*: Essential oils such as oil of bitter almond and oil of mustard are not present in the natural state in the plant material. Instead they are present in a glycosidic form (called amygdaline in bitter almond). Crushing brings about contact with emulsion, an enzyme present elsewhere in the seed. This results in hydrolysis yielding the essential oil, which is eventually separated by distillation. Bitter almonds are first expressed when they yield about 30% fixed oil. The pressed marc is then macerated in water to initiate enzymatic action. This mixture is distilled to yield about 1% essential oil.

5. *Expression*: Some volatile oils such as essential oil of lemon cannot be distilled without decomposition and are usually obtained by expression or by other mechanical means.

Ecuelle's process is a newer mechanical method of separation of the volatile oil from citrus sources. Here the fruit is placed in a device lined with spikes and rolled in such a way that the glands present in the peel are punctured just at the level of the epidermis. The oil globules pass to the center of the device from which it is collected by draining from the bottom. In earlier days, citrus oils were separated manually by the sponge process in which the peel is separated and placed in warm water to make it more soft and pliable. It is then inverted to rupture the oil glands and the rind placed in contact with a sponge. The oil is absorbed into the sponge until saturation, which is then expressed to obtain the essential oil. Such oil is highly priced as it is labor intensive.

6. *Enfleurge*: This method is applicable to the isolation of essential oils that are present in very small quantities and also are heat labile. Hence, it is commercially not feasible to isolate them by the usual method of distillation or expression. Enfleurage makes use of a bland, odorless fixed oil to absorb the delicate essential oil. This fatty material is spread over flat glass plates on which the flower petals are placed in contact for a few hours. The fat absorbs the fragrant volatile oil. The charge is replaced with fresh material until the fat is fully saturated. The volatile oil taken into the fat is then extracted by treating it with appropriate solvent such as alcohol. This method was formerly used extensively for the production of rose oil, jasmine oil, etc., for perfumery.

7. *Solvent extraction*: In today's perfumery industry, most of the modern essential oil production is accomplished by solvent extraction using volatile solvents such as petroleum ether, hexane, methanol, ethanol, etc. The plant material is brought in contact with the solvent at temperatures not exceeding 50°C. The solvent is then separated by filtration and evaporated under reduced pressure. Such oils are called absolutes or concentrates and resemble very closely the natural fragrance of the plant material. This is because temperature does not exceed 50°C and is maintained for the whole extraction period. Hence, the extracted oils have more natural aroma unmatched by distilled oils.

8. *Super critical fluid extraction*: This is a relatively newer method in which carbon dioxide at a hyper critical state is the solvent. At hyper critical pressure of 200 atmospheres, and at 33°C, CO_2 gas reaches a state where it is a super fluid having both the properties of a liquid and a gas. At this state it has greater diffusion and hence acts as an excellent solvent in which the essential oil is completely extracted intact. The solvent is eventually removed by reversing the super critical conditions, when gaseous CO_2 is regenerated and removed with much greater ease than any other solvent. Though expensive, in this method there is no solvent residue and the yield and quality of essential oil are good. It is a clean and environment friendly option for the isolation of number of plant products of medicinal, flavoring, and cosmetic interest. Super critical fluid extraction has also been successfully used for the extraction of a number of alkaloids, diterpenes, fixed oils, pigments, and sesquiterpene lactones. It has been adapted for the isolation of several essential oils such as those of calendula, peppermint, pepper, myrrh, and eucalyptus.

Identification

Essential oil identification and estimation of its quality is an important and integral process of its qualitative analysis. Their high economic value and extensive usage by various industries help in ensuring its quality, which is a significant aspect of its quality control.

Today GC is an invaluable tool in the identification of essential oils. A complete constituent profile of essential oils is done by GLC analysis and GC-MS is used for the identification of essential oil constituents.

Following are some of the routine tests employed in their identification:

1. *Sensory tests*: Examination of colour, viscosity, clarity, and odor of an essential oil will give a preliminary indication of its quality. For example, Otto of rose is viscous at lower temperatures due to the congealing of natural waxes present in it. A highly mobile rose oil at low temperature may not be genuine. Similarly, golden green-coloured geranium oil indicates its purity. Simple odor evaluation of essential oils is an effective way to detect their quality and sensory perception because odor detection is considered a highly skilled task.

2. Other physical parameters such as specific gravity, optical rotation, and refractive index are important for establishing the authenticity of an essential oil.

3. TLC Test: TLC is an important separation technique for the detection of volatile oils. TLC of the oil is developed in solvents such as hexane-ethyl acetate (19:1), hexane-chloroform (1:1), toluene-ethylacetate (8:2) using heat-activated TLC plates. Activation is done by spraying with Vanillin-sulphuric acid (0.5 g vanillin in 2 ml concentrated sulphuric acid with 8 ml methanol) and heating at 105°C for full colour development. Mono and sesquiterpene components of the oil are detected by grayish red spots.

4. A GC analysis of an essential oil shall reveal valuable information about its quality. GC chromatogram is a linear graph that charts the presence and distribution of the volatile components of an essential oil. Every detected component of the oil is traced in the form of a peak in the graph. This GC chromatogram is unique for each essential oil and it may be compared with that developed for an authentic sample of the oil. Though the GC profile of essential oil from the same source may vary at different times, with expertise it is possible to identify the quality of an oil from its GC profile. GC with accompanying MS identifies the individual components, along with their relative percentages.

Resins

Resins are amorphous solid products of a complex chemical nature. They are a heterogenous group with certain well-identified physical, chemical, and solubility characteristics. Resins are formed in schizogenous or schizolysigenous ducts or cavities by cells, which secrete a fluid composed of substances constituting gums, essential oils, and resins. Resin is held in solution by volatile terpenes, which are secreted in association with it. Thus resins are often associated with essential oil (turpentine, copaiba), with essential oil and gums (myrrh, asafetida), or with balsamic acids—benzoic and cinnamic acids (Benzoin, Storax) or are present as glycosides with sugars (Jalap, Podophyllum). Resins from which the associated essential oil is removed are called rosins.

They may be preformed in plants as normal physiological products and their yield is enhanced when an injury is made to the plant tissue. Many resins such as benzoin are formed only in response to injury. Resins may be present in idioblast cells (ginger oleoresin), multicellular internal glands (Clove), external glandular trichomes (Cannabis), tubular ducts with secreting epithelium (Fennel, Pine wood) throughout the tissue (Guaiacum heart wood) or they may be formed from plant juices by the agency of insects (Shellac in glands on the lac insect). Resins may be oxidation products of terpenes.

Plant resins have a long history of use and because of their physicochemical properties and associated uses, resins were used as medicine, in paper sizing, and in the production of varnishes, adhesives, food-glazing agents, incense chemicals, and as source of raw materials for organic synthesis. While most of these uses are replaced by synthetic substitutes for resins, some resins still hold a valued role in pharmacy for their medicinal and unique physicochemical properties. Medicinally used resins have been associated with anti septic, carminative, astringent, stimulant, diuretic and laxative properties.

Resin production is widespread in nature, but only a few families are of commercial importance. These include the Anacardiaceae, Burseraceae, Dipterocarpaceae, Guttiferae, Hammamelidaceae, Leguminosae, Liliaceae, Pinaceae, Styracaceae, and Umbelliferae.

Properties

Resins when separated and purified are often hard transparent or translucent hard, brittle solids or slightly soft semi-solids. They are heavier than water and by the action of heat they soften and fuse, yielding clear, adhesive fluids. Specific gravity of resins varies from 0.9–1.25. They are usually transparent when pure and become opaque when water is present. They burn with a characteristic smoky flame. Resins are insoluble in water and rarely soluble in light petroleum and more or less soluble in alcohol, ether, acetone, chloroform, carbon disulphide, chloral hydrate solution, fixed oils, and volatile oils. On evaporation, solutions of resins deposit a varnish-like thin film.

Chemically, resins are constituted of a complex mixture of resin acids, resin alcohols, resin phenols, esters, and inert resins The element nitrogen is not included in the composition of resin components.

Resin acids (abietic acid in colophony, commiphoric acid in myrrh) represent a large proportion of diterpenoid oxyacids, combining the properties of carboxylic acids and phenols. They occur both in the free state and as esters. They are soluble in aqueous solutions of alkalis forming soap-like solutions or colloidal suspensions. Their metallic salts are called resonates and these are extensively used in the manufacture of soaps and varnishes.

Resin alcohols or resinols (benzoresinol in benzoin, storesinol in storax) occur in the free state or as esters in combination with simple aromatic acids such as benzoic, salicylic, cinnamon, and umbellic acids. Complex molecules of high molecular weight called resinotannols (siaresinotannol in benzoin, peruresinotannol in balsam of tolu) precipitate ferric salts similar to tannins.

Resenes are complex neutral substances without characteristic chemical properties. They do not form salts or esters and are insoluble in and resist hydrolysis by alkalies.

Depending on the predominance of constituents, resins may be classed as acid resins (Colophony, Guaiacum), ester resins (Benzoin, Burgundy), or mixed resins (Mastich, Shellac).

Extraction and isolation

General method of separating resins is dependant upon the plant part associated with the resin, its preferred use, composition and its physical properties. While resins directly collected from the plants are natural resins (mastich, benzoin), those prepared from the plant parts by processing are called prepared resins (Podophyllin, Jalap resin).

1. Mostly resins have been collected from woody plants by methods collectively called tapping. While some resins are formed without injury, many are formed pathologically in

response to an external stimulus. Yield of even those resins that naturally ooze out of the plant can be enhanced by making an injury. Insects puncture the plant tissue as in the case of ammoniacum resin causing an abundant exudation from the stem.

2. Hence it has been a common practice to first bruise the plant tissue using a sharp instrument. This stimulates the flow of the resin from the injured tissue, which is directed to flow into containers. The injury and collection is continued to cover the entire surface of the tree by which time the flow slackens. Quality of resin collected from the first year is usually different from that collected from a tree on the point of exhaustion. Sustainable collection practices are preferred due to the damage caused to the tree.

3. When the resin is associated with a large quantity of volatile oil, it is processed for separation of the same as in the case of colophony. Crude turpentine tapped from the trees is warmed with water to remove floating unwanted plant debris. It is then distilled when the volatile oil—oil of turpentine distills—over along with water. The melted resin is then taken for solidification. This constitutes amber or colophony resin.

4. Resins such as Guaiacum were collected by burning one end of the felled tree trunk. This generates a copious flow of the resin from the entire wood tissue. It may also be collected by extracting the wood pieces with alcohol.

5. Resins like mastich lose a part of their volatile oil content by atmospheric evaporation as they get solidified after oozing out of the plant tissue.

6. Oleoresins like Canada turpentine, Copaiba are collected as such and volatile oil is an important part of their composition and use.

7. Resins like that of podophyllum rhizome are collected by pouring an alcoholic extract of the powdered plant material into acidulated water. Because of its insolubility in water the resin precipitates. It is collected by filtration or centrifugation, washed with water and dried.

8. The resin may be associated with the fruit as in the case of dragon's blood, it having exuded and hardened between the imbricated scales found on its surface. The fruits are beaten and shaken together to separate the scales of red resin. They are then mixed with water and the separated resin is made into balls or pressed into moulds.

9. Resinous crust deposited by lac insects on the twigs of trees is similarly collected by breaking them away from the plant part. It is then purified by treating with water or dilute alkaline solution after which the separated resin is evaporated to dryness in thin layers.

Identification

Resins may be identified based on their physical and chemical properties. In addition, they may be identified by individual chemical tests to detect the presence of specific chemical constituents.

1. Throw a small piece of resin in water. Resins being heavier than water sink in it.

2. Take a few fragments of the resin in a spatula and show it in the flame. Resins soften, fuse, and melt giving a sticky liquid. On further heating, they burn with a smoky flame.

3. Test of solubility: Treat a piece of the resin with water and heat. It does not dissolve. However, they dissolve in most organic solvents such as alcohol, ether, chloroform, and acetone.

4. Balsams rich in acids turn blue litmus red.

5. When solutions of the resin in ether or acetone are evaporated on a glass slide, they leave a thin film. Oleo gum resins like myrrh change colour to violet when the film is exposed to fumes of nitric acid or bromine.

6. Test for colophony:

   i. Dissolve a small quantity of the powdered resin in 5 ml acetic anhydride. Add one drop of sulphuric acid. Formation of purple colour changing to violet indicates the presence of colophony.

   ii. To 1 ml of a solution of the powdered resin in petroleum ether add 2 ml of copper acetate solution. Formation of an emerald green colour in the organic layer confirms the presence of colophony.

7. Balsams may be identified by the presence of crystals of cinnamic acid. When a small piece of the drug is warmed and pressed into a thin film between two glass slides, on cooling, crystals of cinnamic acid may be seen embedded in a transparent mass when viewed under a microscope.

8. Test for cinnamic acid containing resins: When a little of the crushed resin is warmed with dilute sulphuric acid and potassium permanganate, fumes of benzaldehyde emanating, indicate the presence of resins such as benzoin, balsam of tolu, and balsam of peru.

9. Test for guaiacum resin: Dissolve a small portion of the resin in alcohol and add a drop of 2% solution of ferric chloride. Due to the presence of Guaiaconic acid the solution attains a blue colour. This test is also answered by male fern resin and balsams, which give a light green colour changing to brown.

10. Test for umbelliferone: An alcoholic solution of Galbanum resin gives a brilliant blue fluorescence when poured into an alcoholic solution of ammonia, as it contains free umbelliferone. Asafetida (0.5 g) gives this test (as umbelliferone is formed form ferulic acid and resorcinol) when it is boiled with 5 ml concentrated hydrochloric acid and 5 ml water. The cooled filtrate is to be treated with an equal volume of alcohol and twice the volume of ammonia.

APPLICATIONS OF CHROMATOGRAPHY TO PHYTOCHEMICAL ANALYSIS

Chromatography refers to a broad range of physical methods for the separation and/or analysis of complex mixtures of compounds. Plant drugs being constituted of multitudes of phytochemical groups, chromatographic techniques find immense application in their separation, processing, purification, and in qualitative and quantitative analysis. Developments in the field of chromatography have facilitated parallel rapid advancement in our understanding of complex phytochemical profiles of valuable plant drugs. It has been one of the most useful techniques of general application not only to the field of phytochemical analysis, but also to a host of other biochemical processing sectors requiring rapid and efficient resolution of complex mixtures of chemicals.

Basically chromatography involves separation of components of a mixture due to their preferential distribution between a stationary phase and another "mobile" phase that moves through it. Separation is effected due to differential rates of migration of the components of the mixture because of their different adsorption/desorption affinity for the stationary phase as it is carried across by the mobile phase. As a result, different rates of affinity of the components to the phases effect their separation as they are flushed through by the mobile phase over the stationary phase. In other words, subtle differences in a compound's partition coefficient result in differential retention on the stationary phase effecting their separation.

Having originated in the mid 19th century as a form of separation of coloured dyes and plant pigments, chromatography literally means "colour writing." It has since then developed into many newer forms of much utility for a wide range of separation processes in chemical analysis. Today chromatography and the various automated instrumental analytical methods developed based on its principle comprise a unique and specialized branch of "Separation Science." All of these techniques facilitate resolution of mixtures into components due to adsorption/partitioning/ion exchange.

The innumerable techniques based on chromatography ultimately serve either preparative or analytical purposes. Chromatography is preparative when there is quantitative separation of components of a mixture and it is analytical when it aids qualitative identification of the mixture components post separation or estimation of their relative proportions.

The chromatographic identification, isolation, purification, and quantification of phytoconstituents is essentially carried out by a combination of four types of methods. They are:

- Paper Chromatography (PC)
- Thin Layer Chromatography (TLC)
- Column Chromatography (CC) and
- Gas Chromatography (GC)

PAPER CHROMATOGRAPHY	GAS CHROMATOGRAPHY
• Filter paper is both support and stationary phase	• Liquid stationary phase held onto a column
• Separation mostly by partition, if not by adsorption when water is the mobile phase	• Separation by partition between liquid stationary phase and gaseous mobile phase
• Largely used for qualitative work, a small extent for preparative isolations in quantities sufficient for quantitative analysis	• Instrument-enabled procedure for both qualitative and quantitative analysis, lesser extent used for preparative separations
• Detection of separated compounds with or without spray reagents	• Method of choice for analysis of any volatile compound or volatile derivatives of nonvolatile compounds
• Preferred method for analysis of sugars, phenyl propanoids, most flavonoids, organic acids, glucosinolates, hydrolysable tannins, non-protein amino acids and alkaloids	• Preferred method of analysis of essential oil constituents, plant acids, tobacco, and a host of others

Figure 7.1. Chromatographic techniques widely used in phytochemical analysis

THIN LAYER CHROMATOGRAPHY	COLUMN CHROMATOGRAPHY
• Thin layers of sorbent on inert support is stationary phase	• Liquid stationary phase held onto a column
• Separation mechanism is chiefly adsorption (to a lesser extent partition)	• Separation by partition between liquid stationary phase and gaseous mobile phase
• Used largely for qualitative and semi-quantitative work. Quantitative analysis done on HPTLC. Preparative separations yield quantities sufficient for structural characterization.	• Instrument-enabled procedure for both qualitative and quantitative analysis, lesser extent used for preparative separations
• Detection with or without spray reagents including those too drastic for use in PC. Fluorescence quenching compounds also detected.	• Method of choice for analysis of any volatile compound or volatile derivatives of nonvolatile compounds
• Invaluable supplement to GC, CC and HPLC	• Preferred method of analysis of essential oil constituents, plant acids, tobacco, and a host of others
• Economic, versatile and easy for analysis of a vast range of compounds using a broad range of mobile phase solvents	

Figure 7.1. Continued

Paper Chromatography (PC)

Experiments that led to the development of chromatographic methods traceable to the early 19th century works of C.S. Schonbein, F. Goppelsroeder, R.E. Liesegang, and A. Martin used paper as the stationary medium. Martin and his collaborators used filter paper strips as carriers for the analysis of amino acid mixtures. Soon the technique was being used for all classes of natural products. Despite the introduction of more successful methods such as TLC, PC remains the method of choice for the analysis of water soluble compounds such as carbohydrates, amino acids, nucleic acid bases, organic acids, and phenolic compounds.

The mixture whose components are to be resolved is placed as a spot near one end of a rectangular filter paper strip. It is made to dip into a solvent mixture contained in a closed chamber saturated with the solvent vapor, such that the spotted mixture stays above the level of the solvent in the chamber. As the solvent moves up the paper by capillary effect, the components move along at different rates based on their partition coefficient between the solvent and the aqueous hydration shell of the paper cellulose fiber. After completing the development, the paper is dried and the position of the separated components visualized by the use of suitable developing agents.

PC is a form of planar chromatography as the stationary phase is planar in nature. The filter paper is both the support and the stationary phase. The technique may be modified as descending chromatography; when the arrangement is such, the solvent moves down the paper. When it moves from the center toward the circumference of a circular paper strip, it is radial PC. Two-dimensional chromatography refers to the technique when the PC is developed in two different solvents successively, the second solvent run in a direction perpendicular to the first solvent.

Electrochromatography is a form of charge based separation in which a filter paper strip is impregnated with a buffer supported in the center. Either ends of the paper dip into solutions in which electrodes are immersed. A spot of mixture to be separated is placed on the paper and electrical voltage applied across the electrodes. According to their charge, solutes move toward oppositely charged electrodes. Amino acid mixtures may be effectively separated using this technique.

PC involves separation based on either partitioning or adsorption. When the solvent is water-immiscible or partially soluble in water such as butanol, phenol, amyl alcohol, the separation is based on partitioning between the solvent and the water of hydration of cellulose fiber of the paper. Amino acids, alkaloids, phenols, anthraquinone derivatives, steroids, volatile terpenes, and sugars are separated on paper by partitioning.

When the solvent is water, adsorption forces bring about separation. Glycosides, nucleic acids, organic acids, and phenolic compounds may be separated using water as solvent.

Two-dimensional chromatography is especially applicable for the separation of amino acids and flavonoids. Choice of solvent is dependent on the nature of the constituent and its relative polarity, and resolution of mixtures on the chosen solvent may be improved by altering its acidity using ammonia, acetic acid, hydrochloric acid, etc. Alternatively, filter papers may be modified to reduce polarity of cellulose by impregnating it with silicic acid or alumina, hence making them more amenable for separation of nonpolar compounds such as lipids. Good separations on PC are indicated by well-defined, compact spots. The quantity of substance present determines the size of the spot in a particular solvent and this is used as the basis of quantitative evaluation.

For preparative purposes, thicker sheets of paper are used. Compounds separated from the mixture after development on PC can be eluted individually from the chromatogram by treating the cut-out spots with appropriate solvent and estimated by measuring its absorbance or fluorescence in the visible or UV region. PC may be used effectively for the quantitation of several alkaloids, anthraquinones, and volatile oils in extracts of their source herbs.

One of the significant advantages of PC is the reproducibility of R_f values. R_M (Log1/ Rf-1) is a more constant parameter for analysis of a series of structurally related compounds, such as flavonoids, glycosides, so much so it is possible to relate it effectively to chemical features such as number of hydroxyl groups attached. This even aids estimation of R_f values of an unknown member of a compound series.

Phenyl propanoids, lignans, all classes of flavonoids except isoflavones and xanthones, hydrolysable tannins, topolones, carotenoids, organic acids, glucosinolates, non-protein amino acids, amines, alkaloids, and sugars can be analyzed by PC.

Thin Layer Chromatography (TLC)

First referred to in 1938 by Russian workers Izmailov and Shraiber, the method known as TLC today was used by American Chemists Meinhard and Hall in 1949 for separation of volatile oil components. Work of Kirchner and his associates and demonstration of its extensive utility by Stahl in 1958 gave impetus to the development of this technique.

TLC is one of the most popular and widely used separation techniques for all classes of natural products. Its versatility, speed, and sensitivity have established it as an analytical tool in modern pharmacopoeias.

TLC is also planar chromatography in which thin layers of sorbent (absorbing media) are coated on to a suitable support such as glass plate, plastic sheets, or aluminum foil. The mixture to be resolved is dissolved in a suitable solvent and applied as a spot, a short distance away from the edge (width side) of the plate. This side of the plate is dipped (a small angle away from the vertical) in a suitable solvent mixture without its surface reaching the applied spot. The whole set up is enclosed in an airtight chamber, such that it is saturated with the solvent vapor. The solvent rises up the plate due to capillary action and the solvent front travels up the plate to about 85% of its length. The plate is removed, the position of the solvent front marked, and the solvent allowed to evaporate. Depending on the nature of the sorbent and the solvent, mixture components get separated by either adsorption or partition (straight or reversed phase). Position of the separated components on the plate may be identified visually (coloured compounds), under UV light or by spraying with a suitable chromogenic agent.

Silica gel or silicic acid is the most popular and widely used sorbent. It is slightly acid in nature and is mixed with a binding agent such as calcium sulphate to hold it firmly to the supporting base. Silica gel of very fine particle size will adhere well even without a binder. Other sorbents used for different types of compounds are alumina (acid, basic, and neutral), celite, calcium hydroxide, kieselguhr, Magnesium silicate, Magnesium phosphate, polyamide, sephadex, PVP, cellulose, and ion exchange resins.

Fluorescent materials such as sodium flourescien, hydroxyl sulphonate, and rhodamine dyes may be included in the sorbent to facilitate detection of solutes, which quench the background fluorescence. When exposed to UV light (366 nm), these spots appear as dark spots against a greenish-yellow fluorescent background. Inorganic materials like uranyl acetate, manganese zinc silicate, zinc cadmium sulphate, zinc silicate, alkaline earth metal tungstates, and tin strontium phosphate may be included along with the sorbent to facilitate detection of fluorescent quenching compounds at UV 254 nm.

TLC plates may be pretreated with silver nitrate (argentative TLC) or cellulose for separations of isomeric compounds. In reverse phase chromatography, silica gel is treated with dichlorodimethyl silane making the sorbent layer hydrophobic. It is used for the separation of fatty acids, triglycerides, carotenoids, cholesterol esters, steroids, etc.

Like PC, TLC can also be used two dimensionally. Other modifications include electrophoretic separations, quantitative TLC (of spots by densitometric estimation based on UV/Vis absorption), autoradiography (for radioactive substances), and bioautography (biological detection of antibiotics).

Ready-mixed powders with binders are commercially available for making TLC plates of reproducible sorbent thickness. They need to be made into a slurry with water, before being laid on the plate. The films set quickly on air drying and they may be activated at about 105°C for 30 minutes prior to use. Commercially ready-to-use plates pre-coated with fine film of a range of sorbents (with or without fluorescent indicators) are now available.

The usual size of commercially available TLC plates is 20 × 20 cm. Microplates on microscope size support material are also available. Small strips of 10 × 2 cm may be conveniently cut out for use in qualitative detection. Film thickness of such pre-coated plates is characteristically of 250 μm thickness. For preparative separations, layers of thickness ranging from 0.5–10 mm may be used. Generally 1–2 mm thickness will suffice and plates are used in the sizes of 20 × 20 cm or 20 × 40 cm. Though resolving power of preparative plates may not be as good as regular analytical plates, it may still be conveniently prepared in lab for the isolation of quantities of components sufficient for complete structural characterization using IR, NMR, MS, etc.

Solvents used for TLC must be pure (free from admixed other solvents and water) and it is usual to use single or mixture of solvents in different ratios. The solvent mixture to be used for TLC development is arrived at by trial and error experimentation based on solubility characteristics of the compounds vis-a-vis the properties of the adsorbent and the mechanism effecting separation. Solvent selection is therefore one of the most important steps for the successful separation of compounds.

When silica gel, acidic alumina, magnesium silicate, or magnesium phosphate is the sorbent used; adsorption is the chromatographic mechanism effecting separation. A range of compounds such as steroids, amino acids, amine alcohols, hydrocarbons, lipids, bile acids, vitamins, alkaloids, and aflatoxins may be separated on these sorbents. Partition is the mechanism involved with sorbents such as cellulose, kieselguhr, and reversed phase silica gel. Compounds are partitioned between the water of hydration of cellulose fibers and solvents used for development. Commonly used solvents include n-hexane, cyclohexane, petroleum ether, ether, chloroform, ethyl acetate, butanol, isopropyl alcohol, ethanol, methanol, etc. Mobile phase used on silica gel plate often contain small quantities of ammonia solution, diethyl amine, acetic acid, dimethyl formamide, and pyridine.

Detection of compounds post development on TLC may be done by visual (with or without spray reagents) or UV examination. Depending on the nature of compounds, selected spray reagents are used for their detection. UV examination is usually done at 254 and 366 nms.

The developed TLC plate is either sprayed with the reagent or it is dipped it in. 50% sulphuric acid is most widely used for visualization of organic compounds (which on heating are seen as brown or black charred areas). Solutions of sulphuric acid-acetic anhydride (1:4) and Leibermann burchard reagent are used to detect steroids after heating at 140°C for 20 minutes. Vanillin-sulphuric acid reagent is used for detection of terpenes. Dragendorff's reagent for alkaloids, p-anisaldehyde (with sulphuric acid and ethanol) is used for sugars, steroids, phenols, and terpenes, 2,6-Dichlorophenol-indophenol for organic acids, iodine for unsaturated fatty acids, phosphomolybdic acid in ethanol, or antimony trichloride in chloroform for steroids and flavonoids, 10% copper sulphate for sulphur containing glycosides and phosphotungstic acid for triterpenes.

TLC has become one of the most popular, simplest and most widely used separation technique applicable to the analysis of a vast range of compounds ranging from amino acids, sugars, fatty acids, alkaloids, lipids, vitamins, steroids, isoflavones, xanthones, and multiconstituent essential oils in addition to a range of plant pigments, nucleotides, and proteins.

High-end TLC techniques such as centrifugally accelerated TLC, over pressure layer chromatography are current innovative adaptions of conventional TLC for use in specific separations.

HPTLC is a sophisticated, advanced and an automated version of TLC, which combines the simplicity and precision of TLC with the speed and efficient quantitation, which modern instrumentation provides. It employs high-performance pre-coated silica gel plates, which give more efficient and reproducible separation than conventional grades of silica. Very small accurately measured volumes may be applied at a predetermined rate on exact locations at measured distances from neighboring spots if any. Development time is much smaller. Upon development, the spots may be evaluated by comparison with reference standards and also quantified with greater sensitivity and precision than is possible with conventional TLC.

Development of finger print profiles of plant extracts being one of the most salient quality control requirements in herbal drug standardization, HPTLC aids development of such profiles for multi constituent herbal drugs and formulations. Such profiles form important tools in the establishment of the identity of the plant as they are reproducible when performed under similar conditions of experimentation.

Merits of TLC over other chromatographic techniques

1. Economy in solvent and materials needed for development is its greatest advantage.
2. The short development time enables rapid separations compared to PC, with even time for equilibration being minimal.
3. Separated spots are more compact and better resolved from one another compared to PC.
4. Being simple, versatile, and easy to use, TLC is often used to develop solvent systems for and to monitor progress of separations for CC, GC, and HPLC.
5. There are available a wide range of ready-to-use TLC plates, pre-coated with different sorbents to choose from for any given analysis.
6. Using the right combination of sorbent and solvent, any type of separation is possible on TLC.
7. Multiple samples may be developed simultaneously, making it an extremely useful tool for routine analysis of a number of samples.
8. A highly sensitive technique, it can detect and separate even trace quantities of compounds from smaller quantities of mixture compared to PC.
9. TLC profile can act as a fingerprint record, making it suitable for monitoring identity and purity of drugs and also for detecting adulterations and substitutions.
10. TLC also gives semi-quantitative information about major phytoconstituents thus enabling an assessment of overall drug quality.
11. Reagents too drastic for PC such as concentrated sulphuric acid may be used for visualization in TLC.

Column Chromatography (CC)

Chromatographic separation performed with the stationary phase packed in a column as against being planar is column chromatography. The sorbents used in CC are taken in a column and the mobile phase instead of moving up by capillary action comes down due to gravity against the resistance of the sorbent. The mixture to be fractionated is introduced on the column in a small volume of organic solvent. While in TLC the solvent run is terminated and the compounds separated on the plate identified in their positions on the planar phase, in CC, the solvent is allowed to run out of the column (elution) from the bottom, till the compounds are carried along separated from one another.

One of the oldest forms of chromatographic techniques, compound separation is effected by partition and the stationary phase is held onto a sorbent as the mobile phase moves down. Solute resolution is controlled by changing the mobile phase, the interaction between the mobile and stationary phase overall effecting solute separation. The separation of compounds is influenced by the displacement effect of one compound with another and partitioning between phases is independent of concentration and presence of other solutes.

Sorbents of high polarity such as silica gel are used with others like reversed phase silica, ion-exchange resins and size exclusion chromatography phases being used for specific separations. Mobile phase is a miscible solvent mixture of constant ratio-isocratic elution, or of different changing proportions—gradient elution—as the elution continues. In the mobile phase, resolved compounds are collected in fractions. These upon concentration are analyzed by TLC to identify the separated compound(s). Choice of stationary phase and mobile phase for partition chromatography by column is made from a preliminary TLC analysis of the mixture to be resolved. In general, the solvents should be pure, non-viscous, and depending on the nature of the mixture, mobile phase may be selected from a whole range of nonpolar to polar solvents. Polar compounds may be separated using polar stationary phase and nonpolar mobile phase. Conversely, nonpolar solutes may be best separated using a nonpolar stationary phase and a polar mobile phase. In practice, after the range of solvents to be used for separation is selected, the mobile phase composition is adjusted as required, while the elution progresses. Purpose of chromatography may be fractionation of a total extract, further resolution of separated fractions, purification of isolated compound mixtures, or resolution of closely similar solutes.

Several modified forms of CC, used today include:

- Gel filtration chromatography, which is based on molecular size separation
- Ion-exchange chromatography, which separates compounds based on their charge and partitioning effect
- Affinity chromatography, which separates compounds based on the molecular shape due to the functional groups they carry
- Vacuum Liquid Chromatography in which a slight negative pressure is applied at the point of eluent collection to speed up elution
- Flash chromatography, which uses mobile phase passing down the column quickly due to applied positive pressure over it
- High performance liquid chromatography (HPLC) in which the conventional cylindrical column is replaced by narrow columns. Here the stationary phase is bonded to a porous polymer held in a capillary sized stainless steel column and the mobile phase is forced through under pressure.

Of all these forms, HPLC has become one of the most extensively used chromatographic techniques for all types of compound (that are soluble and nonvolatile) separations including phytochemicals. It is a highly sensitive and efficient separation technique especially applicable to analysis of nonvolatile compounds such as alkaloids, lipids, sugars, higher terpenoids, and phenolic compounds. The eluate is closely monitored by a range of detecting systems. UV/VIS detection is most commonly employed. HPLC is a fully automated technique employing highly efficient pre-packed columns and it is one of the latest chromatographic techniques of wide applicability in plant drug identification and analyses. However, it is of limited applicability to preparative separations.

Despite the availability of several sophisticated modifications of CC, the conventional CC has still not been replaced by any other technique for large-scale isolations of compounds. It is however time-consuming and much larger quantities of sorbents and solvents are needed. Mobile phase flow is to be optimized for efficient separation of compounds because very slow and very fast elution does not bring about optimal separations.

With solvent ratios, nature of elution, sorbent selection optimized, CC still forms a reliable and practical option for routine separations of carotenoids, mixtures of alkaloids, and in general for the separation of virtually any category of compounds from their mixtures.

Gas Chromatography (GC)

It is an extensively used method of column chromatography for qualitative and quantitative analysis of complex mixtures of volatile substances that can be vaporized without decomposition. It was initially proposed by Martin and Synge in 1941 and later in 1952 developed by Martin and James for the separation of volatile fatty acids. Today it is of wide applicability in the analysis of a vast array of organic and inorganic compounds in complex mixtures.

Compound separation in GC is effected between a liquid stationary phase and a mobile gaseous phase. Highly sophisticated, fully automated instruments are available for routine analysis of scores of compounds.

In conventional GLC, columns of glass or metal, either straight or coiled, variable in length from 1–20 m of about 5 mm internal diameter, are coated internally with an inert material of uniform and small particle size to give a relatively larger surface area. Stationary phase liquids such as silicone oils, paraffin, apiezon oils, high boiling point alcohols and their esters, propylene glycols, etc., are dispersed over the stationary phase. Special columns, which serve the double purpose of both support and stationary phase such as cross-linked styrene-like polymers, are also used. Nowadays capillary columns of fused silica of bore diameter varying from 0.15–0.5 mm with column length up to 60 m, either directly coated with stationary phase or with a support holding the stationary phase are used for speeding up analysis and for better resolution.

Mobile phase is an inert gas such as helium, hydrogen, nitrogen, or argon. Compound separation is determined by the flow rate of the gas (ranging from 10–50 ml/min).

The whole arrangement of the column is such that it is heated to provide suitable operating temperatures, which could vary from 150–400°C for different types of compounds. Sophisticated GCs could be programmed to achieve a gradient temperature rise. This enables better separation of different classes of compounds, in a single run without the need for long waiting period for the elution of strongly retained compounds.

The sample dissolved in a volatile solvent like ether in volumes as small as 1 µl is injected into the column. The compounds present in the mixture volatilize as soon as they come in contact with the stationary phase (at the temperature of the column) and get swept across the column by the gaseous mobile phase. Based on their relative partitioning between the stationary liquid phase and the mobile gaseous phase, the volatilized compounds are carried across the column and out of it, by the gas, separated from one another. Hence, they elute out of the column at different time intervals and could be detected by a range of detectors used along with GLCs. These detectors, detect and measure the compounds eluting out based on a property that is characteristic for the compound or by measuring an altered property of the effluent gas due to the compound being admixed with it.

Whatever the property measured, detectors record the presence of the compound in terms of the volume of carrier gas required to elute it or as retention time, that is, the time taken for the sample to elute out since being injected. GC detectors are mostly of flame ionization or electron capture type. The variables that can be controlled to bring about effective separation are the stationary phase and the operating temperature. This is in accordance with the temperature of volatilization of compounds. Volatile oils require 150–300°C, steroids require 250°C, and pesticides require 400°C, and so on. Even nonvolatile compounds such as sugars, flavonoids, cardio active glycosides, etc., may be converted into volatile trimethyl siloxy derivatives or as volatile methyl esters (nonvolatile plant acids). These can then be injected into the column and thus separated and detected.

GC is an efficient tool for qualitative detection and reference compounds co-injected with mixture to be resolved, aid in the quicker identification of mixture components. For quantitative analysis, area of the peak recording the presence of the compound on the chromatogram is measured and it is proportional to the quantity that is present in the mixture.

Tentative compound identification may be effected without reference compounds on a GC coupled to MS. This high-end scientific instrument measures the mass spectra of the compound eluting out of GC. The ion fragmentation data of MS is matched against a library of data on known compounds, providing clues on the nature of the compound. Known compounds are identified by an exact match of data, while for unknown compounds, the fragmentation patterns provide clues to its structural features.

Though used routinely for analytical work, larger preparative columns (approximately 60 m in length, 1–2 cm in diameter) can be used for preparative separation of larger quantities (up to 20 ml) of mixtures.

GC is widely used for routine analysis of volatile oils, plant acids, opium, tobacco, tropane alkaloids, cannabis resin, sapogenins, cardiac glycosides, cocaine and its metabolites in body fluids, pesticide residue estimation, etc.

CONCLUSIONS

Phytochemical analysis today includes the use of sophisticated analytical instrumentation by which direct identification of phytoconstituents from fresh plant parts, extracts, exudates, essential oils, and formulations is a straight forward task. However, the complex multi constituent composition of plants makes isolation and purification their active principles, still a challenging issue. An introduction to general principles of phytochemical analysis and to simple methods of extraction, isolation, and identification of some phytochemical classes is presented here. Chromatography being an invaluable and indispensable aid to the separation and analysis of complex mixtures of compounds, four basic chromatographic techniques of wide applicability in phytochemical analysis have been discussed.

REVIEW QUESTIONS

Essay Questions

1. What is phytochemical analysis? Outline the general principles involved.
2. Present a comparative account of column chromatography and gas chromatography.
3. Discuss the properties, method of extraction, separation, and identification of alkaloids.

Short Notes

1. Extraction and identification of lipids
2. Properties and identification of flavonoids
3. Extraction and isolation of volatile oils
4. Properties and extraction of resins
5. Paper chromatography
6. Merits of TLC

8   Plant-Derived Pure Drugs

CHAPTER OBJECTIVES

Introduction

Isolation, Identification and Estimation of Selected Plant-Derived Pure Drugs

INTRODUCTION

Up to mid-19th century, the beginning of the era of natural products, plant-derived drugs remained structurally ill-defined. Plant active constituent isolations from crude drugs were successful when the yield was sufficient and the compounds were more amenable to the then available methods of isolations. However such isolations were not possible for most biologically active crude drugs with unstable and/or poor-yield constituents. Also compound characterization required considerable quantities of the isolated constituents. The advent of modern instrumentation and newer techniques in separation science, such as chromatography, made active constituent isolation and identification much simpler as it became possible to complete compound characterizations on tiny quantities of the isolated material. What followed was considerable progress in the isolation of pharmaceutically important natural products. Plant-derived molecules also served as chemical models or templates for the total synthesis of newer drugs.

Successful introduction of plant-derived drugs including morphine, codeine, papaverine, quinine, atropine, hyoscine, reserpine, digoxin, caffeine, emetine, ergotamine, senna glycosides, vincristine, vinblastine, psoralen, pilocarpine and tannic acid marked the beginning of the era of pure drug molecules, which went on to become the stronghold of modern western medicine. Plants continue to be important sources of drugs as evidenced by the introduction of newer drugs, such as paclitaxel, artemisinin, camptothecin, forskolin, sanguinarine etc. The technology involved in the isolation of commercially important phytopharmaceuticals in many cases is patented information. Availability of analytical techniques and sophisticated instrumentation in the last few decades has made it possible to devise commercially feasible techniques for the extraction of several phytomolecules.

Plant-Derived Pure Drugs in India

In India raw drugs pertaining to some 7,500 medicinal plant species are claimed to be used in traditional medical systems. Many of these drugs are used in folk medicine in contrast to the more systematic and well-validated traditional medicine such as Ayurveda and Siddha which use much lesser number of carefully selected species. It is estimated that in India today more than 80% of the rural population resort to the use of herbal medicines.

The production of plant-derived pure drugs in modern India may be traced back to the establishment of the first phytochemical industry by the then British Raj at Mungpoo, Darjeeling. Quinine was manufactured from cinchona bark in three such state-owned factories. Six decades since independence, large-scale production of plant-derived pure drugs has become an important segment of Indian pharmaceutical industry. Morphine, codeine, papaverine, thebaine, emetine, quinine, quinidine, digoxin, caffeine, hyoscine, hysocyamine, xanthotoxin, psoralen, colchicine, rutin, berberine, vincristine, vinblastine, nicotine, strychnine, brucine, ergot alkaloids, senna glycosides, pyrethroids and podophyllotoxin are being manufactured in India today. Technology for the large-scale production of etoposide, teniposide, L-Dopa, ajmaline, ajmalicine and β-acetyl glycyrrhetic acid has been developed in our country. The Indian pharmaceutical industry is a major contributor to the national economy as 95% of the domestic demand for pharmaceuticals is met through indigenous production. Its export capability makes it a strategic trade sector in the Indian economy. India exports generic drugs to Commonwealth countries, Africa and even to the highly regulated US and European markets. It is one of the top 14 pharmaceutical manufacturing countries in the world with a market of US $2.5 billion. Imports are limited to a few life-saving drugs like anti-cancer, cardiovascular and anti-hypertension and other newer drugs not yet cleared for indigenous production. At present there are 12,000 manufacturing units of which 2,900 are large scale and the remaining small scale units. Of the large-scale units 45 belong to multinational companies. The Indian pharmaceutical industry thus represents a highly successful technology-based industry that has witnessed tremendous growth since the 1970s when our patent laws were changed. With the imposition of the TRIPS agreement, there have been concerns over its continued growth. Development of plant-derived pure drugs has been quite daunting in the face of other hurdles like dwindling supply of raw materials, lack of patent protection for indigenous traditional drug knowledge etc. However India has well lived up to the challenges and is responding to the change in patent laws. The Indian pharmaceutical industry is now moving towards the development of advanced level process and product R&D capabilities.

ISOLATION, IDENTIFICATION AND ESTIMATION OF SELECTED PLANT-DERIVED PURE DRUGS

Ephedrine

Source

It is the principal alkaloid of the species of Ephedra (Ephedraceae) and was first isolated from Ma Huang, one of the oldest known drugs. Identified as *Ephedra vulgaris* var *Helvetica*, Ma Huang consists of the entire plant or tops of various Ephedra species including *E. sinica* and *E. equisetina* from China, *E. gerardiana*, *E. intermedia* and *E. major* from India and Pakistan.

The plants are small bushes with slender aerial stems and minute leaves giving the appearance of being effectively leafless. The plants typically contain 2% to 5% of alkaloids according to species; 30% to 90% of the total alkaloids is (–) ephedrine. Related structures include the diastereoisomeric (–) pseudoephedrine and the demethyl analogues (–) norephedrine and (+) norpseudoephedrine are also present. In *E. intermedia*, the proportion of pseudoephedrine exceeds that of ephedrine. The root also contains a number of macrocyclic alkaloids (ephedradine) and ferruloyl histamine which have hypotensive properties.

Uses

A sympathomimetic amine, the effects of ephedrine are similar to those of adrenaline. It is orally active and has a longer duration of action than adrenaline. Due to its bronchodilator effect, it is used in the relief of asthma and hay fever. Its vasoconstrictor action on mucous membranes makes it an effective nasal decongestant. Ephedrine is of considerable value as a circulatory stimulant in surgical shock, as a mydriatic and in Addison's disease. Pseudoephedrine is also widely used in compounded cough and cold preparations and as a decongestant. In indigenous medicine in Asia, ephedras are used as anti-inflammatory drugs.

Description

Ephedrine occurs as a waxy solid or as crystalline particles. Its IUPAC name is (R*,S*)-2-(methylamino)-1-phenylpropan-1-ol and has the molecular formula $C_{10}H_{15}NO_1$. It has a bitter taste, is odourless or has a slight aromatic odour. In warm weather it slowly volatilizes. The anhydrous substance melts at 36°C and the hemi-hydrate melts at 42°C. It is a weak base, with a pKa of 9.6. Ephedrine decomposes with light. Solutions in oil can have a garlicky odour. It is soluble in water (1 in 20) and in alcohol, chloroform, ether, glycerol, olive oil and in liquid paraffin (Windholz, 1983).

Ephedrine and its optical isomer pseudoephedrine are structurally very similar to methamphetamine. In illicit drug laboratories simple dehydrogenation is used to make methamphetamine from ephedrine. Ephedrine exhibits optical isomerism and has two chiral centres, giving rise to four stereoisomers. By convention the pair of enantiomers with the stereochemistry (1R,2S and 1S,2R) is designated ephedrine, while the pair of enantiomers with the stereochemistry (1R,2R and 1S,2S) is called pseudoephedrine.

Ephedrine is a substituted amphetamine and a structural methamphetamine analogue. It differs from methamphetamine only by the presence of a hydroxyl (OH). Amphetamines, however, are more potent and have additional biological effects.

The isomer which is marketed is (–)-(1R,2S)-ephedrine. Ephedrine hydrochloride is a white crystalline powder. Most of the L-ephedrine produced today for official medical use is made synthetically as the extraction and isolation process from the plant source is tedious and no longer cost effective.

Isolation

1. The plant material is ground to a fine powder, passed through #40 mesh and percolated with 80% alcohol until the percolate is colourless.

2. The percolate is concentrated to a syrupy fluid on a rotary vacuum evaporator. It is diluted with equal volume of water, rendered alkaline with ammonium hydroxide and filtered.

3. Extract the filtrate with chloroform and heat the residue on the filter under reflux with chloroform.

4. Combine the chloroform extracts, concentrate to a small volume and set aside overnight for spontaneous evaporation.

5. A greenish fragrant gelatinous residue that is formed is dissolved in a small volume of hot water and treated with dilute hydrochloric acid until exactly neutral to litmus.

6. The solution is carefully evaporated to dryness and the residual alkaloidal salt is purified by recrystallization from absolute alcohol.

7. Base ephedrine is regenerated from a solution of the alkaloidal salt by first alkalinizing with ammonium hydroxide.

8. It is then extracted with chloroform, which is further evaporated to yield white rosette crystals of ephedrine that are easily broken up into coarse needles.

Identification

1. *Chen-Kao test*: To 1 ml of a solution of the substance add an equal volume of an alkaline solution of copper sulphate (0.1 ml of 10% $CuSO_4$ and 1 ml of 20% NaOH). The solution turns violet due to the formation of a violet-coloured complex between ephedrine and copper sulphate in alkaline medium. While only ephedrine and pseudoephedrine give a violet colour, norephedrine and norpseudoephedrine and related compounds give a bright blue-coloured precipitate.

2. *Simon's test*: To 1ml of a solution of ephedrine in water add an equal volume of Simon's reagent (sodium nitroprusside in a basic buffer). Formation of a bright blue colour that deepens on standing is obtained. This is characteristic of an amine.

3. *Pesez's test*: A small quantity of ephedrine dissolved in 2 ml concentrated H_2SO_4 develops a pink to red colour when 3 to 4 drops of 40% formaldehyde are added. Upon warming the colour changes to wine-red.

4. A slightly alkaline solution of ephedrine when warmed with a drop of a 1% solution of ninhydrin gives a violet colour soluble in amyl alcohol.

5. *Erdmann's reagent*: Solutions of ephedrine with a mixture of sulphuric and nitric acids (Erdmann's reagent) give a yellow ring below and a pink ring with a smoky pink layer on the top.

6. *Mayer's reagent*: To 1ml of a solution of ephedrine add Mayer's reagent. The solution becomes cloudy on standing.

7. *Wagner's reagent*: To 1ml of a solution of ephedrine add Wagner's reagent. An orange precipitate is formed.

8. Solution of ephedrine with phosphor molybdic acid gives a greenish-yellow heavy precipitate which turns blue on standing.

9. With phosphotungstic acid solutions of ephedrine give a heavy white precipitate.

Estimation

Several simple UV spectrophotometric methods of assay are available for the estimation of ephedrine in pharmaceutical formulations.

A. Method I

1. 20 g of powdered plant material is shaken frequently with 200 ml of a 1:3 mixture of chloroform and ether.

2. 10 ml of 10% ammonia solution and 1 g of anhydrous sodium carbonate are added and the mixture shaken for 4 h at frequent intervals and allowed to stand overnight.

3. The mixture is carefully packed in a percolator and percolated with the 100 ml ether-chloroform mixture for 4 h and then further percolated with 100 ml ether for another 3 h for complete extraction of alkaloids.

4. The combined percolates are shaken with successive portions of 4 × 20 ml of N/3 HCl.

5. The combined acid extracts are filtered and treated with 1N NaOH solution to a pH of 4 to 5; 10 g anhydrous sodium carbonate and sufficient NaCl are added to saturate the solution.

6. The clear alkaline solution is extracted with four successive portions of 60, 50, 50 and 30 ml of ether and then with 25 ml portions of ether until extraction of the alkaloids is complete.

7. The combined ether extracts are allowed to stand until clear and then decanted through a filter into a beaker. The ether solution is warmed and poured off from any crystals which may separate.

8. The ether is evaporated to a volume of approximately 10 ml and the residual solvent allowed to evaporate in air.

9. The residue is dissolved in excess of 0.1N sulphuric acid, 20 ml distilled water is added and the excess acid back titrated with 0.1 N NaOH using methyl red as indicator.

10. Each 1 ml of 0.1 N H_2SO_4 is equivalent to 0.01651 g of total alkaloids calculated as ephedrine.

B. Method II

1. A solution of ephedrine (5–500 mg) is taken with 10–15 ml of 50% NaOH in a distillation flask and quickly distilled.

2. The distillate is collected in an excess of standard sulphuric acid. Depending on the amount of ephedrine present 50–150 ml of distillate is collected. Neutral reaction of the distillate to litmus gives an indication of the completeness of distillation.

3. The excess acid is back titrated with standard NaOH using methyl red as indicator .1 ml of 0.1 N H_2SO_4 is equivalent to 0.01652 g of anhydrous ephedrine.

C. Method III

1. Dissolve about 500 mg of ephedrine hydrochloride, accurately weighed in 25 ml of glacial acetic acid.

2. Add 10 ml of mecuric acetate TS and two drops of crystal violet TS, and titrate with 0.1N perchloric acid (test solution) to an emerald-green end point.

3. Perform a blank determination and make any necessary correction. Each ml of 0.1N perchloric acid is equivalent to 20.17 mg of ephedrine hydrochloride.

Rutin

Source

Rutin is a flavonoid glycoside first isolated from *Fagopyrum esculentum* (buckwheat) in 1860 by Schunck. The most frequently occurring flavonoid glycoside it was isolated from *Ruta graveolens* in 1942 by A. Weiss. Since then it has been found in almost all higher plants and commercial production is made from *F. esculentum* (Polygonaceae), *Sophora japonica* (Leguminosae) and *Eucalyptus macrorhyncha*.

Buckwheat is a pseudocereal being used as a foodgrain in the Himalayan region and in the hilly areas of Tamil Nadu. *F. esculentum* and *F. tartaricum* are the two high yielding species with the latter being richer in rutin. *S. japonica* is an ornamental plant grown in Kashmir valley and large-scale production of rutin from *E. macrorhyncha* and *E. youmani* is undertaken in Australia and New Zealand.

Uses

Rutin is one of the bioactive flavonoid compounds which are present in substantial amounts in plants. It has a broad range of physiological activities. The only flavone in clinical use, rutin is used as both rutinoside and as its aglycone quercetin. These two are used in combination with ascorbic acid to treat capillary bleeding due to increased capillary fragility as seen in degenerative vascular disease, diabetes, retinitis and allergic manifestation. Rutin and its aglycone are used as protection against harmful radiations including x-rays.

Rutin inhibits platelet aggregation and decreases capillary permeability. It is an antioxidant, anti-inflammatory and inhibits the enzyme aldose reductase found in the eyes and a number of other body tissues. An anti-coagulant, it improves blood circulation. Synthetic hydroxyl ethyl derivatives of rutin are used in chronic venous insufficiency. It is used in the management of chylothorax in dogs and cats. Both quercetin and rutin are used in many countries as medications for blood vessel protection and are ingredients of numerous multivitamin preparations and herbal remedies.

Description

Rutin is a rhamnoglycoside of flavonol quercetin. Chemically it is quercetin-3-rutinoside or 3-[[6-O-(6-deoxy-alpha-L-mannopyranosyl)-beta-D-glucopyranosyl]oxy]-2-(3,4-dihydroxyphenyl)-5,7-dihydroxy-4H-1-benzopyran-4-one.

It occurs as a yellow crystalline powder of melting point 191°C and has a molecular formula of $C_{27}H_{30}O_{16}$. It is highly soluble in a number of organic solvents like methanol, ethanol, pyridine etc. It is poorly soluble in cold water (12.5 g/100ml) but is fairly soluble in boiling water.

Isolation

Buckwheat is the best commercial source for production of rutin in India. The percentage rutin content is maximum at the flowering time of the plant, which is 6% to 6.6% in *F. tartaricum* and 2% to 4% in *F. esculentum*. Rutin content falls during slow drying due to leaf deterioration, while the dried leaves may be stored indefinitely. Procedures for the extraction of rutin differ according to the nature of the plant, scale of operation and they change from time to time as more knowledge of the physical and chemical properties of rutin become available.

It is poorly soluble in cold water, fairly soluble in boiling water and highly soluble in a number of organic solvents like methanol, ethanol, acetone and pyridine. In general hot water, 70% alcohol and 85% isopropyl alcohol are the commonly employed solvents for the extraction of rutin.

Identification

Chemical tests for identification of rutin are based on the properties of phenolic hydroxyl groups of rutinose and of the benzene nucleus. It may be chromatographically identified on a paper chromatogram developed descendingly (25% isopropyl alcohol) as a brown–orange band. Rutin is even conveniently identified by UV, Nuclear Magnetic Resonance (NMR), Infrared (IR) and mass spectroscopy.

1. An aqueous solution of rutin when treated with a solution of ferric chloride gives a dark green colour.
2. An orange–yellow precipitate intensified in colour by alkalies is formed when an aqueous solution of rutin is treated with lead acetate.
3. Similar coloured precipitates are formed by aqueous solutions of rutin with ammonium molybdate and antimony trichloride.

A. Method I

1. To 20 kg of freshly harvested buckwheat leaves taken in a stainless steel steam-heated vessel, add sufficient quantity of 85% isopropyl alcohol (IPA-75 l) to cover the plant material.
2. The solution is brought to boil as rapidly as possible and held at boiling temperature for 10 min.

3. The hot extract is drawn off by pressure through heavy filter sheets. After the second and third similar extractions (each with 45 l of IPA) followed by filtration, the combined extracts are concentrated by evaporation to one-fourth their original volume.

4. The boiling concentrate is then carefully strained through heavy filter sheets, washed with boiling water (2 l) and the filtrate and washings are immediately cooled by the addition of crushed ice (6 l) to bring the temperature to 5°C.

5. The cold solution containing crude crystallized rutin is allowed to stand for 1 h and filtered carefully, after thoroughly washing with small portions of cold water. The obtained rutin is dried to constant weight at 110°.

B. Method II

1. To 10 kg leaf meal contained in a stainless steel vessel, add 200 l of boiling water. The leaf and water mixture is boiled for about 15 min and filtered hot.

2. The spent leaf meal is washed with further 10 l hot water and the filtrate and the washings are collected in open wooden or stainless steel tanks. It is allowed to stand for about 24 h at room temperature.

3. Rutin crystallizes in yellow crystals as the temperature of the solution falls down. The crystals are filtered out and the filter cake washed with cold water.

4. Purified rutin so obtained may be recrystallized from ethanol.

Estimation

Rutin can be estimated colorimetrically by detection of the red colour it forms upon reduction with magnesium amalgam and hydrochloric acid. This is a useful method for the estimation of rutin content in both plant extracts and in pharmaceutical dosage forms.

It may be more simply assayed spectrophotometrically by measuring its absorption in ethanol at 259 nm and 363 nm. The percentage rutin content may be estimated from an absorption curve of a standard rutin solution.

1. *Sample preparation*: Dissolve 0.5 g of the sample in 50 ml HPLC 80% methanol and filter. Take 2 ml of the filtrate in a 50 ml standard flask. Add 2 ml double-distilled (dd) water and 5 ml ammonium molybdate and dilute the mixture to 50 ml with dd water.

2. *Standard solution*: Dissolve 0.02 g of rutin in 50 ml HPLC 80% methanol. Take 1 ml of this solution in a 50 ml standard flask and add 2 ml dd water, 5 ml ammonium molybdate and make up to required volume with dd water.

Measure the absorption of the sample against dd water as blank at 360 nm. Percentage of rutin content in the sample is calculated by

$$\frac{A_{sample} \times C \times 50 \times 100}{A_{standard} \times W \times 2}$$

where A_{sample} is the absorbance of the sample at 360 nm, $A_{standard}$ absorbance of the standard solution at 360 nm, C concentration of the standard solution of rutin, g/ml, W the weight of the sample in g, 2 volume of the sample.

Calcium Sennosides

Source

Calcium sennosides are calcium salts of sennosides A and B obtained from the leaves and pods of *Cassia angustifolia* and *Cassia acutifolia*. Known in commerce as Indian and Alexandrian Senna these plants have been used as natural, safe, time-tested laxatives in traditional as well as modern systems of medicine. In India, senna is extensively cultivated in Tamil Nadu, Andhra Pradesh and Gujarat and is an important plant drug exported from India.

Despite the availability of a number of synthetic as well as natural laxatives, sennosides remain among the most extensively used drugs for both habitual constipation and occasional use. Senna is listed in the World Health Organization's (WHO) list of essential medicines.

Sennosides A and B were first reported by Stoll in 1941 and they are present in greater concentration than other sennosides namely C, D, E, F and G.

Senna leaf suitable for medicinal use should contain not less than 2% dianthrone glycosides calculated in terms of sennoside B. Sennoside content varies from 1.2% to 2.5% in Indian senna and from about 2.5% to 4.5% in Alexandrian senna. Senna preparations in the form of powdered leaf, powdered fruit or extracts are typically standardized to a given sennoside content. Sennosides are isolated from senna as calcium salts as they are better absorbed gastrointestinally.

Uses

Senna is a stimulant laxative and acts on the wall of the large intestine, increasing peristaltic movement. After oral administration, the sennosides are transformed by intestinal flora into rhein anthrone which appears to be the ultimate purgative principle. The glycoside residues in the active constituents are necessary for water solubility and subsequent transportation to the site of action.

Description

Sennosides are dimeric hydroxyanthraquinone glycosides chemically designated as 5,5'-bis(beta-D-gulcopyranosyloxy)-9,9',10,10'-tetrahydro-4,4'-dihydroxy-10,10'-dioxo[9,9'-bianthracene]-2,2'-dicarboxylic acid. With a molecular formula of $C_{42}H_{36}CaO_{18}$, calcium sennosides occur as pale brownish hygroscopic powder, soluble in water and alcohol.

Sennosides A and B are a pair of stereoisomers containing rhein dianthrone (sennidin A and B) as the aglycone. Minor constituents of senna include sennosides C and D, which are also a pair of optical isomers, di-O-glucosides of heterodianthrone sennidins C and D.

Sennoside A and B both hydrolyze to give two molecules of glucose and the aglycones sennidin A and B. Sennidin A is dextrorotatory and B is its mesoform formed by intramolecular compensation.

Isolation

Ever since the isolation of sennosides A and B from senna, the presence of several other constituents has been demonstrated. The purgative action of the leaf drug is attributed to the synergistic effect of several active principals chief among which are sennosides. The total leaf sennosides constituting largely of sennosides A and B are isolated from senna leaves and or pods and then converted to calcium salts.

Isolation of sennosides involves producing purer fractions of anthraquinone glycosides, both free and in the form of glycosides. These are present both free and as magnesium, potassium and sodium salts combined either through a hydroxyl or a carboxylic acid group. The differential solubility of the glycosides, their aglycones and other anthracene derivatives of senna in chloroform is used for their isolation. While the glycosides are chloroform insoluble, the aglycones and others are soluble in it.

A. Method I

1. 300 g of powdered senna are macerated with 850 ml of 5% acetic acid for 24 h in a 2 l stoppered conical flask. Acidification liberates the free aglycones from their glycosides and from their potassium, magnesium and calcium salts.
2. The maceration mixture is then air-dried and extracted exhaustively with chloroform (10 × 600 ml) to remove free anthraquinones as well as many impurities. The absence of a red colour imparted to a small portion of the chloroform filtrate on the addition of a few drops of 5% alcoholic potassium hydroxide indicates complete extraction of hydroxyanthraquinones.
3. The chloroform extracts are combined, evaporated to dryness and weight recorded.
4. The chloroform exhausted marc is air-dried and extracted exhaustively with 600-ml portions (10 times) of warm ethanol until successive extracts show no red or pink colouration with a few drops of 5% alcoholic potassium hydroxide solution.
5. The combined filtrates are evaporated at 40°C in a rotary vacuum evaporator to about one-third the original volume. To this solution, 5% alcoholic potassium hydroxide is added until no further precipitation occurs.
6. The solution is then filtered and the residue washed with cold ethanol to remove last traces of potassium hydroxide and then dried by suction on a Buchner funnel.

7. The residue consisting of the potassium salts of the glycosides is suspended in warm ethanol and the glycosides liberated by slow addition of glacial acetic acid with stirring.

8. The solution is filtered hot and the residue further extracted with warm ethanol. The combined filtrates are evaporated to dryness in vacuo at 40°C, the residue recrystallized from isopropyl alcohol and weight noted.

Preparation of calcium sennosides

The residues from the chloroform and the ethanol extracts are pooled together and slurried in150 ml water. A mixture of 2 g of calcium hydroxide in 5 ml water is added to the slurry to solubilize the glycosides. The pH of the solution is brought to 6.7 using dilute HCl. Add 75 ml of 90% methanol and 200 ml of 100% methanol solution and stir the solution. Filter to separate the formed precipitate of calcium sennosides. Carefully separate the residue on the filter after washing it with a little methanol and dry it in vacuo.

B. Method II

1. 25 g of powdered senna leaflets are extracted with 75 ml benzene for 15 min on and electric shaker, filtered in vacuum and solvent distilled off.

2. The leftover marc is dried at room temperature and extracted with 75 ml of 70% methanol for 30 min on an electric shaker and filtered under vacuum.

3. The marc is reextracted with 50 ml of 70% methanol for 15 min, filtered and the methanolic extracts combined.

4. The methanolic extract is then concentrated to one-eighth volume, acidified to pH 3.2 by adding HCl with constant stirring.

5. It is set aside for 15 min at 5°C, filtered under vacuum and 1g of anhydrous calcium chloride in 12.5 ml of denatured spirit is added with constant stirring.

6. The pH of the solution is adjusted to 8 by addition of ammonia and set aside for 15 min. The precipitate obtained is dried.

Identification

1. *Borntrager's test*: To 0.1 g of calcium sennosides add 5 ml dilute HCl and boil on a water bath for 2 min. Filter, cool and shake the filtrate with 2 ml ether. Separate the organic layer, add a few drops of 10% ammonia and shake vigorously. A rose red colour is seen in the aqueous layer.

2. *Modified Borntrager's test*: To 0.1 g of the drug add 5ml ferric chloride and 5ml dilute hydrochloric acid. Heat for 5 min on a boiling water bath. Cool, shake with ether and add equal volume of ammonia. An intense red colour is formed in the ammoniacal layer confirming the presence of anthraquinone glycoside.

3. Paper chromatography of the glycosides dissolved in alcohol is developed in the lower aqueous layer of a mixture of water, acetone and benzene (2:1:4), the chamber being equilibrated with the upper phase of the solvent mixture contained in a beaker in the chamber. It is developed by spraying with 0.5% magnesium acetate in methanol followed by heating to 100° for 3 to 5 min. Sennosides are seen as distinct orange spots.

Estimation

Calcium sennosides may be estimated by a number of spectrophotometric, spectrofluorimetric and chromatographic (high performance liquid chromatography, HPLC; high performance thin layer chromatography, HPTLC) methods.

Calcium sennosides are extracted into boiling water, which are oxidized with ferric chloride treatment. Subsequent acid hydrolysis releases anthraquinones from glycosides that are extracted into ether. Residue of anthraquinone from evaporated ether solution forms a pink-coloured complex with 1N KOH which is estimated spectrophotometrically.

1. Weigh accurately 10 mg calcium sennosides, transfer into a conical flask, add 25 ml distilled water using a pipette and heat on a boiling water bath for 20 min.
2. Add 2 to 3 drops of water and filter. To 10 ml of the filtrate, add 20 ml 10% aqueous ferric chloride and heat for 15 to 20 min on a water bath.
3. Add 1 ml concentrated HCL and heat till the precipitate dissolves. Cool and extract with ether (4 × 20 ml).
4. Collect the ether layers into a 100 ml standard flask and make up to volume with ether. Mix well and pipette out 10 ml into a clean china dish and evaporate.
5. To the residue add 10 ml 1N KOH, mix uniformly and determine the absorbance at 500 nm using 1M KOH as blank.

Calculate the percentage sennoside content based on the extinction value of sennosides in terms of free anthraquinoines which is 200 at 500 nm.

Caffeine

Source

Caffeine is a purine alkaloid co-occuring with minor isomeric dimethyl xanthines theobromine and theophylline. Its major sources are tea, coffee, cocoa and cola, which owe their stimulant properties to these water-soluble alkaloids. This alkaloid is found in the leaves, seeds and fruits of 63 different species of plants worldwide.

Caffeine was first isolated in 1821 by the French chemist Pierre Jean Robiquet from coffee. Caffeine acts as a stimulant of the central nervous system (CNS), cardiac muscle and respiratory system as well as a diuretic. As such, it is found to delay fatigue.

The widespread occurrence of caffeine in a variety of plants played a major role in the long-standing popularity of caffeine-containing products. The most important sources of caffeine are coffee (*Coffea* spp.), tea (*Camellia sinensis*), guarana (*Paullinia cupana*), maté (*Ilex paraguariensis*), cola nuts (*Cola vera*), and cocoa (*Theobroma cacao*). The amount of caffeine found in these products varies – the highest amounts are found in guarana (4%–7%), followed by tea leaves (3.5%), maté tea leaves (0.89%–1.73%), coffee beans (1.1%–2.2%), cola nuts (1.5%) and cocoa beans (0.03%).

Uses

Caffeine is used medicinally as a CNS stimulant, usually combined with another therapeutic agent, as in compound analgesic preparations. Caffeine has pharmacologic effects on CNS, heart, peripheral and central vasculature, renal, gastrointestinal and respiratory system. Caffeine competitively inhibits phosphodiesterase resulting in an increase in cyclic AMP and subsequent release of adrenaline. This leads to a stimulation of the CNS, a relaxation of the bronchial smooth muscle, and induction of diuresis as major effects. Caffeine-containing products have been consumed for hundreds of years for their pleasant flavour and stimulating effects.

Description

Chemically it is 1,3,7-trimethyl xanthine and has the molecular formula $C_8H_{10}N_4O_2$. Caffeine has a bitter taste, is odourless and occurs as a white powder or as white needles. In its anhydrous form, caffeine contains one molecule of water of hydration; caffeine in solution is neutral in pH. It has melting range of 235–238°C over which it decomposes by sublimation. Its solubility in water is 22mg/ml at 25°C, 180 mg/mL at 80°C and 670 mg/mL at 100°C. It is soluble in solvents such as acetone, ethyl ether, ethanol, chloroform, methylene chloride etc.

Caffeine is obtained from tea dust, as a by-product from the manufacture of decaffeinated coffee or synthetically prepared via several methods, including from dimethylurea and malonic acid.

Isolation

Several methods and different solvents such as dichloromethane, chloroform, ethyl acetate and supercritical carbon dioxide are used in the extraction of caffeine from tea and other sources. Dichloromethane is used for the decaffeination of several conventional teas.

A. Method I

Tea leaves mostly contain cellulose, tannins and chlorophyll apart from caffeine. Dichloromethane is the most widely used solvent for extracting caffeine from tea leaves as caffeine is more soluble in dichloromethane (140 mg/ml) than in water (22 mg/ml). Also its extracting efficiency is 98% to 99%. Caffeine being more soluble in hot water, it is initially extracted into boiling water, which on cooling is shaken with dichloromethane. Tannins partially soluble in dichloromethane are converted to salts by the added sodium carbonate, in which form they move into the aqueous phase. However tannin salts being anionic surfactants tend to emulsify with water. Hence the solution is not to be vigorously shaken.

1. Place 30 g of the tea leaves in a 500 ml beaker. Add 250 ml of distilled water and 5 g of sodium carbonate and stir the contents of the beaker with a glass rod. Boil the contents of the beaker on a hot plate/water bath for 10 minutes.

2. Place a watch glass on top of the beaker to prevent excessive evaporation. Filter the hot solution through a glass funnel plugged with a small piece of cotton into a 250 ml conical flask.

3. Transfer the tea leaves back into the beaker. Add 100 ml of distilled water and again bring the contents to a boil.

4. Filter and combine the filtrate with the earlier lot in the 250 ml conical flask. Discard the tea leaves.

5. When the filtrate is cooled to room temperature, transfer into a 250 ml separatory funnel. Extract with 25 ml of dichloromethane without vigorous shaking.

6. Carefully drain the lower (dichloromethane) layer into a clean 100 ml conical flask.

7. Extract further with 2 × 20 ml portions of dichloromethane, combine the organic layers and run through a bed of anhydrous sodium carbonate packed atop a glass funnel plugged with cotton wool.

8. The moisture-free filtrate is then gently heated on a hot plate to evaporate dichloromethane.

9. The dried residue of caffeine is purified by recrystallization from hot ethanol. Pure caffeine is vacuum dried and weight noted.

B. Method II

1. Briefly, 20 g of tea and 90 ml of distilled water is refluxed for 30 min, and filtered under vacuum. The residue is again refluxed with 50 ml distilled water and filtered.

2. Obtained filtrates are combined, 12.5 ml of 10% lead acetate solution is added, boiled (5 min) and filtered through a Buchner funnel with silica gel layer.

3. The filtrate is extracted four times with chloroform (40 ml). Combined chloroform phases are washed with 5% KOH solution (to remove traces of acetate) and then with distilled water.

4. Chloroform extracts are dried in a rotary evaporator.

5. The crude caffeine is recrystallized using a mixed-solvent system that involved dissolving it with 5 ml hot acetone followed by the addition of hexane until the solution turns cloudy. The solution is cooled, crystalline caffeine collected by vacuum filtration and the weight noted.

Identification

1. *Murexide test*: To a few crystals of caffeine taken in a porcelain dish add 3 to 4 drops of concentrated nitric acid and evaporate to dryness. Add 2 drops of ammonium hydroxide to the residue. A purple colour is obtained.

2. To about 50 mg of caffeine taken in a porcelain dish add a 1 ml hydrogen peroxide and a few drops of 2% HCl. Evaporation to dryness gives a bright red colour which turns purple on addition of a few drops of ammonia solution.

3. *Thin layer chromatography (TLC) identification*: A few crystals of caffeine are dissolved in dichloromethane and spotted on a silica gel plate and developed in the solvent system: ethyl acetate: methanol: water (100:13.5:10). For activation it is first sprayed with potassium iodide solution (1g potassium iodide and 1g iodine dissolved in 100 ml ethanol), followed by spraying with a 1:1 mixture of 25% HCl and 96% ethanol (I/HCl reagent). Caffeine is identified as a dark brown spot discernible in visible light. Standard caffeine may be co-spotted as positive control.

Estimation

Caffeine content of tea extracts and formulations may conveniently be assayed by a number of titrimetric, spectrophotometric, gravimetric and chromatographic methods. HPLC is the method of choice as it is subject to fewer interferences than other methods.

A. Method I (Spectrophotometric assay)

1. *Sample preparation*: 3 g tea sample is taken in a 250 ml beaker and 20 ml boiling purified water is added. It is stirred for 1 min on a magnetic stirrer (500 rpm) and allowed to cool to room temperature.

2. *Standard preparation*: A 1,000 ppm stock standard of caffeine is prepared by dissolving 198.2 mg of caffeine in 200 ml purified water. Working standards are prepared by pipetting 25, 12.5, 10, 7.5, 5 and 2.5 ml aliquots of the stock standard solution into separate 50 ml volumetric flasks and diluting to volume with purified water.

3. Absorbance of the solutions is measured at 260 nm against purified water as blank. Caffeine content is estimated from standard curve plotted from the absorbance values of the standard caffeine samples.

The method could be modified by extracting the tea infusion with dichloromethane. The organic layer is separated and its absorbance measured at 276 nm against dichloromethane blank. Caffeine content is determined from a similar standard curve of a standard solution of caffeine in dichloromethane.

Quinine

Source

Quinine is a quinoline alkaloid sourced from Cinchona bark. Cinchona alkaloids were of great economic importance for use in the treatment of malaria. Despite the introduction of synthetic antimalarials, salts of quinine remain commercially important due to problems of resistance associated with newer antimalarials. Isolated by P.J. Pelletier and J. Coventou in 1817, quinine was the first effective treatment for malaria caused by *Plasmodium falciparum* appearing in therapeutics in the 17th century. It remained the antimalarial drug of choice until the 1940s.

Uses

Apart from being an antimalarial, it has antibacterial, anti-pruritic, mild oxytocic, local anaesthetic, cardiovascular stimulant and analgesic properties. Quinine decreases the excitability of the motor end plate.

Large quantities of cinchona bark and quinine are used in tonic beverages for its astringent bitter taste and stomachic properties.

Description

Quinine is a natural white crystalline, odourless alkaloid readily soluble in ether and chloroform. Slightly soluble in water, it is also soluble in alcohol, carbon disulphide and glycerol. Intensely bitter to taste, its molecular formula is $C_{20}H_{24}N_2O_2$ and has a melting point of 173–175°C. Being a diacidic base, it forms both acid and neutral salt. While neutral salts are formed by the involvement of tertiary N atom in the quinnuclidine ring, acid salts are formed by the involvement of both the nitrogen atoms.

Sulphate salts of quinine are white, odourless, bitter, fine, needle-like crystals which are soluble in water and alcohol.

Sensitive to UV light quinine fluoresces in direct sunlight due to its highly conjugated resonance structure.

Quinine and salts of quinine are laevorotatory and with sodium and potassium alkyl iodide, quinine forms a series of periodides called kerapathite. While quinine sulphate is given orally, quinine hydrochloride may be administered intravenously.

Isolation

Different cinchona species and its hybrids contain 5% to 14% of total alkaloids of which 30% to 60% is constituted of quinine-type alkaloids. The principal alkaloids are the stereoisomers quinine and quinidine and their respective demethoxy derivatives cinchinidine and cinchonine. Other minor amorphous alkaloids have also been reported. Cinchona alkaloids are present in the bark tissue in combination with quinic acid and cinchotannic acid. The absolute and relative proportions of the alkaloids of cinchona bark varies with cultural and climatic conditions and also in relation to the position on the tree from which the bark is removed. In general, the content of total alkaloids is greater in the root bark and at the base of the tree than in the upper parts of the trunk.

1. Bark dried to a moisture content of 12% to 15% is finely powdered and intimately mixed with about 30% of its weight of calcium hydroxide and the mixture made into a stiff paste with sufficient quantity of 5% solution of sodium hydroxide.

2. The mix is transferred to a percolator and extracted to exhaustion with petroleum ether (80°–100°C).

3. The petroleum ether extract is then shaken with successive portions of warm dilute sulphuric acid for complete extraction of alkaloids into the acid layer.

4. The combined acid extracts while still warm are adjusted to pH 6.5 with dilute sodium hydroxide and the solution is allowed to cool.

5. Crystals of crude quinine sulphate which separate on cooling are separated by centrifugation and purified by recrystallization from hot water using finely divided carbon for removing colouring matter.

6. Quinine sulphate is dissolved in warm dilute sulphuric acid and dilute ammonia solution is added with continual stirring until the solution is alkaline to litmus

7. Base quinine is liberated as an amorphous precipitate which upon standing forms a micro-crystalline mass. The mixture is filtered and the residue of quinine is washed free of sodium and ammonium salts and dried at a low temperature.

Identification

1. Quinine in solution in dilute sulphuric, acetic, phosphoric or tartaric acids exhibits a strong blue fluorescence which is very marked in extremely dilute solutions. The hydrochloride and other halogen compounds do not give fluorescence in solution.

2. *Thalleioquin test*: Dissolve a small amount of quinine in dilute sulphuric acid and add 1–2 ml of water. Add 2 to 3 drops of bromine water and shake the mixture. On the addition of a drop of strong ammonia an emerald green colour is produced.

3. A small quantity of quinine when slightly moistened with glacial acetic acid and heated in an ignition tube shows condensation of blood-red drops on the sides of the tube.

4. *Erythroquinine test*: To a solution of quinine in dilute acetic acid, add 1 to 2 drops of bromine water followed by a drop of 10% solution of potassium ferricyanide. On adding a drop of strong ammonia the solution turns red.

5. TLC identification: Apply 5 μl of 1% solution of quinine in methanol on a silica gel G plate along with a similar sample of quinine sulphate reference sample. Develop in a solvent system made up of 40 volumes of toluene, 24 volumes of ether and 10 volumes of diethylamine. Dry the plate at 105°C for 30 min, allow to cool and spray with potassium iodoplatinate solution (50 ml of 5% w/v solution of chloroplatinic acid and 45 ml potassium iodide solution (20%) made up to 100 ml with water). Violet brown-coloured spot, a standard for the test sample well comparable with that of reference sample, is obtained.

Estimation

Quinine and its salts may be assayed by innumerable methods ranging from gravimetry, titrimetry, spectrophotometry, spectrofluorimetry, potentiometry to newer methods such as fluoro-immunoassay etc. Estimation of quinine in cinchona bark can also be done by several methods, principal of which are gravimetry, titrimetry and spectrophotometry.

A. Method I (Spectrophotometric assay)

1. Mix 2g finely powdered bark and 0.5 g of finely powdered calcium oxide (CaO) with about 10 ml water to make a smooth homogenous paste. It is set aside for 10 min.

2. To the above paste taken in a 200 ml standard flask, add 150 ml 95% ethanol and shake vigorously. Set aside for 1 h with occasional shaking.

3. Make up to volume with ethanol, shake and filter through a Whatman filter paper. Collect the filtrate carefully to minimize ethanol evaporation.

4. Pipette 25 ml of the ethanol extract into a 50 m conical flask and add 20 mg bentonite. Shake well and filter.

5. To 8 ml of the filtrate taken in a standard flask, add 5 ml of 0.1 N HCl and make up to volume with water. This is the test solution.
6. Prepare five graded standard stock solutions of pure quinine sulphate in 0.1 N HCl so as to contain 1.6, 3.2, 4.8, 6.4 and 8 mg of anhydrous quinine sulphate. Transfer 5 ml each of the prepared solutions into a series of five 100 ml standard flasks, add 8 ml ethanol into each and make up to volume with water.
7. Determine the absorbance of the test and standard solutions at 380 nm using a solution of acid and ethanol in water as blank. Calculate the percentage of quinine as sulphate from standard curve prepared.

B. Method II (Non-aqueous titration method, IP)

1. Weigh accurately about 0.2 g of quinine sulphate, dissolve in a mixture of 10 ml chloroform and 20 ml acetic anhydride.
2. Determine the end point potentiometrically using glass electrode and calomel reference electrode containing a saturated solution of potassium chloride in water.
3. Perform a blank determination and make any necessary correction.
4. Each ml of 0.1 M perchloric acid is equivalent to 0.02490 g of quinine sulphate.

Piperine

Source

It is the piperidine alkaloid chiefly responsible for the pungency of the fruits of white and black pepper, *Piper officinarum* and *Piper nigrum*, Piperaceae. Isolated by H.C. Oersted in 1819, it is also found in long pepper (*Piper longum* – 1% to 2%) and West African pepper (*Piper guineense*). At least 5 alkaloids structurally related to piperine have been identified in pepper.

Uses

Pepper has been used since ages as a spice and was a much-prized spice of ancient Indian trade. One of the oldest and important spices, it is used as a stimulant digestive in indigenous medicine. Pepper was a much-valued spice used for various medicinal uses in several European countries into which it was exported from India through trade channels.

Piperine itself is added to food products to enhance aroma and flavour. It is also used as a biological insecticide.

Piperine is a much-researched alkaloid known for its anti-inflammatory, anticonvulsant, anticarcinogenic, insecticidal and cytotoxic properties. By inhibiting enzymes crucial for drug and xenobiotic metabolism, piperine enhances the bioavailability of several drugs thus altering their effectiveness.

Description

When isolated, piperine is a pale yellow to yellow crystalline powder with a pungent odour and a burning after taste. Pungency of piperine is estimated at 100,000–200,000 Scoville units. It is slightly irritating to skin and eyes. Piperine is structurally related to capsaicin, the pungent principal of capsicum.

Piperine has molecular formula $C_{17}H_{19}NO_3$ and the IUPAC name is 1-[5-(1,3-benzodioxol-5-yl)-1-oxo-2,4-pentadienyl] piperidine. It is slightly soluble in water (40 mg/L), soluble in alcohol, chloroform, ether and benzene. Piperine has a melting point of 131–135°C.

Isolation

Piperine can be isolated in good yield from ground black pepper (2% to 5%), which is made up of 5% to 9% alkaloids/amides that also include piperidine, piperettine and piperanine. Pungency of pepper is attributed to piperine and piperanine. Though extracted from pepper, it is manufactured synthetically for commercial uses.

A. Method I

The common procedure for the isolation of piperine involves extraction of the ground black pepper using ethanol (95%).

1. Extract 15 g of powdered pepper with 150 ml of 95% ethanol on a Soxhlet extractor for 2 h.
2. Concentrate the extract to 10-15 ml by simple distillation.
3. Treat the concentrated extract with 10 ml of 10% Potassium hydroxide in 95% ethanol (for removal of the resin fraction of the drug).
4. Heat the resulting solution and add water drop wise. A yellow precipitate is formed. Add water drops until no more precipitate is formed.
5. Allow the mixture to stand overnight and collect the solid by vacuum filtration and recrystallize from acetone.

B. Method II

1. Take 10 g of powdered pepper in a 100 ml round-bottomed flask, add 50 ml of dichloromethane and boil the mixture under reflux for 20 min.
2. Cool the flask, filter through a Buchner funnel to remove the powdered material. Wash the residue with 5 ml dichloromethane. Set aside a few drops for identification by TLC.
3. Transfer the filtrate to a rotary vacuum evaporator and remove the excess solvent until a dark brown oil is left.
4. Cool the oily liquid in an ice bath and add 10 ml cold ether. Stir well and remove the remains of solvents by gentle heating on a sand bath.
5. Add further 10 ml ether and set aside in an ice bath for 15 min with occasional stirring.
6. The precipitate of piperine formed is separated by vacuum filtration and washed with ice cold ether (2 × 5 ml).
7. For recrystallization transfer the residue on the filter into a test tube, dissolve in a hot 3:1 mixture of acetone and hexane.
8. Set aside for 15 min at room temperature and then for 30 min in an ice bath. Vacuum filter the formed crystals of piperine and record the melting point.

Identification

Piperine answers all the tests for alkaloids.

1. To 1 ml of an alcoholic solution of piperine add 2 ml of Meyer's reagent. A dull white precipitate is formed.
2. To 1 ml of the above piperine solution add 1 ml of Dragendorff's reagent. An orange red precipitate is formed.
3. To 1 ml of piperine solution add 3 ml of Hager's reagent. A yellow precipitate is formed.
4. To 1 ml of piperine solution add 2 ml Wagner's solution. A reddish brown precipitate is formed.
5. *TLC identification*: Spot the initial dichloromethane extract and the isolated piperine and piperine reference sample (both dissolved in acetone) on a silica gel plate and develop in a solvent system of acetone and hexane (3:2). Air dry the plates and spray with vanillin sulphuric acid and activate the plates at 105°C for 15 min. Piperine is visualized as yellow spots.

Estimation

Several methods of estimation of piperine, such as gravimetry, titrimetry, spectrophotometry, HPTLC, HPLC are reported in the literature. While spectrophotometric methods are largely the official methods many newer methods of estimation involving extraction with super fluid carbon dioxide are also being reported.

A. Method I (Spectrophotometric assay)

1. Take 1 g finely ground pepper of #40 mesh in a 100 ml conical flask. Add 15 ml methanol and heat to boiling on a steam-heated water bath.
2. The solution is filtered hot and the residue is treated with further 4×15 ml quantities of methanol successively for the complete extraction of alkaloids.
3. The filtrates are collected in a 100 ml standard flask and the filter washed with 2×5ml portion of methanol. The rinsings are collected in the same flask and the volume is made up to mark with methanol.
4. After mixing well, 5 ml of the methanolic solution is transferred to another 100 ml standard flask and its volume made up with methanol. This is the test solution.
5. *Standard sample*: A 200 µg/ml solution of reference sample of piperine is prepared in methanol and it is further diluted to yield a final concentration of 4, 5, 8 and 16 µg/ml.
6. Absorbances of the four standard solutions and that of the test sample are measured at 343 nm using methanol as blank.
7. The percentage of piperine in pepper is calculated from the standard curve of reference piperine.

B. Method II (HPTLC method)

1. HPTLC was performed on 10 cm $\times$ 20 cm aluminum-backed silica gel F_{254} HPTLC plates. They are prewashed with methanol, dried and activated for 30 min at 110°C with the plates being placed between two sheets of glass to prevent deformation of the aluminum during heating.

2. 10 µl each of the prepared four standard solutions of piperine and the test solution (from method I) are applied on silica gel plates as 6 mm bands 6 mm apart and 1 cm from the edge of the plate by means of the automatic sample applicator fitted with Hamilton syringe. A methanol blank is applied to the parallel track.

3. Mobile phase of hexane: ethyl acetate: glacial acetic acid (3:1:0.1) is taken in the TLC developing chamber and left to equilibrate for 20 min. The spotted plates are then developed in it to a distance of 90 mm.

4. After developing, the plates are removed and dried in a current of hot air and scanned at 343 nm by means of densitometric scanner under optimized scanning parameters. Peak height and peak area are integrated for the entire track.

5. A calibration curve is plotted using peak area versus concentration of piperine. Piperine content of the sample is determined from the calibration curve from the peak area of the test sample.

Diosgenin

Source

Diosgenin is a steroidal sapogenin obtained by acid hydrolysis of the saponins obtained from a number of species of Dioscorea (Dioscoreaceae). This principal sapogenin is widely used as a precursor in the semi-synthesis of several important steroids. Diosgenin was first isolated from *Dioscorea tokoro* in the 1930s by Japanese workers and it was semi-synthesized to progesterone in 1940. Since then, the cost of progesterone and the oral contraceptives synthesized from it fell drastically. Until 1970 Mexican yam was the only source of diosgenin for steroidal contraceptive manufacture. Following nationalization of the Mexican yam industry, alternative sources of diosgenin and related steroids have been identified. Today total synthesis of several steroids has also become economically feasible. Disogenin exists in some food supplements and herbal medicines and it is reported to lower plasma cholesterol by increasing fecal cholesterol metabolism.

Description

Disogenin is a white to off white crystalline solid, soluble in chloroform (20 mg/ml), acetic acid and other organic solvents. Chemically it is (3β, 25R) – Spirost – 5-en-3-ol and has molecular formula $C_{27}H_{42}O_3$. Crystallized from acetone it has a melting point of 201–208°C.

Isolation

According to species, dioscorea tubers yield 1% to 8% of total saponins. Diosgenin exists in plant tissues in a combined glycosidal form called dioscin which upon hydrolysis yields diosgenin, glucose and rhamnose moieties. Though diosgenin is the principal sapogenin used by industry, most yams contain a mixture of sapogenins in glycosidic form.

Diosgenin is commercially produced by two methods. From the powdered air-dried drug, the saponin dioscin is extracted using ethanol. The extraction of the glycoside is effected from the plant tissues with ethanol and then the saponins are hydrolyzed by acid treatment to liberate the aglycone which is then extracted with a non-polar solvent. Alternatively diosgenin is extracted by treating the plant tissues with an acidified solution and extracting the aglycone with a non-polar solvent. The first method is more commonly employed and fermentation of chopped tubers for 7 days in the presence of squalene prior to extraction facilitates appreciable increase in sapogenin production. Fermentation loosens the saponins from sugars and the sapogenin production is enhanced in the presence of squalene, which is incidentally an important biogenetic precursor for the production of diosgenin.

A. Method I

1. Dried powdered tubers of dioscorea are finely powdered to 100–200 mesh size. 50 g of this is extracted with 300 ml ethanol in a Soxhlet extractor for 4 h.
2. The ethanol extract is concentrated to one-fifth volume on a rotary vacuum evaporator.
3. To the concentrated extract add 200 ml of 2N HCl and boil under reflux for 6 h for the hydrolysis of dioscin.
4. The flask and its contents are cooled under a stream of water and transferred to a separatory funnel. Extract with 5 × 75 ml of petroleum ether (30% to 60°C) and combine the organic layers.
5. Concentrate the extract to about 100 ml and treat with activated charcoal, filter and load on a column of neutral alumina and elute with chloroform: acetone (3:1)
6. Diosgenin is crystallized from the intermediate fractions and it is purified by recrystallization from methanol/acetone.

B. Method II

1. Add 800 ml of 2N hydrochloric acid to 50 g of finely powdered 100–200 mesh dried dioscorea tubers, in a 1 l round-bottomed flask. Mix well and boil under reflux for 2 h with frequent mixing of the contents.
2. The flask and the contents are cooled under a stream of water and filtered through a Buchner funnel.
3. Wash the precipitate free of acid with 500 ml ice cold water. Press the precipitate between folds of filter paper and dry in an oven at 80°C to a dry brown powder.
4. This residue consisting of crude diosgenin, soil particles and undigested tuber cellulose is placed in filter thimbles and packed into a Soxhlet extractor.
5. Subject it to hot continuous percolation with 300 ml of petroleum ether (30°–60°C) for 6 h.
6. As the extraction proceeds, diosgenin begins to crystallize in the boiling flask.

7. After completion of extraction, reduce the volume of the solvent by evaporation on a steam-heated water bath to about 50 ml.

8. Cool the flask in a refrigerator overnight.

9. Separate the crystallized diosgenin by filtration through a sintered-glass funnel and wash with two 10 ml portions of ice cold petroleum ether.

10. Dry the product by heating at 80°C and note the yield.

Identification

1. *Foam test*: To a small quantity of diosgenin add 5 ml water, shake gently and set aside. There is formation of a persistent foam confirming the presence of a saponin.
   Prepare 10 ml of solution of diosgenin in chloroform and perform the following tests:

2. *Liebermann–Burchard test*: To 1 ml, add few drops of acetic anhydride followed by concentrated sulphuric acid along the sides of the test tube. A violet blue ring is formed at the junction of the two layers confirming the presence of a steroid.

3. *Salkowski test*: To 1 ml, add a few drops of concentrated sulphuric acid along the sides of the test tube. A yellow-coloured ring turning to red is observed at the junction of the two layers. This test is indicative of the presence of a steroid.

4. *Antimony trichloride test*: To 1 ml, add a saturated solution of antimony trichloride in chloroform containing 20% acetic anhydride. Formation of a pink colour on heating indicates presence of steroid and triterpenoids.

5. *TLC test*: Spot 20 µl of the prepared solution of diosgenin along with a similarly prepared solution of a standard sample of diosgenin on a precoated silica gel plate. Develop in a solvent system of toluene: ethyl acetate (7:3). Activate it by spraying with anisaldehyde sulphuric acid reagent. A dark green spot (Rf – 0.37) corresponding to diosgenin is seen in both standard and test tracks.

Estimation

Diosgenin content in plant material may be determined by gravimetric, spectrophotometric, GLC, IR, HPTLC and HPLC methods.

A. Method I (HPTLC Densitometry)

1. Reflux 1 g of dried powdered sample of dioscorea with 25 ml 2.5 N HCl for 4 h. Cool, filter and wash the residue with water until free from acid.

2. Dry the residue in an oven at NLT 80°C and extract with petroleum ether (60° to 80°C) in a Soxhlet for 4 h.

3. Evaporate the petroleum ether to dryness and dissolve the residue in 5 ml chloroform and make up the volume to 10 ml with the same solvent. This is the test sample.

4. Prepare standard solutions of diosgenin (2–25 µg/ml) using a reference standard sample.

5. Apply 5 µl each of the standard and test solutions on a precoated silica gel G 60 plate. Develop in a solvent system of toluene: ethyl acetate (7:3) to a distance of 8 cm.

6. Air dry the plate and spray it with Liebermann-Burchard reagent and heat at 120°C until the spot corresponding to diosgenin turns black.

7. Cool and scan the different tracks in a densitometer in reflectance mode at 600 nm. Note the areas corresponding to diosgenin in tracks developed from standard and test samples. Integrate the peak height and peak areas and calculate the percentage of diosgenin in the test sample from the calibration curve (peak area versus concentration) of the standard.

B. Method II (UV Spectrophotometry)

1. To 1 g of the powdered drug add 10 ml of ethanol (70 % v/v). Heat under reflux on a water bath for 30 min. Allow to cool and filter.

2. Rinse the filter. Combine the filtrate and the rinsing solution in a 10 ml volumetric flask, and dilute to 10 ml with ethanol (70 % v/v).

3. Transfer 5 ml of this solution into a 100 ml volumetric flask, and dilute with methanol. Mix well and take 1 ml of this solution into a small porcelain dish and evaporate to dryness. Dissolve the residue in 10 ml of sulfuric acid R. Leave in contact for 1 h. This is the test sample.

4. Standard sample: Dissolve 2.5 mg of diosgenin R in methanol R in a 200 ml standard flask and dilute with the same solvent. Mix well and transfer 1, 2, 3, 4, 5, 6, 7, 8, 9 and 10 ml solutions into individual labeled (S1–S10) porcelain dishes and evaporate to dryness. Dissolve the residues in 10 ml of sulphuric acid R each. Leave in contact for 1 h.

5. Measure the absorbance values of the test and standard solutions at 410 nm against sulphuric acid R. Calculate the percentage content of diosgenin from the standard curve of diosgenin.

Andrographolide

It is a labdane diterpene lactone and the main bitter constituent and active principal isolated from the dried stems and leaves of *Andrographis paniculata* (Acanthaceae). An herbaceous plant native to India and Sri Lanka, the herb commonly called Kalmegh or Chuanxin Han is used in Asian traditional medicine as anti-pyretic, anti-inflammatory and hepatoprotectant. The herb contains 0.5% to 0.9% andrographolide along with other diterpene lactones such as neoandrographolide deoxy dihydroandrographolide and andrographiside and flavonols, oroxylen, wogonin and andrographidines A, B, C, D, E and F.

Andrographolide and related diterpenes are hepatoprotective agents and also possess choleretic, antidiarrhoeal, immunostimulant and anti-inflammatory activities.

Uses

First isolated by M.K. Gorter in 1911, it is commonly used as bitter tonic, febrifuge and hepatoprotective. It is reported to inhibit hepatic microsomal lipid peroxidation. Among the complex mixture of biologically active compounds present in the plant, andrographolide can be used as an analytical marker to determine the quality of plant material from different sources.

Kalmegh forms an ingredient of many patented Indian herbal proprietary preparations for the treatment of liver ailments.

Description

Andrographolide occurs as colourless crystalline powder with an extremely bitter taste. Its molecular formula is $C_{20}H_{30}O_5$, IUPAC name is 3α, 14, 15, 18–tetrahydroxy-5β, 9βH, 10α – labda– 8(20), 12–dien- 16-oic acid γ- lactone. The molecule has two forms of lactone rings. While two are present in the methylene dioxy group, the fifth is present as an alcoholic group of tertiary character. It is sparingly soluble in water, but freely dissolves in acetone, methanol, chloroform and ether. It has a melting point of 230–231°C.

Andrographolide forms white rhombic prisms or plates from ethanol or methanol with a melting point of 218°C.

Isolation

Depending on various environmental factors, different samples of Kalmegh contain andrographolide varying from 0.5% to 1.5%. While leaves contain the maximum amount of andrographolide, seeds contain the lowest. Aerial parts, preferably stems and leaves, are used for extraction.

1. Freshly collected plant material is air dried under shade for a day and then in a hot-air oven at 60°C. It is powdered to #40 mesh

2. 50 g is exhaustively extracted with a 1:1 mixture of dichloromethane and methanol by cold maceration. It is filtered and the extract concentrated to green crystalline mass in a rotary vacuum evaporator.

3. The green-coloured mass is washed several times with toluene to remove most of the colouring matter.

4. Warm it on a hot plate for complete removal of toluene and dissolve in minimum quantity of hot methanol and refrigerate.

5. Separate the crystals by centrifugation and repeat recrystallization from methanol till colourless plates of constant melting point are obtained.

Identification

1. *Baljet test*: To a small quantity of the drug add 2 to 3 drops of alkaline sodium picrate reagent (1:1 mix of 1% picric acid in ethanol and 10% sodium hydroxide in water). An

orange red colour is obtained indicating the presence of the methylene group of the lactone ring.

2. *TLC test*: Dissolve 1 mg drug in 1.5 ml methanol and prepare a similar solution with standard sample of andrographolide. Apply 5μl each of the test and standard samples on a precoated silica gel plate and develop it in a solvent system of chloroform: methanol (7:1). Develop the plate to a distance of 15 cm. Spray with 20% sulphuric acid in methanol and heat at 120°C for 10 min. Andrographolide is visible as a brown coloured spot and it is comparable to that of the standard.

3. Prepare a 0.1 mg per ml sample of andrographolide in methanol and determine the UV absorption by taking an absorption spectrum scan. λ_{max} of andrographolide in methanol is 222 nm.

Estimation

Many methods such as HPLC, HPTLC, gravimetric, spectrophotometric and titrimetric have been reported for quantitative estimation of andrographolides.

A. Method I (Spectrophotometric assay)

This estimation is based on measurement of the absorption of the orange red colour formed due to the condensation of the butenolide ring of andrographolide with picric acid in the alkaline medium of Baljet reagent.

1. 1 g of the dried aerial parts of *A. paniculata* (1 g) is extracted in hot methanol (4 × 50 ml) and filtered.

2. The filtrate is concentrated on a water bath and the concentrate washed with cold toluene (3 × 25 ml).

3. Excess water is added to toluene insoluble fraction and extracted with ethyl acetate (4 × 50 ml) in a separating funnel.

4. Ethyl acetate is evaporated to dryness on a water bath and residue redissolved in 10 ml methanol. This is the test solution.

5. From this solution, 0.2 ml is taken in a 10 ml volumetric flask, 5 ml of Baljet reagent added, mixed well and made up to volume with methanol.

6. *Standard solution*: Dissolve 10 mg of standard sample of andrographolide and dissolve it in 100 ml of hot methanol in a volumetric flask. Transfer 0.5, 1, 2, 4, 6, 8 and 10 ml solutions into 10 ml volumetric flasks. Add 5 ml of freshly prepared Baljet reagent to each of the flasks, mix well and make up to volume with methanol.

7. Measure the absorbance of the test and standard solutions against a blank prepared in a similar manner but without the sample or standard. The absorbance values are plotted against their respective concentrations to obtain the calibration curve.

8. The amount of andrographolides in the sample is calculated from the calibration curve.

B. Method II (HPTLC assay)

1. Standard sample: 1mg andrographolide is taken in a 10 ml standard flask, 7 ml methanol is added and mixed well to dissolve. Make up to volume with the same solvent. Transfer 0.2, 0.4, 0.6, 0.8, 1, 2, 3 ml of this solution into individual 10 ml standard flasks and make up to volume with methanol.

2. Take 0.5 g of dried powdered kalmegh in a 10 ml standard flask, add 7 ml methanol, mix well and filter.

3. Collect the filtrate into a 10 ml standard flask and wash the residue with 2 ml methanol. Make up to volume with methanol. Transfer the solution into a separating funnel and extract with 3 × 20 ml ether.

4. Pass the ether layers through a bed of anhydrous sodium sulphate and evaporate in a porcelain dish. Dissolve the residue in 5 ml of methanol. This is the test solution.

5. Apply 10 μl each of the standard and test solutions onto a precoated silicagel $60F_{254}$ plate and develop it in solvent system, benzene: ethyl acetate (5:5).

6. Air dry the plate and scan it densitometrically using UV reflectance photomode at 220 nm. Determine the andrographolide content of kalmegh from the calibration curve of the peak area versus concentration of the standard sample of andrographolide.

Digoxin

Digoxin is a purified cardioactive glycoside isolated from the dried leaves of *Digitalis lanata* or *Digitalis orientalis* (Scrophulariaceae). It is a secondary glycoside formed during drying, due to partial hydrolysis of the primary glycosides found in the fresh leaves. Several structurally related cardioactive glycosides are found in *D. lanata* and *D. purpurea,* two important sources of these therapeutically important glycosides. The primary glyscosides of *D. purpurea* are called Purpurea glycosides and those of *D. lanata* are lanatosides. While the former are based on three different aglycones with 3 molecules of digitoxose linked to the aglycone, those of lanatosides are based on 5 different aglycones and the digotixose farthest from the aglycone is acetylated. These C_{23} steroidal glycosides exert on the failing heart a slowing and strengthening effect due to which they are used in the treatment of congestive heart failure and atrial fibrillation.

While *D. purpurea* is of historical importance for use in the treatment of dropsy, digoxin, digoxin, lanatoside C and desacetyl lanatoside C (deslanide) are the isolated digitalis constituents currently employed in therapy.

Acting similar to digitalis leaf, digoxin, first isolated by Sydney Smith in 1930, however has a rapid action. It is more rapidly absorbed from the gastrointestinal tract and is more quickly eliminated than digitoxin and is therefore more widely used of the cardioactive glycosides. It is also more hydrophilic than digitoxin and binds less strongly to plasma proteins and is mainly eliminated by the kidneys, whereas digitoxin is metabolized more slowly by the liver.

Uses

Over the past decades, digoxin has become the most widely used drug in the treatment of congestive heart failure. Proprietary preparations of lanatoside A and C are available in various countries but digoxin is more widely used. It is used for rapid digitalization to control ventricular rate in atrial fibrillation and in the management of congestive heart failure. Therapy with digoxin requires careful monitoring as its therapeutic index is very low. Digoxin preparations are commonly marketed under the name of Lanoxin, Digitek, Lanoxicap etc.

Description

Digoxin, $C_{41}H_{64}O_{14}$ – (3β-5β-12β) – [(O-2,6-Dideoxy-β-D-ribohexopyranosyl-(1 → 4)-o-2,6-dideoxy-β-D-ribo-hexopyranosyl) oxyl]-12,14–dihydroxycard-20(22)-enolide, is constituted of aglycone digoxigenin attached to 3 molecules of digitoxose at the C-3 position. It is a white crystalline odourless powder with a bitter taste. Soluble in dilute (80%) alcohol, pyridine or mixture of chloroform and alcohol, it is almost insoluble in ether, acetone, ethyl acetate, chloroform and water (64.8 mg/L). It is very slightly soluble in 40% propylene glycol. Digoxin has a melting point of 248°C and forms radially arranged 4–5-sided triclinic plates from dilute alcohol or dilute pyridine. Its UV_{max} (ethanol) is 220 nm. Acid hydrolysis of digoxin yields 1 molecule of digoxigenin and 3 molecules of digitoxose.

Isolation

The total cardenolide content of *D. lanata* is 1%, about two to three times that found in *D. purpurea*. The presence of acetyl group on the terminal digitoxose renders the lanatosides in general easier to isolate from the plant material and makes crystallization easier. *D. lanata* glycosides are based on 5 aglycones, digitoxigenin, gitoxigenin, gitaloxigenin, digoxigenin and diginatigenin. While the primary glycosides with the tetrasaccharide unit of 2 digitoxose, 1 acetyl digitoxose and 1 glucose are called lanatosides, lanatosides A and C constitute 50% to 70% of the major components in the fresh leaf. These are based on aglycones digitoxigenin and digoxigenin respectively and lanatosides B, D and E are minor components derived from gitoxigenin, diginatigenin and gitaloxigenin respectively. Drying of the leaf is also accompanied by partial hydrolysis leading to the loss of both the terminal glucose and the acetyl group.

1. 100 g of finely ground, dried powdered leaves of *D. lanata* are packed in a Soxhlet apparatus and extracted exhaustively with 80% ethanol.

2. The alcoholic extract is then shaken with petroleum ether (5 × 75 ml) for the removal of plant pigments.

3. The aqueous alcoholic layer is then evaporated to about one-fifth its original volume, when a whitish or slightly coloured crystalline material separates out.

4. Separate it by filtration and wash with ice cold ethanol. To the mother liquor from which the crystals are separated, add equal volume of 80% alcohol and extract with acetone. Discard the acetone layer and further concentrate the aqueous layer for the separation of crystalline material. Repeat the recrystallization till no further crystals are formed.

5. Separate the crystals by filtration and wash with acetone.

6. Purify by repeated recrystallization from methanol.

Identification

1. *Keller–Kiliani test for digitoxose*: Dissolve the drug in 3 ml glacial acetic acid containing 2 drops of 5% ferric chloride solution. Carefully transfer this solution to the surface of 2 ml of sulphuric acid, a reddish-brown layer forms at the junction of the two liquids and the upper layer slowly becomes bluish-green, darkening on standing. This test confirms the presence of a deoxy sugar.

2. *Legal's test*: To a few milligrams of the drug dissolved in a few drops of pyridine add a drop of 2%w/v solution of sodium nitroprusside. A pink or a deep red colour is formed confirming the presence of a 5-membered lactone ring.

3. *Kedde's test*: To 1 ml of the solution of the drug in 70% alcohol, add 2 drops of 2% 3, 5–dinitro benzoic acid in 90% alcohol. Make it alkaline with a few drops of 20% sodium hydroxide solution. A purple colour is produced indicating the presence of an unsaturated lactone.

4. *Baljet's test*: To 1 ml of a solution of the drug in 70% alcohol, add a few drops of alkaline sodium picrate reagent. Formation of an orange-red colour indicates the presence of a lactone.

5. *Raymond's test*: Dissolve a small quantity of the drug in 1 ml 50% ethanol and add 0.1 ml of Raymond's reagent (1% w/v solution of m-dinitrobenzene in ethanol) and 2 to 3 drops of 20% sodium hydroxide solution. Appearance of a violet colour slowly changing to blue is indicative of the presence of methylene group (at C-21 position on the lactone ring).

6. *Tollen's test*: Dissolve a small quantity of the drug in a few drops of pyridine. To this add 1ml Tollen's reagent (0.1 N silver nitrate solution is treated with dilute ammonia solution till the initially formed white precipitate dissolves on further addition of ammonia) and heat gently if required. Appearance of a silver mirror indicates the presence of a monosaccharide.

7. *Xanthydrol test*: To a solution of the drug in 70% alcohol, add 0.5 ml of xanthydrol reagent (0.125% w/v solution of xanthydrol in glacial acetic acid containing 1% hydrochloric acid). Formation of red colour indicates the presence of an unsaturated lactone.

8. *Antimony trichloride test*: To a solution of the drug in 70% alcohol add a solution of antimony trichloride and trichloroacetic acid and heat the mixture. A blue or violet colour is formed.

Estimation

Digoxin content in plant extracts, formulations, body fluids etc. may be determined by innumerable methods of assay based on colorimetry, fluorimetry, gas liquid chromatography, HPLC and radioimmunoassay to name a few.

A. Method I (IP Method)

1. Weigh accurately 40 mg and dissolve it in sufficient 95% ethanol to produce 50 ml.

2. Transfer 5 ml of this solution into a 100-ml standard flask and make up the volume with the same solvent.

3. To 5 ml of this solution, add 3 ml of alkaline picric acid solution (see tests for andrographolides) and set aside in the dark for 30 mins. This is the test. Repeat steps 1 to 3 on a standard sample of digoxin to make the standard solution.

4. Measure the absorbances of both the test and standard solutions at the maximum at about 495 nm against a blank made up of 5 ml 95% ethanol and 3 ml alkaline picric acid solution.

5. Calculate the content of digoxin from the absorbance of the standard of the known quantity taken for the assay.

Glycyrrhizin

Glycyrrhizin is a triterpenoid saponin isolated from liquorice, the dried unpeeled rhizome and root of the perennial herb *Glycyrrhiza glabra* (Leguminosae), a number of commercial varieties of which are cultivated. Much of liquorice is used in the form of a dried extract of the roots and stolons especially in confectionary and for flavouring, tobacco, beer etc. Owing to its sweet taste, liquorice has been long used in pharmacy to mask the bitter taste of drugs. It has been used in several formulations due to its surfactant, demulcent and mild expectorant properties. An important drug of Asian traditional medicine, liquorice, and its constituents, has been extensively investigated.

Liquorice extracts are reported with anti-inflammatory, corticosteroid-like and mineralocorticoid activities. These are used in the treatment of rheumatoid arthritis, Addison's disease and various inflammatory conditions.

Other constituents of liquorice are triterpenoid saponins, glabranin A and B; glabrolide, isoglabrolide, glycyrrhetol; isoflavones; formononetin; glabrone; neolizuritun; hispaglabridin A and B and coumarins. The yellow colour of liquorice is due to flavonoids which are reported to have gastroprotective effects.

Glycyrrhizin is a mixture of potassium and calcium salts of glycyrrhizinic acid, which is the diglucopyranosiduronic acid of glycyrrhetenic acid which has a triterpenoid structure. Much of the activity reported for liquorice and its extracts has been attributed to glycyrrhetenic acid. It is found to inhibit enzymes that catalyse the conversion of prostaglandins and glucocorticoids into inactive metabolites, resulting in increased levels of prostaglandins and of hydrocortisone. This increased prostaglandin activity of liquorice and its constituents is used in the symptomatic treatment of peptic ulcer pain. A semi-synthetic derivative of glycyrrhetenic acid, the hemisuccinate carbenoxolone sodium, is widely prescribed for the treatment of gastric and duodenal ulcers.

Description

Glycyrrhizin or glycyrrhizinic acid, (3β, 20β)–20-Carboxy-11-oxo-30-norolean-12-en-3-yl, 2-O-β-D-glucopyranosyl-α-D-glucopyranosiduronic acid, has molecular formula $C_{42}H_{62}O_{16}$. The sweet taste of liquorice is due to glycyrrhizin, which is reported to be 30 to 50 times sweeter than sucrose. A sweet, white, crystalline powder, its sweetness is slow in onset and tends to linger. It is odourless and has a characteristic liquorice taste described as 'cooling'. Its sweetness is relatively heat stable. Upon hydrolysis glycyrrhizin loses its sweet taste and forms glycyrrhetenic acid and two molecules of glucuronic acid. Glycyrrhizin is freely soluble in hot water, alcohol and practically insoluble in ether. The aglycone acid form is not very water soluble but its ammonium salt is water soluble at pH greater than 4.5. Glycyrrhizin is also obtained as colourless crystals, melting at 205°C and imparts a sweet taste to water in a dilution of 1 in 20,000.

Glycyrrhizin being incompatible with acids, ammonium glycyrrhizinate is used as a substitute for flavouring.

Isolation

Glycyrrhizin content of liquorice varies from 2% to 9% in different samples. Other constituents are 5% to 15% sugars, 1% to 2% asparigine, 0.04% to 0.06% volatile compounds, β-sitosterol, starch, protein and bitter principals such as glycymarin. Several procedures are reported in the literature on the extraction of glycyrrhizin by various organic solvents, purification by ion-exchange and polymeric resins, adsorption, chromatographic separation, supercritical fluid extraction, foam separation, microwave-assisted extraction and multi-stage counter-current extraction. Due to better water solubility and ease of preparation, glycyrrhizin is isolated in the form of ammonium salt from which glycyrrhizin may be precipitated.

A. Method I

1. Macerate 100 g of liquorice root of # 20 mesh in a mixture of 95 ml of distilled water and 5 ml of solution of ammonia for 24 hours.
2. Filter through Whatman filter paper in Buchner funnel under reduced pressure and wash the residue with sufficient distilled water such that the filtrate measures 100 ml.

3. To the filtrate add sulphuric acid slowly with constant stirring until a precipitate ceases to form.

4. Collect the precipitate on a strainer, wash until free from acid, redissolve in water with the aid of solution of ammonia, filter if necessary.

5. Repeat the precipitation with sulphuric acid; again collect, wash and dissolve the precipitate in a sufficient quantity of solution of ammonia, previously diluted with an equal volume of distilled water;

6. Finally, evaporate the clear solution to a thin syrup which is taken on porcelain tiles or sheets of glass for drying in an oven at temperature not exceeding 60°C.

7. Preserve the dry product in well-closed vessels. The prepared ammonium glycyrrhizin is in the form of dark brown or brownish-red odourless scales, having a very sweet taste. At 100°C the scales become darker in colour, and at a higher temperature melt with decomposition; on complete incineration not more than a trace of ash is left.

8. Dissolve the formed ammonium glycyrrhizinate in distilled water and add sulphuric acid in drops till precipitation is complete.

9. Filter and dissolve precipitated glycyrrhizin in minimum quantity of hot water and set to cool. A jelly-like substance is formed. It is washed with diluted alcohol and dried when an amorphous yellow powder having a strong bitter-sweet taste and an acid reaction is formed.

Identification

1. To a small quantity of glycyrrhizin, add 5 ml water, shake vigorously and set aside. Formation of a persistent foam which does not disappear on shaking indicates the presence of saponins.

2. To a small quantity of glycyrrhizin add 1 ml chloroform, 1ml acetic anhydride and 2 ml concentrated sulphuric acid along the sides of the test tube. Formation of a violet colour at the junction of two layers indicates the presence of a triterpenoid.

3. *TLC test*: Reflux 5 mg of glycyrrhizin with 20 ml 0.5 M sulphuric acid. Cool and extract with 2 × 10 ml chloroform. Evaporate the combined chloroform extract and dissolve the residue in 1 ml of 1:1 mixture of chloroform and methanol. Repeat the same for standard sample of glycyrrhizin. Apply 5µl each of the test and standard samples in two different tracks on a precoated silica gel GF_{254} plate and develop in a solvent system of toluene: ethyl acetate: glacial acetic acid (12.5:7.5:0.5). Air dry the plate and spray with anisaldehyde-sulphuric acid reagent and heat at 100°C for 5–10 min. Glycyrrhizin is visible as a dark violet spot in both the test and standard tracks.

Estimation

Several analytical methods based on HPTLC, HPLC and capillary electrophoresis are reported in the literature for the estimation of glycyrrhizin in extracts and formulations.

A. Method I (HPTLC assay)

1. 500 mg of dried powdered liquorice is treated with 2 × 10 ml of 70% ethanol, each time sonicated for 10 min and filtered. The filtrate is taken as test sample.

2. Dissolve 5 mg of standard sample of glycyrrhizin in 50 ml 70% ethanol in a standard flask. This is the standard sample.

3. Apply 5 and 10µl of the test and 2, 5, 7 and 10 µl of standard sample in different tracks on a precoated silica gel GF_{254} plate and develop in a solvent system of butanol: acetic acid: water (5:1: 4-upper layer)

4. Air dry and scan at 260 nm in absorbance mode using a HPTLC scanner.

5. Determine the content of glycyrrhizin in liquorice from the calibration curve drawn for standard sample of glycyrrhizin using concentration versus peak area.

B. Method II (Spectrophotometric assay)

1. 500 mg of dried powdered liquorice is macerated in 70% ethanol overnight, filtered and evaporated to a pasty mass.

2. Transfer 20 mg of this extract into a 10 ml standard flask, dissolve in a solution of phosphate buffer (pH 6.8) : ethanol (7:3) and make up to volume with the same solvent. Filter it through Whatman filter paper (#44) and dilute 1 ml of the filtrate to 10 ml with the same solvent. This is the test sample.

3. Dissolve 10 mg glycyrrhetenic acid in phosphate buffer: ethanol (7:3) solvent in a 10 ml standard flask and make up to volume. Transfer 50, 100, 150, 200, 250 and 350 µl into individual 10 ml standard flasks and make up to volume with the same solvent and label them appropriately as S1 to S6.

4. Determine the absorbance of the standard and test solutions at 254 nm and calculate the content of glycyrrhetenic acid in liquorice from the calibration curve of concentration versus absorbance prepared for the standard.

Hesperidin

Source

Hesperidin is a flavonone diglycoside occurring in most citrus fruits, especially in the peel and the pulp. In this glycoside, hesperitin is bound to disaccharide rutinose. This polyphenolic citrus bioflavonoid is the predominant flavonoid in lemons and oranges. An abundant and inexpensive by-product of citrus cultivation, hesperidin is associated with a number of pharmacological properties. First isolated from the spongy inner portion of the pericarp of oranges by Leberton in 1828, its presence in lemons was identified by Pheffer in 1874.

While hesperidin is a non-bitter flavonoid from sweet orange *Citrus sinensis* and related species, neohesperidin is a bitter glycoside occurring in bitter orange *Citrus aurantium*. It is closely related to other citrus bioflavonoids such as quercetin, rutin and diosmin. Earlier hesperidin along with rutin and other flavonoids with capillary permeability enhancement property were classified as Vitamin P.

Uses

Hesperidin alone, or in combination with other citrus bioflavonoids, is most often used for vascular conditions such as hemorrhoids and varicose veins. It has an anti-inflammatory and pain-relieving effect in these conditions. Hesperidin is available as a dietary supplement with reputedly beneficial effects on veins and capillaries. It may be beneficial as an antioxidant, antimicrobial, immunomodulatory and chemopreventive agent. Hesperidin also regulates hepatic cholesterol synthesis by inhibiting the activity of 3-hydroxy-3-methlyglutaryl coenzyme A (HMG-CoA) reductase. Its deficiency has been linked to abnormal capillary leakiness as well as pain in the extremities causing aches, weakness and night leg cramps. Supplemental hesperidin also helps in reducing oedema or excess swelling in the legs due to fluid accumulation

Description

Hesperidin occurs as a colourless or pale yellow coloured, tasteless, crystalline glycoside with a melting point of 258–260°C. Chemically it is (S)-7-[[6-O-(6-deoxy-alpha-L-mannopyranosyl)-beta-D-glucopyranosyl] oxy]-2,3-dihydro-5-hydroxy-2-(3-hydroxy-4-methoxyphenyl)-4H-1-Benzo-pyran-4-one and has a molecular formula $C_{28}H_{34}O_{15}$. It is freely soluble in alcohol and forma-mide, moderately soluble in ether, slightly soluble in water (1g/50L), methanol, hot glacial acetic acid, almost insoluble in acetone, chloroform and benzene and also soluble in dilute alkalies. On hydrolysis it yields hesperitin together with dextrose and rhamnose.

Isolation

Several classic methods are reported by many workers for the isolation of hesperidin from orange peel and other citrus sources. Due to its insolubility and crystalline nature it may be isolated with relative ease. The yield may vary from 3 to 5 mg/g of the dried peel depending on the species and other factors.

Method

1. 100 g of dried powdered orange peel is taken in a round bottomed flask with 300 ml of petroleum ether (40°–60°C) and boiled under reflux for 1 h.
2. Filter hot through a Buchner funnel and air dry the residue for complete removal of the solvent.
3. Transfer it into another round bottomed flask, add 500 ml methanol and boil under reflux for 2 h.

4. Filter hot and concentrate the filtrate to a syrupy liquid in a rotary vacuum evaporator.

5. To the syrupy liquid add 50 ml of 6% acetic acid and mix gently. The precipitated hesperidin is separated by filtration through a Buchner funnel. It is washed with 6% acetic acid and dried at 60°C.

6. For purification make a 5% solution of the crude hesperidin in dimethyl sulphoxide and warm to 60–80°C on a water bath with stirring. Add equal volume of water and pure hesperidin precipitates as the mixture cools.

7. Collect the precipitated hesperidin by filtration under reduced pressure, wash with warm water and isopropanol. Dry the product in a desiccator to constant weight.

Identification

1. *Ferric chloride test*: To a small quantity of hesperidin taken in a test tube add 3 ml of 5% ferric chloride solution. Formation of a wine red colour indicates the presence of hesperidin.

2. *Shinoda test*: To a few milligrams of hesperidin taken in a test tube add 2 ml methanol and a few bits of magnesium ribbon. Add concentrated hydrochloric acid dropwise. Formation of a bright violet colour indicates the presence of hesperidin.

3. Solution of hesperidin in 5% sodium hydroxide exhibits an orange red colour.

4. To 0.1 g of hesperidin add 10 ml hydrochloric acid, boil on a water bath, cool and filter. Neutralize with 20% sodium hydroxide solution and add 1 ml each of Fehling's solution A and B. Formation of brick red colour indicates the presence of a reducing sugar in the hydrolysis mixture.

Estimation

Hesperidin estimation is reported in literature based on spectrophotometric and HPLC methods, with the latter being the method of choice for its determination in orange juice, body fluids and in herbal dosage forms.

A. Method I (Spectrophotometric assay)

1. Hesperidin sample is dried at 105°C for 3 h, 50 mg is accurately weighed and transferred to a 10 ml standard flask.

2. Dissolve in 0.01 N sodium hydroxide solution and make up to volume.

3. Transfer 2 ml of this solution into a 50 ml standard flask and make up to volume with 0.01 N potassium hydroxide solution. This is the test solution.

4. Determine the absorbance of the test solution at 286 nm and estimate the percentage purity of hesperidin taking 251.7 as the standard extinction of hesperidin.

B. Method II (HPLC method)

1. Shake 10 g air-dried powdered peel with 20 ml dimethyl sulphoxide (DMSO) and filter.

2. Wash the residue with the same solvent and collect the filtrate and the washings in a 25 ml standard flask. Make up to volume with DMSO.

3. Prepare a standard solution (5 mg dissolved in 0.05 ml of DMSO) using reference sample of hesperidin.

4. Perform HPLC analysis of both the test and standard samples using a Spherisorb ODS1 column with mobile phase of 2% acetic acid (A) and acetonitrile (B) used in gradient mode (0–15 min: A 100%; 15–45 min: A 100-70, B0-30; 45–50 min: A 70%, B 30%; 50–55 min: B 100%; 55–60 min: A 0-100, B-100-0; 60–90 min: A 100%).

5. Volume of injection is 20 µl and mobile phase flow rate 1 ml/min, with oven temperature at 40°C and the wavelength of detection 285 nm.

6. Calculate the hesperidin content of orange peel based on the peak area versus concentration data for the standard at comparable retention times for the test and the standard.

Berberine

Source

This alkaloid belongs to a group of modified benzyl tetrahydroisoquinoline alkaloids. A quaternary ammonium salt from the protoberberine group of isoquinoline alkaloids, it is found in many members of the Berberidaceae (Berberis and Mahonia species), Ranunculaceae (Hydrastis and Coptis species) and other families such as Anonaceae, Menispermaceae, Papaveraceae and Rutaceae. Berberine is found in the bark of the root, stem and branches either as the principal alkaloid or in association with other alkaloids such as hydrastine, canadine, berbamine, oxyacanthine, umbellatine, neprotine, nandinine, domesticine and thalletrine.

Uses

Plants containing berberine have long been used in traditional Ayurvedic and Chinese medicine. *Berberis aristata* called 'Daruharidra' is a reputed Ayurvedic drug used as a bitter tonic, stomachic, laxative, anti-pyretic and antiseptic. It is indicated for use in menorrhagia and neuralgia. Berberine has historical usage as a dye for its yellow colour. It is reported to have anti-amoebic, antibacterial and anti-inflammatory properties. Today it is used in clinical practice for bacterial intestinal infections, trachomas and intestinal parasitic infections.

Description

Coloured alkaloid berberine of molecular formula $[C_{20}H_{18}NO_4]^+$ is 5,6-Dihydro-9,10-dimethoxy benzo(g)-1,3-benzodioxolo(5,6-a) quinolizinium. It occurs as a yellow-coloured, bitter-tasting powder soluble in water (1 in 4.5) or ethanol (1 in 100). It is easily soluble in hot water or hot ethanol, slightly soluble in benzene or chloroform, insoluble in ether or light petroleum. Aqueous solution is bitter to taste, alkaline in reaction and optically inactive. Berberine forms well-defined crystalline salts with acids and behaves as a quarternary base forming salts by replacement of the OH group. It forms yellow needles from ether with a melting point of 145°C. From water or dilute ethanol it crystallizes as bright yellow needles which on heating lose the water of hydration and on further heating decompose at 100°C. The hydrochloride salt crystallizes out in small needles when HCl is added to a warm aqueous solution of the alkaloid. It is soluble in about 500 parts of water but is almost insoluble in ethanol or dilute HCl.

Isolation

In Berberis species (*B. aristata, B. glauca, B. vulgaris, B. aquifolium* etc.) berberine alkaloids are principally located in the cortical tissues and the bark of old roots has the highest concentration. Upper parts of the shoot system have a low concentration of alkaloids and in young leaves they are not detectable. Berberine content varies depending on the species and different plant parts. While Berberis species has 0.12% to 2.8%, Hydrastis species has 1% to 5% of berberine. Plants which contain berberine as the principal alkaloid may be processed for its isolation.

1. Weigh 50 g of the powdered plant material and pack it in a Soxhlet extractor. Subject it to hot continuous percolation using 250 ml ethanol for 4 h.
2. Concentrate the ethanol extract in a rotary vacuum evaporator to a pasty residue.
3. Dissolve the residue in minimum quantity of hot water (100 ml). Insoluble resins which separate out are removed by filtration of the hot solution. Reduce the volume of the filtrate by evaporation to about 20 ml.
4. Treat the filtrate with concentrated hydrochloric acid to a pH of 1 to 2. Berberine hydrochloride that crystallizes out is separated by filtration through a Buchner funnel.
5. For purification of the alkaloid it is recrystallized from ethanol using ether for precipitation.
6. Carefully separate the crystals and dissolve in hot water (5–10 ml). Make the solution alkaline by adding a few drops of 10% sodium hydroxide.
7. Add 2 ml acetone and dilute the solution with an equal volume of water. Set aside overnight in a refrigerator for complete precipitation of berberine-acetone complex.
8. Filter carefully and wash the precipitate with ice-cold water and dissolve the air-dried berberine-acetone in ethanol: chloroform (10:1).
9. Heat the solution to boiling and allow it to cool. Separate the crystals of pure berberine by centrifugation and dry in a desiccator to constant weight.

Identification

Berberine gives precipitation with most of the alkaloidal reagents. Some specific tests for identification of berberine are listed below:

1. To a few crystals of berberine dissolved in water, add a drop of bromine water. A bright red colour is produced.

2. To a small quantity of berberine add 0.5 ml of nitric acid. A reddish-brown colour is obtained.

3. To a small quantity of berberine add 0.5 ml of sulphuric acid. An orange-yellow solution is obtained changing to an olive green colour on warming.

4. To a solution of berberine in sulphuric acid add a few crystals of potassium dichromate. A black colour changing to brownish-violet is produced.

5. To 1 ml of a solution of berberine in water add Froehde's reagent (0.5 g molybdic acid or sodium vanadate in 100 ml hot sulphuric acid). A brownish-green colour is produced.

6. To 1 ml of a solution of berberine in water add Mandelin's reagent (1 g ammonium vanadate in 100 ml sulphuric acid). A violet colour is produced.

Estimation

Estimation of berberine in traditional medicine formulations and conventional dosage forms may be undertaken by several spectrophotometric, chromatographic and other methods.

A. Method I (Gravimetric method)

1. Extract to exhaustion 5 g of powdered plant material with 200 ml ethanol in a Soxhlet apparatus.

2. Evaporate the extract to dryness on a water bath and add 50 ml hot water to the residue.

3. Separate the precipitated resin by filtration and concentrate the filtrate by evaporation on a hot plate to about 20 ml.

4. Add 10 ml of 15% sodium hydroxide and add 5 ml of a 2% solution of gum tragacanth and extract with 5 × 20 ml portions of ether.

5. Collect the ether layers into a 100 ml standard flask and make up to volume if necessary.

6. Transfer 50 ml of the ether solution to a beaker and add a saturated solution of picrolonic acid in ether in small amounts until precipitation is complete.

7. Allow to settle and filter carefully over a tared sintered funnel. Wash the residue on the filter with ether to remove excess picrolonic acid. Dry the product at 105°C and note its weight.

8. The yield of berberine multiplied by the factor 0.561 gives the equivalent amount of berberine. Calculate the percentage purity from the known weight of the plant material.

B. Method II (Spectrophotometric assay)

1. Weigh accurately 50 mg of berberine and prepare a stock solution of 100 µg/ml in water.

2. Transfer 5 ml to a 10 ml standard flask and make up to volume with water.

3. Determine the absorbance of the solution at 345 nm.

4. Calculate the percentage purity of berberine using 722 as the specific absorptivity of berberine at 345 nm.

Tannic acid

Source

Tannic acid or gallotannin is a commercial prepared form of tannin, a collective term applied to a group of complex polyphenolic secondary metabolites. These are present in localized structures associated with different plant parts. Tannins are distributed in both Angiosperms and Gymnosperms and are more common in dicotyledons than monocotyledons. Some important sources of tannins are oak (*Quercus* sps), wattle (*Acacia* sps), *Eucalyptus* species, willow (*Salix caprea*), pine (*Pinus* species) and Myrobalans (*Terminalia chebula* and *Terminalia belerica*).

The ability of these plant-derived polyphenolic substances to convert animal skin to leather or their use in 'tanning' led to these being referred to as tannins. They are rarely representative of a single chemical entity as their composite structure is composed of acid units and their derivatives such as gallic acid, ellagic acid, chebulic acid, catechu-tannic acid etc. Tannins are high-molecular-weight compounds ranging between 1,000 and 5,000 and rarely give sharp melting points due to their complex nature. The chemistry of tannins has been most extensively investigated and they are said to be constituted of an accumulation of a substantial number of phenolic groups within a moderately sized molecule. Associated with a number of 0-dihydroxy and 0-trihydroxy orientation within a phenyl ring, tannins are classified as hydrolysable tannins, condensed tannins and pseudotannins.

Commercial tannic acid is extracted from many sources including gall nuts of the oak tree (*Quercus infectoria*), pods of *Caesalpinia spinosa*, leaves of *Rhus coriaria* among others. Indigenous sources of tannins representing different types of tannic acid are *T. chebula*, *T. belerica*, *Embelica officinalis*, *Cassia auriculata*, *Azadirachta indica*, *Acacia catechu*, *Casurina equistifolia* etc.

Tannic acid or gallotannic acid is found to the extent of 50% to 70% in nut galls (Turkish galls), vegetable outgrowths formed on the young branches of the oak tree. Nut galls are used in the tanning and dyeing industry and earlier in the manufacture of ink. Myrobalans which contain 20% to 40% tannic acid are principally constituted of ellagitannins. Several plants of medicinal interest are found to contain ellagitannins and these are being actively investigated.

Uses

Due to its astringent or protein-precipitating property, tannic acid is used as an antidiarrhoeal and styptic. Formerly it was used in the treatment of burns. It is topically used in the treatment of bed sores, skin ulcerations etc. As an alkaloidal precipitant it is used in alkaloid poisoning. Industrial uses of tannic acid include chemical staining of wood, as a mordant in textile dyeing, iron corrosion proofing and as a clarifying and colour-stabilizing agent in the wine and beer industry.

Description

Tannic acid occurs as yellowish-brown amorphous bulky powder or as flakes or as spongy masses. It has a faint characteristic odour and an astringent taste. It darkens gradually on exposure to air and light. Because of its hygroscopicity it is to be stored in amber-coloured well-closed containers. Commercial tannic acid contains 10% water and does not have a sharp melting point. At 210–215°C it decomposes into pyrogallol and carbon dioxide.

It is soluble in water (1g in 3.5 ml) and glycerol and it is very soluble in alcohol and acetone. Tannic acid is insoluble in benzene, chloroform, ether, petroleum ether, carbon disulphide and carbon tetrachloride.

Commercial tannic acid has a molecular formula of $C_{76}H_{52}O_{46}$. First isolated by Robinson in 1943, tannic acid is not a single homogenous compound, but is a mixture of esters of gallic acid with glucose and its exact composition varies according to its source. For example, tannic acid from Chinese galls (*Rhus chinensis*) yield on hydrolysis, methyl gallate and 1,2,3,4,5-pentagalloyl glucose. Turkish galls on the other hand yield methyl gallate and a mixture of 1,2,3,6- and 1,3,4,6-tetragalloyl glucose.

Isolation

Tannic acid of pharmaceutical grade is commercially obtained from nut galls, which are grown as pathological outgrowths on the stems and branches of the oak tree due to the deposition of eggs of the gall wasp. Galls are obtained in three grades namely blue, green and white. Tannic acid is extracted from these powdered galls by fermenting them and subjecting them to extraction with water. Fermentation facilitates loosening of tannic acid from other constituents. There are several procedures adopted for the extraction of tannic acid from plant material. Common solvents employed for its extraction are ethanol, methanol, ethyl acetate, isopropanol, butyl acetate, absolute alcohol and hot water.

A. Method I

1. Extract about 500 g of the powdered plant material (#40 mesh) by agitation with 2 × 750 ml of methanol for 8–12 h each. Filter.
2. Extract the residue on the filter with further 750 ml of methanol.

3. Combine the methanol extracts and concentrate on a rotary vacuum evaporator to about one-fourth the original volume.

4. Evaporate further on water bath to a sticky mass. Add 1litre of water to this mass and set aside overnight in a refrigerator.

5. Discard the precipitate and filter the supernatant liquid through a fine muslin cloth.

6. Extract the filtrate with 4×25 ml portions of petroleum ether. Discard the petroleum ether layers.

7. Concentrate the aqueous solution to one-third volume and add sodium chloride till the solution is saturated.

8. Transfer carefully into a separating funnel and extract with 4×100 ml portions of ethyl acetate.

9. Combine the ethyl acetate layers and concentrate under vacuum when a brownish-yellow powder of tannic acid is separated.

10. Continue the evaporation on a steam-heated water bath for the complete removal of the solvent and dry the product to constant weight.

B. Method II

1. To about 100 g of the powdered plant material add 400 ml hot water at 80°C and keep on a steam-heated water bath for 2 h.

2. Filter, concentrate the filtrate to about one-third its original volume by evaporation on a hot plate.

3. Extract it with equal volume of petroleum ether (40–60°C) and repeat successive extractions with the same solvent till the petroleum ether layer leaves no residue on evaporation.

4. Separate the aqueous layer and saturate it with sodium chloride, i.e. till there is some deposition of the salt at the bottom of the solution.

5. Extract the mixture with 4×60 ml portions of ethyl acetate. Collect the ethyl acetate layers and concentrate under vacuum when yellowish-brown product of tannic acid is obtained.

6. Evaporate the excess solvent and dry the product to constant weight in a vacuum desiccator.

Identification

Solution of tannic acid precipitates heavy metals, alkaloids, glycosides and gelatin.

1. To a solution of tannic acid in water add a few drops of ferric chloride solution. A bluish-black precipitate is formed confirming the presence of tannic acid.

2. *Gelatin test*: To 5 ml of 1% solution of tannic acid in water, add 1% solution of gelatin containing 10% sodium chloride. A bulky white precipitate is formed.

3. *Phenazone test*: To 5 ml of a 1% solution of tannic acid in water, add 0.5 g of sodium acid phosphate. Warm, cool and filter. To the filtrate add 2% solution of phenazone. A bulky dirty white precipitate is formed.

4. *Goldbeater's skin test*: A small piece of prepared skin mimicking untanned animal hide is soaked in 2% hydrochloric acid for about 10 min. Rinse it off with distilled water and place

it in solution of tannic acid for 5 min. Wash with distilled water and transfer to 1% ferrous sulphate solution. A brownish-black colour on the skin indicates the presence of tannins.

5. *TLC Test*: To 5 ml of a 1% solution of tannic acid in water add 0.5 ml of hydrochloric acid and heat on a water bath for 30 min. Filter. This is the test solution.

For the standard solution, weigh 100 mg gallic acid reference sample and dissolve it in 100 ml water.

Apply both the test and standard solutions to a precoated silica gel plate and develop in a solvent system of chloroform: ethyl formate: formic acid (5:4:1). Air dry and spray with a 1:1 solution of 1% ferric chloride in 10% ethanol and 1% potassium ferricyanide in 50% ethanol.

A black spot exactly comparable to that of standard is seen for the sample.

Estimation

Quantitative estimation of tannins in plant tissue is generally not accurate as other phenolic substances may interfere with the non-specific chemical methods. Also it is not possible to extract completely condensed tannins. Repeated measurements are needed to make an accurate estimation. Chemical assay methods based on functional groups such as Folin-Denis procedure for total phenols and Vanillin-HCl procedure for catechins were used. Currently these are replaced by procedures based on tannin-protein interactions.

A. Method I

1. 20 g of accurately weighed sample of the powdered dried plant material is extracted with 3×30 ml portions of aqueous methanol (1:1).
2. Filter and wash the residue with methanol such that the final volume of the filtrate is 100 ml as collected in a 100 ml standard flask.
3. Take 0.5 ml in a 10 ml standard flask and add 1.5 ml of 12% potassium iodate in 33% methanol. Mix well and cool to 15°C. Make up the volume with aqueous methanol.
4. Measure the absorbance of the solution at 550 nm. Estimate the total gallotannin content based on measurements made on standard sample of tannic acid.

B. Method II

This spectrophotometric method is based on the development of a coloured complex between tannic acid and sodium tungstate. The colour of the complex is stable and is not affected by the presence of phenols, proteins or sugars.

1. Weigh accurately 20 g of powdered material that is passed through #20 mesh. Add 300 ml of petroleum ether, shake well and set aside overnight.
2. Filter and wash with 5×20 ml of petroleum ether. Discard the petroleum ether fractions and air dry the residue.
3. Carefully transfer the residue to a 500 ml beaker, add 200 ml 95% alcohol, shake occasionally and set aside overnight. Filter through sintered funnel.
4. Take 10 ml of the filtrate in a 25 ml centrifuge tube, add 2 ml of a 10% solution of lead acetate and heat on a water bath till the precipitate coagulates.
5. Centrifuge for 3 min, pour off the supernatant and drain as completely as possible. Add 5 to 10 drops of sulphuric acid and mix thoroughly. Add water up to the 20-ml mark in the centrifuge tube and centrifuge again for 3 min.

6. Perform steps 1 to 5 on 2 mg standard sample of tannic acid.

7. To both the centrifuge tubes containing the tannic acid solutions add, 2 ml of sodium tungstate reagent (prepared by heating under reflux a mix of 100 g of pure sodium tungstate, 30 g of arsenic acid, 300 ml of water and 50 ml hydrochloric acid and making up to 1000 ml with water), 10 ml of a 20% solution of sodium carbonate and make up to volume.

8. Measure the absorbance of the colour developed in both the tubes at 760 nm and determine the tannic acid content of the plant material based on the absorbance of the known weight of standard sample.

Eugenol

Source

Eugenol is a phenyl propene extracted from the essential oil of clove, *Eugenia caryophyllus* (Myrtaceae). Though clove is the richest source, it is also found in nutmeg, cinnamon, basil, turmeric, marjoram, bay leaf and many other culinary and medicinal plants. It is the chief aroma chemical of essential oil of clove in which it is present up to 75% to 90%. Other significant sources from which it may be isolated are pimento –80%, cinnamon leaf oil –95% and bay leaf oil –50%. Eugenol is also found in varying amounts in a number of flowers such as rose, acacia, neroli etc.

Uses

A phenyl propanoid, its name is derived from its source *Eugenia*. Eugenol and the essential oil of clove are used in perfumery and flavouring and as an antiseptic and anaesthetic medicinally. Its pleasant, spicy pungent odour makes it valuable in perfumery and flavouring. Cloves have been used since long as a spice and a food preservative. As a complex with zinc oxide, it is used as a prosthodontic in dentistry. Eugenol derivatives are used in perfumery, flavouring and as stabilizers and antioxidants for plastics and rubber. Its antiseptic, anti-inflammatory and antioxidant properties are well reported. Earlier it was used for the production of isoeugenol for the manufacture of vanillin.

Description

Eugenol or 4-allyl-2-methoxy phenol is an aromatic liquid of molecular formula $C_{10}H_{12}O_2$. Its IUPAC name is 2-Methoxy -4(Prop -2 –en-1-yl) phenol. It is a colourless to pale yellow liquid with a strong odour of cloves. It has a boiling point of 256°C and specific gravity of 1.064–1.07. It has a refractive index of 1.54–1.542. Eugenol is stable, combustible and incompatible with strong oxidizing agents. It is slightly soluble in water and fully miscible with organic solvents such as cyclohexane, ethanol, dichloromethane, toluene, benzene, propylene glycol and diethyl ether.

Isolation

Eugenol can be produced synthetically by the allylation of readily available guaiacol with allyl chloride. It is however invariably prepared from its readily available natural sources. It may be separated from its source essential oils by a relatively simple method.

A. Method I (Steam distillation)

1. Powder 10 g of cloves and soak in 150 ml water for about 30 min.

2. Transfer to a distillation flask, add a few porcelain bits, connect to the distillation assembly and heat on a sand bath and heating mantle at a temperature not exceeding 130°C.

3. Continue distillation until about 75 ml of the distillate is collected. The distillate contains both the condensate of eugenol and water.

4. Transfer the distillate into a separating funnel and add 20 ml of dichloromethane. Shake well to extract eugenol from the eugenol-water suspension.

5. Carefully separate the organic layer without any water. Continue the extraction with 15 ml of the organic solvent two more times and pool the organic layers.

6. Pass it through a bed of anhydrous sodium sulphate and collect in a tared 100 ml conical flask. Rinse the drying agent with another 5 ml of dichloromethane and collect it in the same conical flask.

7. Evaporate to dryness on a water bath and note the yield of the product after cooling in a desiccator.

8. To purify the product dissolve it in 30 ml of diethyl ether and transfer into a separating funnel. Extract with 3 × 10 ml of 5% sodium hydroxide solution.

9. Collect the aqueous layers into a clean 100 ml beaker and add concentrated hydrochloric acid until the pH of the solution is 1 (check with indicator paper).

10. Transfer into a separating funnel and extract with 3 × 10 ml portions of dichloromethane. Evaporate the pooled organic layers in a clean tared dish and note the yield.

Identification

Eugenol being a phenol may be identified by simple chemical tests for phenols.

1. Dissolve 5 drops of eugenol in 10 ml of water. Add 3 drops of ferrous chloride solution. Appearance of a bluish-green colour indicates the presence of eugenol.

2. Take 0.5 g of eugenol in a 50 ml beaker. Add 0.1 g of picric acid, 1 ml of benzene and 9 ml of petroleum ether. Mix well and heat until crystals dissolve. The solution turns orange yellow confirming the presence of eugenol.

3. Dissolve 5 drops of eugenol in 5 ml of ethanol. Add a few drops of ferric chloride solution. A blue colour indicates the presence of a phenol.

Estimation

Quantitative estimation of eugenol in volatile oils, extracts, formulations and body fluids may be undertaken by a number of spectrophotometric and HPLC methods. Being a simple phenol, it can be quantified in clove oil by direct titrimetric procedures.

A. Method I

One of the earliest official methods for the determination of eugenol content of cloves involves treatment of oil with a known volume of alkali. Eugenol forms water-soluble salts with alkalis and this water-miscible complex moves into the aqueous phase. The volume of immiscible oil remaining is measured. This subtracted from the volume of oil taken will indicate the volume of eugenol that has moved into the aqueous phase as an alkali salt. The percentage of eugenol may thus be estimated.

1. Take 5 ml of clove oil in a 25 ml burette. Add 5% sodium hydroxide solution up to the '0' mark of the burette. Being denser than water, clove oil remains on the top. Set aside for 3 h.

2. Note the volume of the immiscible portion of the oil directly from the burette. Let it be 'a'.

3. (5-a) × 20 gives the percentage of eugenol in the sample of clove oil taken for analysis.

B. Method II (Spectorphotometric assay)

1. Sample solution: Dissolve 1 ml of eugenol in methanol : chloroform (95:5) taken in a 10 ml standard flask. Add sufficient amount of the same solvent and make up the volume to the mark. Dilute 1 ml of the solution to 10 ml and further dilute 1 ml of this to 1 ml using the same solvent. The resulting 1 µg/ml solution is the test solution.

2. Standard solution: Take 10 ml of standard sample of eugenol in a 100 ml standard flask and make up the volume with the methanol: chloroform solvent. Mix well and from this stock solution prepare 1, 2, 4 6, 8, 20 and 40 µg/ml solutions.

3. Determine the absorbances of the test and standard samples at 281 nm. Prepare a calibration curve of the standard eugenol. Estimate the percentage purity of eugenol based on its absorbance values from the calibration curve.

Menthol

Source

Menthol is a terpene alcohol obtained from diverse mint oils or prepared synthetically by hydrogenation of thymol. It occurs naturally in peppermint oil to the extent of 50% to 60% along with methyl acetate, menthyl isovalerianate and small amounts of other terpenes. Peppermint oil refers to the steam distilled essential oil isolated from the aerial parts of various species of the mint family such as *Mentha piperita*, *Mentha arvensis* and *Mentha canadensis* (Labiateae). *M. arvensis* is extensively cultivated in India, the largest producer of menthol and related products in the world.

The oil composition of peppermint oil is greatly influenced by genetic factors and seasonal variations. Peppermint oil typically produces l–menthol with smaller amounts of stereoisomers d-neomenthol, d-isomenthol and d-neoisomenthol.

Peppermint oil high in ester content is prized for its fine aroma and pleasant taste and is one of the most important and widely used essential oils due to its fine pungent taste which is followed by a cooling sensation. Japanese peppermint oil obtained from *M. arvensis* is high in menthol content and is therefore solely employed for the isolation of menthol. Peppermint oil is extensively employed in pharmaceuticals and oral preparations such as toothpaste, dental creams, mouth washes, cough syrups, chewing gums, confectionary, tobacco, betel nut, cigarettes and in alcoholic beverages. It has stimulant, carminative, counter-irritant and antiseptic properties. Menthol has the characteristic peppermint odour and flavour and gives a cool sensation when applied on the skin.

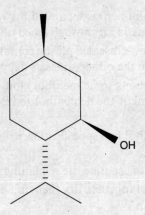

Uses

Menthol is used in foods, topical therapeutic preparations, oral hygiene and dentifrice formulations and tobacco products due to its pleasant minty flavour and the cooling sensation it imparts when in contact with the skin or oral membranes. Menthol is combined with camphor and eucalyptus oil in ointments, cough preparations, nasal sprays and inhalants to relieve symptoms of bronchitis, sinusitis and nasal congestion. This characteristic cooling sensation is produced by interaction with cold receptors rather than the taste buds, so manifestation of the characteristic cooling qualities is not limited to the oral cavity. Menthol produces the sensation of coolness in the oral and olfactory regions only at low concentrations, as higher concentrations induce a burning sensation coincident with some modest degree of desensitization. Menthol has local anesthetic and counter-irritant qualities.

Description

Menthol is 2-(2-Propyl)-5-methyl-1-cyclohexanol. It is a monocyclic terpene alcohol having three asymmetric carbon atoms in the cyclohexane ring, yielding a variety of isomers. While l-menthol constitutes the predominant isomer in natural botanical sources, the racemic mixture dl-menthol is produced synthetically. The *dl* racemate exhibits about half of the cooling properties of l-menthol and finds use mainly in topical skin care products.

Its molecular formula is $C_{10}H_{20}O$. Though known in Japan since ancient times it was first isolated in the west by H.D. Gaubius in 1771. Menthol occurs as white or colourless hexagonal or needle-like crystalline or granular solid, with peppermint taste and odour. It has a melting point of 41–43°C and a boiling point of 212°C. It is slightly soluble in water, very soluble in alcohol, chloroform, ether, petroleum ether and freely soluble in glacial acetic acid.

Isolation

Dried aerial parts of mint contain about 0.4% to 0.8% essential oil of which 40% to 60% is menthol. It is typically isolated from the essential oil of mint by cold freezing, during which menthol crystallizes. The liquid portion is poured off and crystallized menthol is pressed between filter papers and subsequently purified by recrystallization.

Method

1. The volatile oil of peppermint herb is separated by water and steam distillation. The oil is then freed of moisture by passing it through a bed of anhydrous sodium sulphate.
2. The dried oil is then taken in well-sealed plastic containers and frozen to about minus 60°C for about 7 days. Menthol in the oil separates as flaky crystals which are filtered out.
3. The mother liquor still contains some menthol along with menthone and other terpenes. Add 8 g boric acid for 100 ml of the dementholized essential oil and further boil for 3 h to distill off menthone.
4. Convert the borate of menthol by saponification with 50 ml of 15% sodium hydroxide by heating under reflux for 1 h.
5. Cool the resultant solution to separate the remaining menthol.
6. Collect the flakes of menthol together, dry them in a desiccator and note the yield.

Identification

1. Heat a few crystals of menthol taken in a watch glass over a water bath. The entire material volatilizes without leaving any residue.
2. To 0.5 g of menthol taken in a test tube, add equal quantity of camphor or thymol. Liquefaction of the material indicates the presence of menthol.
3. To 0.25 g of menthol, add 5 ml of sulphuric acid and mix well. There is formation of yellowish-red turbidity. Allow to stand for 24 h. Formation of a transparent oily layer with no odour of menthol indicates its presence.

Estimation

Menthol content in peppermint oils, other volatile oils, plant material, formulations and other preparations may conveniently be estimated by GC methods.

A. Method I

1. Weigh accurately 2 g of menthol in a 250 ml conical flask with a ground glass jointed neck. Add 5 ml of a mixture of 4 ml acetic anhydride and 1 ml of anhydrous pyridine and boil under reflux for 30 min.
2. Through the condenser add 30 ml warm distilled water and continue heating for 15 min.
3. Remove from the heat source and cool completely. Disconnect the condenser and rinse it with 15 ml of distilled water.
4. Titrate the contents of the flask with 0.5 M alcoholic potassium hydroxide (KOH) solution using phenolphthalein as indicator. Let the titred value be 'a' ml.
5. Carry out a blank determination to determine the number of millilitres of the titrant required to neutralize the acetic acid produced by 5 ml of the acetylizing mixture. Let the titred value be 'b' ml.
6. (b-a) gives the number of millilitres of titrant equivalent to the acetic acid used up for the acetylation of menthol. Determine the percentage of free menthol from the equivalent factor of 0.5 M alcoholic KOH, which is 0.0781 g.

Guggulipid

Source

Guggulipid is a standardized extract of the oleo gum resin of the mukul myrrh tree, *Commiphora mukul* (Burseraceae), native to India. Shuddha guggulu is a processed form of the resin used in traditional Ayurvedic medicine for the treatment of epilepsy, ulcers, obesity, rheumatoid arthritis and atherosclerosis since 600 BC.

The gummy resin exudate is harvested from the plants' bark through tapping. This product called gum guggulu is used in incense and perfumes for its fragrance. It is processed to separate the essential oil and the gum from the resinous portion.

Chemically guggulu is a complex mixture of steroids, diterpenoids, aliphatic esters, carbohydrates and several inorganic ions. Extracts of the oleoresin contain compounds known to have hypolipidaemic activity such as guggulusterols I, II and III and stereoisomeric guggulusterones (Z and E). Other biologically active constituents include myrrhanol A and myrrhanone – known to have anti-inflammatory activity – and two ferulic acid esters – (Z)-5-tricosene-1,2,3,4-tetraol and (Z)-5-tetracosene-1,2,3,4-tetraol – reported to have anti-tumour properties.

Uses

Research studies showed that guggul is beneficial in cardiovascular disease. Guggulsterones were comparable to cardioprotective drugs propanolol and nifedipine in protecting from myocardial necrosis induced by isoproterenol in rats. Guggul reduced the stickiness of platelets, and is reported to be used in the treatment of hyperlipoproteinemia. Fractions of guggulu rich in guggulusterones are known to have hypocholesterolemic activity. They inhibit cholesterol synthesis in the liver via antagonism of the farnesoid X receptor and the bile-acid receptor. Guggulusterones up-regulate the bile salt export pump (BSEP), an efflux transporter responsible for the removal of cholesterol metabolites and bile acids from the liver. This favours the metabolism of cholesterol into bile acids. Guggulusterones inhibit the activation of nuclear factor kappa B, a critical regulator of inflammatory responses. There are some patents for the use of guggulu in cosmetics.

Description

The oleoresin present in ducts under the soft bark tissue when tapped oozes out as a pale yellow, aromatic fluid that turns into an 'agglomerate of tears or stalactic pieces' that are reddish brown, golden brown or dull green. An average of about 700 to 900 g resin may be collected from each tree. This product called gum guggulu is processed to separate the essential oil and the gummy portion. This is normally done by hot expression at 120–130°C, with a yield of 51%, or by solvent extraction, with a yield of 61%.

The oleo resin of gum guggulu occurs as an off white to pale yellow dusty powder or granules. Like other resins it fuses on heating and forms a milky emulsion with hot water. It mixes well with vegetable waxes, stearic acids and other resins.

It has an acrid odour and a bitter taste. It is soluble in water, alcohol (≥60%w/w) and petroleum ether, ethyl acetate, castor oil, drying oils and turpentine (≥40%w/w). A 1%w/v solution in water has a pH of 5–7. The resin of gum guggulu also acts as a binding agent and there is no need to add a binding agent when it is being formulated into tablets.

The purified resin contains 2% guggulsterones. Guggulusterones when purified occur as white amorphous powder poorly soluble in water and soluble in DMSO.

Isolation

C.mukul is a thorny tree, 4–6 feet tall. It is leafless most of the year and has a dry ash-coloured bark that flakes off easily. For the collection of oleoresin, the tree is tapped by making circular incisions on the main stem no deeper than the thickness of the bark. The yellowish exudate that oozes out dries and it is collected by scraping. The agglomerate mass of the dried material is collected from all the incisions made at a time. It is freed of extraneous plant parts before processing.

1. The collected gum guggulu is taken in four times its weight of hot water and set aside overnight.
2. The next day it is heated gently in iron pans (under dry and sunny conditions using mild heat) with continuous stirring to concentrate the quantity of water to half its volume. Industrially it is heated in steam-jacketed pans under controlled temperatures of 50–60°C. Heating removes most of the volatile material from the oleo gum resin.
3. The hot solution is then filtered through a cotton cloth or mesh. Traditionally further purification is done by processing it with added herbs depending upon the medical condition for which it is being taken.
4. For commercial purposes or for the preparation of standardized extracts, the hot solution is filtered through a #100 mesh and the filtrate further concentrated under vacuum. So concentrated aqueous extract is then lyophilized or spray dried to yield a fine powder.

Figure 8.1 gives the schematic diagram of the steps involved in the fractionation for concentrating guggulsterones. The purified resin is specifically fractionated by solvent extraction to yield standardized extracts or fractions rich in guggulsterones. Its ethyl acetate extract contains 4% to 4.5% guggulsterones. The neutral subfraction contains 4.2% to 4.7% guggulsterones. The ketonic subfraction of the neutral subfraction contains 35% to 40% guggulsterones, from which the 10% E- and Z-guggulsterones are derived.

Estimation

Guggulipid, the purified resin, gum guggulu and preparations containing guggulu extracts may be analysed for the concentration of guggulsterones by thin layer chromatography (TLC) and HPLC/mass spectrometry (MS) and colorimetric methods.

A. Method I (Quantitative)

1. 5 g of accurately weighed sample is extracted with 25 ml chloroform by a sonicator for 20 min, filtered and evaporated to dryness in a tared beaker.
2. Sample solution: Transfer 100 mg of the sample into a 10 ml standard flask and dissolve in sufficient chloroform and make up to the mark. Sonicate the solution and filter through a Whatman filter paper.
3. Standard solution: Disslove 10 mg of standard sample of guggulusterone Z in 10 ml chloroform. Dilute 1 ml of this solution to 10 ml with chloroform (100 µg/ml). Prepare a series of dilutions to get solutions ranging from 10 µg/ml to 60 µg/ml.

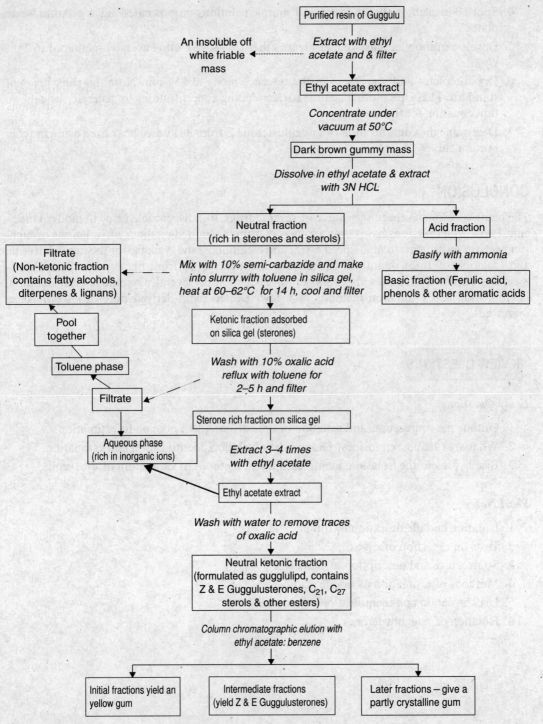

Figure 8.1 Processing of guggulu resin

4. Spot 10 μl each of the standard and sample solutions on precoated silica gel aluminium plates.

5. Develop in mobile phase of petroleum ether (60–80°C): ethyl acetate: methanol (6:2:0.5 v/v).

6. Dry the plates and scan them in fluorescence mode at 254 nm. Note the peak areas of standard. These are plotted against corresponding concentrations to generate the calibration equation for the marker.

7. Determine the concentration of guggulusterone Z from its known peak area using the calibration curve.

CONCLUSION

The plant kingdom has been the source of several drugs of indispensable value to modern medicine. Plant drug isolations have come a long way from the limited methods of isolations of high-yield active constituents to high-speed extraction techniques now available for the rapid detection and isolation of trace quantities of active constituents even from plant parts. Today commercially feasible techniques are available for extraction of several phytomolecules. Isolation, identification and estimation methods of a few selected plant-derived pure drugs have been discussed.

REVIEW QUESTIONS

Essay Questions

1. Outline the source, uses and isolation of ephedrine. Add a note on its estimation.
2. What are calcium sennosides? Discuss their isolation, identification and estimation.
3. Briefly present the isolation, identification and methods of estimation of diosgenin.

Short Notes

1. Isolation and identification of quinine
2. Tests for detection of digoxin
3. Source, uses and description of berberine
4. Methods of estimation of tannic acid
5. Uses, isolation and identification of menthol
6. Isolation of guggulusterones

9   Traditional Herbal Drugs

CHAPTER OBJECTIVES

Introduction	Salient Features of Some Medicinal Herbs

INTRODUCTION

Worldwide re-emergence of utilization of plant-based therapies has opened up a huge potential for the herbal drug industry. There is expansive commercialization of plant-derived products for use as health foods, cosmaceuticals, nutritional supplements and as fast-moving consumer goods. It is time to take classical recipes of ayurveda, siddha, and other indigenous medical systems also to the world market as standardized, approved herbal drugs.

Medicinal plant-related trade in India inclusive of ayurvedic and herbal products has a total turnover of Rs. 2,300 crores, with proprietary preparations accounting for 1,200 crores, other formulations-650 crores and classical ayurvedic formulations contributing to the remaining 450 crores. With the worldwide demand growing annually, the Indian export market for herbal drugs is fast catching up with the domestic market.

The uninterrupted use and popularity of herbal formulations for thousands of years has made the Ayurvedic *materia medica* a valuable resource for modern drug development. Our great biodiversity and immense medicinal plant wealth are our assets and it is time to effectively and sustainably harvest this resource.

In our country approximately 1,000 herbal formulations prepared from around 750 medicinal plants are in regular use today. Traditionally ayurvedic physicians prepared and compounded their own formulations from carefully selected drugs. In the traditional "Guruparampara" form of education, ayurvedic physicians were well trained in the correct identification and processing into herbal drug formulations. They were at liberty to modify the classical ayurvedic formulations as per the regional availability of herbs and in accordance with the disease form in the patient.

Ayurvedic pharmacology has identified an herbs' therapeutic utility based on its inherent qualities (rasa, guna, virya, vipaka, and prabhava) that influence the governing dosha of the individual. According to its own disease classification, the determining factor in herb selection is its quality of altering the tridoshas.

Hence, herbs in a formulation were replaceable with others of similar quality. This led to the usage and nomenclature of herbs based on their therapeutic utility. Thus, many different herbs had a common name and a single herb was referred to by different names. Differences in regional languages and dialects contributed to the so-called controversial drug names of ayurveda. Varying ecological factors such as region, climatic conditions for growth, and so on, contribute to varying properties of the source plants. In addition, interpretations of classical texts into regional languages, actual herb selection by the physician based on the properties of locally available herbs, and his actual clinical experience are some of the reasons for this nonspecific naming of plant drugs. Lapse of centuries and break of continuity led to drugs being identified with one name being replaced with other equivalents due to lack of their availability. For example, classical drugs of the Himalayan region whose supply was limited and seasonal, were often replaced by easily accessible substitute drugs. This was especially so in the case of classical herbal formulations.

Foreign rule, political instability, lack of patronage, and general attitude of our rulers to denigrate claim of Ayurveda as a science, improper communication and transportation and general decadence were some of the factors responsible for lack of sorting out of the name-drug disparity seen with traditional drugs.

The plant drug names were not considered very crucial since the knowledge was transmitted from teacher to student in the traditional education pattern in ancient India. Physicians well aware of different herbs, their habitat, morphology, and properties could thus make their own formulations and plant drug identification was just basic knowledge. Thus, ayurveda and drug formulations were innovative and dynamic with physicians carrying out their own clinical trials on local flora, thus adding newer medicines. Ayurveda also has a long history of incorporating nonnative plants into its *materia medica*, such as Madhusnuhı (*Smilax chinensis*) from China which was incorporated into "Bhavaprakasa nighantu" as a treatment for syphilis.

It is usual to see same preparations described with altered compositions in different treatises, with each of them prescribed for different indications.

Through time, traditional physicians have long since moved into urban locales and thus individual dispensing is today replaced by large-scale production. It is now rare to find ayurvedic physicians dispensing their own medications and both physician and the patient now consider it convenient for their drugs to be readymade and available on the market much like modern medicines. Increasing urbanization, reckless exploitation of flora, massive up-scaling of individually dispensed formulae into commercially processed preparations, have all taken a toll on the quality and efficacy of ayurvedic products that are being manufactured. Today the situation is unlike the erstwhile careful and custom-made preparations, whose quality was implicit. This is worsened by the rampant commercialization seen in herbal drug manufacturing with several haphazard concoctions, cocktails, and combinations of herbs being made into convenient dosage forms. Such combinations are justified on the grounds of the so-called demonstrated pharmacological activities of individual herbs, with no regard for the actual ayurvedic therapeutic basis of drug administration. Such products are being manufactured and even exported, in keeping with the current demand for herbal drugs. These are sold across borders as health supplements and as FMCGs within the country.

Prompt pharmacovigilance enabled with today's worldwide communications network is quick to report the adverse effects of such herbal products. These being attributed to ayurvedic drugs from India or to Indian herbal medicines is a cause for serious concern.

However, the number of adverse drug reactions formally reported or recorded in the National Pharmacovigilance Programme in India is negligible. Though their actual numbers may not be comparable with that reported for pure drugs, lack of knowledge about the concept and importance of pharmacovigilance in ayurveda among ayurvedic practitioners could be a reason.

In this scenario, it is very crucial to disseminate the right information about Ayurveda (and other indigenous herbal traditions) and its therapeutic utility to the scientific community. There is an urgent need to develop herbal drugs as ethical phytomedicines, which are standardized and whose efficacy and safety is well demonstrated

Already countries like China, Korea, Germany, and Chile are fast working to document and enrich their repositories of medicinal plant-related information and are strengthening their herbal industry base. Germany and China are in the lead in providing national health care by beneficially amalgamating traditional and modern medicine. Modern medicine graduates in China are trained in traditional Chinese medicine as part of their formal medical education. It is thus possible for traditional drugs to be prescribed as ethical drugs by modern medical practitioners in these countries.

With such an immense scope and potential for development of herbals as drugs, it is important for students concerned with drug development to have first-hand information and expertise in the identification and properties of herbal drugs.

SALIENT FEATURES OF SOME MEDICINAL HERBS

Punarnava

Punarnava refers to *Boerrhavia diffusa* Linn Family: Nyctaginaceae. The dried, mature whole plant is used in traditional medicine. The plant is an herbaceous perennial growing all over India as a common creeping weed and is specially abundant during the rains.

Synonym

B. repens Linn, *B. procumbens* Roxb, *B. verticillata*

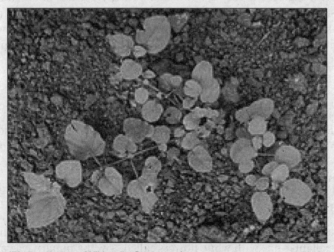

(Photo courtesy: Wikipedia Commons)

Figure 9.1 *Boerhaavia diffusa*

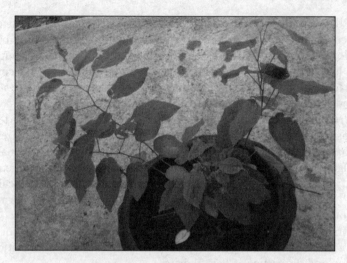

Figure 9.2 *Boerhaavia verticillata*

Common vernacular names

English: Spreading Hogweed, pig weed, red spiderling
Sanskrit: Punarnava
Hindi: Gadhaparna, Sant
Tamil: Mukkarattai
Telugu: Adhikamamidi, giligeru

Morphology

Highly branched stem is greenish purple, swollen at nodes, prostrate, or ascending to a height of up to 1m. Leaves silvery on the undersurface are simple, thick and glabrous. Flower is small pink or white on long axillary peduncled umbellate clusters. Root is stout fusiform with a woody root-stock and has a bitter nauseous taste. Roots of *Trianthema* species are sometimes mistaken for punarnava roots.

Constituents

Major constituent is punarnavoside—a phenolic glycoside, 0.03–0.05%. Others include rotenoids — boeravinones A, B, C, D, and E, Lignans—liridodendron, syringaresinol, some flavones and sterols. Roots contain a purine nucleoside, hypoxanthine-9-arabinofuranoside and boeravine, ursolic acid and β-sitosterol. It contains an insect-moulting hormone, β-ecdysone. In addition, it contains potassium nitrate and other potassium salts.

Traditional uses

Used in Indian traditional medicine since times immemorial, ayurvedic practitioners recognize two varieties of the plant—one with white flowers called "swetha punarnava" and the other with red flowers "raktha punarnava." Ayurvedic formulary "svetapunarnava" as another species is the *B. verticillata*.

The drug is a bitter, astringent, cooling, anthelmintic, diuretic, diaphoretic, emetic, and laxative and tonic.

Whole herb in the form of a juice is given internally as a blood purifier. Dhanvantri has described the white variety in his nighantu as possessing laxative and diaphoretic properties. The red variety is bitter and is considered effective in the treatment of oedema and biliousness. Charaka used it in the form of an ointment in leprosy and skin diseases and as decoction for kidney stone removal. Local applications of the root paste have been recommended in oedematous swellings. The drug being an efficient diuretic relieves oedema and is used in urinary tract diseases. A rasayana or rejuvenating drug, Punarnava is an ingredient of the famous Chyawanaprasha. It is also eaten as a vegetable in curries and soups.

Pharmacology

The root, leaves, and different extracts of the plant exhibit many pharmacological properties. The plant is reported with adaptogenic, hypoglycemic, anti-amoebic and immunomodulant activity. It possesses potent anti-fibrinolytic, anti-inflammatory properties and has demonstrated reduction of IUCD-induced menorrhagia in experimental animals. Punarnavoside is an anti-fibrinolytic agent and liridodendron and hypoxanthine-9-arabinofuranoside are antihypertensive agents (calcium channel blocker). It's anti-inflammatory and analgesic property is comparable to that of ibuprofen. Being a diuretic, refrigerant, and anti-spasmodic, it helps maintain efficient kidney function. It is also a useful haematinic. The plant extracts are attributed with hepatoprotective activity and is effective in cases of oedema and ascites resulting form early cirrhosis of liver and peritonitis. The plant extract has shown differential effects on the GABA levels in various lesions of the brain in experimental rats.

Marketed products

Ayurvedic—Punarnavastaka kvatha curna, punarnavasava, punarnavadi mandura, sukumara ghrta, sathanaghnalepa

Proprietary products—Diabecon, Geriforte, Bonnisan, Evecare, V-Gel, Lukol, Chyawanaprasha, Immunol, Digyton, etc.

Shankapushpi

Shankapushpi refers to *Convolvulus microphyllus* Sieb ex. Spreng, Family: Convolvulaceae according to the ayurvedic dictionary and the Ayurvedic Formulary of India.

Synonym

C. pluricaulis Choisy

In Kerala, however, shanka pushpi refers to *Clitorea ternata* (Family: Papilionaceae) in all medicinal preparations. In Karnataka and Konkan regions, aerial parts of *Canscora decussata,* (Family: Gentianaceae) are used as a substitute for shankapushpi. *Evolvulus alsinoides* (Convolvulaceae) is also mentioned as a substitute for shankapushpi

In general the whole plant is used in the preparation of indigenous medicine.

Common vernacular names

English: Aloe weed
Sanskrit: Vishnukranthi

Hindi: Sankapuspi
Tamil: Visnukarandi
Telugu: Vishnukaranta

Morphology

The plant is a small procumbent herb found in open grassy places almost throughout India, ascending to 6,000 ft., in the Himalayas. It is a fulvous hairy herb, woody at the base and leaves are linear to oblong, small and sub-sessile with trichomes on both surfaces. One to three pink flowers occur together, which are axillary and pedicelled. The sepals are linear to

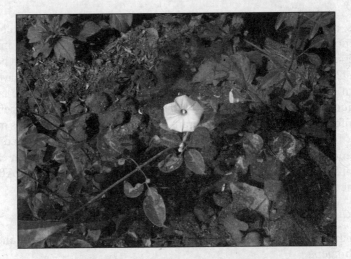

Figure 9.3 *Convolvulus pluricaulis*

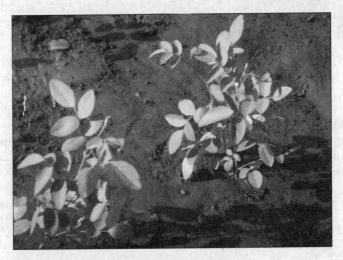

Figure 9.4 *Clitoria ternata*

lanceolate and hairy. Fruit capsules are oblong-globose, pale brown containing tiny brown seeds.

Clitoria ternata is a perennial climber with cylindrical stems and branches with compound leaf bearing 5–7 imparipinnate leaflets. Flowers, blue or white with an orange center, are solitary or axillary, followed by flattened pods containing 6–10 yellowish-brown seeds. It is found throughout India and South East Asia.

Canscora decussata is an erect branching annual of up to 60 cm height found in moist areas all over India up to a height of about 1500 m. Leaves are simple, ovate, opposite and sessile.

Evolvulus alsinoides is a procumbent perennial with a small woody root stock, with simple elliptic-oblong or oblong-ovate leaves, alternately arranged. The flowers are light blue in colour, solitary or in pairs, borne in the leaf axils, giving rise to globose four-valved capsules. *E. alsinoides* is found throughout India up to 1800 m in elevation.

Constituents

The plant contains alkaloids convolvuline, convolamine, phyllabine, convolidine, subhirsine, scopoline, betaine, evolvuline, flavonoids—Kaempferol, kaempferol-3-glucoside, 6-methoxy-7-hydroxy coumarin, long chain fatty alcohols-*n*-hexacosanol, *n*-octacosanol, *n*-triacontanol and dotriacontanol, in addition to 3,4,dihydroxycinnamic acid, sugars-glucose, rhamnose, sucrose and β & γ-sitosterol.

Traditional uses

The plant is considered a bitter tonic, febrifuge, and a vermifuge indicated in dysentery. It is a reputed "medhya rasayana" or a memory-improving drug. The juice of the plant along with those of *Centella asiatica, Beninca hispida, Acorus calamus,* and *Sausserea lappa* is given in psychosis as a psycho-stimulant and tranquillizer. It also promotes digestion, physical strength, and improves skin complexion. It is reported to remedy hypertension.

Leaves of *E. alsinoides* are made into cigarettes and smoked for relief from bronchial asthma.

Clitorea ternata is used as a diuretic and laxative. Root juice is used in chronic bronchitis and is used as a decoction in the irritation of the bladder and urethra. It is used in the treatment of headache in the form of snuff.

Pharmacology

The ethanolic extract of the plant was found to reduce total serum cholesterol, triglycerides, phospholipids and nonesterified fatty acids after oral administration in hyperlipidaemic rats. Besides, high-density lipoprotein was elevated in the animals. The ethanolic extract of the plant when administered to rats through gastric intubation at different time intervals showed enhanced neuro-peptide synthesis. The alcoholic extract of the whole plant depresses the amphibian and mammalian myocardium through negative ionotropic effect. The extract had a spasmolytic activity on the smooth muscles of isolated rabbit ileum and isolated rat uterus. In clinical studies, a decoction of the drug reduced arterial blood pressure. Potentiation of cognitive process (memory) by the drug is reported to be due to an increased supply of proteins to hippocampus, thus enhancing the learning process. It also reduces spontaneous motor activity and fighting response.

Marketed product

Ayurvedic: Brahma ghrta, Agastyaharitaki, Manasmitra Vataka, Gorocanadi Vati.
Proprietary: Abana, Anxocare (heart care)

Lehsun

Lehsun consists of the fresh ripe bulbs of *Allium sativum*, Family: Liliaceae.

Synonym

Porvium sativum Rohb.
   Native to Central Asia it spread to the Mediterranean region and today it is cultivated world-wide. It is commonly found all over India. It grows wild and is also extensively cultivated on account of its use as a condiment and spice. A biennial it is cultivated as a perennial.

Common vernacular names

English: garlic
Sanskrit: lahsuna
Hindi: lahsun
Tamil: vellai poondu
Telugu: tellagadda

Morphology

Allium sativum is a perennial bulbous plant growing to a height of about 2 ft. The plant is strong smelling when crushed and the underground portion consists of compound bulb with many fibrous rootlets. The bulb gives rise to a number of narrow keeled grass-like leaves above the ground. Leaf blade is linear, flat, solid 1–2.5 cm wide, 30–60 cm long with an acute apex.

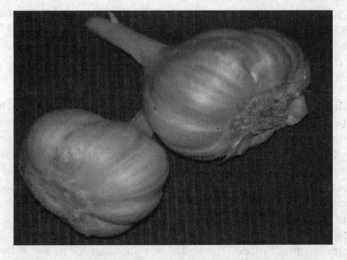

Figure 9.5a Lehsun *(Allium sativum)*

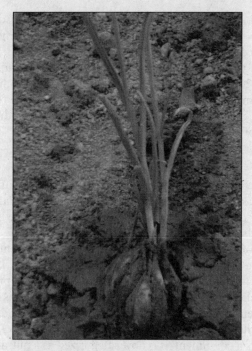

Figure 9.5b *Allium sativum*-herb

Inflorescence is umbellate with variable number of flowers on slender pedicels and fruit is a small loculicidal capsule. The main ovate bulb constitutes garlic and it is made up of 5–15 secondary bulbs, both being surrounded by common, white, dry, scaly leaves. The bulbs may be pink to white in colour with a strong disagreeable odor and a strong characteristic pungent aromatic taste that mellows with cooking.

Constituents

Garlic contains 65% water, 28% carbohydrates, 2.3% organosulphur compounds, 2% protein, 1.2% free amino acids, 1.5% fiber, 0.15% lipid and trace quantities of phytic acid (0.08%), saponins (0.07%) and β-sitosterol. Vitamins B_1, B_2, B_3, B_5, B_6, C, and minerals calcium, iron, magnesium, manganese, phosphorous, potassium, sodium, zinc and selenium are also present.

The organosulphur-rich essential oil of the drug is the chief active constituent and it contains organosulphur compounds—(+)-S-allyl-L-cysteine sulphoxides namely alliin (1%), methiin (0.12%), isoalliin (0.06%) and cyloalliin (0.1%) and -alkyl-L-cysteines – g-glutamyl-S-trans-1-propenylcysteine (0.6%), g-L-glutamyl-S-alylcysteine (0.4%).

Garlic bulbs contain the enzyme alliinase with which alliin comes in contact, when they are bruised or crushed. Thus releases allicin through the intermediate allyl sulphenic acid. 1 mg of alliin is equivalent to 0.45 mg of allicin. Allicin is highly unstable and in the presence of water and oxygen it gets decomposed into polysulphide, which is responsible for the unpleasant odor. Alliicin is the chief precursor of various other compounds found in garlic products such as allyl sulfides, ajoenes, and vinyl dithiins.

The various products of decomposition of allicin include diallyl disulphide, diallyltrisulphide, and the corresponding polysulphides all of which are strong-smelling compounds. (E) Ajoene and (Z) Ajoene are formed from allicin.

Aged garlic extract is prepared by incubating minced garlic in aqueous alcohol (15–20%), which is then stored for 20 months and then concentrated. This product is reported to be very low in organosulphur compound content. Its allicin content is 3% of fresh garlic.

Biological activity of garlic largely depends on its ability to produce allicin, which in turn results in the formation of other active principles.

Uses

As a medicine, garlic has been held in high esteem by ancient physicians of India. Administered in vitiated conditions of kapha and vata, it is a thermogenic stimulant and is administered in fevers, coughs, and other debilitating conditions. Externally the juice is used as a rubefacient in skin diseases and as ear drops in earache and deafness.

Garlic has been used for culinary and medicinal purposes in different regions across the world.

It has also been used to a large extent in western herbal medicine. It is used as a carminative in dyspepsia. Because of its expectorant, stimulant, and disinfectant property, garlic in the form of a juice is used in the relief of cough, colds, catarrh, and rhinitis. It is also used for anti-fertility effects and in the treatment of malignant tumors. Steam distilled oil of garlic is used as insecticide in ring worm and urinary tract infections.

Though largely used as a condiment, it is now categorized as a nutraceutical for its nutritional and medicinal properties.

It is extensively indicated in the management of hypertension and atherosclerosis. Garlic is being recommended as a preventive against age-dependent vascular changes, in mild hypertension, as a hypolipidaemic and in the prophylaxis of atherosclerosis. Several forms of garlic namely fresh bulbs, dried powder, oil macerates, juice, aqueous or alcoholic extracts, aged garlic extracts, odorless garlic products (allinase inactivated) are available for use as dietary supplements.

Pharmacology

There is extensive scientific literature on chemical, pharmacological, clinical, and epidemiological studies related to garlic.

In vitro studies establish its anti-bacterial, anti-mycotic, lipid-lowering, platelet aggregation inhibition, clotting, and bleeding time prolongation and increased fibrinolytic activity. It inhibits milk-clotting activity of papain and the amylolytic—activity of β-amylase.

In vivo animal studies demonstrate garlic's ability to inhibit tumor formation and reduce blood pressure. Garlic powder, fresh garlic, aged garlic extract, and garlic oil is reported with anti aggregative, anti bacterial, anti mycotic, anti viral, larvicidal, and anti hepatotoxic activity. Ethanol extract of garlic is anti-spasmodic and it is anti-inflammatory due to its anti-prostaglandin activity.

The constituents, allicin and ajoene, are shown to bring about inhibition of cholesterol biosynthesis and are also anti-atherosclerotic and anti-thrombotic.

Clinical studies on garlic have demonstrated its hypotensive, firinolytic, anti-atherosclerotic, and hypolipidaemic effect with respect to lowering of total cholesterol, triglycerides and LDL-cholesterol. Clinically it is reported to relieve abdominal distress, flatulence, colic, and nausea and may be given prophylactically to prevent atherogenesis.

Several epidemiological studies correlate cancer prevention to garlic consumption especially with respect to colorectal and gastric cancers.

Marketed products

Traditional: lahsuna, sithadhi oil, tatir tel
Proprietary: appetionic vet, garlic pills, aged garlic extracts

Guggulu

Guggulu constitutes the oleo gum resin of *Commiphora mukul* (Hook ex Stocks) Engl. Syn: *Commiphora wighti* (Arn) Bhandari, *Balsamodendron mukul*, Family: Burseraceae, The plant is native to India and Pakistan and grows wild in dry rocky areas in Rajasthan, Gujarat, Karnataka and Assam. An yellowish oleo gum resin is secreted from the bark of the tree. First mentioned in Atharvana veda, it is also recorded in both Charaka and Susruta Samhitas and is an ancient plant grown exclusively for gum resin because of its medicinal value.

Common vernacular names

English : Indian Bdellium tree
Sanskrit: Kaushika, guggulu, Mahisaksha
Hindi: Guggal
Tamil: Gukkal, matsatchi kungiliyam
Telugu: Gukkulu, maishakshi

Morphology

It is a small bushy shrub or tree, 4–6 ft in height with thorny branches. The leaflets are 1–3 in number and obovate and the tree, however, remains largely leafless throughout the year. The ash-coloured bark comes off in rough flakes exposing the under bark, which also peels off in papery rolls. The tree bears small brownish flowers, slightly ascending branches, and alternate trifoliate leaves. The fruit is a red, ovate, drupe when ripe.

The oleo gum resin from the plant is obtained by incision of the bark during the cold season. It is collected by tapping at regular intervals for some weeks following incision of the bark. The

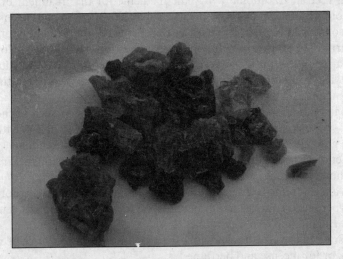

Figure 9.6 Guggulu

oleo gum resin that oozes out is a sticky yellowish fragrant fluid, which turns into brownish yellow fragments with an aromatic balsamic odor and a bitter taste. It is opaque with a dusty surface. Like other resins, it has a low melting point, melts in intense summer heat, and burns in flame. It forms a milky emulsion with hot water. It is processed to remove the essential and gum from the resinous portion.

According to Ayurveda, based on the colour, guggulu is "hemaguggulu"—when of golden yellow colour, "mahisaksam"—dark brown colour, "padmaragabham"—ruby red colour, "bringabham"—deep blue colour and "kumudyudi"—off white colour. Guggulu is to be taken as a drug when freshly collected and its quality deteriorates on storage.

Constituents

It contains up to 8% aromatic essential oil, 30–60% gum and 20–40% resin. The oil constitutes octa nor dammarane terpenes, myrcene, dimyrcene, cuminic aldehyde, eugenol, manusambionic acid, and manusambinone. The sequiterpene fraction of the essential is responsible for the fragrant odor of guggulu. The gummy portion is a highly branched polysaccharide made up of D-galactose, L-arabinose, and 4-methyl ether of D-glucuronic acid. The resin portion contains diaryl furano furanoid lignans-sesamin and related products, a macrocyclic diterpenes such as cembrane A, esters of ferulic acid and of long chain polyhydroxylated saturated hydrocarbons called guggulutetrols—(Z)-5-tricosene-1,2,3,4-tetraol and (Z)-5-tetracosene-1,2,3,4-tetraol, Myrrhanol A and myrrhanone A.

The principal active constituents are considered to be guggulusterones Z and E. These pharmacologically important compounds occur along with guggulu sterols (I-VI), which are di or tri hydroxylated pregnane or cholestane type sterols.

While crude gum guggulu has 2% guggulusterones, its ethyl acetate extract is enriched having 4–5% guggulusterones.

Traditional uses

The crude oleo gum resin called guggulu is used as an incense. Suddha guggulu is a processed form of the resin used in traditional ayurvedic medicine for the treatment of epilepsy, ulcers, obesity, rheumatoid arthritis, and atherosclerosis since 600 BC. The gum resin is a thermogenic given in vitiated conditions of vata. It is used as an astringent, anti-inflammatory, antiseptic, bitter stomachic, carminative, appetizer, and improves digestion. It is used as a lotion for indolent ulcers and as a gargle in tonsillitits, pharyngitis, and ulcerated throat. Guggulu is an ingredient of several ayurvedic formulations both as medicine and as an excipient. Traditionally guggulu is given as a "yog" meaning drug admixture.

It is thus used in combination with several other ayurvedic drugs such as shonti, punarnava, triphala, kaisara, sadanga, amrita, kanchanara, and so on. Its combination with *Inula racemosa* called "pushkara guggulu" is indicated in Ayurveda for chest pain and angina.

In folklore practice, twigs of the guggal tree are as used as tooth brush. Tincture of *Commiphora mukul* is used in homeopathy.

The drug is an ancient remedy given for a range of ailments such as dysmenorhoea, dyspepsia, endometriosis, hypertension, impotence, bronchitis, caries, gingivitis, leprosy, leucoderma, haemorrhoids, urinary calculi, and as a uterotonic.

The resin is also used in varnishes and adhesives, as an important source of raw materials for organic synthesis, or for incense and perfume.

Pharmacology

Ethyl acetate extract of *Commiphora mukul* confers significant protection to albino rats against experimental atherosclerosis. It prevents deteriorating changes in serum cholesterol, triglyceride and plasma fibrinogen levels. Research studies showed that guggul is beneficial in the treatment of cardiovascular disease. Guggulsterones were comparable to cardioprotective drugs, propano-lol and nifedipine, in protecting from myocardial necrosis induced by isoproterenol in rats. It reduces platelet aggregation and is also indicated in the treatment of hyperlipoproteinemia. Oleo resin has anti-arthritic, anti-inflammatory property. Clinical studies indicate it to be a digestive and analgesic.

Fractions of guggulu rich in guggulusterones are known to have hypocholesterolemic activity as they inhibit total cholesterol, LDL, VLDL, and increase HDL/TC ratio.

They inhibit cholesterol synthesis in the liver via antagonism of the farnesoid X receptor and the bile-acid receptor. Guggulusterones up regulate the bile salt e xport pump (BSEP), an efflux transporter responsible for the removal of cholesterol metabolites and bile acids from the liver. This favors the metabolism of cholesterol into bile acids. Guggulusterones inhibit the activation of nuclear factor kappa B, a critical regulator of inflammatory responses. Guggulusterones are reported to increase the activity of dopamine—β-D-hydroxylase.

Myrrhanol A and myrrhanone A have shown anti-inflammatory activity in adjuvant-induced, air-pouch granuloma of mice, and the two ferulic acid esters, are reported to have antitumor properties. Guggulu resin has a curative effect in children with Fasioliasis and Schistosomiasis.

Because of its varied pharmacological effects on lipid metabolism, thyroid hormone homeo-statsis, female reproductive tissues, and endogenous nuclear hormone receptors, guggulu and its constituents are increasingly being used as dietary supplements or fast-moving consumer goods for their anti-obesity and other health-modulating effects.

Guggulipid is a standardized product of ethyl acetate extract of the oleo gum resin guggulu.

Marketed products

Traditional—Yogaraja guggulu, punarnavadi guggulu, pushkara guggulu, shonti guggulu, triphala guggulu.
Proprietary—Diabecon, Koflet, Rumalaya Forte, Reosto, Immunocare, etc.

Kalmegh

Kalmegh refers to *Andrographis paniculata* (Burm f) Wall ex Nees, Family, Acanthaceae.

Synonym

Justicia latebrosa Russ, *J. paniculata* f, *J. stricta* Lam ex Steud.
It grows widely and is cultivated in tropical and sub tropical Asia, South East Asia, and India. The dried aerial parts, preferably the stems and leaves are used in traditional medicine.

Common Vernacular names

English: Green Chiretta, Andrographis
Sanskrit: Bhunimba, Kirata
Hindi: Kirayata, Mahatikta

Tamil: Nilavembu
Telugu: Nela vemu

Morphology

The plant is an herbaceous annual, growing erect to a height of 1 m. The stem is acutely quad-rangular, much branched with simple, opposite, lanceolate, glabrous leaves, about 2–12 cm long and 1–3 cm wide with an acute apex, entire slightly undulate margin with a bractiform short peti-ole. Inflorescence is terminal and axillary in peduncle, 10–30 mm long, with a short pedicel and a small bract. Fruit is an erect linear oblong capsule with small seeds.

The drug made up of dried aerial parts consists of broken, crisp dark green leaves, stems, capsules and occasionally even small flowers. Its odor is slight, characteristic with an intensely biter taste.

Chemical constituents

Principal constituents are diterpene lactones, which occur both free and as glycosides—these are andrographolide, deoxyandrographolide, 11,12-didehydro-14-deoxy-andrographolide, neo andrographolide, andrographiside, deoxy andrographiside, and andropaniside.

Traditional uses

As per Ayurveda, it pacifies pitta and kapha. It is a bitter tonic, febrifuge, and hepatoprotective given as a digestive, for liver and gall bladder protection in jaundice. It is indicated for anemia,

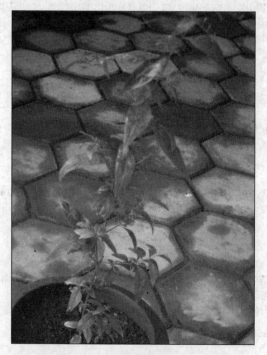

Figure 9.7 *Andrographis paniculata*

bacillary dysentery, bronchitis, coughs, fevers, malaria, mouth ulcers, sores, tuberculosis, and in venomous snake bites. The drug is administered for acne, diarrhea, and general debility. It is said to reduce swelling, skin allergies, and urinary tract infection. Other folkloric usage is for the treatment of colic, pelvic inflammatory disease, bacillary dysentery, bronchitis, chicken pox, eczema and burns.

Pharmacology

Leaf ethanol extract is reported with antibacterial and antifungal activity. Leaf aqueous extract inhibited HIV-antigen-positive H9 cells. Dehydroandrographolide is shown to be inhibitory to HIV–I cells in human lymphocytes. Ethanol extract of the aerial parts is reported to cause non-specific stimulation of immune response, which is more effective than that produced by purified andrographolide indicating it to be a synergistic effect of several constituents.

It is also antipyretic and a 50% ethanol extract is found to be inhibitory to *Plasmodium berghei* demonstrating its anti malarial activity. While the powdered whole herb has shown anti diar-rhoeal activity, deoxy andrographolide, andrographolide and neo andrographolide are reported to show anti-inflammatory activity.

Ethanol extract of the aerial parts has delayed occurrence of respiratory failure and death in experimental mice poisoned with cobra venom. This is found to be due to its muscarinic effect. It has also shown cardioprotective, anti-hyperglycemic, anti-hypertensive, and chemopreventive effects.

Aerial parts and andrographolide are reported to be anti-hepatotoxic and much more effec-tive than silymarin.

Kalmegh is clinically indicated for the treatment of common cold, uncomplicated sinusitis, pharyngotonsillitis, pneumonia, and bronchitis. Reduction in the severity of urinary tract infec-tion brought about by the herb was found to be comparable to that of co-trimoxazole or nor-floxacin. Aerial parts were found to be clinically effective in the treatment of upper respiratory tract infections and urinary tract infections. In bacillary dysentery and enteritis, a combination of andrographolide and neo andrographolide was found to be more effective than furazolidine or chloramphenicol. The herb administration has brought about symptomatic relief from infec-tious hepatitis.

Marketed products

Traditional—Nilavembu kudineer, nilavembu chooranam
Proprietery—Kalmegh liver drops, Air-defense caps, Immunoshield

Ashoka

Ashoka refers to the plant *Saraca asoca* (Roxb.) de Wilde, Family: Caesalpinaceae

Synonym

Saraca indica auct. non Linn.

It is found throughout India in evergreen forests up to an elevation of about 750 m in the central and eastern Himalayas, West Bengal, and South India. One of the most sacred trees of Hindus and Buddhists, their flowers are used for religious ceremonies and temple decorations. It is cultivated as an ornamental and avenue tree throughout tropical India.

Common vernacular names

English: Ashoka
Hindi: Asok
Sanskrit: Gosasokah, Asokah
Tamil: Asogam
Telugu: Vanjalamu, Asokamu

Morphology

It is a medium-sized handsome, evergreen tree up to 9 m height with numerous spreading and drooping glabrous branches. Leaves are paripinnate, 30–60 cm long having 2–3 pairs of lanceolate leaflets, which are oblong, lanceolate, and parallel veined. Flowers are orange yellow in dense corymbs and with great fragrance. Fruits are leathery, flat black pods, compressed seeds —ellipsoid, oblong, compressed. The bark is dark brown with a warty surface and the freshly cut ends are pale yellowish red turning red on exposure to air. Bark is channeled, smooth with circular lenticles and transversely ridged and sometimes cracked.

Chemical constituents

Bark is rich in tannins, constituted of (-) epicatechin, procyanidin, β -2,11'-deoxyprocyanidin B, (+) catechin, (24E)-24- methyl-cholesta-5-en-3-β-ol (22 E, 21Z)-24-ethycholesta-5,22 dien-33-ol,(24 E)-24- ethylcholesta-5-en-3-β-ol, leucopelargonidin-3-O- β –D glucoside, leucopelargonidin, and leucocyanidin. Five lignan glycosides, lyoniside, nudiposide, 5-methoxy-9-β-xylopyranosyl-(−)-isolariciresinol, icariside E3, and schizandriside, and three flavonoids, (−)-epicatechin,

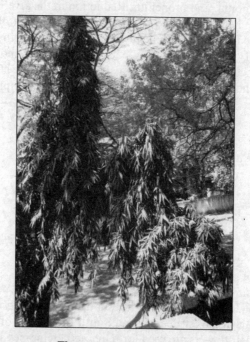

Figure 9.8 *Saraca asoca*

epiafzelechin-(4β→8)-epicatechin, and procyanidin B2, together with β-sitosterol have been isolated form the bark.

The flowers are constituted of mixtures of anthocyanins and other flavonoids including quercetin, kaempferol-3-0-β-D-glucoside, quercetin-3-0-β-D-glucoside, apigenin-7-0-β-D-glucoside, pelargonidin-3, 5- diglucoside, cyanidin-3, 5-diglucoside, palmitic, stearic, linolenic, linoleic, β and γ sitosterols, leucocyanidin, and gallic acid. Seed and pod contains oleic, linoleic, palmitic, and stearic acids.

Traditional uses

Bark, leaves, flowers, and seeds are used in traditional medicine. Bark is bitter, astringent, refrigerant, anthelmintic, styptic, stomachic, febrifuge, and demulcent. It is used as a uterine sedative and tonic, in dyspepsia, colic, ulcers, menorrhagia, leucorroea, and in the cure of pimples. In general, it is given in the treatment of all disorders related to the menstrual cycle.

Leaves are used in the management of gastric distress; flowers are used as a uterine tonic, in hemorrhagic dysentery, syphilis, hemorrhoids, and in diabetes. Seeds are used in treating bone fractures, strangury, and vesical calculi.

Ashoka and its plant parts are used in various traditional and folkloric recipes for vitiated conditions of pitta. Leaf juice mixed with cumin seeds is given for relief from gastric distress. The bark powder is consumed with boiled milk as a uterine tonic and to stop abnormal uterine bleeding and in general it is given in the treatment of all disorders related to the menstrual cycle.

Pharmacology

Bark extracts are reportedly associated with spasmogenic, oxytocic, uterotonic, anti-bacterial, anti-implantation, anti-tumor, anti-progestational, and antiestrogenic activity. They also have a stimulatory effect on the endometrium and the ovarian tissue.

Alcoholic extract of the bark is found to be oxytocic, enhancing the frequency and duration of uterine contractions unlike tonic contractions due to ergot alkaloids.

Extracts of different parts of asoka are found to be antibacterial, anti fungal, anti diabetic, and CNS depressant. Flower extracts have shown anti-cancer activity.

Marketed preparations

Traditional—ashokarista, asokaghrita
Proprietary—Evecare, Menosan, Lucogyl.

Tulsi

Refers to *Ocimum sanctum* Linn. Family: Labiatae

Synonym

O. hirsutum, O. album, O. tometosum, O. viride, O. inodorum, O. monachorum, O. nelsonii, O. vergatum, O. tenuiflorum, O. flexuosum, O. frutescens, Machosma tenuiflorum (L) Heynhold.

The herbaceous annual is found throughout India and parts of north and eastern Africa, Hainan island, Taiwan, and China. Most sacred of all medicinal plants in India, Tulsi is an integral part of all traditional and religious rituals in India. It is cultivated and grown as a pot herb in almost every Hindu household. Two varieties of Tulsi are known—green leaved one called Sri or Vishnu tulasi is more common than the purple leaved Krishna tulasi.

Common vernacular names

English: Sacred basil, holy basil
Sanskrit: Vishnupriya, Tulsi
Hindi: Kala-tulsi, baranda
Tamil: Karuttulasi, tulasi
Telugu: Tulasi

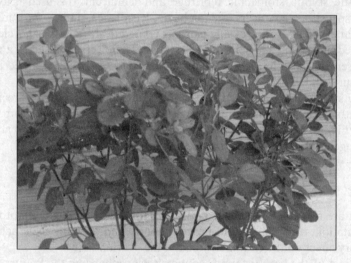

Figure 9.9 *Ocimum sanctum* – Sri Tulasi

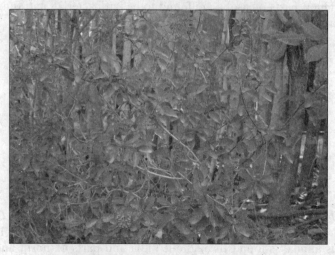

Figure 9.10 *Ocimum sanctum* – Krishna Tulasi

Morphology

It is an erect, much branched softly pubescent undershrub growing to a height of about 1 m. Leaves are simple, opposite, oblong, minutely glanded, 2–8 cm long, 1–3 cm wide with an acute apex and rounded base. Petioles are hairy. Whole herb has an aromatic characteristic taste and a slightly pungent aromatic taste.

Chemical constituents

The plant is reported to contain tannins (4.6%), essential oil (0.4–0.8%)—composed of eugenol (62%), methyl eugenol, α & β – caryophyllene, bornyl acetate, neral, methyl chavicol, linalool and 1,8-Cineole. Composition of the essential oil varies according to geographical distribution and variety. Leaves also contain ursolic acid, campesterol, cholesterol, stigmasterol, β-sitosterol, and β-carotene.

Traditional uses

Ancient knowledge of its diverse medicinal virtues was possibly the reason for its inclusion in all religious and traditional rituals to medicate water. The plant is a bitter, acrid, aromatic, stomachic, demulcent, diaphoretic, expectorant, febrifuge, vermifuge, and digestive. Leaf infusion is given as a stomachic in gastric disorders in children. Root decoction is used as a diaphoretic in malaria and seeds are used in urinary tract infections. It is used in the treatment of arthritis, bronchitis, common cold, diabetes, fever, influenza, peptic ulcer, and rheumatism. It is also indicated in cardiopathy, leucoderma, asthma, vomiting, lumbago, genito-urinary disorders, and ringworm and skin diseases.

Pharmacology

Alcoholic extract of the leaves is reported to be anti-inflammatory, anti-pyretic, anti-spasmodic, hypoglycemic, immunostimulant, anti-bacterial, and anti-fungal in experimental animals. It has shown significant anti-stress effect in several *in vitro* and *in vivo* assays. Animals that received the aqueous extracts in general showed a greater resistance. The seed-fixed oil is analgesic and aqueous extract reportedly potentiated sleeping time induced by hexobarbital. Also the leaf extract was found to be protective against acetyl salicylic acid induced gastric ulcers in *in vivo* studies. It reduces serum thyroxine concentration and inhibits hepatic lipid peroxidation.

Clinical studies have shown that aqueous extract of tulsi relieves labored breathing in asthma and there has been significant reduction of glucose levels by tulsi extracts when compared to control groups. It is also found to be effective in the treatment of viral hepatitis.

Marketed products

Traditional—Tribhuvana kirti rasa, muktadi mahanjana, mukta pancamrta rasa, multadi mahanjana, manasamitravataka.
Proprietary—Organic tulasi, aller-breathe, bio-immune.

Valerian

Refers to underground parts of *Valeriana officinalis* L (Sensulato) Fam: Valerianaceae.

Synonym

V. alternifolia, V. excelsa, Poir, *V. sylvestris* Grosch, *V. edulis, V. flaurei* Briquet (Japanese valerian). About 200 species of valerian are known of which only a few are used medicinally. *Valerian officinalis* includes an extremely polymorphous group of polyploid subspecies having closely similar morphological characteristics. Natural populations of various species and subspecies (*V. officinalis* ssp. *collina,* ssp. *sambucifolia* etc) are found distributed throughout temperate and sub polar Eurasian zones in Belgium, China, France, Netherlands, Nepal, India, and South West Asia. Dilpoid, tetraploid, and octaploid types are cultivated as a medicinal plant in several European countries and in the United States.

Twelve species of Valerian are found in India of which *V. wallichii* DC (Syn: *V. jatamansi* Jones) and *V. hardwickii* are recorded as Indian Valerian. These species are found in the alpine Himalayas.

Nardostachys jatamansii is a related Indian species and an ancient reputed ayurvedic drug of Indo-Greek trade. Used interchangeably with European valerian, the essential oil of this drug is much more agreeable in taste and odor and has been much prized in perfumery world over for its woody aromatic odor.

Common vernacular names

English: Cat's valerian, Garden heliotrope
Sanskrit: Tagara, Kalanusari

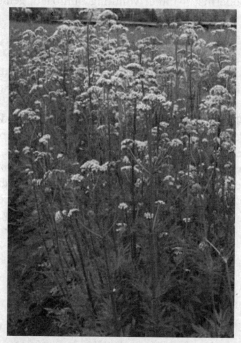

(Photo courtesy: http://www.bluestem.ca/perennials-valeriana-officinalis.htm)

Figure 9.11 *Valeriana wallichii*

Hindi: Mushkbala, sugandhabala, taga-manthoda
Tamil: Grandhi tagarai
Telugu: Tagaramu

Morphology

V. officinalis is a tall, hardy perennial herb with an underground portion made up of a vertical rhizome bearing numerous rootlets and stolons. Stem is hollow, cylindrical, and channeled of about 2 m in height. It is branched in the terminal region bearing opposite exstipulate, pinnatisect, cauline leaves with clasping petioles. Inflorescence is a raceme of cymes whose flowers are small pink or white. Fruits are oblong, four-ridged, single-seeded achenes.

Valerian consists of roots, rhizomes, and stolons carefully dried at temperature not more than 40°C. The erect rhizomes, entire or sliced are yellowish brown and it is accompanied by broken fragments of roots. The dried rhizome occurring as 2–5 cm long, 1–3 cm wide pieces is sometimes crowned by remains of stem bases and scale leaves. It may bear occasional short horizontal branches or scars of roots. Breaking with a short and horny fracture the drug is internally yellowish white. Root fragments are cylindrical, brownish grey externally, striated longitudinally and may bear fibrous lateral rootlets. They are brittle and when broken show a narrow central stele and a wide bark. Normally odorless, the drug develops its characteristic odor during drying and storage due to hydrolytic changes. It has a camphoraceous slightly bitter taste.

Indian valerian largely consisting of dried roots and rhizomes of *V. wallichii*. A tetraploid, it is an erect perennial of about 1 m height with pinnate, divided leaves and bears clusters of pink or white flowers. It has a large root with short rhizomes. The rhizomes collected in autumn from 2-year-old plants is dried and it occurs as yellowish brown pieces 4–8 cm long and 1 cm thick along with some root fragments. The drug is somewhat flattened and has leaf scars and root scars. Internally it shows a dark pith surrounded by visible xylem bundles and thin dark bark. It has a characteristic odor and a bitter camphoraceous odor.

Nardostachys jatamansii yields dried rhizomes attached a to large root stock. The rhizome pieces are short, thick, dark grey with reddish brown remains of leaf petioles. It has an agreeable odor and a bitter aromatic taste.

Constituents

Valerian contains about 0.2–2.8% volatile oil principally constituted of bornyl acetate and bornyl isovalerate. Other significant constituents of the oil are β-caryophyllene, bornyl formate, eugenyl isovalerate, isoeugenyl isovalerate, eugenol, cyclopentane sesquiterpenes—valeranone, valerenal, valerenic acid, and acetoxyvalerenic acid. Volatile oil composition is variable in different sub species of valerian. For example, *V. edulis* and *V. wallichii* lack valerenic acid. Japanese valerian has as much as 8% volatile oil, however, not similar to that of *V. officinalis*.

Valepotriates are another important group of constituents in Valerian species. First discovered from *V. wallichii,* these are non-glycosidic bicyclic iridoid monoterpene epoxy-iridoid esters. Ranging from 0.05–0.67% in different species, >90% of valpotriate content is made up of valtrate and isovaltrate. Smaller quantities of dihydrovaltrate, isovaleroxy-hydroxy dihydrovaltrate, 1-acevaltrate are also found. Valepotriates are unstable due to their epoxy structure and losses occur fairly rapidly on storage or due to improper drying conditions. Such undesirable processing may result in the formation of baldrinal, homobaldrinal and valtroxal as degradation products.

Quartenary alkaloids of about 0.05–0.1% have also been reported from the dried roots.

Nardostachys jatamansii (Syn: *Nardostachys grandiflora*) yields upto 2% volatile oil called spikenard oil, constituted of α-pinene, β-pinene, limonene, dihydroazulenes, α-gurjunene, β-gurjunene, seychelane, β-maaliene, nardol, nardostachnol apart form sesquiterpenes, spiro-jatamol, patchouli alcohol, nor seychelanone, α, β patchoulenes, jatamol A & B, jatamansic acid among others. Terpene coumarins angelicin, jatamansin, lignan and neo lignans such as (+)-hydroxypinoresinol and virolin and terpenoid ester nardostachysin are the other reported constituents of Jatamansii rhizomes.

Nardostachys jatamansii does not contain valepotriates.

Traditional uses

In western herbal medicine valerian has been used as a carminative and digestive aid. It has been used as an anti-spasmodic along with papaverine, belladonna, in spastic conditions of the smooth muscle as in spastic colitis. It is popularly prescribed for its sedative effects. Large quantities of valerian are used in perfumery.

Indian valerian species are indicated in traditional medicine for hysteria, hypochondriasis, and nervous troubles as an ingredient of several ayurvedic formulations.

Folk use indications are for epilepsy, headache, urinary tract disorders, throat inflammation, emmenagogue, anti-perspirant, diuretic and as an anodyne.

Valerian is available in several dosage forms such as expressed juice, tincture, dried extracts, and other galenical preparations. Externally it is used as a bath additive.

Nardostachys jatamansii, commonly called "Jatamansi" referring to the braided external appearance of its roots, has been used for many centuries in indigenous medicine as a sedative in nervous disorders. In combination with other herbs it is given in the treatment of muscle pains, dysmenorrhoea, headache, and in some forms of epilepsy. An ancient and reputed drug of Indo-Greek trade it is a constituent of the Spikenard ointment much regarded by ancient Romans for its medicinal properties. Though used interchangeably with European valerian, the essential oil of jatamansi is much more agreeable in taste and odor and has been much prized in perfumery world over for its woody aromatic odor.

Pharmacology

Aqueous and alcoholic extracts have shown sedative activity with *in vitro* studies establishing the binding of valerian extract constituents to γ–amino butyric acid (GABA) receptors and adenosine receptors (that are barbiturate and benzodiazepine binding receptors). *In vivo* studies have shown that the sedative activity is due to the presence of high concentrations of glutamine in the extracts. It is known that glutamine is taken up by nerve terminals and then metabolized to GABA. Spasmolytic activity is reported to be due to valtrate and dihydrovaltrate, which are demonstrated to act both centrally—in the direct relaxation of smooth muscles, and locally by regulating the entry of calcium into smooth muscle cells.

Clinical data supports the sedative effect of the aqueous root extract. Though the sedative effect is attributed to the sesquiterpene constituents of the volatile oil, it is believed to be a synergistic effect of many constituents.

Thus valerian is indicated for use as a sleep-promoting agent in the treatment of nervous excitation and in anxiety-induced sleep disturbances as a milder alternative to strong synthetic sedatives.

Dried alcohol extract of jatamansii is reported with anti-microbial, anti-oxidant, anti-arrhythmic, dopaminergic, hypnotic, neuroprotective, hepatoprotective, negative ionotropic, and negative chronotropic activity. In experimental animals, it has also shown a beneficial hypolipidaemic effect. Spikenard oil has shown anti-convulsant, hypotensive, and tranquillizing effect. Jatamansi acts primarily upon the nervous system, inducing a natural sleep, without any adverse effect upon awakening, and appears to lack the stimulating effects that a certain number of people experience with Valerian. The most common usage of Jatamansi is as a nervine sedative in the treatment of insomnia, or to treat chronic irritability and nervousness, with exhaustion and debility.

Marketed products

Traditional—Dhanwantartaila, mahanarayana taila, devadarvadyarista
Proprietary—Sundown valerian capsules, valerian root tea, valerian root tincture

Artemisia

Refers to *Artemisia annua* Linn., Family: Compositae,

Synonym

Artemisia chamomila

It is native to Eurasia from south-east Europe to Vietnam and India. It has become naturalized in many countries—Argentina, Austria, Czech Republic, France, Germany, Hungary, Italy,

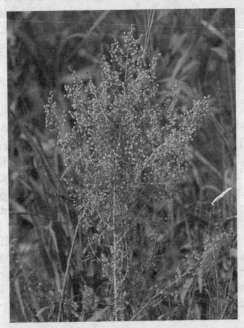

(Photo courtesy: Wikipedia commons)

Figure 9.12 *Artemisia annua*

Poland, Slovakia, Spain, Switzerland, and the United States. It is cultivated on a large scale in temperate areas of China, Vietnam, Former USSR, Turkey, Iran, Afghanistan, and Australia.

An ancient herb of Chinese medicine called "Quingao," it yields artemisinin, a sesquiterpene lactone, currently in great demand because of its effectiveness against drug-resistant forms of malaria. Of about 400 species of Artemisia, artemisinin is found only in *Artemisia annua, A. apiacea and A. lancea*. These plants are the only source of artemisinin with chemical synthesis being too complicated.

In India, it is being cultivated on an experimental scale in temperate and sub-tropical conditions.

Common vernacular names

English: Sweet worm wood, sweet sagewort
Chinese: Quingao

Morphology

Artemisia is an aromatic plant found as a pervasive weed in China. It is thus found both in wild and is also cultivated. It is a single-stemmed, hairless, sweetly aromatic annual growing to a height of 1 m. The stem is erect, ribbed, brownish, or violet brown in colour with very slender and glabrous branches. Leaves are fern-like, 3-pinnatisect, 3–5 cm long, 2–4 cm wide with upper leaves being 2-pinnatisect, smaller and sessile. Inflorescence is a compound raceme with the tiny flower heads being inconspicuous greenish or yellowish, globose, 2–2.5 mm in diameter having a camphor-like scent. Flowers are hermaphrodite, disciform, and made up of outer filiform florets (female) and inner disc like bisexual florets. The involucre of bracts around the flower head are over lapping and hairless. Outer bracts are green, linear-oblong with inner bracts shiny and oval in shape. Fruit is a yellow to brownish, small and thin-walled cypsela, 0.6–0.8 mm long, with a shiny surface marked with vertical grooves and bears a single seed. Oil glands are present on leaves, stems, and florets.

Constituents

The plant yields a sweet-smelling essential oil of about 0.01–0.5% composed of camphor (44%), germacrene (16%), trans-pinocarveol, β-selenin (9%), β-caryopyllene (9%), artemisia ketone (3%), α-terpinene, β–phellendrene, 1,4-cineole, 1,8-cineole, β–thujone, nerol, α–phenanthrene, citral, chamazulene, and citronellal. The concentration and composition of the volatile oil is dependant on the drug source with the Chinese chemotype being rich in irregular monoterpenes like artimisia ketone and Vietnamese chemotype being rich in germacrene and camphor.

Search for effective anti-malarials in the 1970s resulted in the isolation of artemisinin, a bitter sesquiterpene lactone. Called "Quinghaosu," chemically it has a 1, 2, 4-trioxane structure with a unique endo-peroxide bridge without a nitrogen containing ring system. The endoperoxide moiety is essential for activity. It is isolated in the yield of 0.06–0.16% from the aerial parts with artemisinic acid (0.4%), dihydroartemisinin, arteannuin A & B (0.1%) as the other sesquiterpene constituents.

The plant contains several methylated flavonoids—artemetin, chrysosplenetin, quercetagetin, eupatorin, and castian.

Traditional uses

The plant has been used in Chinese traditional medicine, where for centuries it has been used in the treatment of malaria, fevers, skin diseases, jaundice, and haemorrhoids in combination with other herbs.

As an herbal tea and infusion, the herb is an affordable and effective anti-malarial in the tropics and countries such as China and Vietnam where it is commercially available. Leaves are used as an anti-periodic, anti-septic, digestive, and febrifuge. Leaf infusion is used internally to treat fevers, colds, and diarrhea. Externally the leaves are given in the form of a poultice for headache, nosebleeds, boils, and abscesses. Seeds are used in the treatment of flatulence, indigestion, and night sweats. Essential oil obtained on steam distillation of the fresh aerial parts is widely used in the pharmaceutical, cosmetic, and flavoring industries.

Pharmacology

Artimisinin isolated from the leafy tops is selectively toxic to the asexual erythrocyte stage of various species of the malarial parasite like *Plasmodium falciparum*, *P. vivax* both *in vivo* and *in vitro*. It is effective against chloroquine-resistant strains of the parasite even at nanomolar concentrations. Several clinical trials have shown it to be 90% effective and more successful than standard drugs. It has been used in China for the treatment of malaria, especially cerebral malaria. Artemesinin and its semi-synthetic derivatives act as blood schizonticides. Artemether (methyl ether), arteether (β-ethyl ether) and artesunate (12 α-succinate), are the semisynthetic derivatives widely used as anti-malarials in the form of tablets, intramuscular, intravenous, and rectal applications.

Sodium artesunate and sodium artelinate are more water soluble and can be given orally or by injection. Artemisinin is given in combination with other anti-malarials like lumefantrine, amodiaquine, and mefloquine. It is also found to be effective against several species of rodent malarial parasite.

The sequiterpene enriched extract of Artemisia aerial parts is reported with anti-ulcerogenic activity and the essential oil is apoptotic to hepatocarcinoma cells (SMMC- 7721) *in vitro*. Anti fungal, insecticidal, and anti-convulsant activity of the essential oil is also reported. Artemisinin and flavonoid quercetagetin have shown inhibitory activity in several human tumor cell lines.

Artemisinin is reported to be a selective phytotoxin and it is also reported with anti-viral activity. Artemisinin, dihydroartemisinin, and arteether have demonstrated suppressed humoral immune response in experimental animals.

Artesunate is found to be inhibitory to chronic myeloid leukemia cells and breast cancer cells *in vitro*. It is also found to be anti-angiogenic.

Marketed products

Herb Pharm

Chirata

Refers to *Swertia chirayita* (Roxb ex.Fleming) Karsten, Family: Gentianaceae

Synonym

Swertia chirata (Wall) CB Clarke.

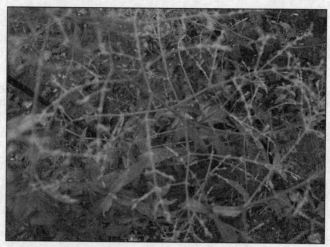

(Photo courtesy: Satheesan.vn, Wikimedia Commons)

Figure 9.13 *Swertia chirayita*

The plant is found in temperate Himalayas at 1200–1300 m altitude from Kashmir to Bhutan and Khasi hills in Meghalaya. The whole plant was held in high esteem and has been used as medicine for centuries in ancient India.

Common vernacular names

English: Brown or white chiretta
Sanskrit: Kairata, Kirata-tikta, nepalinimbah
Hindi: Chirayata, nepalinum
Tamil: Cirattakuchi
Telugu: Nela vemu

Macroscopy

Chirata is an erect annual herb of 80–110 cm long with a stout robust stem, which is rounded in the lower part and branching toward the top. It is about 6 mm thick, yellowish brown, glabrous and slightly winged. Leaves are 7–9 cm long, 3.5–4 cm wide, sessile, elliptic, acute, and seven veined flowers; tetramerous are greenish yellow with two glands on each lobe of corolla. Capsule is sessile, oblong with minute, irregularly ovoid seeds. Root is small, 5–10 cm long, twisted tapering with few rootlets. Its large continuous pith, both of the stem and the root, dark in colour separates easily thus helping to distinguish it from other species of this genus. The whole plant is collected after flowering, dried and bundled before being sent to the market. The dried drug consists of dried brownish stems with root and leaves intact. The powdered plant material is odorless and extremely bitter in taste.

Stems form the major portion of the drug and though the entire plant is used in traditional medicine, root is described as more powerful in terms of its properties.

Constituents

The drug contains not less than 1.3% bitter principles constituted of amarogentin (0.04%) and amaroswerin (0.03%). Other important constituents are xanthone derivatives—more than 20 in number such as chiratol, methyl beliidifolin, decissatin, 7-O-methyl swertianin, mangiferin, swertianin, swertinine, chiratinine, triterpenoids—masilinic acd and its trisaccharide ester swercinctoside, chiratenol, gammacer-16-en-3β-ol, 21-α-H-hep-22(29)-en-3β-ol, swertenol, episwertenol, pichierenol, kairatenol, oleanolic acid, gammacer-16-en-β-ol, swertanone, swertenol, ursolic acid, secoiridoid glycosides- swertiamarin, gentiopicroside, alkaloids- gentianine, gentiocrucine, enicoflavine, Triterpene alcohol – taraxerol, β-amyrin, lupeol.

Traditional uses

The entire plant and the roots are used as bitter tonic in the treatment of fever and for curing skin diseases. For its bitter, cooling and light properties, it is given in combination with other drugs in diarrhea, anemia, liver dysfunction, and bronchial asthma.

Pharmacology

The widespread use of the drug in traditional medicine reflects its pharmacological importance. Extracts of the drug are reported with anthelemintic, anti-tubercular, anti-fungal anti-inflammatory, anti-convulsant, cardiostimulant, CNS depressant, hepatoprotective, hypnotic, laxative, vermifuge and anti cholinergic properties. Seco iridoid glycosides have hypoglycemic and antipyretic properties.

Marketed products

Traditional—Mahasudarsana kvatha, Sudarsana curna, Kiratatiktadi kvatha, Bhunimbadi kvatha, Tiktapancaka kvatha, Kiratadi taila
Proprietary—Zandu sudarshan, pigmento, atic care, ayush -64, diabecon, mensturyl syrup, melicon ointment are proprietary preparations.

CONCLUSION

The present market for herbal products is growing exponentially and there is a huge demand for standardized, approved products of established safety and efficacy. This huge demand, dwindling plant resource wealth, reckless exploitation of natural plant wealth despite strict curtailing regulations in place, and the lack of precise regulatory control over the available vast range of plant based products are driving the extensive commercialization of the herbal drug market. Plant identification is critical and knowledge of the source, varieties, important constituents, traditional and clinical uses is an essential prerequisite for herbal drug development. Salient features of some traditional herbal drugs have been presented.

REVIEW QUESTIONS

Essay Questions

1. Present a comparative account of herbal drugs, Andrographis and Artemisia.
2. Write an essay on the salient features of Lehsun.
3. Discuss the significance of Guggulu as a herbal drug supplement.

Short Notes

1. Ayurvedic drug names–the disparity
2. Shankapushpi
3. Tulasi
4. Valerian
5. Punarnava

10 Herbal Cosmetics

CHAPTER OBJECTIVES

Introduction

Trade in Herbal Cosmetics

Indian Market

Herbals in Cosmetics

Importance of Herbals in Hair and Skin
Care Products

INTRODUCTION

The word cosmetic is derived from Greek meaning 'beautify and arrange' referring both to its cleansing and beautifying property. Cosmetics are defined as preparations designed to beautify the body by direct application. They are intended to be applied to the human body for cleansing, beautifying, promoting attractiveness or altering the appearance without affecting the body's structure or function.

According to the Drugs and Cosmetics Act of India, 1940, cosmetic may be defined as any substance intended to be rubbed, poured, sprinkled or otherwise applied to a human being for cleansing, beautifying or promoting attractiveness.

The concept of beauty and cosmetics is as ancient as mankind and civilization. The history of cosmetics spans at least 6,000 years of human history. Decorating the face and body is an activity that is among the oldest, most widespread and persistent of human behaviours. The ancient science of cosmetology is believed to have originated in India and Egypt, with the earliest records of cosmetic substances and their application dating back to Circa 2500 and 1550 B.C. to the Indus Valley civilization. There is evidence that highly advanced ideas of self-beautification and innumerable cosmetics were used both by men and women in ancient India. Many references to the use of natural preparations for cosmetic purposes are found in classical poetry and literature of ancient civilizations of India, China and other parts of Asia. Such cosmetic practices were intertwined with daily routine, all directed towards the larger goal of achieving longevity and good health. The use of cosmetics thus traceable back to prehistoric times has spread to all races and continents. Throughout history, cosmetics have been used by people for camouflaging flaws, improving overall appearance and enhancing attractiveness.

Despite the belief of certain societies such as in post-medieval Europe that usage of cosmetics was immoral, the use of cosmetics became freely accepted and is today universal. The empirical preparation of cosmetics being as old as medicine and pharmacy, increasing scientific interest in the principles involved has, in recent times converted the craft into an exact science. The stress was in creating preparations of great uniformity, stability and aesthetic attractiveness. Lending itself to the field of pharmacy, the result was carefully compounded preparations such as the vanishing cream in the late 19th century. The cosmetic industry has gone through a state of change with greater stress on dermatopharmaceuticals or therapeutically active cosmetics. Today cosmetic science is a combination of many disciplines. In the west cosmetics were scientifically prepared in France in the 1900s spawning a huge industry which has grown in leaps and bounds.

Today cosmetics are considered a necessity and not a luxury. The desire to appear physically attractive and young is universal what with the world having become a global village with satellite-assisted communications and wide-coverage television channels. The widespread consumerism, flourishing fashion/film industry fuelling the desire for good looks and expanding economy in general account for the high usage of cosmetics. A pleasing appearance drawing attention to one's personality is considered essential as it enhances self-esteem and build's an individual's morale. Conforming to an accepted standard of outward agreeableness has become imperative in today's competitive world and society in general.

The importance of cosmetics has grown tremendously in today's society with the motivation to use them being also skin health preservation. In view of the current extent of industrialization, raising levels of environmental pollution, improper food habits and unhealthy lifestyles, cosmetics have become absolutely essential to maintain healthy appearance of hair, skin etc.

TRADE IN HERBAL COSMETICS

The 21st century saw the development of large cosmetic companies and the value of the industry is growing to billions of dollars. The manufacture of cosmetics is currently dominated by a small number of multinational corporations that originated in the early 20th century, but the distribution and sale of cosmetics is spread among a wide range of different businesses. Cosmetics like any other designer product are now sold on brand image with consumers paying not only for the product but also for the brand. Western brands like Revlon, Elizabeth Arden and Asian ones like Biotherm, Amorepacific, Shahnaz, Lotus and Biotique are a few of the leading brands.

The market volume of the cosmetics industry in the United States, Europe and Japan is about € 70 billion per year. The cosmetic industry in Germany generated sales of € 12.6 billion at retail sales in 2008. The German cosmetic industry is the third in the world, after Japan and the United States. In Germany, this industry has grown nearly 5% in one year, from 2007 to 2008. Its exports reached € 5.8 billion in 2008, whereas the imports of cosmetics totaled € 3 billion.

The worldwide cosmetics and perfume industry currently generates an estimated annual turnover of US$ 170 billion (according to Eurostaf, May 2007). Products that claim to renew cells, minimize pores and restore hydration have created an US $83 billion worldwide market.

Europe is the leading market, representing approximately € 63 billion, while sales in France reached €6.5 billion in 2006, according to FIPAR (Fédération des Industries de la Parfumerie, the French federation for the perfume industry). France is another country in which the cosmetic industry plays an important role, both nationally and internationally. According to data from

2008, the cosmetic industry has risen constantly in France for 40 consecutive years. In 2006, this industrial sector reached a record level of € 6.5 billion. Famous cosmetic brands of France include Vichy, Yves Saint Laurent, Yves Rocher and many others.

In the European cosmetic market, the Italian cosmetic industry has an important share with an overall contribution of € 9 billion in 2007. Unlike the predominantly make-up and facial care products of the US market, the Italian cosmetic market as in other European countries is significantly represented by hair and body care products.

With the entry of internet companies, several cosmetic manufacturers are now able to sell their products online, even in countries where they lack a physical marketing presence. This has largely aided in the rapid expansion of the cosmetic market worldwide. The global resurgence of interest in plant-derived drugs and other products and disillusionment with harsh synthetic chemicals in cosmetics have shifted the consumer market towards herbal cosmetics. Cosmetics containing herbal ingredients and/or natural products are now in popular demand. The beauty business is overwhelmingly taken over by the herbal cosmetics industry as organic and Ayurvedic recipes gain precedence over chemical concoctions. Many cosmetics of today originated in Asian countries, especially the herbal-based cosmetics and today India is a leading presence in the cosmetic business.

INDIAN MARKET

According to the Associated Chambers of Commerce and Industry of India (ASSOCHAM) the projected market size of the cosmetics industry is currently estimated at Rs.10,000 crores. It is expected to double to Rs.20,000 crores by 2014.

In India, the economic boom of the 1990s and victorious emergence of Indian women in international beauty pageantry events has witnessed a spiralling increase in cosmetic consumption in the country. The growing cosmetic sector has managed to reach even the rural markets. The Indian cosmetic industry had rapid growth growing at a CAGR of around 7.5% between 2006 and 2008. Enhanced purchasing power of the average Indian and greater fashion consciousness could be behind the continued growth of the Indian cosmetic industry from 2009 to 2012.

The Indian cosmetics market – defined as skin care, hair care, colour cosmetics, fragrances and oral care segments – stood at an estimated $2.5 billion in 2008 and is expected to grow at 7%. Today the success of Indian cosmetic players such as Himalaya, Dabur, Lotus, VLCC, Biotique, to name a few, forecasts the large potential growth of this sector.

In 2009, the cosmetics industry registered sales of INR 356.6 billion (US $ 7.1 billion) despite the global economic recession. The Indian cosmetic market, traditionally a stronghold of a few major Indian players like Lakme and Ponds, has seen a lot of foreign entrants to the market within the last decade. The size of the Indian cosmetics industry globally is US $274 billion, while that of the national industry is US $4.6 billion. Leading cosmetics brands in the country today are Lakmé, Revlon, Oriflame Cosmetics S.A, The L'Oréal Group, Chambor, Maybelline, Avon Products, Inc., Make-up Art Cosmetics or MAC Cosmetics, ColourBar Cosmetics and Street Wear.

Several cosmetics manufacturers in India who catered to the domestic market are slowly expanding into the international market due to the greater global demand for herb-based cosmetics from India.

HERBALS IN COSMETICS

The growth of the cosmetic industry in the west was the result of meticulous study of the age-old cosmetic preparations by cosmetic chemists. There is elaborate literature on the scores of chemical ingredients used and their physicochemical properties, and cosmetics were classified according to their effect or purpose or alternatively according to their physical/chemical composition. Research was essentially directed at developing products with better presentation, stability, uniformity in composition and virtual assurance of relatively innocuous character of the finished product. From the simple vanishing cream of the late 19th century to the sea of foundation creams available in the market today, the cosmetic industry has come a long way to the current multi-billion dollar industry that it is.

On the other hand, India's ancient and rich herbal tradition represents a treasure house of knowledge on cosmetic utility of plants. Ayurvedic medical treatises such as Charaka Samhita, Sushruta Samhita, among many others, contain elaborate references on groups of herbs used for a glowing complexion, herbs used in several skin diseases etc. Aside from such references in our literature on the elaborate usage of herbs for self-adornment, the healing and cosmetic properties of thousands of herbs including those on the kitchen shelves is common knowledge in Indian households. Turmeric, sandal paste, castor oil, honey, neem, saffron and henna that are a part of everyday routine in traditional living are today well-known cosmetics. From rainwater to seaweed, the amazing healing quality of nature has been realized. Rainwater according to herbal therapists is the best skin toner, honey is the best moisturizer and seaweed has a revitalizing effect on the skin.

With this global awakening of interest in the gentle, yet powerful healing virtues of herbs, herbal ingredients are increasingly being incorporated into cosmetic bases. Most herbs used in herbal cosmetics are included based on traditional usage, i.e., experience rather than by experimental investigation. But then worldwide usage of herbs in cosmetics and scientific evaluation of cosmetic potential of thousands of herbs is now unravelling their better physiological effectiveness. Several herbals are now used in medicinal care aside from their use in cosmetics.

Why Herbs in Cosmetics?

The appropriateness of the use of herbs in cosmetics is well reinforced by the following facts:

- Plants possess a vast and complex arsenal of phytochemicals able not only to calm or smooth the skin but actively restore, heal and protect it.

- Herbal extracts have antioxidant property mostly attributed to the presence of carotenoids, flavonoids and polyphenols.

- Flavonoids impart ultraviolet (UV) protection and metal-chelating properties in addition to antioxidant property.

- Herbal constituents such as allantoin exhibit topical anti-inflammatory property due to which they block the anti-inflammatory changes associated with cutaneous ageing, thus helping reverse signs of skin ageing.

- Herbs with topical anaesthetic and anti-pruritic property such as capsaicin in capsicum and menthol in mint are used against dermatitis, sunburn and acne.

- Some herbal constituents are associated with anti-cellulite property such as xanthine alkaloids, caffeine and theophylline from tea. Via beta adrenergic stimulatory action they are known to stimulate the breakdown of fat.
- Hair loss is prevented by the normalization of the keratinization of cells by plant-derived constituents like azelaic acid found naturally in wheat, rye, barley due to their effect on the hornification process of the epidermal cells.
- Herbal materials are much preferred for use as excipients such as carrier oils, cosmetic bases for their emollient, moisturizing, skin toning, bleaching properties.
- Tannin-rich plant extracts due to their astringent or skin-constricting effect may be used in skin conditions associated with infection and inflammation.
- Herbs in cosmetics work slowly but effectively over a period of weeks or even months.
- Herbal cosmetics are viewed as having better physiological activity such as healing, enhancing and conditioning properties.
- They influence biological functions of the skin and provide nutrients such as antioxidants, vitamins, various oils, hydrocolloids, proteins and terpenoids necessary for healthy skin or hair.
- Herbs are well known for their action in controlling scabies, itching, acne, dermatitis, ringworm, skin eruptions, allergic rashes, warts and other skin complaints.
- Since the 1990s cosmetic manufacturers have adopted the term 'cosmeceuticals' to refer to over-the-counter (OTC) products containing plant-based active ingredients such as ascorbic acid, retinoic acid, alpha hydroxyl acid, co-enzyme Q, other nutraceuticals and pharmaceuticals claiming to have both therapeutic and cosmetic benefit.
- These active ingredients are associated with increased skin elasticity, delayed skin ageing, reduced wrinkles, protection against UV radiation and inhibition of degradation of skin collagen.
- Essential oils when incorporated into cosmetics impart a pleasant aroma, shine or conditioning effect in hair care products, emolliency and improved elasticity of the skin.

Incorporating Herbs into Cosmetics

Categories of cosmetics available range from skin-care creams, lotions, powders, perfumes, lipsticks, finger nail and toe nail polish, eye and facial make-up, towelettes, permanent wave setters, hair colours, hair sprays, gels, deodorants, sanitizers, baby products, bath oils, bubble baths, bath salts, butters etc. Make-up is a subset of cosmetics referring primarily to coloured products intended to alter the user's appearance. Based on the purpose of usage cosmetics may be either decorative or care cosmetics.

Based on physical state cosmetics can be grouped into following major categories:

- *Solids*: Talcum powders, face packs, masks, compact powders, cake make-up etc.
- *Semi-solids*: Creams, ointments, liniments, wax base creams, pastes etc.
- *Liquids*: Lotions, moisturizers, hair oil, conditioners, shampoos, cleansing milk, mouth washes, deodorants, liniments, sprays etc.

Manufacturers use a wide variety of herbs in their herbal cosmetics. For extemporaneous use herbal crude drugs may be used fresh, as aqueous extracts, juices, dried powders, infusion, decoction, tincture etc. For large-scale manufacture of products intended to have a longer shelf life, herbs are mostly used in the form of concentrated extracts. These are prepared using aqueous, hydroglycolic, alcoholic solvents, liquid carbon dioxide, essential oils and other distilled extracts.

Thus herbs can be utilized for cosmetics in three forms:

- Total extracts, applied mainly according to the historical tradition of their use.

  Aloe vera gel from the leaves of Aloe species are used as such and as stable proprietary preparations made from the gel for use in cosmetics especially for its wound healing, emollient and conditioning effect for use in hair and skin care cosmetics.

  Green tea is rich in polyphenols and polysaccharides. Its whole extract is extensively used as sunscreen as it absorbs UV A and B rays and is a powerful antioxidant. The polysaccharides enhance fibroblast cell proliferation making it valuable as an anti-ageing agent in cosmetic formulations

- Selective extracts prepared to concentrate specific active fraction of the plant.

  A lipophilic extract of liquorice rich in triterpenoid saponins such as glabridin is a useful cosmetic ingredient on account of its skin-whitening, anti-inflammatory, antimicrobial, melanogenesis inhibitory and antioxidant properties. Due to its antioxidant and regenerative properties it is an important ingredient in several body care and cosmetic products.

  A polyamine-rich extract of wheat germ is used in cosmetics for its anti-ageing property.

  Flavonoid- and terpene-rich extracts of ginkgo due to their antioxidant, anti-inflammatory and cell-regenerative properties are used for their anti-ageing, photo-protective, anti-cellulite advantages in skin care cosmetics.

- Single molecules extract derived purified such as resveratrol, glycyrrhizin, rutin, lawsone, vitamins, coenzyme Q_{10} are used more based on their tested specific activity.

  Resveratrol belonging to a class of polyphenols called stilbenes found in the skin of red grapes is found to reduce wrinkles, stimulate collagen and elastin and is anti-inflammatory and antimicrobial. Likewise rutin, a furano cumarin from buck wheat, is an antioxidant, hair and skin conditioner.

Preparation of herbal cosmetics follows the same procedure as cosmetics with the incorporation of the herbal materials along with the basic ingredients needed for the preparation of the cosmetic in question. It requires appropriate alteration in the ingredient composition such as use of suitable emulsifying agents towards preparing the desired product of specified parameters. Modification of methodology of preparation like avoidance of excessive processing is essential to retain the bioactivity of the botanicals to ascertain its availability after application. Based on evaluation of parameters such as organoleptic characteristics, pH, viscosity, stability towards light, refrigeration etc. manufacturers ensure the quality of the products.

IMPORTANCE OF HERBALS IN HAIR AND SKIN CARE PRODUCTS

Recent extensive research on the physiological effects of herbal extracts and isolates aided by *in vivo* and *in vitro* experimentation on the level of the ultra structure of the skin and the hair shaft are unravelling their specific activities. This is not only adding more and more numbers of tested herbs being used as cosmetics, but is also expanding our understanding of the cosmetic worthiness of time-tested herbs used traditionally since ages. In view of their profound modulatory effects upon maintenance of hair and skin health, herbals are being increasingly included as medicinal products.

Herbs are known to act as cleansers, moisturizers, reconstructors, acidifiers, nourishers, tonics, colourants, emollients, antimicrobials, wound healers and a natural source of vitamins, minerals and trace elements needed for the preservation of health of our body integuments.

Herbs Used in Hair and Skin Care Cosmetics

Cosmetics for hair care are numerous ranging from shampoos, gels, sprays, conditioners, massage oils, colourants, wave setters etc. Shampoos are the largest group of hair care cosmetics. There are a range of products available for different types of hair.

Shampoos are hair care products used for the removal of oils, dirt, skin particles, dandruff, environmental pollutants and other contaminant particles that gradually build up in hair. They are generally made by combining a surfactant such as sodium lauryl sulphate and/or sodum laureth sulphate with a co-surfactant like cocamide propyl betaine in water to form a viscous liquid. Other essential ingredients include sodium chloride to adjust the viscosity, a preservative and a fragrance.

The word shampoo is derived from the Hindi word 'Champo' referring to an Indian traditional head massage that contained several natural oils and fragrances in an alkali mix. It was first introduced in Britain by a Bihari entrepreneur Sake Deen Mohammed in 1762. Soon the meaning of the word shifted from head massage to hair cleansers. Earlier ordinary soap was used for washing hair. Due to the dull film it left on the hair, herbs began to be added and the first commercially available shampoo was available from the turn of the 20th century.

Conditioner literally means those additives that improve the quality of another substance. Though for centuries natural oils have been used to condition human hair, modern hair conditioner was first created at the turn of the 20th century by Ed Pinand for softening men's hair, beard and moustaches. There are several categories of substances used for their specific skin and hair conditioning effect. They include moisturizers, reconstructors, acidifiers, detanglers, thermal protectors, glossers, essential fatty acids and surfactants. Several herbal materials known to bestow these advantages are used as conditioners. They are incorporated in shampoos and in skin care products and also sold as supplements to these products.

Hair colours have been in usage since ancient times and many colourants are today available to colour different hair types. Consumer interest is however directed towards safe and effective hair colours of natural origin. Herb-based hair colourants are the most saleable ones available today.

Thus herbs are basically incorporated into hair care cosmetics for cleansing, conditioning and colouring properties.

A list of some important herbs for various uses follows.

Hair Cleansers

Acacia concinnia DC (Mimosacea)

Commonly called *Shikakai* or soap pod, this is a climbing shrub native to Asia, common in the warm plains of central and south India. The fruit is known in India as *shikakai* 'fruit for hair' referring to its use as a traditional shampoo.

Cosmetic use

In order to prepare the traditional shampoo, the fruit pods are dried, ground into a powder, then made into a paste which is worked through the hair. It is mild, having a naturally low pH and does not strip hair of natural oils. Usually no rinse or conditioner is used since shikakai also acts as a detangler. This ancient product is probably the world's original pH-balanced shampoo. The resulting shampoo is gentle, mild, naturally low pH and is a genuine alternative to surfactant-based shampoos found today.

A. concinna extracts are used in natural shampoos or hair powders and the tree is now grown commercially in India and Far East Asia.

Pods of *Acacia concinna* (Leguminosae) contain several saponins known for their foaming property, including kinmoonosides A-C, triterpenoidal prosapogenols named concinnosides A, B, C, D and E, together with four glycosides, acaciaside, julibroside A1, julibroside A3, albizi-asaponin C and their aglycone, acacic acid lactone.

Extracts of the ground pods have been used for various skin diseases. An infusion of the leaves has been used in anti-dandruff preparation. Leaves and pods are rich in alpha-hydroxy acids that serve as exfoliating and moisturizing agents.

Thus *Acacia concinnia* pods are effective as hair cleanser, conditioner and for dandruff control, all in one.

Sapindus mukorossi, S. trifoliatus (Sapindaceae)

Sapindus is a genus of about 12 species of shrubs and small trees in the Sapindaceae (soapberry family). Also known as soap-nut tree, its fruits are called *Reetha*, soap nut, soap berry and wash nut. It is one of the most important trees of the tropical and subtropical regions of Asia.

Soapnuts from the *Sapindus mukorossi* tree have the highest saponin content. Soapnuts traditionally used as hair shampoos are today an eco-friendly alternative to detergent chemicals. Due to their gentle insecticidal property soapnuts have been used for removing head lice. Recent studies have also reported the tumor cell inhibiting activity of soap nut saponins. They have been used for varied medical conditions as an expectorant, emetic and contraceptive and for relief from migraine.

Cosmetic use

Traditionally in India it is used as a shampoo by bruising the whole nuts which are soaked in warm water. The foamy liquid is then pressed out by squeezing and applied on the hair. It lathers richly and is considered an ideal hair wash preferably after an oil massage on the hair. Dried powder is also used either singly or along with shikakai, fenugreek and fragrant herbs.

Main chemical components are saponins, sapindoside A and B, kaempferol, quercetin, B-sitosterol, palmitic, stearic, oleic, linoleic and eicosenoic acids and glycerides.

Sapindus trifoliatus popularly known as three-leaf berry is the South Indian soap nut.

Trigonella foenum-graecum (Fabaceae)

Commonly called fenugreek or methi, it is cultivated worldwide as a semi-arid crop and is a common ingredient in dishes from Pakistan and the Indian subcontinent. India is the largest producer of fenugreek with Nepal, Bangladesh, Pakistan, Argentina, Egypt, France, Spain, Turkey, Morocco and China being the other major producing countries.

Cosmetic use

The crushed seed mixed with oil and massaged into the scalp is recommended for glossy hair. An infusion of the seed, used as a skin lotion, is said to be good for the complexion.

Methi seeds are a rich source of the polysaccharide galactomannan. They are also a source of saponins such as diosgenin, yamogenin, gitogenin, tigogenin and neotigogens. Other bioactive constituents of fenugreek include mucilage, volatile oils and alkaloids such as choline and trigonelline.

Hair Conditioners

Aloe vera (Liliaceae)

Related species are grown in several parts of the world for the purgative juice and the mucilaginous gel their leaves contain. The mucilage from the leaves is collected after it has been drained of the aloetic juice.

Cosmetic use

The gel popularly called Aloe vera gel is extensively used as an external application for skin irritations, burns, sunburn, wounds, eczema, psoriasis, acne and dermatitis. Due to its astringent qualities it is used in massage therapy. One of the most extensively and popularly used cosmetic ingredient, when used with other ingredients it soothes the skin and stimulates cell regeneration.

Calendula officinalis (Asteraceae)

Called calendula or pot marigold, this is probably native to southern Europe. It is a short-lived aromatic herbaceous perennial. Flowers were used in ancient Greek, Roman, Middle Eastern and Indian cultures as a medicinal herb as well as a dye for fabrics, foods and cosmetics.

Cosmetic use

A number of ingredients used in cosmetics and personal care products are made from *Calendula officinalis*, such as, extract of the whole plant, flower extract, flower oil and seed oil.

Of the calendula-derived ingredients, the flower extracts are the most commonly used in cosmetics and personal care products. They may be used in the formulation of a variety of products, including skin and eye products, hair products and bath products. Flower and seed oil function as skin conditioning agents. *C. officinalis* has been used orally and on the skin in traditional herbal medicine, often because of its reported anti-inflammatory activity.

Important components of *C. officinalis* include triterpene saponins, flavonoids, and carotenoids, which give the flower the orange and yellow colours. The petals and pollen of *C. officinalis* contain triterpenoid esters and carotenoids flavoxanthin and auroxanthin (antioxidants, and the source of the yellow-orange colouration). The leaves and stems contain other carotenoids, mostly lutein (80%) and zeaxanthin (5%) and beta-carotene.

Rosmarinus officinalis (Lamiaceae)

Commonly known as Rosemary, this is a woody, perennial herb with fragrant, evergreen, needle-like leaves and white, pink, purple or blue flowers, native to the Mediterranean region. A member of the mint family, rosemary is used as a decorative plant in gardens and has many culinary and medical uses. The leaves are used to flavour various foods, like stuffings and roast meats. Oil distilled from the leaves called rosemary oil is an important perfumery raw material and the herb is burnt as incense.

Cosmetic use

Rosemary oil has a clear, refreshing herbal smell. It is traditionally known to support circulation, especially to the scalp by strengthening and supporting weak capillaries and is beneficial for hair growth. Used in both hair and skin care cosmetics it also promotes a healthy complexion. Due to its rubefacient effect, oil of rosemary has a toning and binding effect on sagging skin. It relieves skin congestion thus improving its function. Rosemary oil is extensively included in anti-ageing skin creams. It is the preferred ingredient of shampoos and cleansers as it improves skin tone, relieving puffiness and swelling possibly due to its diuretic influence.

Apart from iron, calcium and pyridoxine, antioxidants – carnosic acid and rosmarinic – and camphor (constituting 20% of its dry weight) are the bioactive constituents of rosemary. Caffeic acid, betulinic acid, ursolic acid, rosmaridiphenol and rosmarinol are the other important constituents.

The oil is attributed with analgesic, astringent, diuretic, rubefacient, stimulant and tonic therapeutic properties in skincare.

Chamomilla recutita (Asteraceae)

German Chamomile and *Chamomilum nobile* (Roman Chamomile) are the two varieties of chamomile, one of the most ancient medicinal herbs known to mankind. Traditional uses of chamomile as an anti-inflammatory, antioxidant and astringent are well known. In the form of an aqueous extract or as herbal tea, it was used as a mild sedative and as an anxiolytic.

Cosmetic use

Essential oils of chamomile are used extensively in cosmetics and aromatherapy. Chamomile is processed in many forms as extracts, infusions or essential oils and is included in cosmetics for its anti-inflammatory property.

The plant contains 0.24% to 1.9% volatile oil composed of a variety of separate oils. Approximately 120 secondary metabolites have been identified in chamomile, including 28 terpenoids and 36 flavonoids. The principal components of the essential oil extracted from the German chamomile flowers are the terpenoids α-bisabolol and its oxide azulenes, including chamazulene and acetylene derivatives. Other active ingredients are flavonoids, apigenin and bisabolol (inhibit inflammatory leukotrienes).

Urtica dioica (Urticaceae)

Commonly called stinging nettle or common nettle, it is a herbaceous perennial flowering plant, native to Europe, Asia, northern Africa and North America, and is the best-known member of the nettle genus Urtica. The plant has many hollow stinging hairs called trichomes on its leaves and stems, which act like hypodermic needles injecting histamine and other chemicals that produce a stinging sensation when in contact with humans and animals. The plant has a long history of use as a medicine and as a food source. Nettle leaf is an herb that has a long tradition of use as an adjuvant remedy in the treatment of arthritis in Germany.

Cosmetic use

Used externally, modern herbalists use stinging nettle in the form of a purified extract as a hair tonic and growth stimulant and also in anti-dandruff shampoos. Nettle tea is also considered an effective hair tonic that may bring back the natural colour of the hair also making it glossier.

The stinging nettle is rich in minerals, vitamins A, B group and C along with protein, high amounts of chlorophyll, formic acid, caffeic acid and malic acid, serotonin, glucoquinones, lecithin and lycopene.

Simmondsia chinensis (Simmondsiaceae)

This is grown commercially for jojoba oil, a liquid wax ester, extracted from the seed. A shrub native to the Sonoran and Mojave deserts of Arizona, southern California and northwestern Mexico, it is the sole species of the family Simmondsiaceae and is also known as goat nut or wild hazel. The oil makes up approximately 50% of the jojoba seed by weight. The wax esters are made up of a disproportionately large amount of docosenyl eicosenoate.

Cosmetic use

Jojoba oil is easily refined to be odourless, colourless and oxidatively stable, and is often used in cosmetics as a moisturizer and as a carrier oil for speciality fragrances. It is found as an additive in many cosmetic products such as lotions and moisturizers, hair shampoos and conditioners. Or, the pure oil itself may be used on skin or hair.

Hair Darkeners

Lawsonia inermis (Lythraceae)

Commonly referred to as henna, this flowering plant is native to southern Asia, tropical and subtropical Africa, and the semi-arid areas of northern Australia. Use of henna leaves as a dye for skin, hair, finger nails, leather, wool etc. is a well-known practice since antiquity.

Cosmetic use

Henna has been used as a cosmetic hair dye since ancient times in India, the Middle East and Africa. For skin dyeing, a paste of ground henna (either prepared from a dried powder or from fresh ground leaves) is placed in contact with the skin from a few hours to overnight. The colour that results from dyeing can fall into a broad spectrum, from auburn, orange, deep burgundy, chestnut brown to deep blue-black. Henna invigorates and strengthens hair while giving it volume and protecting it from climatic aggressions. Henna deposits on the surface of the hair a coloured film which fortifies and gives body to the finest hair. An excellent hair conditioner, it is also an effective anti-seborrheic.

Henna's colouring properties are due to lawsone, a naphthaquinone dye that has an affinity for bonding with protein. Lawsone is primarily concentrated in the leaves, especially in the petioles of the leaf. Sugars, fraxetin, tannin, gallic acid, resin and coumarins are the other constituents of henna.

Commercially packaged henna, intended for use as a cosmetic hair dye, is available in many countries, including India, Middle East, Europe, Australia, Canada and the United States.

Phyllanthus emblica (Phyllanthaceae) syn. *Emblica officinalis*

Commonly called Indian gooseberry, it is well known for its edible fruit known as amla. Dried and fresh fruits are renowned for their extensive traditional medicine use in Ayurveda and Unani medicine. Other plant parts such as fruit, seed, leaves, root, bark and flowers are also used in traditional medicine. The primary ingredient of the ancient and now popular 'chyawanaprash' – a rasayana or rejuvenator polyherbal Ayurvedic formulation, amla is rich in tannins. Because of this it is also widely used in inks, shampoos, textiles (as a mordant for fixing dyes) and hair oils.

Cosmetic use

Amla has been traditionally used in India to nourish hair and prevent premature graying of hair. Widely used as a cosmetic in India in the form of shampoos and hair oils, it is an accepted hair tonic in traditional recipes for enriching hair growth. The amla fruit is reputed to have the highest content of vitamin C of any natural-occurring substance. The other major chemical constituents of amla are phyllemblin, gallic acid, ellagic acid, pyrogallol, some norsesquiterpenoids, corilagin, geraniin, elaeocarpusin, and prodelphinidins. Rich in minerals and amino acids, amla reportedly has thrice the protein content and 160 times the apple content in comparison to apples. Amla juice has 20 times more vitamin C than orange juice.

Hibiscus rosa sinensis (Malvaceae)

The flower of this evergreen flowering shrub native to East Asia is commonly called 'hibiscus' or 'shoe flower'. Bearing large red flowers in the original variety, different varieties of the shrub with flowers varying in colour from white to shades of red are widely grown.

Cosmetic use

Flowers and leaves are commonly used in homemade hair conditioners and shampoos for their softening and conditioning effect on the hair. Mucilage from the flowers and leaves are used for preparation of hair oils due to their hair toning and darkening characteristic. Traditionally the mucilage is separated by crushing the flowers and leaves in a mortar along with water and squeezing the mass. The mucilage is then blended into coconut oil or sesame oil by heating. The hair oil is used also for dandruff control. Some baby shampoos and healing lotions also contain hibiscus leaves.

Fresh or dried flower petals are consumed as an herbal tea and are also an ingredient of several commercially available herbal tea mixes.

The principal constituents of *H. rosa sinensis* flowers are flavones such as quercetin-3-diglucoside, quercetin-3,7-diglucoside, cyanidin-3, 5-diglucoside, quercetin-3-sophorotrioside, kaempferol-3 xylosyl glucoside, cyanidin-3-sophoroside-5-glucoside. The other constituents are cyclopeptide alkaloid, cyanidin chloride, hentriacontane, riboflavin, ascorbic acid, thiamine, taraxeryl acetate, beta-sitosterol and cyclic acids – sterculic and malvalic acids.

Camellia sinensis (Theaceae)

Extensively grown as a cultivated crop for production of the popular beverage tea from its leaves and leaf buds, it is the subject of much scientific research for its influence over human health. Of the several varieties of tea commercially available and consumed world over, green tea is being promoted for use in hair care cosmetics.

Cosmetic use

Rich in tannins tea leaves are used to fix hair colourants such as henna on to the hair shaft. Due to its stringency it is used as hair conditioner and colourant both in extemporaneous shampoos and it is also an ingredient in popular herbal hair colourants.

Tea is rich in polyphenols well known for their antioxidant activity. While the whole extract is promoted as a sunscreen, its polysaccharide components are recognized for their anti-ageing effects.

Eclipta alba L Hassk (Asteraceae) Syn. *Eclipta prostrata* (L.)

It is commonly known as False Daisy and Bhringraj. Bhringraj means "King of Hair" and it is considered a rejuvenating herb in Ayurveda. Its profound biological effects including hepatoprotective activity are reported in literature. In traditional medicine the plant is rubbed on the gums for toothache and applied with a little oil for relieving headache and with sesame oil in elephantiasis. A black dye obtained from bhringraj is also used for dyeing hair and tattooing. Its traditional external uses are in athlete's foot, eczema and dermatitis and topical application to the scalp to address alopecia (hair loss). The leaves have been used in the treatment of scorpion stings.

Cosmetic use

A thick slurry of the leaves crushed in water is filtered and mixed with sesame or coconut oil. Other ingredients such as amla, brahmi, curry leaves, fenugreek, henna or hibiscus may be included before heating the oil for complete blending of the herbal ingredients into the oil. This when filtered and scented with the desired fragrance is a popular household hair oil. Hair oils containing bhringraj, amla and brahmi are today important commercial brands used extensively for their hair dyeing effect.

E. prostrata was shown to significantly decrease the amount of time it took for hair to begin regrowing and to fully regrow in shaved albino rats. In these experiments, hair growth initiation time was reduced to half on treatment with the extract, as compared to control animals. Quantitative analysis of hair growth after treatment with bhringraj exhibited greater number of hair follicles in anagenic phase which were higher as compared to those in the control animals.

This herb contains mainly coumestans – wedelolactone (I) and demethylwedelolactone (II) –, polypeptides, polyacetylenes, thiophene-derivatives, steroids, triterpenes and flavonoids.

Arnica montana (Asteraceae),

Commonly known as mountain arnica, leopard's bane, wolf's bane or mountain tobacco, it is a European flowering plant with large yellow flowers grown in herb gardens and has long been used medicinally.

Cosmetic use

A. montana flower extract available commercially is an important herbal ingredient of a variety of personal care formulations such as skin care products, skin fresheners and hair care products like shampoos and conditioners. Cosmetic effects of the flower extract include enhancing the appearance of dry or damaged skin by reducing flaking and restoring suppleness.

Hair Nourishers/Growth Stimulants

Cocos nucifera (Arecaceae)

Commonly called the coconut palm it is the only accepted species in the genus *Cocos*. Widely grown throughout the tropical and subtropical regions of the world, its fresh kernel and kernel oil are an essential part of the diet of the people in the regions in which it is grown. The edible, tasty and mineral-rich endospermous fluid of tender coconuts is considered an invigorating drink and is used as a vehicle in some extemporaneous herbal preparations of indigenous medicine.

Different parts of the coconut palm find multiple domestic, commercial and industrial uses in the form of various products made from them.

Cosmetic use

Coconut oil is considered an ideal hair nourisher in India since ages and it is an essential base or carrier oil in several hair oils and preparations meant for application on the hair. An excellent emollient, lubricant and skin moisturizer, coconut oil is an important base ingredient for the manufacture of soap. Coconut oil-based soaps, being harder despite retaining more water (compared to other oils), are preferred sometimes as they enhance the overall soap yield. These soaps are also more soluble in hard water and salt water and lather better. A basic coconut oil soap is clear when melted and a bright white when hardened.

Categorized as a hair and skin conditioning agent, emollient and fragrance ingredient, coconut oil is used in several hair and skin care cosmetics. Coconut oil makes a good massage oil as it is readily absorbed by the skin. Finely powdered coconut shell could be added to skin scrubs as it effectively exfoliates dead skin. Lauric acid from coconut oil could be converted to sodium lauryl sulphate, a shampoo and shower gel detergent.

Sesamum indicum (Pedaliaceae)

Its seeds popularly called sesame yield a pale yellow oil upon expression. Sesame oil and sesame seeds have been consumed by humans for thousands of years. Crude expressed sesame oil can be used as a food item with little or no refining. Sesame oil is consumed primarily as a cooking and salad oil and is an important flavour in Asian food. Asian sesame oil is made from roasted seeds and is amber in colour.

Cosmetic use

This highly nourishing oil has immense healing properties. Its use has been extensively mentioned in ancient Ayurvedic text for over thousands of years. It is considered a hair nourisher, natural sunscreen and has hair-darkening properties thus preventing premature greying of hair.

Excellent for dry scalp and hair growth treatment, regular warm oil massage is the traditional prescription for controlling dryness and flakiness which also increases penetration of oil in the scalp, resulting in enhanced blood circulation, thereby promoting hair growth.

Classified as hair and skin conditioning agent, binder, surfactant, emulsion stabilizer and viscosity builder, it is extensively used in cosmetics and personal care products.

Sesame oil and derived ingredients such as hydrogenated sesame seed oil, sesame oil unsaponifiables and sodium salt of sesame oil-derived fatty acids are components of several cosmetic formulations. They are included in the composition of hair care and make-up products, sunscreen lotions, skin cleansers, moisturizers and lipsticks among others.

Centella asiatica (Apiaceae)

Commonly called Brahmi, mandukparni and Indian pennywort, it is a small, herbaceous, annual plant native to India, Sri Lanka, northern Australia, Indonesia, Iran, Malaysia, Melanesia, Papua New Guinea and other parts of Asia. Brahmi has great value in Ayurvedic medicine as a memory enhancer and a brain tonic. It is used to treat Alzheimer's disease, memory loss, insanity, insomnia and other mental illnesses. It is widely used for its effect in blood circulation thus promoting efficient function of the liver, lungs and the kidneys.

Traditionally Brahmi was used to treat skin problems including psoriasis, eczema, abscess and ulceration. In Ayurveda it is considered a rejuvenator for the entire body and is commonly used as medicated oil. This oil has a beautiful sweet fragrance and natural green colour and is calming and soothing.

Cosmetic use

Brahmi oil is a natural herbal hair rejuvenator and promotes positive memory functioning. Brahmi is used to stimulate skin-cell regeneration and growth. An essential component of many herbal oils, its antioxidant properties allow the proper nourishment to reach the hair roots and thus promote their growth. It is also used in many massage oils, conditioners and shampoos. Having a fruity, fresh herbal aroma, Brahmi oil can be blended with sandalwood and other essential oils for a relaxing experience.

Panax ginseng, (Chinese ginseng) Panax quinquifolium (American ginseng) (Araliaceae)

An ancient Chinese herb, the world famous 'man root', it is considered an adaptogenic herb and is widely promoted as an aphrodisiac. It is preciously cultivated for its great commercial value in the United States, Canada, China and Korea. One of the most highly imported drugs in world trade, roots and rhizomes of Ginseng, as it is commonly called, constitute a highly venerated herb in herbal medical practice. Well known for its anti-ageing property, the crude drug in the form of extracts is included in cosmetics for its rejuvenating property on the skin and hair.

Cosmetic use

Classed as a skin-conditioning agent, emollient, hair conditioner, skin protective and tonic, the root extract is used in all kinds of cosmetic products such as lotions, creams, soaps, bath preparations and perfumes. Ginseng oil and extracts (probably both American and Asian) are used in cosmetics for their rejuvenating and anti-ageing property. They activate the skin metabolism and blood flow, reduce keratinization, moisturize and soften, alleviate wrinkling and enhance skin whiteness.

Lavandula angustifolia (Lamiaceae)

Commonly called lavender or English lavender formerly *L. officinalis*, it is a flowering plant native to the western Mediterranean, primarily the Pyrenees and other mountains in northern

Spain. English lavender is commonly grown as an ornamental plant. It is popular for its colourful flowers and its fragrance. The flowers and leaves are used either in the form of lavender oil or as herbal tea.

Cosmetic use

Essential oils distilled from members of the genus *Lavandula* have been used both cosmetically and therapeutically for centuries. Lavender essential oil, when diluted with a carrier oil, is commonly used as a relaxant with massage. Lavender flower petals and oil are popular ingredients of handmade soap, lotions and eye pillows. In combination with other oils such as thyme, rosemary and cedar wood, it is used in alopecia areata or hair loss. One study showed evidence that this combination might improve hair growth by as much as 44% after seven months of treatment.

L. vera is primarily constituted of linalyl acetate and linalol.

Serenoa repens (Arecaceae, Palmae) Syn: *Sabal serrulata*

Commonly called saw palmetto, it is a small, scrubby dwarf palm tree native to North America and grows primarily along the Atlantic coast in Georgia and Florida. Saw palmetto berries were used by the American Indians to treat genitourinary tract conditions and also as a tonic for nutritional supplementation.

The active ingredients are believed to be found in the plant's brown-black berries and in the form of an extract it is the most popular herbal treatment for benign prostatic hyperplasia. It is also popular as an herbal remedy for a type of hair loss and baldness called androgenic alopecia, or male- and female-pattern baldness.

Cosmetic use

Saw palmetto extract has been suggested as a potential treatment for male pattern baldness. This type of hair loss is typically the greatest at the top of the head or around the temples. Much of saw palmetto's popularity as a remedy for hair loss and baldness, however, is based on how it is believed to work rather than on evidence that it actually does. It is reported to inhibit 5-alpha reductase and is used in hair care gels, creams etc.

Saw palmetto berries contain 1.5% of pleasant-smelling oil constituted of 63% free fatty acids such as capric, caprylic, caproic, lauric, palmitic and oleic acids. Ethyl esters of these fatty acids, beta sitosterol and daucosterol are the other reported constituents of the oil. The berries are also comprised of carotenes, lipase, tannins and sugars.

The lipid-soluble components of the berries are extracted and purified, yielding the pharmacologically active portion of the oil. This medicinally used extract contains about 85% to 95% fatty acids and sterols. It is rich in fatty acids and phytosterols. A lipophilic extract of saw palmetto is being used clinically to treat benign hyperplasia.

Portulacca oleraceae (Portulacaceae) (Lunia-Hindi, Paruppu keerai-Tamil)

Common purslane, pusley, pigweed or hogweed, as it is commonly called, is an annual succulent native to the Indian subcontinent and now widely distributed across the continents actually as a wild weed. Pusley is widely grown in many Asian and European regions as a staple leafy vegetable and long used in salads and as a medicinal. This leafy vegetable is a rich source of vitamin A (1320 IU/100 g provides 44% of RDA), vitamin C, protein and omega-3 fatty acids. Carotenids,

B-complex vitamins such as riboflavin, niacin, pyridoxine, dietary minerals such as iron, magnesium, calcium, potassium and manganese are also present. Other reported bioactive constituents are noradrenaline, calcium salts, dopamine, DOPA, malic acid, citric acid, glutamic acid, aspartic acid, nicotinic acid, glucose, fructose and sucrose.

Cosmetic use

Extract of the whole plant is used in several skin care products for acne control. Its high vitamin A content known for powerful antioxidant activity makes it an ingredient in botanical extracts included as damage control agents in skin care.

Anti-Dandruff Herbs

Azadirachta indica (Meliaceae)

Commonly called Neem or Indian lilac it is a tropical evergreen tree widely distributed in southeast Asia. Called Nimba in Sanskrit, it is a highly reputed medicinal tree in the Indian traditional medical systems of Ayurveda and Siddha. Extensively used for its insecticidal properties in storage grains, all parts of the plant namely the leaves, fruits, flowers, seeds, seed oil, bark, roots are considered medicinal and form part of several traditional medicines of repute. The tree is considered sacred and it is associated with many traditional seasonal rituals in the Indian subcontinent. Extensive scientific research on the plant parts have revealed powerful biological activities that range from antibacterial, antiviral, anti-inflammatory, anti-hypertensive, hypoglycemic, hepatoprotective, anti-fertility effect to potent anti-HIV properties. In folk medicine a paste made out of neem leaves and turmeric is considered an effective protective against several skin diseases. Advocated for use in the treatment of infectious diseases such as chicken pox, measles etc. even fanning the wounds with neem leaves is considered beneficial. In traditional Indian medicine neem seed oil has been effectively used since centuries for topical skin disorders such as eczema, psoriasis, rashes, burns, abrasions etc.

Cosmetic Use

Today neem oil and neem extracts find extensive use in branded herbal cosmetics and other personal care products. Due to worldwide demand for natural molecules as mediators of health, these natural cosmetics find inclusion especially in skin care products due to their powerful antimicrobial efficacy. Neem bark and leaves in the form of extracts form part of several medicinal and cosmetic products. Neem seed oil after the process of refining loses its unpleasant smell and can be used to manufacture cosmetics.

Neem and its products are important ingredients of skin and hair care cosmetics for their powerful antibacterial, antifungal properties due to which they may be used for dandruff control and to relieve itch, rashes, skin redness etc. Neem oil is also an excellent skin moisturizer and is included in medicated and cosmetic soaps and shampoos. Neem leaf extracts are thus included in face and body lotions and creams, herbal face packs, fairness creams, hand creams and as a natural moisturizing base in skin care formulations. Neem products are reputed to be suitable for all skin types.

All parts of the plant continue to receive extensive phytochemical and pharmacological investigation. Neem leaves and seed oil are rich in several groups of phytoconstituents principal among which are limonoids, flavonoids and their glycosides, coumarins etc. Azadirachtin is a potent insecticidal agent isolated from it.

Arctium lappa (Asteraceae)

Commonly called greater burdock, edible burdock, lappa or beggar's buttons, it is a biennial plant cultivated in gardens for its root used as a vegetable.

Cosmetic use

An oil extract of the roots is used for scalp conditions (dandruff and hair loss). It improves hair strength, recovering its vitality and shine. Modern studies have shown that burdock root oil extract is rich in phytosterols and essential fatty acids required for promotion of hair growth. Classed as a skin conditioning agent, it is included in skin care cosmetics for its anti-inflammatory property.

Seeds contain arctigenin which has shown potent in vitro antiviral activities against influenza.

Acorus calamus (Araceae)

Commonly known as Sweet Flag or calamus, or Vaz it is a tall perennial wetland monocot. A reputed Ayurvedic medicinal herb, it grows throughout India in marshy places. Indigenous to India, A. calamus is now found across Europe, southern Russia, northern Asia Minor, southern Siberia, China, Indonesia, Japan, Burma, Sri Lanka, Australia, as well as southern Canada and the northern United States.

The root and its essential oil are used for their sedative, digestive, expectorant and stimulant properties and considered efficacious in facilitating speech development functions in childhood in native medicine.

Cosmetic use

Its sweet aroma makes the essential oil of the roots of acorus a valued commodity in the fragrance industry. Classified as a skin conditioning agent, the oil and the root extract are used as a fragrant inclusion in hair and skin care products.

The rhizomes contain calamediol, tanning substances and vitamin C. Two new selinane-type sesquiterpenes, acolamone and isoacilamone, have been isolated. Other constituents reported are asarone, asarone in oil, calamenol, calamene, calamenone, eugenol and methyl eugenol. The leaves contain also essential oil, tanning substances and vitamin C. The sweet flag oil contains two new sesquiterpenic ketones named as calamusenone and a new tropone. The essential oil present in a concentration of 2% to 4% in the rhizome contains a number of sesquiterpenes and asarone, a compound related to myristicin.

Salvia officinalis (Lamiaceae)

The common sage or culinary sage is a short-lived semi-woody shrub. A small evergreen plant with woody stems, grayish leaves and blue to purplish flowers it is native to southern Europe and the Mediterranean region.

Leaves are used extensively in the kitchen to add a unique flavour to salads, egg dishes, soups, stews, meats and vegetables.

Cosmetic use

Sage is used as an ingredient in soaps, cosmetics and perfumes. Smeared on the skin, sage is a useful insect repellent. Modern research has confirmed antiseptic, estrogenic, anti-inflammatory, and antimicrobial properties in extracts from sage. As a cosmetic ingredient it is classed as anti-dandruff, antimicrobial, antioxidant, astringent, cleansing, deodorant, skin conditioning, skin protecting, soothing agent and tonic.

In cosmetics and personal care products, the ingredients derived from the whole plant, leaves, flowers, stems and roots are used in the formulation of a variety of products including bath products, shaving creams, fragrance products, shampoos, and cleansing products.

Skin Whiteners

Skin whitening refers to the practice of using chemical substances to lighten skin tone by lessening melanin concentration. Melanins are dark-coloured pigments produced by special skin cells called melanocytes. Whitening agents act at various levels of melanin production in the skin. Several of them are competitive inhibitors of tyrosinase, a key enzyme in melanogenesis. Certain others inhibit enzyme maturation or prevent transport of melanin-carrying granules from melanocytes to surrounding keratinocytes.

These melanin-inhibiting ingredients are used alone or in combination with a sunscreen or a retinoid in the form of topical lotions or gels. Several plant-derived and synthetic chemicals are being used in these treatments and are also being incorporated into skin care cosmetics. In medical literature, hydroquinone is considered the primary topical ingredient for inhibiting melanin production. It is used topically from 2% to 4% concentrations singly or in combination with tretinoin (0.05% to 0.1%). A powerful inhibitor of melanin, hydroquinone lightens skin tone by disrupting melanin pigmentation. At higher concentrations of 4%, it could be a skin irritant especially when used in combination with tretinoin.

Some alternative lighteners are natural sources of hydroquinone such as those listed below:

Arbutin

Arbutin (hydroquinone-beta-D-glucoside) which can inhibit melanin production is present in *Mitracarpus scaber* extract, *Uva ursi* (bearberry) extract, *Morus bombycis* (mulberry), *Morus alba* (white mulberry) and *Broussonetia papyrifera* (paper mulberry). Pure forms of arbutin are considered more potent for effecting skin lightening (alpha-arbutin, beta-arbutin, and deoxy-arbutin). Beta-arbutin is also known by its more common name of bearberry extract.

Sourced from the leaves of bearberry, cranberry, mulberry and some types of pears, arbutin and its source plant extracts are considered safe and natural alternatives to pure chemical skin depigmentation agents. The skin-lightening property of arbutin is reported in medical literature with such usage being controlled by patents. Out of the two structural conformations of arbutin, the α-form is relatively more stable and thus preferred as a skin lightener.

Kojic acid

A fermentative by-product of malting rice in the manufacture of Japanese rice-based wine, kojic acid is reported in some studies to be a melanin inhibitor. Due to its susceptibility to colour change and loss of activity on exposure to air or sunlight, the more stable kojic acid diplamitate, also an effective antioxidant, is used in cosmetic formulations.

Azelaic acid

An ingredient of grains such as wheat, rye and barley, azelaic acid is being used topically in 10% to 20% concentration. It is considered an effective treatment for acne and skin discolouration.

Vitamin C

Vitamin C and its various forms such as ascorbic acid, magnesium ascorbyl phosphate etc. are considered effective antioxidants for the skin and help to lighten it. One study found it to raise glutathione levels in the body. Another study found that brownish guinea pigs given vitamin C, vitamin E and L-cysteine simultaneously lead to them having lighter skin. Several natural sources of vitamin C such as amla used in cosmetics also serve the purpose of skin whitening.

Toxicity-free skin-lightening products are both expensive and in great demand. Japan and Pacific countries are fertile markets for good-quality skin-lightening products from Europe.

Skin Conditioners/Moisturizers

Prunus amygdalis (Rosaceae)

Native to the Middle East and South Asia, almond is also the name of the edible and widely cultivated seed of this tree. It is considered one of the earliest domesticated tree nuts. The oil from the nuts is produced mainly in Italy, France, Spain and North Africa. The two varieties of the tree yield sweet and bitter almonds. Commonly called badam in India, it is a popular edible nut used extensively in Indian cuisine.

Cosmetic use

A renowned beauty aid since the times of ancient Romans, almond oil is an excellent emollient and helps to retain skin moisture balance. It is reputed to enhance complexion and add a healthy, youthful glow to the skin. The skin and hair care benefits of almond are attributed to the vital minerals and vitamins it contains. It is easily absorbed and is most effective for combating dry and irritated skin. It cures dryness, irritation, itching and inflammation. It is also a remedy for dark circles, fine lines, chapped lips and body rashes. Because of its fine texture, the oil will not leave a greasy feeling on the skin and does not block pores. As a result of its moisturizing quality, it is now being used in many soaps and moisturizers. Almond oil has also been known to facilitate hair growth. It smoothes hair cuticles and provides nourishment to the hair. It strengthens hair and gives it a natural shine. It forms an excellent massage oil as it is easily absorbed and is a great lubricant. It is a natural moisturizer, and therefore suitable for all skin types. Almond oil is an effective and popular carrier oil for essential oils in aromatherapy for its soothing effect and calming pleasant aroma.

Almond oil contains 40% to 55% of fixed oil, about 20% proteins, mucilage and emulsion. It contains a considerable amount of olein, with smaller quantities of glycosides of linoleic and other acids. Rich in vitamins A, B1, B2, B6 and E it acts as great nourishment for the skin.

Citrus Limoni (Rutaceae)

The source of lemon fruits, it is a small tree cultivated in several countries across the globe. Being Indian in origin, lemons were unknown in Europe till the 12th century. Numerous varieties and hybrids are widely cultivated for the oil. Peel of lemons and the essential oil separated from it are used in flavouring and as a cosmetic.

Cosmetic use

While lemon oil is used as a fragrance ingredient and as a flavouring agent, several products made from the peel such as peel oil derived by solvent extraction after removal of the essential oil, peel powder, peel water and peel extract are used in cosmetics. While the peel powder is an effective absorbent and viscosity-controlling agent, peel extract and peel oil are classed as skin conditioners. They are used in cosmetics and personal care products, including bath products, soaps and detergents, skin care products, cleansing products, eye make-up, fragrance products and hair care products.

Whole lemons are macerated by incubation with *Lactobacillus lacti.* The fermentative process that is initiated causes the release of valuable chemicals from the peel. This subsequently processed product, the lemon peel bioferment, is an antioxidant, bactericide and inhibitor of melanin synthesis. Similar to hydroquinone, it has high anti-tyrosinase activity. This ferment is then further processed to remove the potential allergens, citral and geraniol. The resulting ferment is said to have both anti-tyrosinase and antioxidant activity. Lemon peel bioferment is used in skin-lightening products and anti-ageing skin care products to improve and lighten age spots and irregular skin pigmentation.

Ginkgo biloba (Ginkgoaceae)

A unique tree species native to China, ginkgo is the oldest living member of the Gymnosperms and the only survivor of Gingkoaceae, all other species being found only as fossils. Today it is widely planted as an ornamental and cultivated for drug use in Korea, France and the United States.

Standardized extracts of the leaves are marketed for use against cerebrovascular disease and senile dementia. Ginkgo may exert beneficial effects by improving brain blood circulation and assist with other symptoms such as vertigo, tinnitus and hearing loss.

Cosmetic use

Extract from the leaves of *G. biloba* tree have antioxidative function and improve capillary circulation making it a very useful herb in cosmetology. By scavenging free radicals and peroxide in skin tissues it delays skin ageing. Classified as a skin-conditioning agent *G. biloba* extracts are used in anti-ageing skin care products at a concentration of 0.01% to 0.05% in which it is added to lotions, creams ointments, masks, cleansers etc.

Active constituents of Ginkgo are characterized as mixtures of terpenoids and flavonoids. The dried leaves contain 0.1% to 0.25% terpene lactones, comprising five ginkgolides (A, B, C, J and M) and bilobalide.

Carthamus tinctorius (Asteraceae).

Commonly called safflower, this highly branched herbaceous thistle-like annual is commercially cultivated for vegetable oil extracted from the seeds. It is a very ancient crop plant as revealed from the safflower-based dyes found in textiles of Egyptian mummies dating back to the 12th century.

Safflower seed oil is flavourless and colourless, and nutritionally similar to sunflower oil. An edible vegetable oil it used as cooking oil and in salad dressing. Having an extensive history of use in food, it is commonly found in mayonnaise, salad dressing, frozen desserts and speciality breads. Linoleic acid, which is considered to be an essential fatty acid, is a major component of this oil.

Cosmetic use

Safflower seed oil is included in topical skin care lotions, moisturizers, bath products etc. as its lubricant effect gives a soft and smooth appearance to the skin. Dried flowers of safflower are used as a natural textile dye.

Carthamin, a quinine-type dye, is the pigment responsible for its natural red colour. This dye used as a food additive and in cosmetics is coded as CI Natural Red 26. Safflower pigment is used for imparting yellow, mustard, khaki, olive or even red colours to textiles.

Carica papaya (Caricaceae)

Commonly called papaya it yields a fruit of the same name. The sole species in the genus *Carica*, the tree is native to the tropics of the Americas, perhaps from southern Mexico and neighbouring Central America.

The latex obtained from the unripe fruit is the source of the proteolytic enzyme papain. It is applied topically in countries where it grows for the treatment of cuts, rashes, stings and burns. Papain ointment is commonly made from fermented papaya flesh and is applied as a gel-like paste.

Cosmetic use

Papaya is frequently used as a hair conditioner, but should be used in small amounts. Because of its exfoliating property it is used in some skin care products.

Papaya fruit is rich in vitamins A, B_1, B_2, niacin, ascorbic acid and β-carotene. Papaya skin, pulp and seeds also contain a variety of phytochemicals including natural phenols.

Rosa damascena, Rosa centifolia (Rosaceae)

R. damascena is the source of the damask and cabbage rose grown commonly for the distillation of its essential rose oil. Also called attar of rose or rose absolute, it is extracted from the petals of various types of rose. While rose ottos are extracted through steam distillation essential oil obtained from rose by solvent extraction or supercritical fluid extraction is called rose absolute. The latter is more commonly used in perfumery. Despite its high price and the availability of synthetic substitutes, natural rose essential oil is still in great demand in perfumery. Bulgaria produces about 70% of all rose oil in the world. Other significant producers are Morocco, Iran and Turkey, as also China.

Cosmetic use

Rose oil has been credited with antiseptic, disinfectant, slightly tonic and soothing properties. It is found to be helpful in cases of skin redness or inflammation, and where moisturization and regeneration is needed. Being an expensive essential oil, it is used only in very high-grade perfumes. For cosmetic and perfumery purpose, rose water, the aqueous portion of the distillate of rose petals, is widely used. Rose oil is considered ideal for most skin types, especially for mature, sensitive or dry skin.

β-damascenone, β-damascone, β-ionone and rose oxide are the principal constituents imparting the characteristic scent to rose oil. Present in less than 1% of the content of rose oil, these constituents make up more than 90% of the oils' odour content due to their low odour threshold. Proportion of β-damascenone in rose oil is the marker for its quality.

Zea mays (Poaceae)

The source of maize kernels or corn used in cooking as a vegetable or starch, this constitutes a staple food in many regions of the world. Maize is a major source of starch. Cornstarch (maize flour) is a major ingredient in home cooking and in many industrialized food products. Corn is one of the most commonly grown foods in the world. The seed can be eaten raw or cooked and the mature seed can be dried and used whole or ground into flour. Corn oil, obtained from the seed, is an all-purpose oil that is frequently used for cooking and in salad dressings.

Cosmetic use

Corn is the source of several products of use in cosmetics and personal care products. The most common corn-derived ingredients used in cosmetics include corn oil, corn starch, corn cob meal, corn cob powder, corn fruit, corn germ extract, corn germ oil, corn oil unsaponifiables, corn gluten protein, corn kernel extract, corn kernel meal, corn seed flour, corn silk extract, hydrolyzed corn starch, hydrolyzed corn protein, corn acid, corn glycerides and potassium cornate. These ingredients are used in the formulation of skin care, hair care, bath products, eye and facial make-up, lipsticks and hair dyes and colours. While hydrolyzed corn starch is used as a skin-conditioning agent, hydrolyzed corn protein is used as hair-conditioning agent.

Corn contains vitamin B1 (thiamine), folate, vitamin C, phosphorus, vitamin B5 (pantothenic acid), vitamin A (more in the yellow corn), manganese and several antioxidants including ferulic acid and phenolics.

Medicago sativa (Fabaceae)

Known as alfalfa or Lucerne, it is the most cultivated forage legume in the world. A perennial flowering plant in the pea family it is cultivated in the United States, Canada, Argentina, France, Australia, the Middle East, South Africa and many other countries.

Alfalfa is rich in several essential vitamins such as the complete spectrum of B vitamins, vitamins A, D, E and K. Iron, niacin, biotin, folic acid, calcium, magnesium, phosphorous and potassium are adequately present in it and when burnt, ashes of alfalfa are rich in calcium. It is high in protein content (25%) and is a good source of chlorophyll.

Cosmetic use

Alfalfa extracts are used in skin care products as antioxidants due to their nutritional content.

Anti-Infectives

Melaleuca alternifolia (Myrtaceae)

Commonly called tea tree it is native to the northeast coast of New South Wales, Australia. Tea tree oil, or melaleuca oil, is a pale yellow colour to nearly colourless and clear essential oil with a fresh camphoraceous odour taken from its leaves. Scientifically investigated only recently, it is attributed with antiviral, antibacterial, antifungal and antiseptic qualities.

Cosmetic use

Traditionally tea tree oil has been used as a topical application for the relief of several skin conditions. Its effective antibacterial, antifungal, antiviral activity as also its efficacy in scabies and against head lice is recently reported. It is demonstrated to be more effective than permethrin (synthetic insecticide used against body mites) against head lice.

While topical application of tea tree oil is comparable to that of 5% benzoyl peroxide in the treatment of common acne, shampoo with 5% tea tree oil is highly inhibitory to dandruff. Tea tree oil is commercially available as a cosmetic blended into creams or lotions for topical application. It is extensively promoted for use in a variety of dermatological conditions such as boils, abscesses, dandruff, bed sores, rashes etc. Principal components of tea tree oil are α-pinene, β-pinene, sabinene, myrcene, α -phellandrene, α -terpinene, limonene, 1,8-cineole, γ-terpinene, p-cymene, terpinolene, linalool, terpinen-4-ol and α -terpineol.

Curcuma longa (Zingiberaceae)

Turmeric is a rhizomatous herbaceous perennial native to tropical South Asia. No longer known in the wild state, it is cultivated extensively throughout the warmer parts of the world, especially in India and China. Turmeric has been used as both spice and medicine in traditional Indian medicine for over 2,500 years. Knowledge about its medicinal value could be the reason for its inclusion as a food ingredient and in auspicious traditional rituals and ceremonies. Turmeric is a household remedy for local application to cuts and wounds and other inflammatory and painful conditions. Use of turmeric in the treatment of jaundice and other liver disorders is well known.

Cosmetic use

In India, turmeric has been used for centuries as a natural cleanser; the powder is mixed with milk to bring a healthy glow to the skin. In the form of a paste (made by rubbing the prepared rhizome on a hard wet surface) turmeric is used as a facial cosmetic possibly for its antimicrobial effect. Such an application is believed to improve skin appearance by eliminating superfluous hair and easing out wrinkles.

Today turmeric and its derived chemicals are extensively included in cosmetic formulations. It is reported with many cosmetic and therapeutic benefits. The chief colouring principals of turmeric are diaryl hepatanoid derivatives primary of which is curcumin. Turmeric powder, extracts and curcumin are reported to have powerful antioxidant, anti-inflammatory, choleretic, immunomodulatory and antimicrobial properties. It is recommended for use in the treatment of eczema and acne as it moisturizes skin and accelerates healing. On account of its wound-healing potential it is widely included in skin care cosmetics.

Turmeric contains about 5% curcuminoids, 5% essential oil, 25% of which is zingiberene and a minor proportion of bioactive polysaccharide fraction.

Ocimum tenuiflorum (Lamiaceae) Syn: Ocimum sanctum

Tulsi or Holy Basil is an aromatic plant cultivated for religious and medicinal purposes and for its essential oil. Tulsi in Sanskrit means 'the incomparable one' and it is a sacred plant worshipped in India. Tulsi has been used for thousands of years in Ayurveda for its diverse healing properties. It is mentioned in the Charaka Samhita, an ancient Ayurvedic text. Tulsi is considered to be an adaptogen and is regarded in Ayurveda as a kind of 'elixir of life' as it is believed to promote longevity. Tulsi extracts are used in Ayurvedic remedies for common colds, headaches, stomach disorders, inflammation, heart disease, various forms of poisoning and malaria. Tulsi is recommended to be taken in many forms as whole leaves in water, herbal tea, dried powder with ghee etc. Its antioxidant, analgesic, radioprotective property is reported in litera-ture. It has antioxidant properties and can repair cells damaged by exposure to radiation.

Cosmetic use

Essential oil is mostly used for medicinal purposes and in herbal cosmetics, and is widely used in skin preparations due to its antibacterial activity. Classed as a fragrance ingredient and skin-conditioning agent it is used in anti-acne preparations. Tulsi extracts are used as a prime ingredi-ent in herbal cosmetics, including face packs, creams and many other products.

Some of the main chemical constituents of tulsi are oleanolic acid, ursolic acid, rosmarinic acid, eugenol, carvacrol, linalool, β-caryophyllene (about 8%),[12], β-elemene (c.11.0%) and andgermacrene D (about 2%).

Psoralea corylifolia (Fabaceae)

Babchi is an important plant in the Indian Ayurveda and Siddha systems of medicine, and also Chinese medicine. The seeds of this plant contain a variety of coumarins including psoralen. The seeds have a variety of traditional medicinal uses. The seed and its essential oil are used as an anthelmintic and in the treatment of leucoderma and epilepsy.

Cosmetic use

Babchi as an extract is used in anti-aging formulas because of its anti-inflammatory and antibac-terial properties. It shows promise as a skin care ingredient particularly as an acne fighter and due to its antioxidant and skin-whitening properties.

P. corylifolia extract contains a number of chemical compounds including flavonoids (neoba-vaisoflavone, isobavachalcone, bavachalcone, bavachinin, bavachin, corylin, corylifol, corylifolin and 6-prenylnaringenin), coumarins (psoralidin, psoralen, isopsoralen and angelicin) and meroterpenes (bakuchiol and 3-hydroxybakuchiol).

Symphytum officinale L (Boraginaceae)

Commonly called comfrey, it is a perennial herb with a black, turnip-like root and large, hairy broad leaves that bears small bell-shaped flowers of various colours. It is used in organic garden-ing as a fertilizer. One of the most common uses of comfrey extract is in skin treatment. The plant contains allantoin, a nitrogenous crystalline substance that is a cell proliferant, which is thought to stimulate cell growth and repair while simultaneously depressing inflammation. Comfrey is restricted to topical use and should never be ingested, as it is toxic and carcinogenic due to the presence of pyrrolizidine alkaloids.

Cosmetic use

Topical application of comfrey due to its anti-inflammatory properties is recommended only for short-term use if the amount of pyrrolizidine alkaloids is less than 100 micrograms per applica-tion. The allantoin in the plant is thought to help replace and repair cells in the body through its proliferant properties. As a cosmetic and bath herb, with continuous use, it regenerates aging skin.

Mucilage, steroidal saponins, tannins, pyrrolizidine alkaloids, inulin, vitamin B12 and pro-teins are the other constituents present.

Skin Rejuvenators

Santalum album (Santalaceae)

Indian sandalwood is a medium-sized hemi-parasitic tree found in India, Nepal, Bangladesh, Sri Lanka, Australia, Indonesia and the Pacific Islands. The Indian sandalwood is a threatened species. It is indigenous to South India, and grows in the Western Ghats and a few other mountain ranges like the Kalrayan and Shevaroy Hills. Sandalwood is an age-old article of commerce cultivated, traded and utilized in traditional rituals, as a fragrance article, medicine, for its essential oil and high-prized exquisite-smelling timber. Due to its fine and delicate aroma, the long waiting period before it can be harvested, huge market demand and the high price it commands, sandalwood has been recklessly exploited to the point of veritable extinction.

S. album has been the primary source of sandalwood and the derived oil. The use of *S. album* in India is noted in literature for over 2,000 years. It has use as wood and oil in religious practices. It also features as a construction material in temples and elsewhere. In traditional medicine, sandalwood has been used for thousands of years as an antiseptic, anti-inflammatory, antispasmodic, astringent, diuretic, disinfectant, emollient, expectant, hypotensive and sedative agent.

Cosmetic use

Sandalwood oil is an essential oil obtained from the steam distillation of chips and billets cut from the heartwood of the sandalwood tree. Sandalwood oil is used widely as a base note and fixative in modern perfumery and cosmetic production. The oil is highly valued for its deep woody aroma. It is a base note that helps to hold the scent of other lighter oils that tend to dissipate quickly. Sandalwood is central to the making of traditional attars in India. It is used as an ingredient in fragrant products such as incense, perfumes, aftershaves and other cosmetics. Sandalwood oil is used in perfumes, cosmetics and sacred unguents.

Sandalwood oil contains more than 90% sesquiterpenic alcohols of which 50% to 60% is the tricyclic α-santalol. β-santalol comprises 20% to 25%.

Echinacea (Asteraceae)

This is a genus of herbaceous flowering plants in the daisy family. The nine species it contains are perennials native to the prairies and eastern United States, and are easily recognizable by their pink/purple daisy-like flowers with orange/brown centres. *E. purpurea, E. angustifolia, E. pallida* are species used medicinally and in cosmetics. Echinacea has been approved by the German Commission E for the treatment of colds and chronic infections of the respiratory tract and lower urinary tract. It has been used as therapy in chronic candidiasis. Externally, it has been approved for treatment of poorly healing wounds and chronic ulcerations. Echinacea increases resistance to infection and is used as a stimulant to the immune system. It is also used for the treatment of eczema, burns, psoriasis and herpes. As an immunostimulant, echinacea is used in the treatment of chronic respiratory infections, prostatitis and polyarthritis (rheumatoid arthritis) and inflammatory skin conditions.

Cosmetic use

Different plant parts such as leaves and root, in the form of extracts, expressed juice etc. are used in skin care because of its antioxidant activity. Classed as a moisturizing, tonic and skin conditioning agent it is used in skin care cosmetics for its antibacterial and anti-inflammatory activity.

The chemical compositions of different species of echinacea vary. All species have phenols such as cichoric acid and caftaric acid in *E. purpurea*, echinacoside in greater levels in *E. angustifolia* and *E. pallida* roots than in other species. When making herbal remedies, these phenols serve as markers for the quantity of raw echinacea in the product. Other chemical constituents that may be important in echinacea health effects include alkylamides and polysaccharides.

Rhodiola rosea (Crassulaceae)

Commonly called the golden root or rose root, the plant grows in the cold regions of the world. In Russia and Scandinavia, *R. rosea* has been used for centuries to cope with the cold Siberian climate and stressful life. The plant has been used in traditional Chinese medicine. *R. rosea* extract is mainly used in the form of capsules, tablets or tinctures.

Cosmetic use

The root extract is classed as an emollient, skin protecting, antioxidant, cosmetic astringent and skin-conditioning agent and used in several popular herbal cosmetics.

The dried rhizomes yield an essential oil with a total of 86 compounds identified. Geraniol was identified as the most important rose-like odour compound besides geranyl formate, geranyl acetate, benzyl alcohol and phenylethyl alcohol. Its oxygenated metabolite rosiridol is an aglycon of rosiridin, one of the most active constituents of rhodiola in bioassay-guided fractionation of rhodiolathe extract.

Vetivera zizanioides (Poaceae)

Commonly known as vetiver, it is a perennial grass native to India. In western and northern India, it is popularly known as khus. Though it originates in India, vetiver is widely cultivated in the tropical regions of the world. The world's major producers include Haiti, India, Java and Réunion.

Unlike most grasses, which form horizontally spreading, mat-like root systems, vetiver's roots grow downward, 2–4 m in depth. A fragrant grass, vetiver grass is grown for many different purposes. The plant helps to stabilize soil and protects it against erosion, Vetiver oil is derived from the plant's spongy, white net of roots, which are steam distilled after having been dried and chopped, producing the essential oil. Oil of vetiver used since centuries in India in incense and perfumes is now much prized for use in aromatherapy. Its pleasant scent and calming effect make it a good massage oil or a bath oil. Folk usage recommends it in the treatment of insomnia, depression and anger. A natural insect repellant and antiseptic, vetiver oil has also been used as a herbal remedy in arthritis and rheumatism.

Cosmetic use

This oil has been used in aromatherapy since ages. It is also an important ingredient of perfumes, soaps and cosmetics. Due to its excellent fixative properties, vetiver is used widely in perfumes as a scent and fixative. It is a constituent in 90% of western perfumes, more commonly in fragrances for men.

Due to its antibacterial activity, this oil can be used effectively for healing external wounds. Vetiver oil is known to eliminate skin blemishes and help accelerate healing. For this reason, this oil is indicated for application in a number of skin problems, such as acne, burns and skin marks. Vetiver oil and related products are included in leading brands of massage oils, bath oils, bath salts etc.

Oil of vetiver has over 100 identified components and α-vetivone is the chief constituent. Best quality oil obtained from 18–24-month-old roots is slightly viscous and amber brown in colour. Perfumery industry categorizes its odour as deep, sweet, earthy and balsam-like.

Vitis vinifera (Vitaceae)

This is the source of grapes. Grapes can be eaten raw or they can be used for making jam, juice, jelly, wine, grape seed extract, raisins, vinegar, and grape seed oil. Concentrated extracts prepared from whole grape seeds are reported to have a range of beneficial effects such as in wound healing, tooth decay, osteoporosis, skin cancer, radioprotection etc. Having received a lot of research interest grape seed extracts contain a high concentration of vitamin E, flavonoids, linoleic acid and proanthocyanidins.

Cosmetic use

Biochemical and medical studies have demonstrated significant antioxidant properties of grape seed oligomeric proanthocyanidins. Chemical constituents such as proanthocyanidins, polyphenols, flavonoids and anthocyanins, all of which are very potent antioxidants that help diminish the sun's damaging effects and reduce free-radical damage. Grape extract has also been shown to have wound-healing properties and hence included as supplementation for sunscreen protection. Its topical application in association with other antioxidants reportedly reduces skin cancer biomarkers. Presence of resveratrol, a powerful antioxidant in red grapes, is responsible for the health benefits of grape juice and thus red wine. *In vitro* studies on human skin equivalent biomodels demonstrated enhanced synthesis of healthy collagen, elastin and overall improvement of other skin structural components. Grape seed oil obtained by expression is an important cosmaceutical included in many skin care products.

Grape seed oil has some amount of tocopherols (vitamin E), but is notable for its high contents of phytosterols, polyunsaturated fatty acids such as linoleic acid, oleic acid and alpha-linolenic acid.

Honey

Honey is a naturally occurring sweetener produced by bees of the genus Apis. It is produced by bees from the nectar of certain flowering plants. Primarily consumed as food, honey is highly regarded as a cosmetic ingredient.

Cosmetic use

Honey is added to cosmetics and personal care products as a humectant, a flavouring agent and as a skin-conditioning agent. Also it is reported to have antioxidant and anti-inflammatory properties. Honey is used in the formulation of a wide range of products including baby and bath products, eye and facial make-up, fragrances, colouring and non-colouring hair products, personal cleanliness products and suntan and sunscreen products.

Honey is a mixture of glucose, fructose, sucrose and other naturally occurring sugars. It generally has a moisture content of 14% to 18%.

CONCLUSION

Use of plants and other natural materials for modifying one's appearance thus enhancing physical attractiveness is age old. Today's already rapidly growing cosmetic industry, which is almost synonymous with herbal cosmetics, is a vast global industry with huge growth potential. Apart from increasing interest in plants used for cosmetic purposes in various societies since ages, current scientific focus is unravelling systematic evidence for their cosmetic utility. Results from such scientific experimentation demonstrate the physiological effectiveness of herbs, thus proving their therapeutic worthiness resulting in such tested herbs being included in medicinal care products. More and more cosmaceuticals are being isolated and identified for their therapeutic/cosmetic benefits. Herbal extracts from neem, turmeric, tea tree oil etc. are being accepted for use in ethical dermatological products for their clinically tested effects.

Further research actively undertaken in premier research laboratories and institutes across the world will definitely add more such tested herbs to medical and cosmetic use. Thus the potential for herbals in cosmetics is just beginning to open up with tremendous scope for plant-based products in the cosmetics of tomorrow.

REVIEW QUESTIONS

Essay questions

1. Write an essay on the worldwide trade in herbal cosmetics. Add a note on the Indian cosmetics market.
2. Discuss the cosmetic value of herbs used for hair cleansing and conditioning properties citing appropriate examples.
3. What is skin whitening? Describe the natural sources of skin whiteners and moisturizers.

Short notes

1. Significance of the usage of herbs in cosmetics.
2. Forms of incorporating herbs in cosmetics.
3. Hair nourishers and growth stimulants.
4. Anti-infective cosmetic herbs.
5. Herbs as skin rejuvenators.

11

Plant Biotechnology

CHAPTER OBJECTIVES

Introduction

Milestones in the History of Plant-Tissue Culture

Scope of Plant-Tissue Culture Techniques

Media Requirements for Plant-Tissue Culture

Plant Growth Regulators

Types of Cultures

Plant Cell Immobilization

Bio Transformation

Transgenic Plants and Their Applications

Secondary Metabolite Production in Plant-Tissue Culture Systems

INTRODUCTION

Biotechnology refers to the technology-based utilization of biological systems for generation of products to improve quality of human life. Such utilization has been happening since thousands of years in terms of agriculture (raising food crops), food production (baking, brewing, dairy products), and more recently in medicine (antibiotics from soil microorganisms). Developments in the late 20th century have expanded it, to include technological advancements such as genetic engineering, microbial, plant and animal cell and tissue culture, artificial plant hybridization, bio informatics, and so on. Such technological advances in life sciences have found applications in areas including health care, agriculture, medicinal plant cultivation, industrial plant-based products, and environmental management.

Plant biotechnology includes applications of technological tools in plant sciences. Several significant achievements in plant biology such as cell and tissue culture, regeneration of whole plants from somatic cells, genetic recombination, and other such achievements have resulted in applications such as rapid plant propagation, developing uniform healthy plant saplings, somatic hybrids from naturally incompatible species, germ plasma storage, improved transgenic plants, harvesting plant secondary metabolites from cultured plant cells, and so on.

Aseptic culturing of plant cells, tissues, and organs under conditioned physical and chemical environment *in vitro* gave interesting insights into basic and applied areas of experimental botany including plant secondary metabolism. Extensive exploration of various possibilities of applying this technique to practical use has made it into a promising branch of science with commercial applications in agriculture, horticulture, forestry, and drug development.

MILESTONES IN THE HISTORY OF PLANT-TISSUE CULTURE

Tracing the history of plant-tissue culture, one can identify the series of land mark discoveries in this field to be originating from the proposal of cell as the basic unit of form and function of an organism.

- Schleiden and Schwann in 1839 propounded the cell theory and visualized its autonomy and potential to regenerate into a whole organism.
- Vochting's classical experiments in 1878 demonstrated the polarity of plant cuttings to regenerate shoots or roots depending on their relative position on the stem.
- Classical experiments of Gottleib Haberlandt, a German botanist in 1902 on isolated single plant cells demonstrated their growth in size in basic salt solution (Knops Media) supplemented with sucrose. He is now considered the "Father of Plant-Tissue Culture" and he had rightly proposed the ability of plant cells to resume uninterrupted plant growth and even form artificial embryos from vegetative cells.
- Successful growth to maturity of nearly mature embryos of radish species on simple media of mineral salts and sugar solution by Hanig in 1904, established the foundation of later successful embryo culture technique.
- Laibach in 1929 reared embryos from nonviable seeds of artificial hybrids of *Linum* species on nutrient medium, opening up possibility of culturing aborted embryos of several hybrids.
- Van Overbreek in 1941 succeeded in culturing young embryos on media supplemented with embryo sac fluid-coconut milk.
- As suggested by Haberlandt, his student Kotte and Robbins, both working independently, cultured growing root tips in 1922.
- Modifying media composition, White in 1934 managed to continuously maintain tomato root tips in culture for about 34 years. His media constituted of inorganic salts, sucrose, and yeast extract, which was later replaced with vitamins B6, B2, and nicotinic acid. Recognition of importance of B vitamins in plant growth was an important milestone, as was the first identification of use of Indole acetic acid (IAA) for enhancing growth of *Salix* cambium by Gauthret in the same year (1934).
- IAA was earlier discovered in 1926 as a plant growth regulator by Fritz Went. In 1939 White reported similar results with *Nicotiana* species hybrid tumor tissue as had Nobecourt with carrot cultures in 1937. Media used by Gauthret, White, and Nobecourt went on to become the basic tissue culture media used in later years up to this day with modifications.
- Skoog in 1944 and Skoog and Tsui later in 1951, identified the importance of vascular tissue in inducing cell division in tobacco pith cells in media supplemented with adenine and phosphate.

- Jablonski and Skoog found that pith tissue could grow even without the presence of vascular tissue when DNA was added to the media. In 1955 Miller and workers isolated the first cytokinin called kinetin from DNA of herring sperm. These experiments on tobacco pith cultures showed that high concentrations of IAA and such auxins promoted rooting and high concentrations of kinetin initiates shooting and bud formation in cultures. At equal concentrations, the tissue grows in an unorganized manner forming callus tissue.

- In 1962 Murashige and Skoog showed that growth of tobacco tissue is enhanced 5 times when media salt concentration was 25 times as much as Knops media. Today Murashige & Skoog (MS) medium has great commercial application in tissue culture.

- In 1953 Muir was successful in growing individual cells mechanically separated from cultures shaken to disperse aggregates of callus tissue. These cells from *Tagetes* and *Nicotiana* species underwent division on a filter paper nursed with established callus culture underneath.

- It was possible to observe cultured single cells growing in hanging drops of tissue-conditioned media, due to the work of Jones and his group in 1960.

- In the same year, Bergmann developed a technique for cloning large numbers of single cells of higher plants by filtering suspension cultures. This formed the basis of the plating technique widely used later for cloning isolated single protoplasts.

- From isolated cells of colonies of hybrid from *Nicotiana glutinosa* and *N. tabacum*, Vasil and Hildebrandt regenerated whole plantlets in 1965.

- Instead of cells from actively growing tissues in cultures, mature mesophyll cells from *Macleaya* species were successfully cultured by Kohlenbach in 1966.

- In the same year, Steward reported induction of somatic embryos from free cells in carrot suspension cultures. Thus, so far the prediction of Haberlandt to regenerate whole plants from single cells was realized by way of shoot and root differentiation or embryogenic development from cultured tissue cells. Such a possibility of regenerating whole plants from single somatic cells found great applicability in both plant propagation and later in genetic engineering.

- Further detailed studies by Bingham, Saunders, Reisch, Bhojwani, Green, Philips, and Vasil from 1970–1980 revealed that while it was easy to raise somatic embryos from plants like carrot, cereals, and legumes do not respond similarly. Regeneration potential was reported to be genetically controlled and proper genotype selection and physiological state of explant were important factors.

- With successful growth of plant cells in suspension in a liquid medium, began attempts to generate plant-derived chemicals *in vitro*. First large-scale production of plant secondary metabolites from cultured plant cells was reported by Tulecke, Nickell, and Routien in 1956–58 on *Ginkgo*, *Rose*, and *Lolium* species. Despite problems of slow growth, genetic instability, intracellular accumulation of generated compounds and the like, work of Kaul and Staba in 1967 and Zenk in 1978 showed generation of secondary metabolites in cultures in much larger quantities than whole plants.

- Shikonin, a red-coloured dye from tissue cultures of *Lithospermum erythrorhizon* was the first product to be commercialized.

- Next the technique of immobilization of secondary metabolite generating plant cells was developed by Brodelius and his group in 1979. Larger quantities of plant cellular mass could be used for longer periods making harvesting of the generated secondary metabolites much easier than from suspension cultures.

- Ball in 1946 raised whole plants of *Lupinus* and *Trapaeolum* from shoot tip culture. This technique found extensive practical application in terms of rapid propagation of large number of genetically identical plants from a very small portion of an explant. This soon became a regular method of propagation of orchids and many other plant species including flowering and fruiting plants began to be cloned. Genetic variation found in plants raised from cultured cells was beneficially utilized for specifically raising resistant, high yield, or novel variants/strains with respect to secondary metabolite composition.

- Nay and Street by regenerating plants from frozen carrot cells in 1973 gave impetus to the idea of freeze preservation of valuable germplasm.

- Morel and Martin in 1952 cultured virus free shoot tip meristem of virus infected Dahlia plants and generated disease free plants. Today this technique of micrografting to raise pathogen-free plants from infected stocks is of great agronomic and horticultural importance.

- *In vitro* culturing of pollen grains together with excised ovules resulted in *in vitro* or test tube fertilization of ovules by the germinated pollen due to the work of Maheswari and Kanta in 1960–1962. This technique was successfully used to overcome sexual incompatibility between species and genera and also to produce rare hybrids.

- By growing large numbers of androgenic haploid plants from cultured pollen grains of *Datura innoxia* in 1966, Guha and Maheswari opened up the possibility of introduction of newer varieties of rice, wheat, and tobacco.

- A significant breakthrough in plant-tissue culture was isolation of protoplasts from plant cells by enzymatic cell wall degradation by Cocking in 1960. These naked cells without cell wall could be fused to generate somatic hybrids as reported by Carlson in 1972 with tobacco species. The reconstituted cell was shown to regenerate a new wall and continue with cell division. Isolated protoplasts were shown to be totipotent and with protoplast fusion, it was possible to generate genetically altered somatic cells or hybrids. By raising whole plants from such somatic hybrids, it became possible to generate agronomically useful variants or hybrids. Today protoplast fusion techniques have become much more technologically sophisticated with contributions from advances in genetic engineering.

- Isolation of restriction endonuclease enzymes by Smith and Nathans in 1970 and reverse trasncriptase by Baltimore enabled insertion of foreign genes into native DNA of plant cells thus enabling their genetic modification.

- This heralded a new research area of genetic engineering, and by 1972 *in vitro* recombinant DNA virus was reconstructed by Paul Berg. This tool made possible construction of human insulin using recombinant bacteria.

- Observation of crown gall disease causing gram negative soil bacteria *Agrobacterium tumefaciens* in gall forming plants by Zaenan and group in 1974 led to the demonstration of the transfer and integration of a large plasmid from the bacterium into the plant cell genome. This induced the formation of excessive epidermal cell growth and hence, gall formation.

- Due to the work of Chitton et al., in 1977 and Barton et al., in 1983 it became possible to insert heterologous DNA into this bacterial plasmid, which was transferred by it into plants thus producing a genetically altered plant. This gave birth to the production of transgenic plants pioneered by the generation of transgenic tobacco plants by Horsh et al., in 1984. Several other gene transfer methods such as bolistic gene transfer, eletroporation, microinjection, and particle gun were introduced and many genetically improved plant varieties with economically useful traits were developed.

As predicted by Haberlandt, experiences with plant-tissue culture greatly expanded our understanding about the "inter relationships and complementary influence to which cells are exposed to within a multicellular organism." This was reflected in extensive commercial applications in several areas of life sciences including production of improved crop varieties, biotransformation of secondary metabolites, proptoplast generated somatic hybrids, genetically transformed transgenic plants, rapid propagation of genetically uniform plants, and germplasm storage.

SCOPE OF PLANT-TISSUE CULTURE TECHNIQUES

Future scope of plant-tissue culture in terms of applications in agriculture and horticulture is enormous. In our country, it is being extensively worked on toward developing improved crop varieties to feed our burgeoning population, improve dwindling forest cover, micro propagate for rapid propagation of precious trees like bamboo, teak, sandal wood, eucalyptus in addition to medicinal, aromatic, horticultural, and ornamental plants.

Following are some of the areas of utilization of plant-tissue culture techniques:

Clonal Propagation

Developing large numbers of identical plantlets by using shoot tip or auxillary bud culture of the plant variety with the desired traits, shall supplement the present methods of sexual and asexual propagation methods. Such micropropagation is of specific use for plants difficult to propagate by these conventional methods. It offers high multiplication rates and is an effective method of conserving endangered plant species. It is being tried in our country for sandal wood, high curcumin turmeric, ginger, dioscorea, citrus, papaya, and cardamom.

Somaclonal Variation

Plantlets from tissue culture give rise to morphological variation compared to the original source plants. These variations may be of economic importance, when desirable variants are suitably selected. This is especially valuable in plant-breeding programs in sexually reproducing crop plants with limited variability and to induce variation in vegetatively propagated species. Somaclonal variation has been successfully exploited in producing better variants of wheat, rice, maize, alfalfa, tomato, tobacco, sugarcane, cardamom and the like. In our country, variants of lemongrass, turmeric, ginger, cardamom, sugarcane, and mustard have been released. High yielding somaclonal variants of medicinal plants include those of *C. roseus, Nicotiana rustica, Coptis japonica, Anchusa oficinalis, Lithospermum erythrrorhizon*, and *Hyoscyamus muticus*.

Embryo Culture

Aseptic isolation of embryos at different developmental stages from ovules, immature seeds, polyembryonic seeds either inviable or abortive is called embryo culture. *In vitro* embryo culture is used to regenerate healthy plants from non-viable embryos, to overcome seed dormancy, to obtain rare and novel hybrids, propagate rare plants, and raise haploid plants. It is used for recovering hybrids of several economically important plants like ground nut, cotton, flax, rice, barley, and tomato. This is because, hybrid embryos from inter-generic and inter-specific crosses result in sterile seeds and extensive use of embryo rescue may be made using embryo culture techniques.

Artificial Seeds

Formation of simply organized embryo-like structures originating in culture from somatic cells either spontaneously or through growth regulators is called somatic embryogenesis. This is a versatile technique used for micropropagation and when somatic embryos are coated appropriately they form artificial seeds. These may be sown in the field directly and this technique increases germination of hybrid embryos. It is possible to generate artificial seeds of maize, carrot, alfalfa, and cotton among many others. Somatic embryo cultures may be stored for a longer duration through cryopreservation. In India some *Brassica* species are conserved by embryo rescue. Somatic embryogenesis has been induced in medicinal plants such as *Atropa belladonna, Brassica oleraceae, Carica papaya, Citrus sinensis, Nicotiana tabacum,* and *Saccharum officinale.*

Pathogen-Free Plants

In vitro culture of shoot meristem measuring less than 0.1 mm in length is called meristem culture. It is employed in the *in vitro* clonal propagation of plants from shoot tips, leaf sections, and calli. By this technique it is possible to generate virus-free plants in culture from meristem of infected plants. This is especially applicable to those propagated vegetatively as unlike seeds (which do not carry viruses), the pathogens are transferred directly to the regenerated plants. Garlic, pineapple, banana, sugarcane, and potato may be raised as virus free plants from infected lots by meristem culture. Apart from raising virus free plants, it is also used for micropropagation and germplasm storage.

Androgenic Haploids in Crop Breeding

Anther or pollen culture *in vitro* gives rise to plants with haploid number of chromosomes. While naturally occurring haploids are rare as reported in *Datura, Nicotiana, Coptis,* and *Arrhinium* species, tissue culture–raised haploids are of great economic importance in plant-breeding programs and in mutation studies. By themselves sterile, they may be made to form homozygous diploids by colchicine treatment. Ever since Bourgin and Nitch (1967) raised the first mature haploid plants of Nicotiana, so far androgenic haploids have been raised in more than 200 species belonging to about 88 genera and 34 families. Haploids are used in crop improvement of wheat, barley, rye, maize, potato, tomato, sunflower, and peanut.

Germplasm Storage

Conventional methods of germplasm storage follows seed storage at 10–20°C at reduced moisture in sealed containers. Germplasm deteriorates under such conditions in plants such as rubber, neem, cocoa, jackfruit, mango, and litchi. For these and for seedless plants like tapioca, sugarcane, and sweet banana, germplasm storage may be in the form of cryopreservation of *in vitro* cultures of shoot tips, roots, somatic embryos, tissue, and pollen. Germplasm storage of endangered plants, primitive cultivars, and wild relatives of crop plants is undertaken to avoid erosion of plant genetic resources. Through cryopreservation, such as *in vitro* gene banks shall ensure availability of valuable germplasm to breeders to develop new and improved varieties. Many categories of endangered plants and living fossils like Ginkgo, Cycads, Metasequoia, and Cyathea apart from several Orchid species and medicinal plants Rauwolfia, Dioscorea, and Aconitum have been successfully conserved by tissue-culture methods.

Protoplast Fusion

Fusion of two protoplasts—plant cells whose rigid cell wall has been removed—facilitates fusion of their DNA, cell organelles, bacteria, and virus. This process of somatic hybridization following isolation, culture, and fusion of protoplasts is a very significant milestone in plant-tissue culture. The unique properties of protoplasts, their ability to regenerate a cell wall and resume further cell division, and their totipotent nature has opened up further extensive possibilities in terms of plant regeneration and cell wall formation studies, genetic manipulation, and somatic hybridization. It gives a novel breeding technique to enable crosses between species and even genera. Since both nuclear and cytoplasmic material is transmitted, somatic hybridization has a much greater scope of introducing genetic variability to achieve resistance to diseases, pests, abiotic stress tolerance, improved growth characteristics, and even enhanced plant size and improved secondary metabolite constitution of the progeny.

In addition to being a gateway for fundamental and applied research, protoplast fusion has been exploited for somatic hybridization in several plants of Solanaceae such as *Nicotiana, Datura, Petunia, Solanum,* and *Lycopersicum* in addition to many more families.

Literature abounds in references to novel inter-specific, intra-specific and intergeneric hybrids made from protoplast fusion. Genetic transfer of desirable characteristics by protoplast culture furthered by recombinant DNA technology has made possible insertion and expression of desired genes in a recipient cell. Through this the flower colour of Petunia could be changed and Nicotiana hybrids became resistant to tobacco mosaic virus.

Transgenic Plants

Plants raised from cells genetically engineered to carry genes not native to the species are transgenic plants. There has been exciting progress in developing improved novel traits in many crop plants. The first transgenic tobacco plant was developed in 1983 followed by cotton, soybean, mustard, maize, and so on. There is a large-scale cultivation of insect-resistant transgenic crops, few of which are boll worm–resistant cotton, corn borer–resistant maize, and herbicide-resistant soybean. A large number of transgenic plants are of economic value due to their enhanced stress tolerance, resistance to bacterial, viral, and fungal pathogens, improved nutritional quality, therapeutic protein content, ability to generate antigenic proteins for use as vaccines, ability to form biodegradable plastics, or accumulate larger quantity of novel secondary metabolites. Multiple benefits of transgenic crops include flexible crop management, beneficial crop variants (e.g., β-carotene-enriched rice grains) and crops of higher produce.

Secondary Metabolite Production

The various techniques of plant-tissue culture have made possible medicinal plant improvement through genetic engineering, selection of higher yielding strains, generation of novel metabolites in culture, isolation of biosynthetic enzymes, and production of secondary metabolites of plant cells in much higher yields than in intact plants. Plant-tissue culture could thus be a significant source of phytochemicals used as pharmaceuticals, food additives, fragrance chemicals, and pesticides. Cell-suspension cultures have been used to generate a large number of alkaloids, steroids, volatile oils, saponins, cardiac glycosides, anti-cancer agents, insecticides, and volatile terpene constituents. Novel plant products not made by whole plants have been formed in cultured cells from precursors added to the media. Large-scale production of plant products similar to microbial fermentative production has generated scores of compounds in culture such as berberine, ajmalicine, fucin, colchicine, anthraquinones, quinine, jasmine, diosgenin, morphine, codeine, camptothecin, nicotine, glycyrrhizin, and stevioside among others.

MEDIA REQUIREMENTS FOR PLANT-TISSUE CULTURE

Plant-tissue culture basically involves growth of an excised plant organ or tissue called explant on a suitable nutrient medium under aseptic culturing conditions. Clean work areas with sufficient space for housing basic equipment like growth chambers, inoculation cabinets, shakers, centrifuges, autoclaves, ovens, microscopes, weighing equipment and so on in designated washing, media preparation, aseptic transfer and culture incubation areas are the infrastructural requirements.

Intact plants are photosynthetically active and fix atmospheric carbon dioxide with the help of water and sunlight thus producing carbon as source of basic energy. Required mineral nutrients are derived from the soil through the roots and plants synthesize a vast array of vitamins and other necessary biomolecules needed to support their structural and functional development. Plant cells growing in culture are not autotrophic with respect to carbon and it is essential to include a carbohydrate to provide the needed elements C, H, and O in the medium. Other nutritional requirements of cells in culture are similar to that of whole plants.

Media requirement for culturing plant cells *in vitro* depends on the plant species, plant organ, type of culture, and its purpose. There is no single universal medium catering to all types of cultures and different early workers have used their own media according to their work. These media were composed of simple salts, a sugar with different qualitative and quantitative combinations of various nutritive mixtures or extracts. Several ready-to-use media are now available such as Murashige and Skoog media and these are in general suitable for most plant-tissue-culture experiments. These are admixtures of chemically defined substances and are known as "synthetic media." Alternatively media needed for a specific work may be constituted based on a published recipe with added chemical ingredients and may also be supplemented with natural mixtures such as casein hydrolysate, coconut milk, malt extract, yeast extract, tomato aqueous extract, water melon juice, and so on. Thus, media composition is variable according to the type of culture work. For example, alkaloid production in cultures sometimes requires media different from that needed to support the growth of cells. In many cases, elicitors or precursors are required to be added to improve metabolite production.

When we study the composition of media that supported successful plant cell culture trials, it is essentially composed of the following:

Inorganic Substances

Plant cells in culture are required to be provided with a continuous supply of 12 inorganic elements. Elements—Nitrogen, Phosphorous, Sulphur, Calcium, Potassium, and Magnesium—required in quantities greater than 0.5 mM/L are macro elements. Micro elements—Iron, Manganese, Copper, Zinc, Boron and Molybdenum—are needed in concentrations less than 0.5 mmol/L.

Nitrogen provided in the form of $(NH_4)^+$ or $(NO_3)^-$ can be provided in an organic or inorganic form each of which has a specific influence on *in vitro* morphogenesis. It is a constituent of amino acids, proteins, chlorophyll, and some growth hormones. Nitrogen is an important element contributing to overall pant growth both *in vivo* and *in vitro*. It is usually added up to 60 mM.

Phosphorous added as phosphate salt is needed in about 1.25 mM for cell division and for energy transfer and energy storage in plants.

Sulphur is provided as sulphate or from amino acids included in media such as cysteine, methionine, homocysteine, and glutathione. It is utilized for protein synthesis and required in concentration of around 1.5 mM.

Calcium in the form of calcium salts like calcium chloride in the concentration of about 3 mM is essential. It is involved in cell hormonal response to light, temperature, and so on. Calcium is needed for incorporation of phospholipids within the plant cell membrane and being an important component of cell walls, it is essential for cell membrane integrity.

Potassium in the form of potassium salts provided in the concentration of about 20 mM is required to be provided because it is needed for normal cell division and in the synthesis of chlorophyll, protein, and in the reduction of nitrates.

Magnesium in the form of magnesium sulphate in 1.5 mM concentration is to be provided. It is a co-factor of several enzymes and it is also a component of the chlorophyll molecule.

Microelements usually provided in trace amounts are needed as co-factors/catalysts or as inducers of enzyme synthesis.

Organic Substances

Theoretically, cultured plant cells are equipped to synthesize the needed biomolecules, vitamins, and other growth elements. However these are supplied in the media for providing maximal/optimal conditions for growth. In general, sucrose in 2–5% concentration is the carbon source. Glucose, fructose, maltose, galactose, mannose, and lactose may also be used. Sucrose plays an important osmotic role in the medium and is required for several metabolic activities.

Amino acids as l-forms play an important role in morphogenesis and serve as sources of reduced nitrogen. Glycine is commonly used and tyrosine supports shoot initiation. Arginine facilitates rooting and amides glutamine and asparigine enhance somatic embryogenesis.

Though plants can synthesize their own vitamins, depending on the nature of plant species and nature of culture, vitamins B_1, B_3, B_6 and myo-ionositol, pantothenic acid, vitamin C, vitamin D and vitamin F have been used in different culture media. B_1 is an important co-factor in carbohydrate metabolism, B_2 improves shoot formation, and prevents explant browning. Vitamin D has a growth-regulatory effect and vitamins C and E act as anti-oxidants. Myo-ionositol, a member of B vitamin complex, is a natural plant constituent and a crucial precursor in biosynthesis of pectin and hemi-cellulose needed for cell wall synthesis. It is also known to support the action of auxins.

Complex nutritive mixtures such as casein hydrolysate (30–300 mg/L), coconut milk (10–20% v/v), yeast extract (50–500 mg/L), tomato juice (30%), and malt extract are added to medium in specific cases to support culture growth.

Non nutritional Media Ingredients

Gelling agents are used to make the media semi-solid for it to provide support to the explant without which it may submerge and deprive the growing cells of the needed oxygen. Agar (0.8–1%), agarose (0.4%), and gelrite—a bacterial polysaccharide (0.1–0.2%) are usually used as they withstand sterilization by autoclaving and are liquid while hot and semi-solid when cool.

Water-soluble antibiotics, carbenecillin (500 mg/L), cefotaxime (300 mg/L), and augmentin (250 mg/L) are included in the culture medium to prevent problems of contamination.

PLANT GROWTH REGULATORS

They are groups of plant hormones, widely distributed in higher plants and known to exert profound influences on the growth and development of plants. They exert their effect at very low concentrations and regulate a range of cell activities such as cell growth, cell division, differentiation, morphogenesis, dormancy, and senescence. Following the discovery of their crucial role in shooting and rooting of plant cells in cultures, they became essential additions to culture media. They are used in vegetative propagation, micropropagation, and in tissue culture. Their requirements in culture vary with tissue and their endogenous levels in cells. Variations in relative proportions of plant growth regulators in tissue culture media affect metabolism. Also there are several interesting reports of enhanced secondary metabolite production due to modulation of growth hormone levels of the media.

Auxins

Auxins are a group of compounds associated with stem and internode elongation, tropism, apical dominance, adventitious root production, fruit setting, rooting, and in similar functions in whole plants. They promote production of other hormones. Indole acetic acid (IAA) is a major auxin found in actively growing tissues with many of its potential precursors reported from several plants. In tissue culture, auxins at low concentrations are required for cell elongation and root initiation, and at high concentrations, they suppress morphogenesis. Several synthetic auxins are being widely used, and the most commonly used ones in tissue culture are IAA, Indole-3-butyric acid (IBA), and Naphthalene acetic acid (NAA) for rooting and along with cytokinin for shoot proliferation. 2,4-Dichlorophenoxy acetic acid (2,4-D) and 2,4,5 -trichlorophenoxyacetic acid are used for callus initiation and growth in somatic embryogenesis. Naphthoxy acetic acid (NOA) and p-chlorophenoxy acetic acid (p-CPA) are the other auxins used.

Auxins have been reported to enhance ergot alkaloid production in submerged culture and also anthraquinone production in *Morinda citrifolia* cell suspension cultures.

Cytokinins

Kinetin was the first cytokinin to be isolated from the DNA of herring sperm, and zeatin was the first plant cytokinin isolated from coconut liquid endosperm. Since then it has been reported from maize and several other plants. Cytokinins influence cell division and shoot formation. These have a synergistic effect with auxins and ratios of these two hormones affect plant growth. They counter apical dominance induced by auxins and along with ethylene promote leaf, flower, and fruit abscission. Cytokinins are used in tissue culture for cell differentiation, shoot proliferation, shoot morphogenesis and formation of adventitious buds. With several more, such as Isopentenyl adenine (IPA) and dihydrozeatin being identified, Benzyl aminopurine (BAP), fufuryl aminopurine (kinetin), and Thidiazuron (TDZ) are used in plant-tissue culture. TDZ is effective at low concentrations to stimulate shoot formation. Cytokinins have been shown to increase biosynthesis of berberine and condensed tannins and rhodoxanthin in *in vitro* cultures of their source plants.

Gibberellins

The first gibberellins was isolated form a fungus—Gibberella fugikuroi. At present about 90 gibberellins are reported from plants and they are named GA_1, GA_2, GA_3, etc. They are synthesized by leaves and stored in immature seeds and fruits. Gibberellins cause internodal cell elongation and induce seed germination and seedling establishment. Gibberellins have been extensively studied with respect to their effects on many medicinal plant species such as Eucalyptus, Hops, Citrus, Coriander, Datura and Nicotiana, Vince, Tea, Digitalis, Sienna, and Buck wheat. In plant-tissue culture, they are used rarely and GA_3 when used is reported to induce plantlet generation form adventive embryos in culture.

Ethylene

It is a gaseous growth regulator and emitted especially from storing plant-tissues and ripening fruits (produced by all higher plants in almost all tissues). It is known to influence leaf abscission and fruit ripening and is associated with the triple response of shoot growth, root growth, and differentiation. Ethylene has limited solubility in water and hence diffuses out of cells after being formed, into the plants' environment. Some young tissues like seedlings make more ethylene much faster than it can be diffused out. Hence there will be inhibition of leaf expansion with further growth, exposure to light, ethylene production decreases, thus promoting leaf expansion. It is used routinely for enhancing flow of rubber latex. Ethylene and related compounds such as 2-chloroethyl phosphonic acid are investigated for their effects on plant-tissue culture. It is reported with variable effect on cell morphogenesis *in vitro*.

Growth Inhibitors

Several plant compounds are reported with growth inhibitory effect in plants. These affect leaf and fruit abscission, dormancy, seed germination, and bud opening. Abscisic acid isolated from a fungus *Cenospora rosicola*, is used in embryo culture and to promote morphogenesis.

Brassinosteroids, jasmonates, stringolactones, karrikins, and polyamines are some of the other identified plant growth regulators.

TYPES OF CULTURES

There are multiple methodologies being followed for different types of plant cell/tissue culture techniques. The current know how in this area is such; it is not only possible to culture free cells, genetically alter them, induce cell divisions, and elicit secondary metabolite production; plant cells cultured from plants with desired combination of traits may be somatically fused to form artificial hybrids, plantlets regenerated, and whole plants could be raised from it. Cell culture allows study of plant cell metabolism and effect of various substances on cellular responses and also enables clonal propagation of genetically identical plants. Thus, depending on the purpose, cultures may be categorized as organ, tissue, and cell cultures.

Organ Culture

Aseptic culturing of isolated plant organs or those obtained from callus differentiation is called organ culture. It is possible to culture virtually any plant part such as root, leaf, stem, flower, seed, and cotyledon. These are cultured for plantlet regeneration or to induce callus formation. Cultured organs can be made to generate secondary metabolites in higher yield than intact plants, for example, leaf cultures of *D. purpurea* and *D. lanata*. In cases as in leaf cultures of Vinca and Rauwolfia, a variety of constituents not found in intact plants are produced. Similarly, leaf and root cultures of *C. ledgeriana* accumulated quinine and quinidine not found in cell suspension cultures. Root cells genetically transformed through bacteria such as *Agrobacterium tumefaciens*, when grown in a medium devoid of growth hormones, give rise to numerous fine hairy roots. Such transformed hairy root cultures of several medicinal plants reportedly accumulate much higher yields of normal secondary metabolites as well as compounds not associated with intact plants. For example, Solasodine content in *S. laciniatum* cultures was four times over intact plants. Hairy root cultures of *P. ginseng* reported more effective production of ginsenosides over ordinary root cultures. Similarly valepotriate yield was four times over whole roots in *V. officinalis* hairy root cultures. Ginseng hairy root cultures have reportedly transformed added digitoxigenin to novel stearate, palmitate, and myristate esters.

Tissue Culture

Excised plant-tissues such as root tips, shoot tips, leaf primordia, ovaries from pollinated or unpollinated flowers, ovules, anther, embryos, nucleus and endosperm are cultured *in vitro* for plant cell physiological/morphological studies, clonal propagation, plant hybridization, and in plant breeding programs.

Cultured plant-tissues are grown on hormone-controlled media to induce callus formation. Callus actually refers to wounded tissue that an intact plant produces when there is injury. In tissue culture, proliferating mass of unorganized/undifferentiated parenchymatous cells arising from an explant is called callus. Such callus cultures could be maintained for prolonged periods by repeated sub-culturing. They may thus be made to form an extended area of tissue or form a friable mass, which can be dispersed into a suspension culture.

Callus cultures may be utilized for plant regeneration, preparation of single-cell suspensions, protoplast isolation, and in genetic transformation studies. Callus derived cultures from medicinal plants are being much investigated and form an important source of plant secondary metabolites. Explant or the plant part that generates the callus is crucial in determining the nature of secondary metabolites formed in culture.

Single-Cell Culture

Culturing single cells derived from callus cultures or by mechanical or enzymatic isolation from plant material is called cell culture. Since they are totipotent and carry the required genetic information, by hormonal manipulation they may be induced to form roots, shoots, and thus regenerate into a complete plant in culture. Alternatively, when isolated single cells are placed in a conditioned medium, they undergo repeated division, multiply, and result in callus formation. When single cells are cultured in a conditioned liquid medium, they are called suspension cultures. In this way it is possible to culture them in large volume bioreactors similar to micro organisms and they can be maintained in continuous culture for the production of a range of high value, low volume phytochemicals. Unlike microbes, cell proliferation rates are much lower and they have a tendency to grow as aggregates. Also being fragile, dispersing aggregates in large volume liquid cultures requires special low-shear mixing techniques to prevent cell rupture. Free cell suspension cultures can be grown using the following techniques:

Batch Culture

It is a suspension culture of smaller volumes ranging from 100–250 ml, being agitated continuously to break aggregates of cells. Cells grow and multiply in medium constituted of limited amount of nutrients, after a lag period of cell acclimatization. Following an exponential growth and division phase, due to exhaustion of a nutrient, they fall into the stationary growth phase. As no further medium is added in each batch of cultured cells, it is a "closed" system and is generally used for initiating single-cell cultures. Such cultures may be subcultured by transferring aliquots into fresh medium. Such repeated culturing may generate a fine suspension of cells.

Continuous Culture

Here cells are grown in suspension in media that is limited in quantity with respect to one nutrient. Since cell growth is limited by this nutrient, before its exhaustion, fresh medium is added to this limiting nutrient. Growth of cells in culture is thus continuous. When the old medium is withdrawn, if cells are separated and added back to culture, it is a "closed continuous culture." However, with addition of medium, there is withdrawal of suspension, without adding back cells, it is an "open continuous culture." Here the medium input and culture harvest are so balanced that cells are in a constant submaximal growth rate continuously. When media addition is determined by constant level of a particular nutrient, the culture is a "chemostat." If, however, media addition is intermittent, as and when the turbidity of the culture is enhanced due to an increase in number of steadily growing cells, it is called a "turbidostat" culture.

Protoplast Culture

Protoplasts are cells without cell walls. Though they may be isolated directly from any plant part such as young leaf, root, stem, seedling, pollen grains, petals and embryo sac, leaf mesophyll cells and cells from suspension culture are convenient for protoplast isolation. Several enzymatic and mechanical means are employed for stripping the cells of their cell wall. Such protoplasts, almost spherical in shape may be cultured by plating them on agar. The pinocytic activity, that is, the ability to take up extracellular material and totipotency make them ideal research tools for both fundamental studies in cell biology and applications based on somatic hybridization and genetic engineering.

PLANT CELL IMMOBILIZATION

Cultured plant cells in suspension usually demonstrate an inverse relationship between growth and primary or secondary metabolism. Secondary metabolite formation usually does not reach optimum levels until the growth rate of the culture decreases substantially during the stationary phase. In other words, secondary metabolite generation could be maintained for extended periods if stationary phase cells are held in productive metabolic state. Large-scale production of secondary metabolites by plant cell culture is associated with problems such as lower growth rate, low product yield, genetic instability of cell lines, cell fragility, and intracellular accumulation of generated products. Some of these drawbacks may be minimized by immobilizing the cultured cells on an inert support system. To facilitate release of intracellular products, the cell membrane may be permeabilized using surface-active chemicals such as DMSO, phenetyl alcohol, chloroform, triton X-100. Alternatively, physical methods such as ultrasonication, electroporation, and ionophoretic release may also be used.

Such immobilized cells

- can be used as reusable biocatalysts for longer periods of up to 60 days
- are nondividing and hence, such stationary phase cells are in productive metabolic state for this entire duration
- are not subject to genetic changes and there is no cell division
- are protected from the shear stress of agitation due to stirring, rotation, tumbling, or shaking required for cells in suspension
- are not associated with viscosity, agitation, and aeration problems of suspension cultures
- show increased product accumulation and extended bio synthetic activity
- are sometimes induced to spontaneously release products normally stored within cells in suspension
- may effectively bring about biochemical conversions of precursors added to the extracellular medium
- reduce processing costs due to ease of product harvesting from the media

Cultured cells may be immobilized by several strategies such as:

- entrapment within preformed structures or inert support material such as alginate beads, polyurethane foam, fibre glass mats, polyester fiber, etc.
- enclosure within hollow fibre or flat semi-permeable membranes
- precipitation resulting in cell entrapment within a lattice of polymers such as agar, agarose, etc.
- ionic network formation with alginate, polyacrylamide, κ-carrageenan, and alginate in the form of calcium alginate is used extensively for plant cell entrapment by ion exchange reaction
- formation of photo cross linkable bonds with resins such as polyethylene glycol, polypropylene oligomers as pre polymers,
- microencapsulation

Surface immobilization on to a support matrix is ideal for secondary metabolite generation, as the cells are entrapped within it and then grow as a continuous tissue-like structure on its surface. The cells are cemented together by a mucilagenous material secreted by the entrapped cells. This natural tendency of plant cell to aggregate improves synthesis and accumulation of secondary metabolites.

A successfully immobilized plant cell system if viable for long periods is a highly cost-effective method of secondary metabolite generation especially if these are secreted extracellularly. This is because product harvest is much easier than from intact plant organs or from suspension cultures. Such immobilized systems may be cultivated in large reactors specifically designed for the process of large-scale production of plant secondary metabolites. Immobilized cells thus can also be used much similar to immobilized enzymes to facilitate bioconversion of compounds added to the medium

Some successful examples of plant cell immobilization are

- higher serpentine accumulation by *Catharanthus roseus* cells over suspension cultures;
- 50 times more capsaicin generated by *Capsicum frutescens* cells;
- 40% greater diosgenin production by immobilized *D. deltoidea* cells;
- double sanguinarine yield by *Papaver somniferum* cells;
- enzymatic conversion of β-methyl digitoxin to β-methyl digoxin by *Digitalis lanata* cells;
- biotransformation of codeinone to codeine by *P. somniferum* cells;
- Moringa cells immobilized with higher level of glucosinolates; and
- higher anthraquinone production by *Morinda citrifolia* cells.

Despite several successes in experimental trials on immobilized cell systems, the technique is still not a very feasible option for commercialization for harvesting secondary metabolites because of issues such as

- Secondary metabolite yield is enhanced only when its generation in media is independent of cell growth.
- Large-scale production is feasible only when the formed product is released into the medium.
- Cell membrane is to be permeabilized by chemical or physical methods, which may reduce cell viability.
- Product extracellular degradation is a possibility.
- Support matrix used to immobilize cells may pose an additional diffusion barrier for product release.
- Due to tendency of plant cells to aggregate, process engineering problems such as culture sedimentation, blockage of openings, etc., develop in large-scale reactors.

BIO TRANSFORMATION

Chemical change brought about by biological systems such as cells, organelles, enzymes, or cell free extracts resulting in compound conversions or *de novo* synthesis from added precursors is called bio transformation. Microbial biotransformations have enabled the highly cost-effective manufacture of several medicinally important steroids from plant-derived steroid precursors which are a few steps away from the desired compound.

Similarly, plant cells are able to perform special biotransformation reactions on organic compounds added to the medium. They bring about glycosylation, hydrolysis, esterification, methylation, demethylation, dehydrogenation, epoxidations, and isomerizations, which can even be stereospecific. They can be used to chemically alter natural or synthetic compounds added to the media and thus generate known or newer compounds. Compounds not found in the plant from which the cell culture was made are also formed.

Such selective modifications of pure compounds by plant cells into defined final products are one of the most promising areas of plant cell culture. It's potential lies in the fact that specific structural modifications on added compounds can be performed much more easily by cultured plant cells than by chemical synthesis or by microbes. There is a huge scope for generation of novel compounds and to transform routine low-value chemicals to high-value pharmaceuticals. There are several successful reports of plant cell biotransformations.

- Cell suspension cultures of *Digitalis lanata* have effected 12β-hydroxylation of digitoxin (a secondary glycoside of *D. purpurea*) converting it into digoxin—a therapeutically more useful cardotonic drug. This has resulted in large-scale production of β-methyl digoxin from β-methyl digitoxin in *D. lanata* cultures. This was a commercially feasible alternative to poor yields seen in normal cultures of *D. purpurea* and *D. lanata*. The fact that such cultured cells can efficiently glycosylate, hydroxylate, and acetylate steroid precursors is being commercially exploited in making newer cardenolides from added precursors. Leaf, root, and callus cultures of *D. lanata* were shown to rapidly transform progesterone to pregnane, thus accumulating a higher quantity of digoxin over normal suspension cultures.

- Vincristine and vinblastine are anti-cancer drugs in high demand, but produced in very poor yields by the source plant *Catharanthus roseus*. The plant produces vinblastine in higher proportion than vincristine, which is in greater demand due to its better anti-cancer activity. In the plant, these alkaloids are shown to be biogenetically derived by the oxidative coupling of monomeric indoles catharanthine and vindoline (Fig. 1), with vindoline occurring in a higher proportion. Cell culture attempts to generate a higher yield have resulted in the generation of a mixture of monomeric alkaloids with poor yield of coupled useful dimeric alkaloids. This was because of inability of the cultures to produce vindoline, one of the monomers needed for the coupling.

- It can be seen from the figure that peroxidase enzyme is crucial for the coupling of monomers vondoline and catharanthine. Using commercial horse-radish peroxidase enzyme, the cell-free extract of *Catharanthus roseus* cells containing catharanthine (among other monomers) was made to generate 3,4-anhydrovinblastine (52.8%) and vinblastine (12.3%) from added vindoline (synthetic or isolated from plants). This possibility was a great leap forward in the production of these anti-cancer alkaloids.

- Today further improved methods of chemical or microbial (N-demethylation) coupling of catharanthine and vindoline as also conversion of vinblastine into more useful vincristine are available. These have therefore contributed to better commercial utilization of cell culture monomers of *C. roseus* cultures using techniques of biotransformation.

- It is known that the lignan podophyllotoxin is semisynthetically converted to etoposide and teniposide—much valued anti-cancer drugs. *Podophyllum peltatum* cultures have been found to biotransform precursor synthetic dibenzyl butanolides to lignan derivatives. Similarly, cell suspension cultures of *Forsythia intemedia* have been shown to effect useful

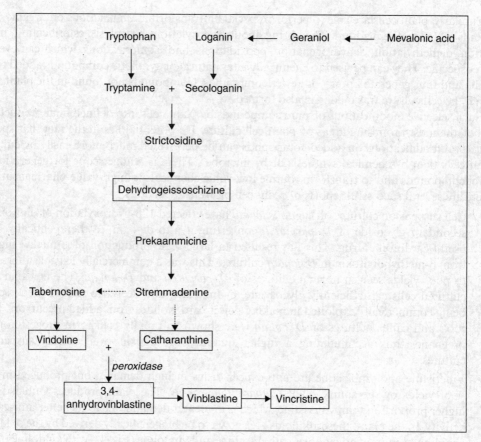

Figure 11.1 Biogenesis of Vincristine and Vinblastine

hydroxylation and oxidation reactions, bringing about biotransformation of added podophyllum lignans.

- Arbutin is a skin-whitening agent much prized for use in cosmetic preparations. It has been found that *R. serpentina* cells in culture accumulate high levels of rauffricine—a glucoalkaloid as against reserpine. When hydroquinone is added as a precursor to the culture medium, the cells glycosylate it and transform it into arbutin and hydroquinone diglycoside at a very high yield (9.2 g/L of arbutin) within 3–4 days of culturing. Several other phenolic compounds are reportedly glycosylated by plant cell cultures.

- Cell cultures of *N. tabacum* are demonstrated to selectively hydrolyze the R-configurational monoterpenes like bornyl acetate and isobornyl acetate thus bringing about stereospecific conversion into borneol and isoborneol—important aroma chemicals. Likewise, geraniol and nerol are transformed to citral and neral respectively. Several such monoterpene transformations are reported in literature.

- Cell cultures of *C. roseus* hydroxylated coumarin to form 7-hydroxy coumarin. This in turn was methylated by cell cultures of *Ruta graveolens* to yield analogs of herniarin, marmesin and other novel compounds.

- Biotransformation reactions mediated by plant cells may be optimized for large-scale production starting with screening for and selecting high-yield strains capable of effecting economically important biotransformations.

Hairy Root Cultures

Callus-derived cells sometimes fail to generate secondary metabolites and even when they do so in many cases the initial spurt in secondary metabolite production slowly declines and comes to a halt. However, on organogenesis, they continue to accumulate secondary metabolites. Since in whole plants production and storage of secondary metabolites is regulated by and associated with different developmental stages, organ culture appears to be a more feasible alternative to continuous large-scale production of plant secondary metabolites.

It is to be observed that many valuable and much needed phytopharmaceuticals are predominantly accumulated in bark and root tissue. Roots are an important storage organ for a variety of edible and nonedible phytochemicals. This observation led to attempts to maintain continuously growing root cultures.

It was found that many dicotyledonous plants, when infected with the soil bacteria *Agrobacterium rhizogenes,* are genetically transformed due to the integration of a root inducing plasmid of the bacteria into the plants' genome. Due to this, there is proliferative formation of roots at the site of infection. Similarly, *in vitro* transformation of cultured cells from plants that accumulate secondary metabolites in roots initiated proliferation of fine fibrous roots in culture. These were formed not only in the absence of a growth regulator; they also showed a very high growth rate and did not show geotropism. They showed a high degree of lateral branching and the profuse growth is accompanied by an accumulation of secondary metabolites. For example, hairy root cultures of *Hyoscyamus muticus* when grown in batch root cultures showed a 2500–5000 fold increase in bio mass within 3 weeks and generated tropane alkaloids in yields comparable to normal plants.

Similarly, "hairy root" culture of *Valeriana officinalis* var *sambucifolia* made valepotriates four times in yield compared to normal roots. Secondary metabolite yield in hairy roots of *Lupinus* species (Isoflavonoids), *Peganum* species (serotonin), *Datura stramonium,* and *Duboisia myoporoides* was much more than that made in suspension cultures. Production of artemisinin from transformed root cultures of *Artemisia annua* has been extensively studied. Co-culture of hairy roots and microbes are reported to produce unique secondary metabolites. For example, *Hordeum vulgare* hairy root culture infected with Vesicular Arbuscular Mycrorrhizal (VAM) fungi *Glomus intra radices* produced a new terpenoid glycoside. Many industrial scale reactors able to house and culture such hairy root cultures are being experimented with, to upscale the success seen in laboratory level trials.

TRANSGENIC PLANTS AND THEIR APPLICATIONS

When the plant genome is altered by artificial introduction of one or few genes responsible for a desired trait, it is referred to as genetic transformation. Such genetically altered cell, when manipulated to develop into a whole plant, due to its totipotency, results in a transgenic plant. Though not all plants are amenable to such a transformation, this technology has resulted in the development of improved and novel varieties of some plant species. Unlike in conventional hybridization, the whole genome is not disturbed as only a few genes are inserted and hence, the time taken for establishment and multiplication is much lesser.

Ever since the introduction of tobacco as the first transgenic plant in 1983, several economically important plants like cotton, maize, soyabean, papaya, and the like are among about 18 transgenic crops introduced so far. Lot of research work undertaken since then has enhanced the understanding of regulation of gene expression and enabled recognition of regulatory sequences involved in differential expression of gene activity. With today's technological knowhow, it is possible to isolate desired genes and integrate them into the genome of living plants, such that the genotype of the recipient plant is altered and also expressed.

When simplified, the steps involved in the generation of transgenic plants are

- isolation of desired gene from the donor organism;
- selection of a vehicle or vector that is to carry the gene;
- restructuring the vector before gene is inserted into it;
- gene insertion into the vector;
- transformation of the recipient cell through the vector;
- selection and identification of transformed cells;
- regenerating plants from such cells; and
- lab to field transfer of the regenerated plants and their sustenance.

Molecular biology techniques such as DNA isolation, gene restructuring, cloning, vector construction, identification of gene areas and what they code for, identification and selection of transformed cells are crucial to generation of transgenic plants. Likewise tissue culture techniques such as co-cultivation, protoplast fusion, organogenic differentiation, and lab to field transfer protocols are also important for their successful development.

Gene Transfer Strategies

Understanding the process of crown gall formation through *Agrobacterium tumefaciens* has shown that virulent strains of this bacteria are able to introduce a part of their genome material into the plant cell. This results in not only successful integration and transformation of the plant cells, but also prompt replication of bacterial genes, along with the plant genome. This is however possible only in dicots having a wound response mechanism. This natural ability of the bacterium to transform plant cells led to the development of effective vectors for introducing foreign genes into higher plants.

These are of 2 types—co-integrating vectors and binary vectors. They are based on a small circular non-chromosomal DNA of the virulent strains of *Agrobacterium tumefaciens* called Ti-plasmid. Only a portion of this plasmid is introduced into the host cell and they carry genes for the synthesis of opines and phytohormones. This portion, the T-DNA carries prokaryotic promoters that enable it to be expressed in eukaryotic organisms. T-DNA is identified by specific repeat border sequences on either side and any piece of DNA inserted between these two borders gets introduced into the plants' genome. A certain length of base pair regions lying just outside the right border of T-DNA is important for transferring it into plant cells. Thus being responsible for virulence of the bacteria, it is called the "vir" region. When the entire wild type Ti-plasmid with a small fragment between the border sequences replaced by the desired gene is used as vector, it is called a co-integrating vector. The replaced fragment represents oncogenes that code for synthesis of phytohormones—cytokinin and auxin in the transformed cells, making them proliferate uncontrollably. This may interfere with recognition of morphologically normal transformed plants. Hence, when they are replaced, the Ti-plasmid is disarmed and so used in plant genetic transformation.

While the "vir" regions are important for transferring genes into the plant cells, they need not be physically linked to the T-DNA. Hence, these are carried separately on a plasmid disarmed with respect to the oncogenes. Another plasmid without the "vir"-regions, carries the desired foreign genes between the border regions. These two vectors or binary vectors are used for transformation of the plant cell genome, thus overcoming problems of manipulating the large-sized native Ti-plasmid.

The desired gene (DNA) to be inserted into the T-DNA is first inserted into an *E-coli* plasmid with DNA sequences homologous to those between the border regions of the T-DNA. Once cloned, such a carrier vector with the desired DNA is transferred from *E-coli* to *Agrobacterium* (having the disarmed Ti-plasmid) by conjugation using a helper plasmid. In the bacterium, this carrier vector is first unable to replicate. However, recombination happens between it and the disarmed Ti-plasmid and the so combined plasmid, having both the inserted gene as well as the native "vir" gene continues to remain in the bacterium. This is then used for transfecting plant cells.

In the case of binary vector, the "vir" gene of T-DNA (with the desired gene inserted) is replaced with a plasmid replication region so that it can replicate both in *E. coli* and *Agrobacterium*. It is cloned in *E. coli* and transferred to *Agrobacterium* having the disarmed Ti-plasmid with "vir" genes. Now the *Agrobacterium* has both vectors and it is used to transfect plant cells.

Plant Cell Transformation

The bacterium having the vector with the desired gene is put in the media having the sterilized and freshly cut plant explant which may be colyledon, leaf, hypocotyl, or stem meristem. The bacteria is able to transfect the explant cells after which the medium is treated with antibiotics to phase out bacterial cells.

Transformed Cell Selection

Transformed plant cells are selected based on several strategies such as identification based on selection of marker genes inserted into the transformation vectors.

Growth and Regeneration of Plantlets

Media composition and culturing conditions are altered to encourage growth of only transformed cells. Such cells are then manipulated to undergo organogenesis for plantlet regeneration. Shooty or rooty cultures are formed depending on whether the gene insertion has replaced the auxin or cytokinin loci on the phytohormone gene.

Lab to Field Passage

Plantlets so formed are carefully transferred from media to very small lots of sterilized soil samples under appropriate lighting and other conditions within the laboratory in an area earmarked for such nursing protocols. After a certain period of acclimitization based on the plant species, the tended saplings are shifted to green house conditions with close supervision. After observation under such controlled conditions, further grown plantlets are finally transferred to the field.

Though initially applicable only to dicots, today the technique may be used even with monocots by adding phenolic compounds, such as acetosyringine, that act as inducers of vir-genes, to the cultivation medium having both the bacteria and plant cells. These compounds elicit wound response in the explant thus enabling infection of the monocot cells by the bacterium and so even transformation.

Plant viruses capable of introducing their genome into plant cells can be used for generating transgenic plants of vegetatively propagated plants. Today several chemicals are known to induce DNA uptake by plant cell protoplasts. Also many mechanical methods of DNA transfer into plant cells such as electroporation, microinjection, and particle bombardment, are added to the arsenal of gene transfer methods.

Applications of Transgenic Plants

- With advancements in our understanding of the genetic basis of plant diseases, genetic engineering has been effectively utilized for developing plants resistant to various plant pests and thus diseases.

- Also plants resistant to newer herbicides used to control weed growth have become a possibility due to strategies such as over producing the enzyme that confers herbicide resistance to the plant.

- Plant cells transformed by bacterial genes from a bacterium lethal to insects have produced transgenic plants resistant to insect pests, for example, Boll worm–resistant cotton plants. Many such genetically transformed economically important plants are now insect resistant. This reduces cost spent on pesticides and enhances the yield, as plants are healthy and also act as biopesticides.

- Milder forms of viral strains may be used to transfect host plants to develop resistance to more virulent strains of virus much similar to vaccination to protect it, for example, papaya against papaya ring spot disease.

- Genes responsible for plant pathogen defense mechanisms are identified and made to over express in plants making them resistant to a range of bacterial and fungal pathogens.

- Similar over expression of genes coding for compounds released in response to abiotic stress such as drought, temperature extremes, and nutrient deficiency are used to develop transgenic plants that can better tolerate such adverse conditions.

- Fruit ripening may be delayed to enable the intact transfer of fruits to distant locations over a longer duration. This can be done by transgenic plants whose ethylene-producing genes have in-built trigger genes that slow down natural ethylene production by the fruits.

- By manipulating enzymes involved in the biosynthesis of several phytochemicals, plant yield with respect to these economically important compounds may be greatly increased. Such experiments have been tried on Taxus species to enhance taxol yield.

- Transgenic tobacco plants bearing gene coding for mannitol dehydrogenase from *E. coli* produce high levels of mannitol. Transgenic potato bearing the gene coding for cyclodextrin glucosyl transferase from *Klebsiella* produces tubers rich in α- and β-cyclodextrin, which is used as a drug solubilizing agent in pharmaceutical dosage forms.

- Transgenic rice able to generate vitamin A as a result of having three additional genes that code for enzymes controlling carotenoid biosynthesis has been developed.
- Genes coding for many therapeutic and diagnostic proteins having been identified, transgenic plants with such genes may be used as sources of monoclonal antibodies, blood plasma proteins, growth hormones, cytokinins, etc.
- Likewise, if antigenic proteins can be produced in plants, they will become sources of vaccines as well.

These modifications may be possible when few genes have to be manipulated. However, plant secondary metabolite biogenesis happens due to a complex and multiple cascade of metabolic reactions, controlled by multiple enzymes. It may still be a long time before we have transgenic plants acting as biochemical factories generating the needed quantity of secondary metabolites.

SECONDARY METABOLITE PRODUCTION IN PLANT-TISSUE CULTURE SYSTEMS

Plant secondary metabolites are biosynthetically derived from primary metabolites—those having an essential role in basic cell metabolism and are not essential for the survival of the individual plant cell. Though being non nutritive and not directly required for growth, they play ecologically significant role in how plants deal with their environment and are important for the survival of the plant as whole. Their distribution may be restricted to specific taxonomic groups and are present in plants in smaller quantities compared to primary metabolites. They are biosynthesized in specialized cell types at distinct developmental stages. Many of them are phytoalexins, that is, produced in response to external physical, chemical or microbiological stimuli. Thus, they may be rapidly synthesized and rapidly destroyed in response to pathogen invasion. Several secondary metabolites are of great economic importance as pharmaceuticals, flavor or fragrance chemicals, pesticides, and so on.

Advances in plant-tissue culture studies have greatly contributed to our understanding of plant secondary products. They have resulted in the identification of more than 200 specific enzymes and this has been invaluable for the study of biosynthetic pathways. Apart from being a source of known compounds, plant-tissue cultures are also known to accumulate newer compounds not found in plants. It has become possible to use plant-tissue culture for bringing about useful chemical conversions on precursor compounds. There has been an increasing interest toward producing plant secondary metabolites by cell cultures to overcome many problems associated with their industrial production from whole plants.

From the time when James Bonner reported rubber bioproduction by guagule plant-tissue cultures in 1940 and Tulecke and Nickells' demonstration that plant cell biomass could be grown in multi gallon containers in 1950, we have come a long way. A great deal of work especially in Japan and Germany has gone into attempts to generate pharmaceuticals in culture. At least 50 categories of products from plant-tissue culture have been investigated for the feasibility of their generation in large quantities. At least 70 compounds are known to accumulate in plant-tissue culture in concentrations equal to or exceeding that of the parent plant, for example, Catharanthus alkaloids (>1% dry weight), Nicotine and diosgenin (>3.5%), trigonelline and ginseng saponins (>5%), rosemarinic acid (15%), Morinda anthraquinones (18%), proanthocyanins (up to 40%), and Vomelenine alkaloid (>50%) compared to the plant.

Despite extensive research to make possible commercial production of plant secondary metabolites in culture, so far only shikonin, ginseng, and taxol are being commercially produced by tissue culture. Even in successful cases of plant secondary metabolite production in cultures, overall, the technology of growing large quantities of plant cell biomass for biotechnological production of plant secondary metabolites is not yet cost effective.

While several factors such as slow growth of plant cells, their low/variable secondary metabolite yield, genetic instability are quoted, huge volume of work undertaken on plant cell culture have thrown light on many other aspects involved and the problems it poses.

A brief glimpse at the lessons learnt from studies on plant secondary metabolite production:

Shikonin Production

Shikonin was the first phytoconstituent to be commercially produced from tissue culture. It is a nathaquinone dye with anti-bacterial, anti-inflammatory properties and has been used in the treatment of burns, wounds, and hemorrhoids. A valuable vegetable dye, it gives a spectrum of colours ranging from red, purple, to blue. It is obtained from *Lythospermum erythrorhizon,* a plant that has been extensively harvested to the verge of extinction in its native habitat in Japan, China, and Korea. The plant takes 3–4 years to yield roots before they can be collected and the shikonin content of the reddish purple roots is only 1–2%. In 1983, Scientists at Mitsui Petrochemical Company developed a commercially successful tissue culture process for the production of shikonin from cell cultures of *Lithospermum erythrorhizon.* Such a product derived from tissue culture was commercialized for sale as a natural colour in soaps, lipsticks, and other cosmetic products.

Commercialization of shikonin production was possible largely because of selection of high-yielding cell lines and optimizing culture conditions to enhance yield to 15% of the biomass. Thus cost of production became economically feasible considering the fact that the plant population is declining in its native countries, making tissue culture technique the method of choice for its production.

Selecting high yielding cell lines is an important first step to enhance productivity. This is because the explant that initiates a cell culture is heterogenous with respect to metabolic productivity of its component cells. When cultures are derived from cells grown from it, due to various genetic and other conditions, they are exposed to in cultures and clusters of cells show great variation in secondary metabolite accumulation. There will be high- and low-yielding cells and therefore selecting and cloning high yielding cells in media that maximizes product formation is very important. Such selected cell lines must be genetically stable over several cycles of aggregate sub culturing and/or single cell cloning. In some cases as in *Datura innoxia* suspension cultures, it has been observed that gross chromosomal changes occur in the cultured cells. Cells were noted to be tetraploid, haploid, or of variable ploidy in different proportions. While sometimes as in protoplast-derived *Hyoscyamus muticus* cultures, the haploid plants were richer in hyoscine than diploid plants, maintenance of uniform genetic characteristics among high yielding cells is a significant prerequisite.

The fact that media composition is the most important determinant for optimum production of secondary metabolites has been illustrated by the pioneering work of Zenk, Fujita, Tabata, Gamborg, Blaydes, and Nitsch among others. In general, it was observed that both in the whole plant and in culture, cell growth and secondary metabolite production do not often happen together. When media composition is conducive to optimum cell growth, secondary metabolite production starts happening in the late stationary phase when the growth has become static. Thus came about the two-culture system, where the first culture media's composition was optimized to support cell growth. Once the optimum level of biomass got accumulated, the cells were transferred to a different medium that is favorable for product yield. First used by Zenk et al., in 1977 for indole alkaloid production by *Catharanthus roseus* cells, it was also used for shikonin production. Here the change was from growth supporting Linsmaier and Skoog medium to nitrate rich White's medium. The type of nitrogen affected shikonin production and the nitrate had to be the sole source of nitrogen. Even little replacement with others such as ammonium salt greatly reduced shikonin production.

The right media composition that supports production of secondary metabolites varies with different cultures and even different metabolites of a particular cell line. For example, for maximum ajmalicine production by *C. roseus* cell cultures, glucose concentration is critical at 500 mM, whereas for optimum tryptamine production, the media has to have lower glucose concentration of 100 mM.

Many cell cultures can be optimized for growth, and secondary metabolite production in a single medium. For example, LS medium supplemented with 10 times the usual copper concentration increased berberine production by 20–30% in cell cultures of *Coptis japonica* without adversely affecting biomass production.

Catharanthus Alkaloid Production

Catharanthus roseus is the source of important anti-cancer drugs, vincristine and vinblastine, which are produced in very low yields requiring huge quantities of the whole plant and extensive chromatographic processing for their isolation. Root suspension cell cultures of *C. roseus* produced alkaloids when the media concentration of growth hormone 2,4-D was reduced. Several workers have reported the influence of relative hormonal content of the medium upon secondary metabolite production.

In general, an increase in auxin level, such as 2,4-D, stimulates cell proliferation and reduces secondary metabolite production. Cytokinins reportedly enhance secondary metabolite accumulation and gibberellins in general inhibit it.

Thalictrum minus cell cultures showed good cell growth in the presence of 2,4-D and showed enhanced berberine production with ethylene or NAA and BAP or a cytokinin. On the other hand, cardenolide content in *D. lanata* cultures decreased with ethylene.

Cinchona Alkaloid Production

Several Cinchona species are sources of the anti-malarial drug quinine and anti-arrhythmic drug quinidine and other related alkaloids. Quinine remains an important anti-malarial drug and economic production of quinine and related alkaloids from tissue culture is of high commercial value. There has not been much success, however, in their production in cell culture as was the case with morphine and codeine. Cell cultures of *Cinchona ledgeriana* and *Papaver somniferum* accumulated alkaloids other than the commercially important ones. It was found that *C. ledgeriana* suspension cultures induced using sterile shoot cultures of plantlets germinated from surface sterilized seeds could accumulate important alkaloids, but cell growth was very slow and could not be sustained beyond 5–8 sub cultures. Transformed roots could to a certain extent accumulate alkaloids but they too had variable productive capacities.

Similarly, with *P. somniferum* lack of organized laticiferous tissue was found to be responsible for negligible morphine biosynthesis. However, when cultured cells were manipulated to undergo organogenic differentiation, forming latex-accumulating cell types, there was some morphine accumulation.

In the same way, transformed cultures of *Mentha citrata* and *Mentha piperita* accumulate terpenes when they are made to undergo shoot differentiation. The terpene formation is associated with formation of leaf-bearing shoots and even presence of oil glands on leaves. Several other volatile oil-bearing plants have reportedly not accumulated terpenes because of noncompartmentalization of the formed metabolites. In cultures of *Lavandula angustifolia*, even the formed monoterpenes disappeared after sometime because of lack of storage structures, like tichomes, vittae, or glands. It can be seen that culture morphology strongly influences the ability of the tissue to biosynthesize secondary products. Many secondary metabolites appear to require an organized structure indicating a regulatory hierarchy in which the morphology is a dominant factor. Thus, biosynthetic capacity seems to be localized in specific cell types within the organ.

Effect of Other Culture Conditions

Secondary metabolite production is greatly influenced by other culture conditions that need to be identified and optimized for maximum production. Intensity of light and wavelength used has an influence over secondary metabolite production. In cultures of *Dioscorea deltoidea,* while blue light stimulated alkaloid production, red light decreased it. Similar reports are associated with cell culture accumulation of cardenolides, flavonoids, and betacyanins. *Catharanthus roseus* cultures when grown under dark conditions accumulated more of serpentine and ajmalicine than in light. When calli were grown under white light, first ajmalicine got accumulated, but when they were exposed to red or blue light there was a constant ajmalicine content and serpentine content was lower.

Presence of gases, oxygen and carbon dioxide in the culture environment has an important role in secondary metabolite production. A higher dissolved oxygen in the media stimulated greater serpentine accumulation in *C. roseus* cultures. Likewise, formed carbon dioxide and accumulated ethylene, if not quickly removed from the culture head space, inhibited ajmalicine production in these cultures.

UV irradiation induces production of important dimeric alkaloids in *C. roseus* shoot cultures.

Elicitors

Since many secondary metabolites are generated in plants in response to external stimuli that may be physical, chemical, or microbial, in cultures, many fungal, yeast extracts and a number of organic and inorganic compounds have been found to induce secondary metabolite formation in cell and organ cultures. It appears that these elicitors may be giving the right stimulus to cells in cultures for the initiation of secondary metabolite production.

Adding *Verticillium dahliae* spores to cell cultures of *Gossypium arboreum* greatly enhanced gossypol yield. Likewise, in *C. ledgeriana* cultures there was an increase in anthraquinone production. In *Pimpinella anisum* cultures, coumarin synthesis was initiated by addition of *Phytophthora. P. somniferum* cell cultures accumulate sanguinarine when treated with a homogenate of the fungus *Botrytis.*

Addition of yeast extracts to *Thalictrum rugosum* cultures enhanced berberine content four times. Similarly, in *Orthosiphon aristatus*, there was a stimulation of rosmarinic acid production. *Rhizoctonia solani* increased production of sesquiterpenes in *Agrobacterium rhizogenes* transformed hairy-root cultures of *Hyoscyamus muticus*.

Supplementing media with sodium chloride, potassium chloride, and sorbitol individually increased catharanthine accumulation in cells of *C. roseus*. Addition of vanadyl sulphate increased production of catharanthine, serpentine, and tryptamine. Likewise addition of phenyl alanine to *Lavendula* cultures enhanced rosmarinic acid production. Copper sulphate addition to *Lithospermum erythrorhizon* cultures stimulated greater shikonin production. Colchicine application to *Valeriana wallichii* root cultures showed a 60-fold increase in valepotriates. Thiosemicarbazide promotes saponin biosynthesis over phytosterol production in *Panax ginseng* cultures.

Most cultures respond to an elicitor when included during the growth phase of the cells. For example, *Papaver somniferum* cell cultures are to be treated with solubilized chitin 6 days after culture initiation for optimal production of sanguinarine. Likewise, cultures of *Eschscholtzia californica* cultures had to be treated with yeast extract on the 6th day after culture initiation, for maximal production of benzophenanthridine alkaloids.

Cell Permeabilization

One of the major challenges facing large-scale production of secondary metabolites in culture is the tendency of the cultured cells to accumulate the biosynthetic products intracellularly. There have been attempts to permeabilize cell walls of the cultured cells to enable release. This has been tried with DMSO, making media acidic and even with physical treatments such as ultrasonication and short electrical pulses. An ideal permeabilization technique has to be reversible and should not affect cell viability.

Product Harvest from Media

Periodic removal of secondary metabolites accumulated in media is necessary to prevent unwanted degradation of products or feedback inhibition of the proceeding biosynthesis. Several extraction techniques like two-phase liquid cultures are in use. Here an additional immiscible liquid acting as a solvent for the formed metabolite is added to the culture liquid by which it goes into solution into this liquid. Being immiscible it can easily be separated and product harvested. For example, *C. ledgeriana* cultures were treated with Amberlite XAD-7—a resin, to selectively phase out formed anthraquinones in culture. Such periodic removal by solubilizing it in the second phase enhances further production. Several such newer immiscible liquid phases such as dimethyl siloxane are being experimented upon.

CONCLUSIONS

Plant biotechnology includes applications of technological tools in plant sciences. Several significant achievements in plant biology such as cell and tissue culture, regeneration of whole plants from somatic cells, and genetic recombination have resulted in applications such as rapid propagation, developing uniform healthy plant saplings, somatic hybrids from naturally incompatible species, germ plasm storage, improved transgenic plants, and so on. Observation that plant secondary metabolites accumulate in cultures in quantities larger than in intact plants, opened up possibilities of exploring such production as an economically viable alternative to their conventional extraction from whole plants. Resulting extensive work has thrown light on the many facets of plant secondary metabolism. Plant growth and its sustenance is now understood to be based on a wonderfully complex and dynamic interaction between the plant cell milieu and its environment. Plants are revealing themselves to be highly sensitive organisms as well, able to gauge their environment and adapt themselves physiologically and biochemically in accordance to external stimuli. Secondary metabolites are bio-synthesized by complex and multiple cascade of metabolic reactions triggered by several different enzymes. They are so made, in specialized cell types at distinct developmental stages. Presence of morphologically organized structures both for their synthesis and storage appear essential in many plants. Hence, though there have been spectacular advancements in crop improvement with profound implications in agriculture, forestry, and horticulture, development of transgenic plants producing required large quantities of secondary metabolites is still a distant possibility. As of today, however, few pharmaceuticals of interest like shikonin, ginseng, and taxol are being industrially produced in plant-tissue culture. Also, cultured plant cells are being used to effect economically useful chemical conversions on added precursors.

Still, many more hurdles are to be crossed and many more discoveries awaited before plant cells could be used as factories to generate the needed phytopharmaceuticals.

REVIEW QUESTIONS

Essay Questions

1. Outline the significant milestones in the development of plant-tissue culture as a technology.
2. Explain the steps involved in the production of transgenic plants. Add a brief note on significant applications.
3. Discuss the factors influencing the production of plant secondary metabolites in culture.

Short Notes

1. Scope of Plant-tissue culture
2. Role of Plant growth hormones in plant-tissue culture
3. The technique of hairy root cultures
4. Merits and demerits of plant cell immobilization
5. Bio transformation in the *in vitro* production of Vinca alkaloid

12 Intellectual Property Rights—Traditional Knowledge and Plant Drugs

---

CHAPTER OBJECTIVES

Introduction

Events in History that Led to IP Regime

Recent International Developments
in IP Arena

TRIPS Agreement

Controversies Surrounding TRIPS
Agreement

Indian Patent Law

Issues Pertaining To Herbal Drug
Patenting

INTRODUCTION

The term "property" refers to ownership or appropriation of an object by an individual to the exclusion of rest of society. This right, fostered and protected by law, entitles one to the exclusive use, enjoyment and disposal of the object, and others accept this and are duty bound not to interfere with this right. The concept of ownership of tangible physical assets such as land, dwellings and other goods is intricately linked to man and civilization.

Intellectual property (IP), on the other hand, refers to the intangible products of human intellect. In today's world, due to the commercial value of the intellectual creation, it is vested with the status of property. This concept of ownership of mankind's creations is not new. Greater awareness of its economic value has resulted in the creation and protection of IP in the form of statutes in the latter half of the present millennium. Its value and significance is enormous, especially when viewed in the context of the kaleidoscopic social, cultural and technological changes and the resultant economic development the world over. While knowledge and creativity are being recognized as the cornerstones of corporate development, effective protection and jurisprudence of IP is considered the key to nurture socio-economic progress, thus promoting national social endeavors. IP rights created and protected by statutes are meant to foster creativity by providing the necessary incentives to the creator of the IP.

IP law confers on the owner the proprietary rights over his products and authorizes him to take action against the infringement on his right. The IP, like any other property, can be assigned, mortgaged and licensed. In order to get protection, the owner has to satisfy the conditions imposed by the statutes. It has to be registered with a competent authority and protection is given for certain duration. After the expiry of the period, it becomes public property and anybody is free to use it. The modes of acquisition of IP may be by agreement or by inheritance.

IP laws are concerned with the creation, vesting and use of IP rights, and they relate to various creations including literary and artistic works, inventions, symbols, images, designs and names used in commerce. While inventions and products pertinent to industrial commerce are covered by the industrial property rights, literary and other artistic creations (such as literature, music, cinema and other visual arts, sculpture, architectural designs) come under copyright protection.

EVENTS IN HISTORY THAT LED TO IP REGIME

The concept of putting identification marks related to source on the articles of trade, especially merchandise taken across geographic borders is very ancient. Prehistoric earthen pots, coins, stone tablets, etc., mention such a practice, and there are claims from several parts of the world of having literary references to the practice of bestowing special privileges on innovators.

- Republic of Venice is credited with framing a law in the year 1474 in its economic policy that provided grant of exclusive rights to inventors for limited periods of time. These were part of efforts to regain trading ground lost by Venice to Turks.

- In France, inventors solicited privileges from the King in return for handing over the same to the King's offices after expiration of the privilege period. Modern statutes on such privileges were introduced in France in 1791.

- In 1641, a patent for a new process of salt making was granted in Massachusetts in North America.

- The Statute of Anne enacted in the British Parliament in 1710 gave legal protection for consumers of copyrighted works by curtailing the term of copyright, preventing monopoly on book selling.

- At the height of industrial revolution, when the impact of patents was being seriously felt in England, the US constitution drafted its US patent law. During the colonial period and Articles of Confederation years (1778-1789), many states of the US adapted their own systems of patents. In 1790, the American Patent Bill signed by George Washington laid the foundation to the modern American patent system. The first patent was granted under the Act in the same year for a potash production technique.

- Since then, the US patent and Trademark Office has recorded and protected inventions such as the electric lamp of Thomas Alva Edison, telephone of Alexander Graham Bell, etc.

- Thus, the patent system has protected the inventors by giving them an opportunity to profit from their labors and has benefited the society by systematically recording new inventions and releasing them to the public after the inventors' limited rights have expired.

- The patent system, however, started to come under attack, and the Sherman Antitrust Act in the US in 1890 was the result of concerns over big businesses monopolizing. However, after the economic depression of the late 19th century, the reviving economy saw the resurgence of interest in patenting.
- The advent of industrial revolution and the powers brought with newer technologies saw the countries competing in trade to gain supremacy. World War II highlighted the toll of warfare on nations, and thus, innovations and technological benefits resulting from them appeared more alluring than the short-lived supremacy gained through wars.
- In the scenario of technological supremacy and economic benefits accrued from innovations in general, innovators were not willing to let out their invention unless there was monetary gain.
- To provide governmental support to creative endeavors, nations came up with the idea of balancing the interests of inventors to secure a monetary gain for their creation with the interest of the society in benefiting from the creation.
- Thus was born the system of patenting by which a set of exclusive rights are granted by an established governmental authority to an inventor for a limited period of time in exchange for public disclosure of the invention.
- Post–World War II, many countries such as Japan built their economic and industrial base and potential through extensive use of their IP. The Asian nations also are now utilizing their IP system for developing their industrial base, exports and, thus, economic growth.

As technology is an important asset in trade, investment and economic development, its development is largely dependent on strong IP protection, thus creating newer ways of making products of creative activity reachable to public. Ensuring effective use and protection of IP is of great economic significance as IP is an important resource for sustainable economic development.

The advent of sophisticated technologies has made the act of piracy and counterfeiting much easier. Strict enforcement of IP laws is therefore needed to provide an environment conducive to investment.

Thus, industrial property and patent information have an important role to play in determining the direction of researches in industries, businesses, government and academic institutions to encourage invention and innovation. Hence, globally IP rights are assuming an increasing importance in trade relations and national growth.

RECENT INTERNATIONAL DEVELOPMENTS IN IP ARENA

Being intangible, IP is existential only on account of the legal rules and laws that enforce it. Due to the unique and fragile nature of IP rights and their possible exploitation the world over, nations making progress industrially and scientifically took cognizance of the need to protect these rights by bringing about the necessary legislations in their respective countries and by international cooperation.

- The Paris Convention for the Protection of Industrial Property in the year 1883 was the first international effort by 14 member states that recognized protection for patents, trademarks and industrial designs (ID).
- Following the Berne Convention in 1886 for the Protection of Literary and Artistic Works, the International Copyright Act of 1886 was passed to facilitate the member states help

their nationals with international protection of their right to control use and sale of their literary, artistic and creative works.

- In 1893, these two independent bureaus merged to form the United Nations Bureaux for the Protection of Intellectual Property (BIRPI).
- Following the establishment of the United Nations (UN) in 1945, an organization known as General Agreement on Tariff and Trade (GATT) was set up in 1948 to reshape the world economy after the Second World War (1939-1942). It provides a forum to regulate tariff rates on the world scale.
- To bring more powers to GATT, the United Nations Commission on International Law (UNICITRAL) and the United Nations Conference on Trade and Development (UNCTAD) were set up by the UN.
- Agencies governing the Paris and Berne conventions moved form Berne to Geneva to be closer to the UN. In 1970, BIRPI became World Intellectual Property Organization (WIPO), and in 1974, it became a specialized agency of the UN system of organizations with a mandate to administer the IP matters recognized by the member states of the UN.
- GATT was a multilateral body formed to lay down the code of conduct in the area of international trade and is a contractual agreement among the countries that provides a general framework for discipline on tariffs and non-tariff measures. Its main objective was to minimize the tariff rates and remove the impediments coming forward in the way of international trade.
- With exponential growth in world trade and rising merchandise exports, in order to ease the trade barriers among the member countries, under the auspices of GATT, series of international negotiations were held. These dealt with regulation of UN tariffs, anti-dumping, countervailing practices, geographic quotas, etc.
- Due to inability to reach an agreement, the latest round of negotiations which started in 1991, based on the Dunkel's draft, were held between 1986 and 1994, at Uruguay. This led to the creation of the World Trade Organization (WTO).
- The WTO agreements, as a result of negotiations between the members, led to the establishment of a multilateral trading system encompassing trade in goods and services. There was strong lobbying on the part of US for the inclusion of IP rights in the multinational trade negotiations to stop the perceived excessive trade losses to economies of the developed world. This led to the inclusion of Trade Related Intellectual Property Subjects (TRIPS) agreement that was supposed to be aimed at protecting the IP rights, thus rewarding creativity and inventiveness.
- While India expressed fear of monopolistic powers being wielded by these economies in the name of patents, developing countries were still compelled to surrender their economies before developed countries.
- After the Uruguay round of negotiations, GATT, a non-UN organ, became WTO which was to administer TRIPS. Thus, WTO enforced TRIPS agreement as a package deal, with member countries having to accept all the agreements *in toto* without the option to opt out of any of the provisions without quitting WTO itself.
- India, by signing the Uruguay round of GATT negotiations, thus became a member of WTO, and TRIPS agreement was added to the agreement establishing WTO as annexure I-C. All the member countries were under obligation to implement the provisions of

agreement on TRIPS. They were also obliged to bring their domestic laws in consonance with the provisions of this agreement.

TRIPS AGREEMENT

This comprehensive and influential international agreement establishes minimum standards on IP rights. By providing more stringent patent protection, TRIPS will help to generate increased profits for patent holders on new technologies, which are largely with industrialized countries and multinational corporations. Industrialized countries account for over 90 per cent of global research and development and the US alone accounts for almost half of it.

WTO's TRIPS agreement is an attempt to narrow gaps in the ways IP rights are protected around the world, by bringing them under international rules. It establishes minimum level of protection that each government has to give to the IP of fellow WTO members. This strikes a balance between the long-term benefits and possible short-term costs to the society. In the long term, the society is benefited as IP protection encourages creativity and invention and also they enter the public domain upon expiration of period of protection.

TRIPS agreement covers the following:

- Basic principles of trading system and application of international IP agreements
- Ways and means of effecting IP protection
- Means of enforcement of these IP rights by countries in their territories
- Effective and expeditious IP-related dispute settlement between WTO members
- Transitory arrangements to be made before the introduction of the new system
- Lists out categories of IP that are to be protected

Main provisions under TRIPS agreement relating to patents require the following:

- Member countries to provide product patents in all fields of technology without any exception
- Providing a minimum uniform period of 20-year protection
- Grant of compulsory license – which is an obligation by the patentee to issue license for the patent on his terms, subject to certain terms and conditions, upon order of a controller – on the basis of individual merits of the case, such as lack of availability to public at a reasonable price, etc.
- The burden of proof of a process patent that leads to production of a patented product is to be placed on the process patentee
- Availability of patent rights to products irrespective of whether they are locally produced or imported
- Providing protection to micro-organisms and micro-biological processes
- Enactment of an effective system for the protection of new plant varieties

The objectives of TRIPS are enshrined as promotion of technological innovation, and transfer and dissemination of technology to the mutual advantage of producers and users of technological knowledge in a manner conducive to the social and economic welfare and to a balance of rights and obligations.

While making it mandatory for the WTO member countries to implement TRIPS, it allows certain flexibilities enabling necessary amendments to national IP laws in accordance with the health care needs of the respective developing and least developed countries. TRIPS, in its objectives, also lays down that enforcement of IP rights should not themselves be barriers to legitimate trade.

Though the objective of TRIPS was projected as reduction of distortions and impediments to international trade, it actually succeeded in bringing about effective and adequate protection of IP rights, especially to the following categories listed out in its agreement:

- Patents
- Copyrights
- Trademarks
- Geographic indications (GI)
- Trade secrets
- Integrated circuits (ICs) layout designs
- ID

Patent

It is a grant made by the government to an inventor, conveying and securing him the exclusive right to make, use and sell his invention for a term of 20 years. It is granted for an invention that is new and useful. Invention may be a new or improved product or process that is capable of industrial application. Novelty is a fundamental requirement for grant of patent and it should not include "prior art" or knowledge already existing in the public domain. What constitutes prior art has been a matter of debate as the later sections of the chapter reveal. The Colonial Indian Patent and Designs Act, 1911 was re-enacted as the Indian Patents Act, 1970. Various amendments made from 1999 to 2005 were the result of extensive consultations by the government with several expert groups and trade representatives. In its present form, it is both TRIPS compliant and also provides measures and safeguards that will not be detrimental to research and development activities in the country.

Copyright

According to the Webster's Dictionary, copyright is defined as the exclusive right to reproduce, publish and sell matter and form of a literary, musical or artistic work. Aimed at fostering creativity and ingenuity, it is a property right that grants exclusive rights to do or authorize others to do certain acts in relation to original literary, dramatic, musical and artistic works, cinematographic films and sound recordings. Literary works also include computer programs, labels and compilations including computer databases. Copyright is a form of IP, which, though intangible, manifests ultimately in the form of a tangible property (music on recording media such as DVDs, CDs, paintings on a medium, cinematographic creations on photographic films, etc.).

Fundamentally, copyright law exists to prevent others from taking unfair advantage of a person's creative efforts. The object of copyright law is to facilitate, encourage and motivate artists, composers, designers and software programmers, etc., to create original works by rewarding them with excusive rights for a limited period. The owner of the copyright has exclusive rights to make multiple copies of his work. It prevents others form making copies of the copyrighted material. India is signatory to the International Copyright Conventions, and provisions of these conventions give copyright protection to works of Indian nationals in all the member countries that are signatories to these conventions. Likewise, foreign authors from these countries are entitled to copyright protection in India. Indian Copyright Act, 1957, amended in the years 1984, 1994 and 1999, provides for exclusive rights to authors and other owners of original works. Under the Act, the Copyright Enforcement Advisory Council (CEAC) constituted by the Department of Education, Ministry of Human Resource Development, the Government of India, is concerned with the enforcement and review of the Indian Copyright Act. Special cells for copyright enforcement have so far been set up in 23 states and union territories in India. Registered copyright societies for respective different classes of works are set up for collective administration of copyright.

Trademark

It is a sign or symbol or a picture, label, word or words that are used by a person on his goods or articles intended for sale to distinguish/identify them from the goods or articles of others. It is recognized as a very valuable form of IP as it is associated with quality and consumer protection in relation to a product or service. It is essentially a product of competitive economy where more than one person competes for the manufacture of the same product. This necessitated the need for marking of each manufacturer's goods by a symbol that distinguishes it from similar goods made by others. Essentially a property law, it grants the trademark owner exclusive right to protect his mark by virtue of priority in adoption, long, continuous and extensive use.

Trademark is used as a product differentiator and is a valuable marketing tool in today's competitive markets. Good trademarks are associated with quality, security and even sense of belonging in the minds of consumers for that product. Trademarks like Tata, Godrej, etc., embody the goodwill of the company and institution they represent.

Trademark Law in India is contained in the provisions of Trademark Act, 1999. The object of this Act is to confer protection to the user of the trademark on his goods and prescribe conditions for acquisition and legal remedies for enforcement of trademark rights. The earlier Trade and Merchandise Act, 1958 has been repealed, and the Trade Marks Act, 1999 was passed after taking into consideration developments in trading and commercial practices in the country since liberalization. Trademark protection under TRIPS is of significance to the Indian pharmaceutical industry which was in the practice of receiving protection for drug names closely resembling the International Non-proprietary Name (INN). As per Section 13 of the amended Trademark Act, 1999, the World Health Organization (WHO) approved INN for a potential new chemical entity cannot be registered for protection as a trademark. Post-TRIPS era, there are several trademark-related litigations in India.

Geographic Indications

These identify goods as originating in the territory or a region or a locality in that territory, where a given quality, reputation or other characteristic of the goods is essentially attributable to that particular geographic location. Kanjeevaram silk sarees, Basmati rice, Darjeeling tea, Kashmir carpets, Sivakasi crackers, Scotch whisky, etc., are some examples. Law relating to GI intends to protect the interest of producers or manufacturers of such goods, also preventing consumers from being deceived by the falsity of geographic origin. It is a form of IP whose protection helps in the economic prosperity of such goods and ultimately promotes goods bearing such GI in the export market. Right conferred on GI prevents competitors from commercially exploiting the respective rights to the detriment of the owner of that property.

In India, the GI Act was found necessary to protect Indian GIs from being misused in other countries. To seek redressal as in the case of basmati rice and Darjeeling tea [India had to fight infringement cases against these Indian GIs (see Box items 1–3)], these GIs had to be protected in India first. Hence, in December 1999, the Indian Parliament passed the Geographical Indications of Goods (Registration and Protection) Act, 1999, as this was a pre-requirement without which there would be no obligation under the WTO for other countries to extend reciprocal protection. This Act seeks to provide for the registration and better protection of the GIs relating to goods in India.

Industrial Designs

Design, in the view of patent law, is that characteristic of a physical substance which, by means of lines, images, configuration, etc., casts an impression of uniqueness and character in the mind of the observer. Design is thus a conception, suggestion or idea of a shape and not an article. Under TRIPS, the original designs relating to features of shape or configuration of an article are protected. This protection covers whole or part of a product's appearance to the eyes, resulting from the features, lines, contours, colours, shape, texture and/or materials of the product itself and/or its ornamentation. This protection does not cover the working or operations of the products. The main objective is to protect novel designs made with the object of applying to particular articles to be manufactured and marketed commercially. It is chiefly meant to prevent other manufacturers from using or reproducing the protected design.

In India, protection to product designs and appearance is covered under Design Act, 2000. To be protected, the design must primarily be aesthetic and the owner on registration is assured an exclusive right against unauthorized copying or imitation of the design by third parties. The Indian Act grants protection for 10 years for a registered design.

Integrated Circuits

These include semi-conductor chips fabricated of transistors, resistors, capacitors and their interconnections. These tiny, single-piece layout designs of ICs are creations of the human mind, products resulting out of an enormous amount of time and money. There is a continuing need for the creation of new layout designs that reduce the dimensions of the existing ICs and simultaneously increase their functions. ICs are utilized in a large range of products such as watches, TVs, automobiles, washing machines and sophisticated data processing equipment. The protection of IC refers to the protection of the layout design of the circuit and allows the owner of the design to prevent unauthorized reproduction and distribution of such designs.

With India's capability in software and hardware designing being recognized globally, in order to be TRIPS compliant, the Semi Conductor Integrated Circuits Layout Design Act, 2000 was enacted to offer protection to original or inherently distinctive layout designs not yet commercially exploited.

Trade Secrets

This is a relatively newer form of IP and ideologically does not fall in the line of IP rights. This is because while all other forms of IP protection require disclosure of information to public in return for protection, this is a special and privileged protection *enabling non-disclosure* of corporate secrets. In doing so, the economic value of the enterprise holding it is much enhanced. This protection is for information such as formulas, patterns, training programs, methods, techniques, etc., that are vital to the operation of the business. Trade secret is an IP of which a business organization is the lawful owner or custodian of the same, so that the information is not used by others without their permission or consent for commercial exploitation (e.g., the formula for Coco-Cola is the most guarded trade secret in the world). Trade secret is thus both a type of IP and a strategy for protecting a firm's IP.

In India, there are no statutes dealing with trade secrets. It is common law based and Section 27 of the Indian Contract Act, 1872 provides some remedy by barring disclosure of information acquired as a result of a contract.

Plant Varieties

Protection of plant varieties is the most recent inclusion in TRIPS. Research and development in agriculture led to the creation of new plant varieties which were covered by rights commonly referred to as breeder rights. Though Article 27.3(b) of TRIPS agreement excludes plants from patentability, it provides protection of plant varieties either by patents or by an effective "*sui generis*" system (meaning self-generating) system. This means that a country can decide on any system, provided it grants effective plant breeder's rights. Under this, plant varieties are protected based on the criteria of novelty, distinctiveness, uniformity and stability. India, like many developing countries, has chosen the *sui generis* option over patenting of plant varieties. Accordingly, it passed the Protection of Plant Varieties and Farmers' Rights Act in August 2001. The purpose of this was to provide for the establishment of an effective system for protection of plant varieties, protection of the rights of farmers and breeders, and encouraging the development of new plant varieties and thereof. The key element of the Act is protection of IP rights for plant varieties by a registration process. Through such registration, both breeders and farmers of plant varieties are protected and given rights. It also gives rights to researchers, the government and the public.

CONTROVERSIES SURROUNDING TRIPS AGREEMENT

It is a fact that TRIPS agreement was the result of relentless efforts made by the developed countries. Despite the well-designed TRIPS objectives aimed at protecting and rewarding creativity and inventiveness, recently its enforcement the world over has precipitated some emerging issues that are both controversial and biased, favoring possibly only the powerful players in the WTO.

- IP rights are meant to encourage creativity, rewarding human intelligence. However, traditional knowledge (TK), which is the accumulated result of human intelligence over centuries, is denied IP status, whereas small simple acts of human creativity such as designs and such other forms are given protection and exclusive rights.
- Discrepancies over what is patentable and what is prior art is the most debated issue. It is interesting to note that on one hand, TK is considered prior art for purposes of non-inclusion as IP. On the other hand, it is argued that TK-related facts can be patented in

countries that do not have TK – guggulu is patented in the US because such knowledge is not prior art there. Thus, prior art is subject to connotation to suit convenience.

- According to the provisions of TRIPS, "patent rights should be given to products irrespective of whether they are locally produced or imported." This provision of TRIPS is in defense of the patented drugs being produced by alternative processes in India. When the same argument of TK not being prior art in US is applied for the knowledge of the process of making innovator drugs in India, which is not known here, it is not prior art; and hence, the process is patentable. But that is not possible as per TRIPS. It is thus quite obvious that word play and clever rephrasing of facts into meanings can make anything patentable or non-patentable, especially if it suits the economic needs of the country. Of course, to push this through, lobbying is needed.

- Normally GI is an IP that can be protected to prevent the use of these names, *if they indicate that they originate from a specific geographic origin that is not the real place of origin of the product.* For example, using the term Kashmir carpets to the carpets made elsewhere misleads the consumer into believing that they are of the same quality associated with the original quality which is unique to Kashmir carpets because of some specific quality attributable to them. Depending on the GI, the specific quality could be attributable to something unique to the geographic location, such as soil, climate, traditional method of production, etc.

- However, TRIPS agreement provides an "enhanced" minimum level of protection for GIs that identify wines and spirits. By this, wines and spirits cannot use GI even *if they do not imply that they originate in a place other than the true place of origin.* Thus, nobody can use the word "champagne" as the word does not indicate that it is not made in France. On the contrary, the words "chai" (referring to Darjeeling tea) and "mulligatony" soup (referring to a traditional South Indian pepper soup) are being used freely, with the former being used for a special brew made by the famous Starbucks Company of the US. We are not in a position to prevent the use of the word "chai" because it does not have the special enhanced protection like wines and spirits of France. The reason behind is powerful lobbying by France in a big way to ensure that its markets are protected. Hence "lobbying" is an available recourse for the inclusion of special category (within TRIPS) of any particular product to the exclusion of other similar categories. Each country has to "lobby" for its own cause as the world body can not take up the cause of a developing country on its own.

- In the same way, "trade secrets" and "disclosure of information" are not ideologically IP. TRIPS agreement has made exception to even the definition of IP by including trade secrets for IP protection. The justification of IP system is rewarding inventiveness with exclusive rights in exchange of the usage of the invention for the benefit of society. Holders of trade secrets are entitled to protection, though there is no mandatory disclosure of information. Even such a category gets special protection under the very IP system which by definition grants privileges in return for disclosure of information that will be of use to society. Here, an exception was made to include a category which neither fits into the criteria of being an individual act of creation nor is of any benefit to the society. The special protection is given only to further the economic interest of trade secret holders.

- The whole system of IP found international protection and acceptance under WTO due to the persistence and promotion by developed nations. Hence, only those categories that are in their economic interests have somehow managed to get included under TRIPS. It is up to the developing nations and countries holding TK to find ways and means of seeking protection for TK in order to prevent unjust exploitation of this wealth of knowledge by the very same instrument of IP rights which was supposed to protect it.

- It is argued that since IP rights are for individual rights, TK, being a collective right, is unable to seek protection. While the collective rights of bigger nations get managed to get protected, TK holders' rights are waiting to be to be adequately protected. Meanwhile, cases of biopiracy of TK by bigger corporates of developing countries are being fought against at huge costs to these nations holding the TK.

- Ethical objectives are made with respect to pharmaceutical patents for the high medication prices they enable their proprietors to charge. This is unaffordable to poorer sections of the society.

- Questions are being raised regarding the rationale behind the high prices and exclusive patent rights required by pharmaceutical companies to recoup the large investments needed for research and development of these drugs. It is unfortunate that several new drugs so introduced at the end of long and expensive clinical trials are withdrawn hastily against new evidence of toxicity or adverse effects.

- Patenting seems to help misplaced pharmaceutical R&D priorities of making slightly improved treatments for lifestyle disorders as against developing life-saving drugs for the diseases that are devastating large parts of the world.

- Costs of patent litigation exceed their investment value as seen in the software industry. Similarly, infringement costs are exorbitantly expensive as was the case for fighting for revoking the US patents for neem and basmati by India.

INDIAN PATENT LAW

Ancient Indian Innovations Happened Without the Need for Patents

The wealth of scientific heritage of ancient India – considered as the cradle of world civilization – encompasses innovations in diverse fields of human knowledge and creativity, such as astronomy, mathematics, medicine, surgery, architecture, alchemy, metallurgy, etc. This is apart from substantial literary and other works of grammar in Sanskrit, now identified as the most suitable language for computer software. India gave the world the number system and the number zero. Algebra, trigonometry and calculus came from India, and the value of pi was first calculated in the 6th century BC, long before the time of European mathematicians. We were the most agriculturally advanced nation, built the worlds' first reservoir and dam for irrigation, and were pioneers in rhinoplastic surgery. The list is long, and in every sphere of human activity, we have been innovators and pioneers.

These were the contributions of a highly advanced civilization that had no need for the concept of IP protection. Due to common philosophical underpinnings, Indian socio-cultural ethos was able to go beyond the realm of individual glorification and personal benefits. Realization of larger values in life by even common folk enabled them to go beyond such partisan concerns. Such strong spiritual values were the founding pillars for the larger-than-life missions of visionary Indians.

Colossal works of human endeavor such as the resplendent architectural designs of magnificent ancient Indian temples and mammoth monolithic works are a standing testimony to the grandeur and peak of human achievement without a skirmish over vain personal credit and glory. These were the results of the hard work and intellectual contribution of generations of people working over several centuries. Often the dream of an architect or a king is realized a few generations later. Several profound works of art, literature and even the medical treatises are not attributable to a single author. Unlike today's practice of each vying to take credit for their share of contribution, these ancient works were compilations of multiple authors spanning over centuries.

Thus, history has minimal references to the royal patronage under which such massive achievements could be made. Names of master sculptors, architects, and thousands of other creators and artisans are conspicuous by their absence.

This was a society that could look beyond personal emancipation, and hence, concepts such as "creator's rights" and "exclusive benefits" were much below the domain of ancient Indian knowing and creativity.

Events later in history like foreign invasions and colonial rule have ravaged India and transformed it to the point where young Indians today are not even aware of the depth of knowing that was ours.

Imprints of submission, imperial dominance and its fallout on our societal values, culture and economy have left us as poor imposters of ideas and values form the West. Most of our legal and other administrative laws and regulations are styled on the lines of what our rulers left us. Hence, they are complex by intent to serve our rulers' prerogative of delaying, if not denying justice as and when it suits their priorities.

Patent Law in Modern India

Our patent law was no exception and was modeled on the same lines as those enforced in our country by the British to further its trade objectives and use the Indian market. Pre-independence, our patent paws were modeled on the lines of the British Patent Act of 1852 without proper policy-based objective of the IP system that is unique to the needs of our country.

Post-independence, the government directed a review of the prevailing patents and designs legislation in India by T. B. Chand Committee in 1948. Consequent to this and the recommendations of Justice Rajagopala Iyyengar Committee in 1957, the Indian Patent Law enacted in 1856 by the British Empire was revised and amended in 1970 to suit the industrial need of our growing newly independent nation. The Act along with the rules came into force in 1972.

Transformation of Indian pharmaceutical industry (1970–1995)

In the scenario of relative inaccessibility, unaffordability or non-availability of essential life-saving medicines, most of which had to be imported, the committee recommended the provision of process patenting system of drugs. Thus, the Patents Act, 1970 abolished product patents for food and pharmaceuticals and restricted grant of patents in these fields only to process patents. Simultaneous passage of Drug Price Control Order in 1970 gave greater governmental control over drug prices.

The term of process patents was restricted to 7 years from the date of application or 7 years from the sealing of patent against 14 years from the date of application for other fields. It provided for "automatic compulsory license" or "license of right" by which anyone is free to practice an invention, if it is in public interest.

According to Gopakumar G. Nair, former president, Indian Drug Manufacturers' Association (IDMA), "The Patents Act 1970 incorporated very well thought out, highly effective, safe-harbor provisions, though considered controversial in the global context, for early generic introductions of patented New Chemical Entities (NCEs) in India and essential life saving medicine based on them."

This was great stimulus for the Indian pharmaceutical industry, which from 1970 to 1995 went about developing innovative processing methods for manufacturing patented NCEs. Because of process patenting, it became possible to develop economic versions of therapeutically equivalent generics to a number of patented drugs. This "reverse engineering" initiative enabled India to be nearly self-sufficient in manufacturing of patented drugs. Once the international patents for these drugs expired, India moved aggressively into the international market with generic drugs, thus becoming a substantially large manufacturer and exporter of bulk drugs/active ingredients with its vibrant generic drug industry. India became a net exporter of pharmaceuticals, occupying the 3rd largest position in terms of volume and 14th largest in terms of value. With the effective amendment of Indian Patent Law in 1970, India moved from being a huge importer of exorbitantly costly essential medicines to becoming a self-reliant manufacturer and exporter of life-saving medicines.

Introduction of IP agenda during the Uruguay round of GATT talks in 1986, and the later Dunkel Draft, evoked concerns about the future of the Indian pharmaceutical industry. There were fears of escalating drug prices initially, largely because of misconception and lack of awareness of the IP system.

Post-TRIPS changes (1995–2004)

Once India became a member country of WTO in 1994, it was compelled to honor TRIPS agreement. Being a developing country, a grace period of 10 years from 1995 to 2004 was given to enable transition for complying with TRIPS requirements. Despite initial apprehensions, India began equipping itself as a TRIPS-compliant nation by several national expertise developing efforts. Efforts at initiating education and training in IP rights and dissemination of information regarding IP involving educationists, lawyers, jurists, industry leaders, etc., began. It was identified that of the various categories of IP covered by TRIPS, patents, trademarks and trade secrets play an important role in the development and commercialization of the pharma industry, with copyright, designs and confidential information also being relevant. To become TRIPS compliant, India amended the Patents Act, 1970 three times in 1999, 2002 and 2005. Amendments of significance to the Indian pharma and herbal drug industry are as follows:

1. The Patent (First) Amendment Act, 1999 inserted a new Chapter IV-A that deals with Exclusive Marketing Rights (EMR). EMR means the exclusive right to sell and deal with the patented article or with an article in relation to which an application for obtaining patent has been made. As per TRIPS agreement, developing nations were to extend patent protection to earlier unprotected sectors at the end of the 10-year transition period. By 1995, EMR was to be introduced as a concessionary means to protect the IP of inventors. Being a product patent, EMR gave exclusive marketing rights only to sell the product and not to manufacture as well. This was meant to be stop gap arrangement before product patenting was to come into force from 2005. There were initial fears about the impact of

grant of EMR on our pharma industry. However, criteria to qualify for an EMR as per Chapter IV-A were such that these could be granted only to those products for which tests were conducted after January 1994. Out of 8,500 EMR applications filed, only 14 could be filed, and because of the complexity of qualifying criteria, most of them got rejected.

2. Patent (Second) Amendment Act, 2002 amended the definition for "invention" as a "new product or process involving an inventive step and capable of industrial application." Micro-organisms were made patentable and the term of patent was extended to 20 years from the date of filing application for all fields of invention.

3. It deleted the provision of license of right and reversal of burden of proof (of novelty on the process patentee in infringement suits) was inserted. Deletion of the license of right provision from the 1970 Act is a major factor that is taking India to the global patent arena, since it enables protection of patentee's rights without dilution. With this ushered in the product patent regime in India, as it moved from a process patent system to a product patent system.

4. An important amendment of great significance to the pharmaceutical industry was exemption of exclusive rights for research purposes. As per Article 30 of TRIPS agreement, the member nations can include exemptions that do not unreasonably conflict with normal patent exploitation. A patent grants exclusive rights upon the patentee to prevent unauthorized third parties from making, using, offering for sale, selling or importing the patented product within the territorial jurisdiction of India. However, as per the newly included experimental/research exemption, any person can use the patented product or process for the purpose of experimentation or research, including tutoring pupils. This exemption, known as the "Bolar Provision" in Canada or "Hatch–Waxman exemption" in the US, is meant for academic purposes for further research and experiment. This exemption can be used as a statutory defense against infringement, as the amendment in the Act states that any act of making, constructing, using, selling or importing a patented invention solely for uses related to the development and submission of information does not amount to patent infringement. Thus, Indian generic drug manufacturers can perform further research and development activities on the patented products for preparing for regulatory approval to prepare a generic version *before* a patent expires.

5. Another important amendment of great consequence to the pharmaceutical and herbal drug industry was removal of subsection (g) of Section 3 of the Patent Act which lists non-patentable invention. According to this, "a method or process of testing applicable during the process of manufacture for rendering the machine, apparatus or other equipment more efficient or for the improvement or restoration of the existing machine, apparatus or other equipment or for the improvement or control of manufacture is non-patentable." Removal of this section broadens the scope of patentability of processes or methods that are being developed in relation to manufacture in a pharmaceutical industry. Similarly, even processes for characterization or standardization of herbal drugs and herbal ingredients could become patentable. Standardization protocols developed for multi-component classic and proprietary herbal drugs can thus come under this category.

6. Patent (Third) Amendment Act, 2005: To become fully TRIPS compliant, by the end of the 10-year grace period for developing countries (with no existing product patent regime), the Patent (Third) Amendment Act, 2005 came into effect. This Act omitted Section 5 of

the Indian Patent Act that granted process patents for food, medicines or other drug substances. With this latest amendment, Indian pharmaceutical companies are prohibited to market a generic drug – a drug patented elsewhere – by using a different process. Henceforth, the product patents became available in all fields of invention.

7. Section 2(1)(j) defines an "inventive step" as a feature of an invention that involves "technical advance as compared to the existing knowledge or having economic significance or both and that makes the invention not obvious to a person skilled in the art." Under this category could come newer herbal drug formulations for the diseases assuming epidemic proportions, apart from newer processes for the manufacture of patented drugs of economic significance.

8. Earlier "compulsory license" for certain extreme/urgent situations such as patentee's anti-competitive practices, lack of drug availability in India at an affordable price, public non-commercial use, patented invention not worked in India, etc., continues to exist. Also, there are several built-in measures and safeguards that are not detrimental to the research and developmental activities in the country, especially in the field of pharmaceutical products

9. Earlier Chapter IV-A and Sections 24A-F of the original Act enabling EMR were omitted as product patent regime became operational.

Post-TRIPS (from 2005 to present)

Disproving initial fears about TRIPS agreement implementation, the Indian pharmaceutical industry has vibrantly faced up to the changed scenario. Large visionary corporates like Dr. Reddy's took to drug discovery programs and others began investing in setting up of research facilities and innovative research programs to face the challenges of the product patent regime in the early 1990s.

There has been extensive IP/patent awareness creation with increasing trend in education and training in universities, institutions and law campuses and colleges. Thus, technical and legal professionals in the Indian pharma industry began incorporating IP/patent practices in their knowledge upgradation and work culture. Complying with global IP practices has enabled identification of advantages such as freedom to market analysis and operation, patent landscaping, adoption of non-infringing processes for filing Drug Master Files and Abbreviated New Drug Applications (ANDA), etc. This has enabled much greater technological progress and market penetration, so much so that India's pharma exports are now directed to developed countries such as the US and Europe in the post-TRIPS era.

Having noted the earlier success of the Indian generic industry post-TRIPS, overseas generic pharma corporations have set up research facilities in India and have also made major mergers and acquisitions. The post-TRIPS knowledge-driven pharma research environment is attracting Indian origin pharma professionals back to the country. According to Gopakumar G. Nair, "there is about 30 per cent share for pharma in filing and grant of trademarks and patents. There is a recent surge in filing of ANDA in the USA, thus encouraging co-marketing, colicensing alliances and networking of Indian pharma companies with global pharma corporations." India, which commenced export of bulk drugs and formulations to least developed countries in the late 1970s and 1980s, has now emerged as a major global player post-TRIPS.

Today the country appears well geared to be a successful and single largest pharma player in the global scenario post-TRIPS.

ISSUES PERTAINING TO HERBAL DRUG PATENTING

TK on Herbal Drugs

TK refers to the knowledge, innovations and practices of indigenous and local communities around the world, developed from the experience gained over the centuries and adopted as per the local culture and environment.

TK, especially in well-established civilizations such as India, is the collective result of careful observation, understanding and experimentation of culturally and socially stable societies over long periods of time. Such information faithfully transmitted through generations orally and later textually is a cultural heritage and a veritable storehouse of enormous knowledge related to various fields of human endeavor. Practical management and sustainable utilization of natural resources has been the stronghold of ancient Indian way of life. Our agriculture is a treasure house of information on the development and adaptation of plants and crops to different ecological conditions such as soil, rainfall, temperature, altitude, etc. ·

Several reasons are attributed to the loss/lack of comprehension of the nature of knowledge that ancient Indians possessed. Accepting other forms of knowledge as an understanding of life and its ways from a totally different perspective is needed to appreciate the depth of human knowing that was then available.

Today, however, there is growing appreciation of the value of TK and it is finding increasing applicability and utility to agriculture as well as modern industry. The practical applicability of TK in fields such as agriculture, fisheries, health, horticulture and forestry is now being recognized. It is found to be an immensely valuable knowledge reserve to develop newer drugs, herbal cosmetics, agri-chemicals, non-wood forest products, handicrafts, etc.

Our vast knowledge reserve on herbal drugs in the form of Indian traditional medicine is finding increasing acceptance the world over. It is an invaluable resource as it provides valuable leads for the development of drugs, other useful products and processes.

Thus, TK saves investment in terms of time, money and effort needed for the otherwise large-scale "needle in a haystack" type of screening methodologies (like the National Institute of Health (NIH) screening for marine anticancer drugs) needed to identify potentially useful drugs from plant sources. Thus, it has the potential of being translated into commercial benefits by providing leads for the development of useful products and processes. However, ironically and maybe conveniently (for modern Western science), the very knowledge that forms the basis of modern scientific plant drug screening programs is not regarded as a science. It is unfortunate that the so-called "modern medicine" is regarded as the only authentic body of knowledge against which standard all other forms of knowledge are measured and judged.

Even when seen through the only accepted perspective of modern science, TK from this subcontinent and elsewhere has been the largest contributor of newer drugs to modern medicine. It is for this reason and because of the disillusionment with the approach and attitude of modern medicine that TK systems related to health and drugs are being consciously revived. What has been denigrated by modern science as "superstitious," "mythical" belief systems is being encouraged by world bodies like the WHO as an "alternative" health care option.

The world over, there is a frantic quest for newer drugs from traditionally used herbs. Multinational drug companies (proponents of modern scientific methods) too are vying with each other to squeeze out maximum economic benefit from TK audaciously, without even the need to recognize TK as scientific knowledge. Cases of biopiracy against TK are a standing testimony to this blatant plagiarism.

With the IP system imposed on the global economy by the powerful developed nations, individual rights have been enshrined at the cost of the collective rights of TK holders, just because it serves the interests of these nations and goes against the unwritten dictum that "anything that comes from the West is science and anything that comes form the East is superstition."

TK Outside IP Protection – The Fallout

Though TK represents collective IP of communities or indigenous groups, with all its seemingly equitable and just objectives, TRIPS agreement does not include TK for IP protection. Prime reasons quoted for this glaring omission are the following:

- Possession is the most important basis to claim IP protection. TK, it is said, being a product of collective experience without an individual act of creation, is not recognized as IP.
- TK, being available for long periods of time, does not meet the criteria of "novelty" or "non-obviousness," i.e., it is "prior art" – already available in the public domain.

On the contrary, not all categories under TRIPS protection are acts of individual creation. Trade secrets refer to information possessed by a firm which is protected. Such experimental data, design manuals, R&D reports, etc., that are protected may not be the result of individual act of creation. In this case, a firm or a corporation is seeking protection for the information which is also collective.

To the question of prior art, although TK is already available in certain parts of the world, it is not universally known. It is not prior art as it was never patented and so cannot be said to have entered the public domain.

Impact of the non-inclusion of TK under TRIPS has precipitated the following.

Biopiracy

While TRIPS enshrines the rights of inventors and creators, instead of protecting TK, the current IP regime has facilitated its commercialization by individuals or entities, completely leaving out the original holders of the knowledge out of the loop of benefit sharing. Many patents have been granted in the US and UK to foreign bioprospectors on medicines and products that evolved out of TK. For example, India was affected due to this biopiracy and had to fight it out in international courts to revoke patents granted to the "use of neem as fungicide," "turmeric as a wound healing agent" (Box items 1 and 2) and on "basmati rice for its special flavor and taste." In response to such concerns about such misappropriation of TK, defensive arguments such as "TK is prior art in India but not in the US, hence patentable there" have been evoked, thus demonstrating how the definitions and provisions of TRIPS are modifiable to suit convenience.

Need to prove TK as prior existing knowledge

In countries such as the US, prior existing knowledge does not include information orally passed down generations. Journal publication and database information alone constitutes prior art. Ironically, thus, the burden of *making TK come into the definition of "prior existing knowledge"* is on countries holding the TK. They are now resorting to document the vast storehouse of information in regional languages into multilingual digital libraries that can be accessed by patent examiners before granting TK-related patents.

Box item 1

US patent on turmeric

US patent number 540504 on "the use of turmeric in wound healing" was granted to two scientists of University of Mississippi Medical Center. This was challenged by CSIR, India that requested the US Patent and Trademark Office (USPTO) to re-examine the patent as turmeric has been used for thousands of years for healing wounds and rashes, and hence, its medicinal use was not novel. USPTO upheld the objections and revoked the patent.

Box item 2

European patent on neem

European patent number 0436257 was granted to the US Corporation W. R. Grace and the US Department of Agriculture (USDA) for a "method of controlling fungi on plants by the aid of hydrophobic extracted neem oil." A group of Indian non-governmental organizations (NGOs) and representatives of Indian farmers legally opposed the patent, submitting evidence that the fungicidal effect of extracts of neem seeds has been known and used for centuries in Indian agriculture to protect crops. With the claim of being non-novel, the patent was revoked.

Box item 3

European patent on Indian wheat

EP number 445929 was granted to American seeds multinational Monsanto for the wheat variety "invented" by crossing a traditional Indian wheat "Nap-Hal" with another soft wheat variety. Nap-Hal germplasm was accessed by the company from UK collection. The patent granted in 13 countries gave Monsanto monopoly rights over the traditional characteristics of the Indian wheat variety and it also covered biscuits, flour and dough produced from this wheat. This enabled the company to take legal action against the Indian farmers trying to breed wheat with similar genetic traits. This patent was legally challenged by Greenpeace and Indian farmers, following which the patent on this wheat variety was revoked.

Patenting life forms

The entire idiom of Western legal practices and the vocabulary of IP protection law carve out exclusive rights to an individual to exploit creations of human ingenuity. This has resulted in attempts to privatize even community rights over biodiversity (BD) and indigenous knowledge. Such attempts to monopolize or patent life forms such as crops and seeds are raising concerns about removal of control of food production from local communities and farmers to multinational corporations (Box item 3).

Biotrade – an ecological concern

There is a marked imbalance in the system of IP rights due to insistence of monopoly rights only to the field of technology and denying it to the vast pool of knowledge reserve of indigenous communities that have so far managed the natural resources. This has generated a global push to privatize BD. Many countries and the large businesses they support increasingly want control over these resources and the knowledge associated with them for commercial purposes. The IP regime has greatly facilitated such drives. Thus, against the threat of depletion of global biological reserves, there is a large "biotrade," i.e., movement of biological reserves between countries, companies, academic institutions and individuals, which is a cause of serious concern. Booming global trade in herbal products, demand for exotic herbs and other natural materials, and associated rampant commercialization have thus made economy, a driving factor, tilting even governmental decisions in favor of biotrade in the name of profitable overseas trade and research ventures.

This is causing a disruption in the relationship between the TK generators and their resources, leading to the disintegration of the very processes by which the knowledge evolved and is kept alive.

BD appropriation

In the resultant scenario of fast vanishing natural resources, the IP regime has raked up the conflict of the rules of division and appropriation of BD. BD refers to the variability of life forms within an ecological zone. It has become increasingly important because of the scientific and commercial interest attached to it with a range of different groups including indigenous people asserting their claims and rights to it.

The imminent threat to global BD resulted in the Convention on Biodiversity (CBD). Member countries under this international convention have enacted BD laws to protect national BD reserves and to provide a comprehensive framework for the conservation and sustainable use of biological resources. The IP right framework enacted on biological reserves will also have significant social and human impact as biological resources are not only economic resources but also constitute the primary food supplies of the nation. Despite disparate resistance to incursion on indigenous rights to local resources, communities are increasingly losing control over their resources as industry supported by governments is establishing greater control over plant genetic resources and the associated knowledge through the use of IP rights.

Non-conducive environment to research on herbal drugs

Lack of IP protection and the huge cost of infringement suits are not conducive to research on traditional herbal drugs. There is little financial incentive to explore traditional medical claims of herbal drugs for therapeutic efficacy. Current scientific drug discovery research is based on "single molecule–single receptor–single activity" approach of activity screening. Such methods of experimentation on herbs and their activity studies are unable to bring out the actual panoramic dimension behind herbal drug pharmacology. For example, isolation of a single chemical entity from an efficacious anti-diabetic traditional herb, if found to be not safe leads to unjustified apprehensions about the safety of the herb. What is needed is development of lateral analysis protocols tailored to evaluate multiple pharmacological effects of polychemical herbal drugs. Unless there is sufficient financial incentive and protection to fund such research efforts, herbs and herbal drugs will not receive the needed research attention.

Global Initiatives to Secure TK to Rightful Owners

It is well known that indigenous and local communities depend on TK for their livelihood as well as to sustainably manage and exploit their ecosystem. The WHO estimates that up to 80 per cent of the world population relies on traditional medicine for primary health care. Thus, on one hand, organizations such as Food and Agriculture Organization (FAO), the World Bank and the United Nations Environmental Program now encourage the use of TK in sustainable rural development programs. On the other hand, TRIPS agreement of WTO fails to see it as a knowledge reserve to be protected. In view of the trend towards biopiracy and misappropriation of TK, the international community is debating the consequences of globalization in its various forums. The role of IP regime in relation to TK, ways and means of preserving, protecting and equitably making use of it, has received increasing attention in a range of international policy discussions. IP matters relating to TK were discussed internationally in forums relating to food and agriculture, environment, conservation of BD, public health, human rights, indigenous issues, trade and economic development. Though at the international level, there is significant support for opposing the grant of patents on non-original inventions, the current IP regime fails to develop a system of reward or protection for TK.

The following international bodies touch upon the rights of TK holders:

- The CBD in its preamble and Article 8(j) recognizes "the close and traditional dependence of many indigenous and local communities embodying traditional lifestyles on biological resources and the desirability of sharing equitably the benefits arising from the use of TK, innovations and practices relevant to the conservation of BD and the sustainable use of its components." Under the CBD, a working group in relation to access to genetic resources and benefit sharing (has developed the Bonn Guidelines). These are designed to facilitate access to genetic resources among the member states. Though the guidelines seek to balance the interests of the country of origin of genetic resources with those of the recipient in benefit sharing arrangements, they are basically premised on the commercialization of these resources. With indigenous groups and people's organizations stressing the need for more focused attention on TK, at the Madrid Workshop, the requirement for a working group on Article 8(j) was endorsed.

- Under the auspices of the FAO, the International Treaty on Plant Genetic Resources provides the space for national recognition of farmer's rights. Despite attempts by Asian countries to include farmer's rights in the text of the treaty, the treaty fails to do so and also has controversial provisions on IP rights.

- WIPO, under its Intergovernmental Committee on Genetic Resources, Traditional Knowledge and Folklore (IGC-GRTKF), has created a task force under the committee of experts of the International Patent Classification (IPC) to study the relation and possible integration of a TK resource classification into the IPC. WIPO's 184 member states are negotiating an international legal instrument intended to ensure the effective protection of TK and traditional cultural expressions and to regulate the interface between IP and genetic resources.

- Under the Asia-Pacific Economic Cooperation (APEC), the Intellectual Property Rights Expert Group is making action plans to promote an internationally harmonized IP system.

- Though the TRIPS agreement does not expressly cover patent protection for TK, it contains several provisions including articles 7, 8, 27, 29, 32 and 62.1, which are relevant to the issue of disclosure of the source of TK in patent applications. It provides for plant variety protection through patent protection or a *sui generis*. However, the procedures and schemes by which this may be used to protect indigenous knowledge are yet to be worked out.

- The WTO, TRIPS council was requested by India on behalf of the other Asian countries to harmonize TRIPS agreement with the CBD. The objective is that TRIPS agreement should be supportive of CBD. A submission to amend TRIPS agreement was made to provide for a requirement by a patent applicant (in relation to biological materials) to furnish information on the country of origin of the biological resource, evidence of prior informed consent and that of a fair and equitable benefit sharing arrangement as a condition for acquiring patent rights.

Practically viewing, enforcement wise and implementation wise, there is virtually no attempt at the international level to seriously bring the rightful rights, recognition and protection to TK holders. The protection of genetic resources, and folklore and TK has, however, provoked a long and unrelenting debate between developed and developing nations.

Indian Initiatives for TK Protection – Impact on Herbal Drug Industry

Many developing countries are attempting to promote legislations to protect BD and TK.

The Indian Biodiversity Act, 2002

It focuses on the rights of the state and monopoly IP rights such as patents. The implication is that most property rights will be in the hands of the state and private companies. The Act addresses basic concerns of access to collection and utilization of biological resources and knowledge by foreigners and sharing of benefits arising out of such access. The Act provides for National Biodiversity Authority (NBA) which will grant approvals for access, subject to conditions, that ensure equitable sharing of benefits. The main intent of this legislation is to protect India's BD and associated knowledge systems against their use by individuals/organizations without sharing the benefits arising out of such use and also to check biopiracy. The legislation provides for a federal management structure with the NBA at the apex and the BD management committees at local community level. These are to consult each other in taking decisions relating to the use of biological resources/related knowledge within their jurisdiction. The NBA under 36(5) and 62 sections of the Biodiversity Act, 2002 has drafted the Biological Diversity Rules, 2009 for the protection, conservation and effective management of TK.

Indian Patent (2nd Amendment) Act, 2002

This amendment to the 1970 Act inserted Section 3(p), according to which "an invention, which is in effect traditional knowledge or which is aggregation or duplication of known properties of traditionally known component or components is not patentable." This is of significance to medicinal plant related TK as it cannot be patented. This will thus rule out international filing of patents on Indian medicinal plants by a single international application under the Patent Cooperation Treaty (PCT).

In this context it is to be mentioned that the IP rights policy of the Kerala government released in 2008 proposes adoption of the concept of "knowledge commons" and "commons license" for protection of TK. It seeks to put all TK into the realm of "knowledge of commons" distinguishing this from the public domain.

Another amendment of importance is the deletion of subsection (g) from Section 3 – list of non-patentable inventions. Thus, earlier, before the amendment, "a method or process of testing applicable during the process of manufacture for rendering the machine, apparatus or other equipment more efficient or for the improvement or restoration of the existing machine, apparatus or other equipment or for the improvement or control of manufacture" was non-patentable.

Deletion of this section is of significance to the pharma sector in the following ways:

- It broadens the scope of patentability to include the testing methods or processes that are being developed in support of manufacture in the pharmaceutical industry.
- Newer methods of standardization of phytoconstituents and/or herbal formulations including classical and non-classical herbal drugs could be patented.
- Newer herbal drug formulations, if shown to be much more efficacious than the existing ones, could come under this category for patentability.

This amendment thus encourages newer herbal drug development and also novel analytical methods for standardization of classical and non-classical herbal drugs. Such newer methods of standardization shall enable several of our traditional Ayurvedic, Siddha and Unani drugs to be filed as even ethical drugs. With the booming global herbal drug trade, our vast BD and wealth of TK on medicinal herbs has to be rightly and assertively utilized in developing newer ethical herbal drugs.

Section 10 of the 2nd amendment Act deals with contents of specification of a patent. According to this provision, "the applicant must disclose the source and geographical origin of any biological material deposited *in lieu* of a description." Indication of geographic origin shall facilitate verification of prior art on the medicinal plant or biological material. This will serve as a check on biopiracy.

Section 25 of the 2nd amendment Act deals with opposition to the grant of a patent. This has been amended allowing for opposition to be filed on the ground that "complete specification does not disclose or wrongly mentions the source or geographical origin of biological material used for the invention."

Protection of Plant Varieties and Farmers' Right Act, 2001

This Indian legislation acknowledges that the conservation, exploration, collection, characterization and evaluation of plant genetic resources for food and agriculture are essential to meet the goals of national food and nutritional security, as also for the sustainable development of agriculture for the present and future generations.

The concept of effective benefit sharing arrangement between the provider and recipient of plant genetic resources forms an integral part of the Act. The amount of benefit sharing will be based on the extent and nature of the use of genetic material of the claimant in the development of the variety and also commercial use and sale in the market of the variety. Thus, the Act provides for mandatory disclosure of the geographic location from where the genetic material has been taken and the information relating to the contribution, if any, of the farming community involving such variety. The protection provided to a plant variety bred by a breeder can be cancelled if there is an omission or wrongful disclosure of information. Such a mandatory disclosure will prevent patenting or monopolizing of plant varieties inclusive of medicinal plants to the exclusion of rightful breeders or cultivators.

The Indian Ministry of Environment and Forests

Under its mandate to oversee BD, the ministry issued a circular in 1998 to all universities and research institutes prohibiting the transfer of genetic material outside the country without prior informed consent and proper material transfer agreement.

The Karnataka Community Intellectual Rights Bill, 1994

This is an Act to provide for the establishment of a *sui generis* system in respect of plant varieties in the state of Karnataka. As per this Act, no community-based innovation shall be sold or assigned to foreign-based institutions and individuals except jointly with the state government or its assignees. Any organization or corporation using any innovation for commercial utilization shall pay to the local community the custodian of such an innovation not less than 20 per cent of the gross sales of any product or process incorporating the innovation.

The Kerala Tribal Intellectual Property Rights Bill, 1996

This bill in the draft form seeks similar provisions to be implemented in the state of Kerala.

The Geographical Indication of Goods (Registration and Protection) Act, 1999

The Act is primarily meant to protect the valuable GIs of our country. It may be possible for holders of TK in goods produced and sold using GI to register and protect their TK under this law.

Documentation of TK

Biopiracy of Indian TK was possible because the information regarding the prior existing knowledge of the products was not available to patent examiners. Though large part of our traditional medical knowledge has been meticulously documented in several Indian languages, these are not accessible to patent offices. Also, TK available orally as folk knowledge is not accepted as proof of prior art.

Hence, India has initiated the concept of Traditional Knowledge Digital Library (TKDL) to record details of medicinal plants in an easily navigable computerized database. Such documentation involved conversion of TK information available in ancient manuscripts and that provided by communities to ensure that such information is not lost and is protected by showing that it is prior art. Thus, TKDL is an initiative aimed at providing easy access to traditional Indian systems such as Yoga, Ayurveda and Unani in the form of a digital encyclopedia. The details have been converted into patent application format and include description, method of preparation, claim and the usage of the bibliography. The original Sanskrit texts are translated and presented in French, German, English, Japanese, Spanish and Hindi. Through unit code technology that is language independent, local names of plants are converted into botanical names and Ayurvedic descriptions of diseases into modern medical terminology. The database, which took 200 researchers 8 years to compile by meticulously translating ancient Indian medical treatises, has a total number of 140,000 pages per language. Information retrieval is based on Traditional Knowledge Resource Classification (TKRC) and the IPC to enable easy access to patent examiners. By making the information on TKDL available via access and non-disclosure agreements to six major patent offices, India's global biopiracy watch system is further strengthened, thus preventing the grant of erroneous patent on Indian TK.

WIPO has adopted this digital library as a model for future work on TK databases. Work on such libraries is being conducted by WIPO with a task force of representatives from China, India, the United States Patent and Trademark Office (USPTO) and the European Patent Office (EPO) to examine how such libraries may be integrated into existing search tools used by patent offices.

The Indian Council of Medical Research (ICMR) is in the process of documenting traditional medicinal knowledge belonging to indigenous communities from the Andamans.

Several non-governmental organizations (NGOs) are also involved in documenting TK, some of which are given below.

- Community Biodiversity Register initiated by Foundation for Revitalization of Local Health Traditions and Centre for Ecological Sciences at the Indian Institute of Science, Bangalore

- Honey Bee Network operated by the Society for Research and Initiatives for Sustainable Technologies and Institutions (SRISTI) has documented "green" innovations based on indigenous BD knowledge, creativity and innovation. Further, it has set up Grassroots Innovation Augmentation Network in Gujarat in collaboration with the state government to develop innovations into products and then into enterprises. National multimedia database has also been launched by SRISTI. The Honey Bee Network is an extensive and possibly the world's largest database on grassroot innovations with names and addresses of innovators, either individuals or communities. This database has entries on the traditional uses of medicinal products and the products related to agriculture, pisciculture and sericulture.

While national initiatives are essential to conserve and protect indigenous knowledge and bioresources, an international consensus such as IP protection from TRIPS is highly essential for the rights of TK holders to be claimed and enforced in other countries. TK holders must be able to take an active role in the procedure without shouldering the burden of combating those who seek to obtain patents on their knowledge.

CONCLUSION

In recent times, IP rights have been the single important determinant of the changed trend in global trade relationships between nations. With globalization of culture, trade and communication, the patent system associated with a wealth of technological information has become an important resource for technological development, an aid in technology transfer and, thus, a significant factor in global economic growth. This is because patent information is of economic value owing to its ability to provide industry enterprises with technical information that may be used to commercial advantage. Considered by WIPO as an "engine for growth," the patent system is envisioned to establish an IP-empowered society with raised living standards at all levels of the society. As the IP rights are being considered the driver for innovation and creativity, their correct governance through appropriate national legislations and policies is considered essential for a country's economic and trade programs. Thus, globally, the IP rights are assuming increasing importance in trade, investment, economic relations and national growth. IP protection is conducive to increased investment in countries that provide for such protections. To avail global opportunities, IP system of nations has to be constantly upgraded through legislations and enforcement of IP laws.

Pre-TRIPS, the introduction of process patenting in our country has given the needed impetus for our pharmaceutical industry to be self-sufficient. TRIPS, while enshrining the rights of inventors, fails to protect TK, which is collective IP accumulated over generations. This imbalance in the system of IP rights granting monopoly rights to technology on one hand and denying it to the TK reserve of indigenous communities on the other has generated a global push to privatize BD. Because of the current scientific and commercial interest attached to TK, many developed nations and the large businesses they support increasingly want control over biological resources and the knowledge associated with them for commercial purposes. IP regime has greatly facilitated such moves. Booming global trade in herbal products, demand for exotic herbs and other natural materials, and associated rampant trade have thus made economy, a driving factor, tilting even governmental decisions (in developing nations holding TK) in favor of biotrade in the name of profitable overseas trade and research ventures.

TK about herbal drugs is realized to be an invaluable resource of newer leads for new drug development. The world over, there is a frantic quest for newer drugs from traditionally used plant drugs. Using the instrument of IP rights, large businesses are trying to appropriate TK on herbal drugs in the form of patents without the need to acknowledge and share the benefits with the communities holding such TK. While there are global concerns about securing TK to its rightful owners, its implementation is still far away, unless there is an international consensus, such as its inclusion in TRIPS for IP protection.

To protect its BD and TK, India has brought about legislative changes that are meant to be a check against biopiracy. With the right amendments to Indian Patent Act using in-built flexibilities of TRIPS agreement, the country appears well geared to be a successful pharma player in the global scenario post-TRIPS.

These amendments are also favorable to promote newer herbal drug formulations and development of standardization protocols amenable to herbal drug analysis. Indian TKDL is a digital database documenting TK in several languages, thus making it accessible to patent examiners the world over.

With these initiatives, it is hoped that India will assertively utilize its vast BD and wealth of TK on medicinal herbs to carve out a place for itself in the world herbal market.

REVIEW QUESTIONS

Essay Questions

1. Write an essay on the historical milestones that led to the developments resulting in the IP regime.
2. What is TRIPS agreement? Discuss the categories that are covered under it for IP protection.
3. Why is TK not considered an IP? Discuss the issues arising out of this omission.

Short Notes

1. Controversies surrounding TRIPS agreement
2. Changes in the Indian pharmaceutical industry post-TRIPS
3. Indian Patent Act amendments of significance to herbal drug industry
4. Biopiracy and biotrade
5. TKDL

13 Zoo Pharmacognosy— A Rediscovery?

CHAPTER OBJECTIVES

Introduction

Some Interesting Facts Revealed by
Observation and Research on Animals

Animal Self-Medication—Some
Specific Reports

Animal Self-Medication—Implications
for Humans

INTRODUCTION

The term "zoopharmacognosy" was proposed by Eloy Rodriguez and Richard Wrangam in 1987, to describe the process by which wild animals select and use specific plants with medicinal properties for the treatment and prevention of disease. This was following several anecdotal evidences from many naturalists' observation that animals in the wild resort to plant self-medication to seek relief from disease conditions. Since then several reports on the various behavioral strategies of animals in maintaining health care are being documented world over by behavioral scientists, parasitologists, chemical ecologists, ethnobotanists, herbalists, veterinarians and physicians. A study of such self-help strategies of animals is slowly starting to reveal several facets of life, hitherto unrecognized by modern science. Several of its long held assumptions are being disproved one after another thus reaffirming the tenets of herbalism, folklore and traditional knowledge of well established societies that have all along been denigrated as "claims of a pre-scientific era of witch-craft and superstition."

One of the assumptions of modern western medicine is that deliberate treatment of disease with medicines is a unique human trait. Also the fact that animals *feel* pain was itself *accepted* as late as 1985 at a Seminar Conference of the British Veterinary Association for "recognizing, assessing and alleviating pain in animals." Despite such scanty knowledge about animal physiology in health and disease, know-how of other knowledge systems on animal health and disease treatment has been denied any value.

Tradition of veterinary therapy in India developed as early as Vedic times predating history. There is extensive literature on animal treatment between 1500 and 600 BC when oral knowledge was first put to script.

For example, the Atharvanaveda (VIII, 7, 23) states that "the wild boar knows the herb which will cure it, as does the mongoose." Careful observations of animals in health and disease have given way to a rational and coherent medical system that developed several centuries before the Christian era. There is a large volume of literature in Sanskrit and other Indian languages on procedures for the treatment of horses and elephants then extensively used in war and in peace. Treatises dealing with therapy for camels, cattle, sheep and several other domestic animals stress on the prevention of disease, moderation in animal feeding, and cleanliness, which are now being realized as vital, due to "fresh new observations" of modern day naturalists.

Though observations of animals healing themselves with natural remedies have been documented from several parts of the world, scientists have dismissed assigning such human traits to animals as romantic anthropomorphism.

Such denial can no longer continue in view of the extensive newer reports on animal behavioral strategies aimed at health maintenance. This is because, despite the medical advances of the last century, health issues still loom large among our concerns. Our pathogen targeted antibiotic therapy approach to even known infectious diseases, is creating drug-resistant super microbes! In this scenario, it is now being realized that the wealth of successful strategies created by animals over millennia offers the potential for providing sustainable health care for both animals and us—humans.

SOME INTERESTING FACTS REVEALED BY OBSERVATION AND RESEARCH ON ANIMALS

Wild Animals

A wild animal is a product of natural selection, in which those that have best adapted to their environment have survived to breed. They demonstrate successful strategies for survival that have been honed by natural selection. It is a general observation that wild animals free in their undisturbed habitat not exposed to extremes of environmental changes are in good health, free from contagious diseases. They live within their ecosystem to which their physiology and behaviour are well adopted. This has been of considerable interest to modern human and animal health research programmes, which lay stress on disease rather than on ways and means of health maintenance.

A brief look at some interesting results of observations and research related to wild animals:

- They are able to carry pathogens without themselves being susceptible to disease, i.e., they are often immune to vector-borne diseases and show few clinical signs of illness from parasite infections.

- Disease out break in wild populations is often the result of human intervention such as shrinkage of their natural habitats due to urbanization, and/or pollution, with agrochemicals, industrial wastes, introduction of newer pathogens, global warming, depletion of ozone layer, and so on. Occurrence of disease in wild animal populations has become an indicator of some form of pollution in their ecology.

- Animals appear to select a nutritionally balanced diet and change the diet to suit changes either in their natural surroundings or in their specific physiological requirements. For example, herbivores, like camels, change the shrubs they eat during drought. Likewise birds eat differently in preparation for migration to alter their metabolism to enable fat deposition—energy reserves for food less periods during long flight.

- In the wild, animals seek the needed minerals such as phosphorous, calcium and sodium by making unusual changes to their diet. They seem to have an awareness of the right balance of nutrients they need to get from their diet. Nutrition apart, they clearly eat food that both prevents and cures diseases.

- Animals are surrounded by powerful pharmacological substances found in plants (primary and secondary metabolites), soil and other organisms. They are found to actively utilize them for health maintenance. Even man-eating carnivores consume plants for their powerful medicinal effects.

- Wild animals thus use plants, rocks, mineral-rich waters, sunlight, toxic insects, charcoal and so on for medicinal purposes.

- Animals in the wild, highly adapted to their ecological food reserves, are rarely poisoned in the undisturbed state. Used to a range of plants in their habitat, herbivores are better adapted for dealing with plant poisons than omnivores, which are better than carnivores in this regard. They are observed to consume emetics to induce vomiting reflex. For instance, cats eat grass to vomit.

- They seem to know the right ratio or combination of diets that are needed to counter toxicity of the compounds contained in them. They consume plant parts for nutritional or medicinal value, discarding poisonous plant parts of the same plant.

- Animals rely on natural degradation to overcome changes in plant toxicity over time. For example, rabbit like pikas of North America store plants rich in toxic phenols, while eating those in lower phenol content. Over time due to breakdown of phenol content, the stored plants become less astringent and more palatable and then they are consumed in the long winter months.

- Animals are in mutually beneficial feeding programmes with plants, microbes and other animals. For instance, certain species of ants co-habit with a fungus that breaks down toxic plant compounds, both thus benefiting in the process.

- A wide variety of animals are known to resort to soil or earth eating (Geophagy) to counter gastrointestinal troubles. They appear to select the right soils often going long distances in search of them.

- Animals have a fascinating range of strategies to handle scores of microbes in their surroundings, such as hygiene, behavioral manipulation of body temperature, feed avoidance, consuming anti microbial plant diet, preparing their own anti microbials from plant chemicals.

- Animals in the wild deal with ectoparasites such as fleas, mites, ticks and lice by strategies such as

  1. swatting
  2. grooming-self and one another
  3. using specifically selected plants/insects/animal parts (having aromatic, astringent, analgesic substances) to rub into their skin, lay in their lair or chew and apply such material for ease of release of active principles
  4. exposing to sunlight
  5. rolling in dust, salt, urine
  6. accumulating toxic secondary compounds making their flesh pungent and unpalatable

- Wild animals manage other endoparasites by avoiding parasite hot spots such as feces, consuming clay-rich earth or by specifically feeding on plants with anthelmintic, anti-amoebic, purgative and bitter plants. Even carnivores such as wolves consume constant amounts of certain medicinal plants throughout the year in addition to their regular carnivorous diet.
- Animals deal with wounds, pain and broken bones by appropriate stretching and other physical postures, rubbing of bactericidal plant parts, licking (saliva is antibacterial), self treating using medicinal plant juices, honey and even are known to resort to making their own plaster casts from twigs, leaves and sticks.
- They synchronize their reproduction with food availability and consume fertility modulating plants, labor-inducing plants and even eat plants to tackle pregnancy-related discomforts.
- Animals cope with psychological ills much like humans by isolating themselves.

Domestic Animals

A domestic animal has been artificially selected by humans for certain characteristics such as temperament or appearance. Since they have been bred for characteristics attractive or useful to humans, they are very different from wild animals. Our extensive experience with domestication of animals is bringing up many aspects which seem to better our understanding of animal health.

- Most domestic animals share with us, both the food and diseases of industrialized society. They are prone to allergies (horses allergic to grass), obesity, dementia, neurosis and even show signs of psychological illnesses. They also lose the instinct of avoiding poisons.
- Farm animals selectively bred for "productivity" are reared to add muscle even before their circulation and heart have developed. Chicken thus especially suffer circulatory problems, heart failure and weak bones and are in extreme poor health. Because they are fed with antibiotics, they colonize dreadful resistant forms of bacteria and hence such animals are a potential threat to humans who eat them. However, health of animals meant to be sold as food is of no concern to the breeder. They need to be alive till they are taken for slaughter.
- Wild animals born into captive environments such as zoos are nutritionally compromised. Though they may live longer, they are in poor health suffering from anaemia, fertility problems and eating disorders. They are susceptible to many diseases and usually die of cardiovascular disease.
- In addition to being precluded from hunting, foraging and other forms diet selection avenues, captive wild animals are restricted from social interaction and are thus denied the needed physical exertion that is critical for good health.
- Most intensely reared farm animals such as cattle, sheep and pigs are depressed and hence are prone to many pathologic conditions. Captive parrots and macaws are well known for self-abuse. These social birds used to living in flocks show signs of psychological illness in captivity due to confinement.

ANIMAL SELF-MEDICATION—SOME SPECIFIC REPORTS

The first modern observation of self-medication in non-human vertebrates was put forth by Daniel H Janzen, an ecologist at the University of Pennsylvania. Jane Goodall—a British

Primatologist, Ethologist and Anthropologist, Eloy Rodriguez—a biochemist and Professor at Cornell University, Richard Wrangham, a Harvard University Primatologist, World Wildlife Fund Scientist Holly Dublin, Michael Huffmann and Toshisada Nishida—Primatologists of Kyoto University, Mary Baker—an Anthrolopogist of University of California were some pioneering researchers in the field of zoo pharmacognosy.

Their meticulous long-time observations of animals in the wild, often in unison with several traditional healers, local forest officials and teams of phytochemists, toxicologists has resulted in a lot of scientifically validated data on animal self medication. This has generated a lot of research interest in zoopharmacognosy as it is being realized that it has profound implications for human medicine and animal care. In the words of Huffmann, "With growing chemoresistance to the Western world's current arsenal of antibiotics and anthelmintics (antiparasites), we cannot afford to let that potential source of knowledge disappear."

The most convincing and detailed evidence for the use of medicinal plants in animals so far comes from primates and carnivores. Due to constraints and difficulties of systematic research on wild animals in their natural habitat, what has been observed could just be a very small sample.

A brief look at some specific reports (Table 13.1 gives some more reported observations):

1. Super Anthelmintic Self-Therapy of Chimpanzees

At Gombe National Park and Mahale Mountains National Park in Western Tanzania, Chimpanzees were observed to follow a seemingly puzzling feeding behavior. Within an hour of leaving their sleeping nests, before their first big meal, these animals carefully and slowly selected leaves of specific plants such as *Aspilia rudis*, *A. pluriseta* or *A. mossambicensis* before swallowing them. What was puzzling was, while the chimps chewed and ate most other leaves that were part of their diet, these leaves were taken whole. The animals selected each leaf by feeling it with lips while it remained attached to the stem. The selected leaves were then folded into length wise sections and then swallowed. Phytochemical examination of the leaves revealed the presence of Thiarubrine A. A polyacetylenic intensely red compound, it is highly unstable in light and in gastric pH. Thiarubrines B, C, D, E also have been identified from several other plants known to be antibacterial, antifungal and anthelmintic. *In vitro* and *in vivo* experiments of thiarubrines established their nematocidal activity and the quantity of leaves consumed by the chimps was proposed by Rodriguez and Wrangham to carry the sufficient dose of thiarubrine needed to kill their intestinal nematodes.

Leaves of several other plants such as *Lippia placata, Ficus exasperata, Commelina* sps were among 19 different plants reported to be swallowed whole by chimpanzees. However, these leaves were not shown to contain thiarubrin and obviously the animals were consuming leaves from plant groups with varying chemical composition, many of them with no antiparasitic effect. In other words, there seemed to be no common chemical denominator for these taxonomically diverse plants that were being swallowed whole.

What followed was extensive physical and chemical examination of samples consumed by chimpanzees, their range of nematodes and their life cylces, fecal examination, and so on. A startling observation was made from inspection of fecal samples of chimps that consumed whole leaves. Several worms of *Qesophagostemum stephanostomum* were firmly stuck between intact leaf folds that were excreted out whole in the feces. These worms had to be tugged by tweezers to separate them from the leaf. It was then realized that rough texture and presence of short flexible leaf trichomes had enabled the worms to be stuck to the leaf and remain trapped within the leaf folds as they passed out of the intestine into the feces. So this "velcro" effect—as Huffmann

Table 13.1 Zoopharmacognosy—Some more reported observations

S. No.	Animal	Natural material used/ mode of use	Constituents	Protective against	Reference
1.	Mantled Howler monkeys (*Alouatta palliata*)	Cashew pedicels (*Anacardium occidentale*) - eating	Phenolics - anacardic acid and cardol	Tooth decay	Kakiuchi et al, 1986.
2.	Shell less Spanish dancer nudibranch (*Hexa branchus sanguineus*)	Sponges—it feeds on	macrolides	Fungal infections	Dale H C & Nathan D W 1993
3.	Tobacco hornworm (*Manduca sexta*)	Tobacco leaves (*Nicotiana tabacum*) - eating	Nicotine and other tobacco alkaloids	Bacteria	Dale H C & Nathan D W 1993
4.	Dusky footed wood rats (*Neotoma fuscipes*)	Bay leaves (*Umbellularia caifornica*) –nibble at leaves placed in their stick houses	High content of monoterpenes—1,8, cineole, umbellulone (released from nibbled leaves)	Developmental stages of nest-borne ectoparasites	Richard B H et al, 2002
5.	Wood ants (*Formica paralugubris*)	Conifer (*Picea abies*) resin– bring the solidified resin to their nests	α-pinene, limonene	Invading bacteria and fungi in the nest	Philippe C et al, 2003
6.	Anubis baboons (*Papio anubis*) & Hamadryas baboons (*Papio hamadryas*)	Fruits and leaves of *Balanites. aegyptica* - eating	Diosgenin (as hormone precursor)	Schistosomiasis	Janzen D H, 1978
7.	Capuchin monkeys (*Cebus capucinus*)	Stems of *Piper marginiatum*—fur rubbing	Volatile compounds, pungent alkaloid piperine	Insects, mites etc	Baker M, 1996

called it, was helping the purging of whole worms as the leaves passed undigested through the intestinal tract of chimpanzees. Later, leaf swallowing was observed in 11 different species of chimpanzees (*Pan troglodytes schweinfurthii, P. verus*, etc.), Bonobo monkeys (*Pan paniscus*) and lowland gorillas (*Gorilla gorilla graciers*).

The rough surface texture of the leaves swallowed was the common determinant that hooked worms out. Also the roughness of the leaves swallowed on an empty stomach stimulates diarrhea and speeds up gut motility, further helping to shed worms and their toxins from the body. Huffmann deduced that removal of adult worms, made the larvae emerge out of the tissue, relieving general discomfort.

This was the first meticulous observation to be reported scientifically that showed how chimps were resorting to planned self-medication to rid themselves of resource draining worms.

There have been other reports of Tamarins—squirrel-sized, new world monkeys, swallowing large seeds that effectively dislodge and sweep worms out of their intestinal tract.

2. Bitter Pith Chewing for Anti-Parasitic Effect

In 1987, in the beginning of rainy season, Hufmann and Mohamedi Seifu Kalunde—game officer, Mahale Mountain National Park observed a sick non-feeding female chimpanzee self-medicating. It selected a small shrub—*Vernonia amygdalina* (called goat killer for its extremely poisonous bitter leaf) bent down several shoots, carefully stripped off the outer layers and began sucking and chewing on the exposed inner pith. The plant is used by local people to treat stomachaches, parasitic diseases like schistosomiasis, ameobic dysentery, and so on. This was one of the bitterest plants and healthy chimpanzees seemed to avoid it and took to pith eating only in sickness. Further to this self-medication, the sick animal had an unusually long rest and appeared better the next day, as it had even regained appetite and was feeding as usual.

Phytochemical analysis of the pith revealed the presence of a series of steroidal glycosides (vernosides) and sesquiterpene lactones—vernodalin, vernolide, hydroxyl vernolide and vernodalol. *In vivo* testing of compounds found in the pith revealed powerful anthelmintic action of the steroidal glycosides and the sequiterpene lactones were found to be anti-amoebic, anti-tumor and anti-microbial. The outer bark and leaves, which were carefully discarded by the chimps, were found to contain high levels of venonioside B1, which is extremely toxic to them. Consumption of the powerful anti-microbial, anthelmintic pith had impacted the nodule worm infestation of the animals. Thus bitter-pith chewing like leaf swallowing was seen to be more common at the start of rainy season, when nodular worm infestation is on the rise. Further it was noticed chimpanzees with higher worm loads were more ill and tended to chew more bitter pith than those with lower infestation levels.

This study was the first to document sickness at the time of ingestion of a medicinal plant by a wild animal. Also the animal was followed up to apparent recovery as a result of this self-medication. This has further triggered extensive research on other plants of chimpanzee diet and sesquiterpene lactones in general for possible identification of lead molecules effective against schistosomiasis, leishmaniasis, dysentery and drug-resistant malaria.

3. Bird Nesting and "Anting" to Fight Ectoparasites

About 50 species of birds are known to include fresh plant material inside their nests and roosting environment. Increasing evidence indicates that heavy infestation of nests by ectoparasites affects survivor ship and fecundity of breeding adult birds. When ectoparasite build up is high, sea birds and swallows abandon breeding colonies. Certain birds characteristically place green plant material in their nests that is not intended to be part of the nest structure. The secondary compounds of the placed plant material act to reduce pathogens and ectoparasite populations. Several plant secondary compounds are known to function as insect repellants. Some of them act as arthropod juvenile hormone analogs, which delay developmental stages in ectoparasite transition. Birds therefore seem to preferentially select plant species to protect themselves against pathogens and parasites.

Birds such as European starlings (*Sturnus vulgaris*), Purple Martins (*Progne subis*), and American crows (*Corvus brachyrhynchos*) reportedly place fresh greenery or aromatic inner bark of western red cedar (*Thuja plicata*) in their nests. Greenery use varies geographically within a species.

The rich monoterpene and sequiterpene composition of the volatile oil-bearing plants are shown to be harmful to bacteria, mites and lice. Birds appear to choose the best plants available to fumigate their nests against both microbes and ectoparasites. This they do with their discriminatory ability that can detect specific, volatile, oil-rich plants. In addition to being used for ectoparasite control, these plants also appear to enhance the overall health and weight of the chicks.

House sparrows (*Passer domesticus*) bring neem leaves (*Azhadirachta indica*) to their nests at breeding time. The leaves contain powerful limonoids—several of which are insecticidal, in addition to being anti-bacterial and anti-fungal. Neem reportedly disrupts egg laying in several plant, animal and human pathogenic parasites. In an interesting observation by biologist Sudhim Sengupta in Calcutta, during an outbreak of malaria, sparrows change to lining their nests with quinine-rich leaves of *Caesalpinia pulcherrina* (Guletura, Krishnachura). Birds that nest in small cavities like red breasted nuthatch (*Sitta Canadensis*) apply antiseptic, insecticidal plant resinous secretions around the entrance of the cavity before reusing them.

Even rodents are known to place selected plants in burrows or sleeping nests to possibly act as a fumigant against nest-borne ectoparasites.

"Anting" is another bird behavioral self-help strategy in which they rub crushed ants through their feathers. Sometimes, they let ants crawl over their feather by lying over an anthill with spread out wings. About 200 bird species are known to resort to anting. Birds exclusively use ants that secrete formic acid and such other acrid compounds, which help fight in its ectoparasite defence. It has been demonstrated that anting reduces feather mites in birds resorting to anting. In addition to analgesic formic acid, ants secrete several auxins and β-hydroxy fatty acids that are antibacterial and antifungal. Some bird species are known to rub citrus fruit peel, aromatic leaves, flowers and inanimate objects like naphthalene balls, all of which have antimicrobial, insecticidal property. They are even known to roll in dust and fan out their wings in sunlight to effectively benefit from its UV radiation for sanitation and antibacterial, antiviral effects.

4. Animal Fur Rubbing for Skin Health

Several animals adapt a variety of strategies for skin health and to deal with skin-borne parasites. Many mammals topically apply leaves, arthropods or other aromatic materials to their skin.

Capuchin monkeys (*Cebus capucinus*) are known to rub their fur with several species of citrus fruits, leaves and stems of *Piper marginatum* and *Clemetis dioica* (Ranunculaceae). Such "fur rubbing" is a typical behavior of a variety of primates. Citrus being pungent and stimulating due to its volatile oil composition is known to have analgesic, insecticidal and antimicrobial properties.

Carnivorous white-nosed Coatis (*Nasua narica*) is reported to rub into its fur resin of the tree *Trattinickia aspera*. The resin contained in the resin ducts of the tree oozes out on scratching and it has a pleasant camphoraceous odor. The animals are observed to travel long distances to reach the trees. They scratch the tree wounds to allow the resin to flow out and they were seen to enjoy rubbing it with their paws over their entire bodies. Phytochemical analysis revealed the presence of triterpenes, amyrin, selinene and sesquiterpene lactones in the resin. The animals are possibly using the resin for its soothing stimulant effect or are seeking to get relief due to the insecticidal and parasitic effect of the resin.

Kodiak bears (*Ursus arctos*) reputedly dig up roots of *Ligusticum wallichii* and *L. porteri* called Osha roots by native Americans. The bears chew the root and rub the root saliva mixture into their fur. This is called "bear-medicine" following the human use of the root by the natives as a topical anaesthetic and anti-bacterial for external wounds and bruises. Osha root is reported to contain lactone glycosides, alkaloids, phytosterols, saponins, ferulic acid, volatile terpenes and fixed oil. It is said to have an analgesic and antiviral effect and hence chewing may deliver additional medicinal effect to the bears.

Neotropical Capuchin monkeys of *Cebus* genus are reported to rub and roll over their skin, millipedes that secrete toxic benzoquinones. This is to benefit from the insect-repellant properties of benzoquinones, which will be especially protective against insect attack during rainy season.

Several species of monkeys, lemurs and birds are known to anoint themselves with millipedes.

5. Earth Eating for Stomach Troubles

Consumption of soil, powdered rock, termite-mound-earth, clay and mud is a common feeding behaviour in many animals. Also called "Geophagy", several herbivorous, omnivorous mammals, birds, reptiles and insects are known to indulge in it. It appears to be more common in herbivores, especially in the tropics. Animals and birds seem to take to soil eating when their dietary toxin load is high. In some instances, it is believed that soil eating is for getting the sodium missing in plant diet. The mechanical and pharmaceutical properties of natural kaolinite-based clays are possibly countering the effects of parasites. Clay is known to be a powerful adsorbent and soils rich in clay are specifically consumed possibly to adsorb bacterial or plant secondary compound toxins. Clay is known to absorb intestinal fluids in diarrhoea. Animals are seeking to get relief from gastrointestinal distress caused by infectious parasites.

Chimpanzees, monkeys, tigers, elephants, parrots, deer are a few animals observed to mine for clay-rich, volcanic and other soils for apparently different reasons.

6. Mutually Beneficial Animal-Plant Interaction

South American maned wolf (*Chrysocyon brachyurus*) is omnivorous and feeds on lobeira fruit (*Solanum lycocarpum*), which constitutes 30–50% of its diet. Native to Brazil, the plant is found throughout the wolf"s habitat. The wolves are susceptible to cystinutira, a condition where there is inability of the kidneys to absorb amino acid cystine. As a result, the amino acid tends to crystallize in the bladder and kidneys causing blockage, renal failure and death. Also the animals are prone to giant kidney worm (*Dioctophyma renale*) infection, which can aggravate the already vulnerable renal system. These worms can infect the kidneys and inhibit renal function.

The worm infection compromises the immune response of the wolf to other pathogens and parasites. The animal appears to benefit from the consumption of lobeira by fighting off kidney infection. Rich in phenols, sapinins and tannins, the exact mechanism of protection conferred by loberia is as yet undetermined.

The plant is also benefited as the seeds that have passed through the wolf's digestive tract are spread over larger distances and have higher germination rates than untouched seeds. This is an example of a symbiotic relationship hinting at complex interactions among organisms in general.

ANIMAL SELF-MEDICATION—IMPLICATIONS FOR HUMANS

Recent reports on animal self medication strategies have created a lot of interest and scientists assert that understanding the process has significant implications for humans. While initially it was viewed as a potential source for newer drugs, today it is a rapidly expanding subject relating to animal, environmental and human health care needs. Hence, it is of interest to pharmacologists, veterinarians, ethnobotanists, pharmacists, environmentalists and conservationists. Zoopharmacognosy has opened the option of giving animals in our care the opportunity to select their diet from an offered range of plant remedies. It has especially opened up to the world the apparent ability of the animals to show a cognitive grasp of potential medicines in their environment.

Anecdotal observations of animal ways of health maintenance are revealing the significance of several facts of animal and plant life, some of which were long known in traditional knowledge.

- The underlying principles of animal health maintenance suggest a holistic approach of avoidance, prevention and treatment of diseases. Modern medicine's expectation of conquering disease with pathogen-targeted antibiotics and receptor-binding pure chemicals is a reductionistic approach to health care.
- The active self-help strategies that seem to support the health of animals in wild are not idealizations of nature. They have emerged as the most successful through the test of natural selection.
- An important lesson to be learnt from wild health is that disease avoidance is the result of constant vigilance rather than the resorting to magic bullets after succumbing to it.
- Eating the right foods and natural medicines is based on the animals' body needs and its sensitivity to subtle changes in appetite. The shift of focus for health maintenance, seems to be-eating in accordance with the body's cravings rather than tongue cravings. An intentional role in taking preventive steps before disease sets in seems to be the crux of the matter.
- Scientific experimentation on animal ageing is revealing that life span can be extended by restricting calories intake and that dietary modification is the key to successful ageing.
- All this "newer" information appears to reaffirm the wholistic approach of traditional medical knowledge. Frugality in diet, physical agility and right attitude towards life were considered essential for healthy living in Indian traditional medicine.
- Plant secondary metabolite production is considered to be an evolutionary adaptation of plant defense mechanism. They vary in their proportion in plants according to herbivory and other environmental changes. Tropical plants have a more complex array of secondary

metabolites than temperate climate plants. Nature possibly intended to provide better chemical weapons against greater predation in the tropics.

- Traditional medicine dictum of collection of medicinal plant parts and secretions during specific lunar cycles (optimum chemical composition—right medicinal effect) can no longer be said to be a superstitious practice

- Animal pattern of consumption of plants—edible, moderately toxic and toxic appears to be based on the following generalizations:
  a. Toxic plants are consumed in moderation, when excess is lethal
  b. Some selected plants are consumed at certain times of the year
  c. Some specific plants are safe when first eaten, but not for prolonged feeding
  d. Some plants are safe after processing or preparation
  e. Some plants are safe when taken in combination with others

- From reported evidence, primates and carnivores are using plants for the value of their secondary compounds. Scientists suggest that other mammalian species may be using similar strategies. This phenomenon of innate knowledge of health sustenance could be universal to all life forms.

- It is being realized that all of life is linked at a very basic level with each life form perceiving it in different ways. In many traditional societies, animal behavior was used to forecast changes in the weather or warn of impending natural disasters, thus benefiting from their different sensory perception. Today it is a fact that fish like salmon are very sensitive to minute changes in water chemistry. They do not swim up in rivers polluted with copper or zinc mining.

- Each living organism appears to be bestowed with the needed cognition to sustain its life by dynamically interacting with its environment.

- In the context of zoo phamacognosy, if animals are able to identify the needed medicinal material from their environment, much evolved Homo sapiens—man, is a much greater potential in terms of innate awareness of life and its intricacies.

- Much the same way as domestic animals lose their ability to detect toxins, civilization and industrialization could have taken a toll on the depth of innate human knowing.

- To the risk of "evidence-based knowledge" calling it as unjustified generalization, it may be surmised that realization of this innate life knowledge (which includes life-sustaining health strategies)—the science of life, was being symbolically referred to as "revealed by Gods" in ancient Indian tradition.

- Science with its methods seems to be coming back a full circle to accepting this primeval fount of knowing within.

CONCLUSION

Zoopharmacognosy has become a topic of interest with significant implications for human medicine and animal care. Reports of several anecdotal observations and research experiments related to animal health in the wild, in captivity and on domestication are being increasingly reported in the literature. These are revealing natural ways of handling health and disease, so far unrecognized by modern science. Knowledge of medicinal properties of herbs arrived at by centuries of observation and practice is traceable to times before recorded history in this subcontinent. Hence, observations of animals in disease in the wild, definitely predates this. Tenets of disease prevention, enabling of innate healing, and dietary role in health maintenance, which were the basic precepts of traditional medicine are now being recognized as rationalistic approaches. Zoopharmacognosy is further reaffirming these wholistic methods and it looks like we have much to re-learn along these lines.

REVIEW QUESTIONS

Essay Questions

1. Summarize the salient findings of observations and research on animals in the wild.
2. What is Zoopharmacognosy? Discuss the observations made on Chimpanzees.
3. Write an essay on the implications of animal self-medication in humans.

Short Notes

1. Bird self-medication strategies
2. Geophagy
3. Fur rubbing

Bibliography

Chapter 1

1. Handa SS, *Indian Herbal Pharmacoepia*, SS Chand, New Delhi, 1998, p. 4.
2. Man-Son-Hing M and Wells G, Meta analysis of efficacy and quinine for treatment of nocturnal leg cramps in elderly people. *BMJ*, 310, 1995, 13–17.
3. Jansen PHP, Veenhuizen KCW, Wesseling AIM et al. Randomised controlled trial of hydroquinine in muscle cramps. *Lancet*, 349, 1997, 528–532.
4. Mechoulam R, Breuer A, Feigenbaum JJ et al. Nonpsychotropic synthetic cannabinoids as therapeutic agents. *Farmaco* 46(Suppl) 1991, 267–276.
5. Jenne JW, Two new roles for theophylline in the asthmatic? *J Asthma*, 32, 1995, 89–95.
6. Minton N, Swift R, C Lawlor et al. Ipecacuanha-induced emesis: a human model for testing antiemetic drug activity, *Clin Pharmacol Ther*, 54, 1993, 53–57.
7. Phillipson JD, Natural products as drugs, *Trans R Soc Trop Med Hyg*, 88(Suppl 1), 1994, 17–19.
8. Newman DJ, Cragg GM, and Snader KM, Natural products as sources of new drugs over the period 1981–2002, *J Nat Prod*, 66, 2003, 1022–1037.
9. Jones WP, Chin YW, and Kinghorn AD. The role of pharmacognosy in modern medicine and pharmacy, *Curr Drug Targets*, 7, 2006, 247–264.
10. Pitman NCA, and Jergensen PM, Estimating the size of the world's threatened flora, *Science*, 298, 2002, 989.
11. Cordell GA, and Colvard MA, Some thoughts on future of ethnopharmacology, *J Ethnopharmacol*, 100, 2005, 5–14.
12. Evans WC, *Trease and Evans' Pharmacognosy*, 14th edn, WB Saunders, London, 1996.
13. 'Whatis Herb Standardization.' Available at: http://content.herbalgram.org/abc/HEG/files/MBHerbsfor Health.pdf (PDF).
14. Virender Sodhi. Ayurveda: The science of life and other of the healing arts, In: Pizzorno JE and Murray MT (eds), *Textbook of Natural Medicine*, 3rd edn, Churchill Livingstone Elsevier, St. Louis, 2006, p 317–325.
15. Ten Kate K and Laird SA, *The Commercial Use of Biodiversity*, Earth Scan Publications, UK, 1999.
16. Farnsworth NR, Screening plants for new medicines, Wilson EO and Peters FM (eds), *Biodiversity*, National Academy Press, Washington, DC, 1988, 83–97.

17. Farnsworth NR, Akerele O, Bingel AS et al. Medicinal plants in therapy, *Bull World Health Organ*, 63, 1985, 965–981.

18. John Maddox, When to believe the unbelievable, *Nature*, 333, 1988, 6176.

19. Beniveste J, Dr. Jacques Beniveste replies, *Nature*, 334, 1988, 6180.

20. 'Why Standardized Herbal Extracts?' (http://www.planetherbs.com/phytotherapy/why-standardized-herbal-extracts.html)

21. Berenbaum M, What is synergy? *Pharmacol Rev*, 41, 1989, 93–141.

22. Wagner H, New targets in phytopharmacology of plants, In: Ernst E (ed), *Herbal medicine, a concise overview for healthcare professionals*, Butterworth-Heinemann, UK, 1999.

23. Balick MJ and Cox PA, Plants, people and culture: the science of ethnobotany, Freeman, London, 1997.

24. American Society of Pharmacognosy, http://www.phcog.org/definitin.html

25. Unnikrishnan, PM, The Materia Medica of Ayurveda, In: Darshan Shankar and Unnikrishnan PM (eds), *Challenging the Indian Medical Heritage*, Ahmedabad, Centre for Environment Education & Foundation Books, New Delhi, 2004, p 40–62.

26. Pharmaceutics and Alchemy. Available at: http//:www.nlm.nlh.gov/exhibition/Islamic_medical/Islamic_11.html

27. Traditional and modern medicine – harmonizing the two approaches. WHO Publications, Geneva.

28. Cox PA, Saving the ethno pharmacological heritage of Samoa, *J Ethnopharmacol*, 38, 1993, 181–188.

29. Feyerbend P, *Science in a Free Society*, NLB, London, 1978.

30. Cox PA, Shaman as scientist: indigenous knowledge systems in pharmacological research and conservation, In: Hostettmann H, Marston A, Maillard M, and Hamburger M (eds), *Phytochemistry of Plants Used in Traditional Medicine*. Clarendron Press, Oxford, 1995, p 1–8.

Chapter 2

1. Virender Sedhi, Ayurveda: the science of life and mother of healing arts. In: Pizzorno JE and Murray MT (eds), *Text Book of Natural Medicine*, 3rd edn, Vol I, Churchill Livingstone, Elsevier, St. Louis, 2006, p 317–325.

2. Atreya, Practical Ayurveda: Secrets for Physical, Sexual and Spiritual health, Mumbai, Jaico Books, 2008.

3. Budwar Peth YJB. *Sharangadhai Samhita, Part 1*. Dixit, Pune, India, 1908.

4. Rig Veda, Sec 10 Ch-97, Verses 1-23.

5. Donn Brennan. *Live Better: Ayurveda*, Duncan Baird Publishers, London, 2006. p. 32.

6. Virender Sodhi. Ayurveda: the science of life and other of the healing arts, In: Pizzorno JE and Murray MT (eds), *Textbook of Natural Medicine*, 3rd edn, Churchill Livingstone Elsevier, St. Louis, 2006. p 317–325.

7. Shanti Gowans. *Ayurveda for Health and Well Being*, Jaico Publishing House, Mumbai, 2010, p 17.

8. Unnikrishnan PM. The Materia Medica of Ayurveda, In: Darshan Shankar and Unnikrishnan PM (eds), *Challenging the Indian Medical Heritage*, Ahmedabad, Centre for Environment Education & Foundation Books, New Delhi, 2004, p 40–62.

9. Todd Caldecott, *Ayurveda The Divine Science of Life*, Mosby Elsevier, Philadelphia, 2006.

10. Ashok Majumdar, *Ayurveda – The Ancient Science of Healing*, Mac Millan India Ltd, New Delhi, 1998.

11. Tirtha S. Overview of Ayurveda, In: *The Ayurveda Encyclopedia: Natural Secrets to Healing, Prevention and Longevity*, Ayurveda Holistic Center Press, New York, p 3.

12. Lock Stephen, et al. The Oxford Illustrated Companion to Medicine. Oxford University Press, USA, 2001, p 651–652.

13. Sharma PV. Development of Ayurveda from antiquity to AD 300. In: Chatopadhyaya DP and Kumar R (eds), *Science, Philosophy and Culture*, PHISPC, New Delhi, 1992.

14. Verma RL, Indian –Arab relations in medical sciences. In: Sharma PV (ed), *History of Medicine in India*. Indian National Science Academy, New Delhi, 1992, pp 465–484.

15. Siddiqi MZ, *Studies in Persian and Arabic Medical Literature*, Calcutta, 1959, pp 31–43.

Chapter 3

1. Agarwal SG, Thappa RK, and Dhar KL (1997) Trends in trade of essential oils. In: Handa SS and Kaul MK (eds), *Supplement to Cultivation and Utilization of Aromatic Plants*, RRI, CSIR, Jammu-Tawi, pp 17–46.

2. Arai S, Studies on functional foods in Japan – state of the art. *Biosci Biotechnol Biochem*, 60, 1996, 9–15.

3. Blankson H, Stakkestad JA, Fagertun H, Thom E, Wadstein J, and Gudmundsen O, Conjugated linoleic acid reduces body fat mass in overweight and obese humans, *J Nutr*, 130, 2000, 2943–2948.

4. Calixto JB, Efficacy, safety, quality control, marketing and regulatory guidelines for herbal medicines (Phytotherapeutic agents), *Braz J Med Biol Res*, 33(2), 2000, 179–189.

5. Christie A, Herbs for health, but how safe are they. *Bull World Health Org*, 79(7), 2001, 691–692.

6. De Silva T, UNIDO development programmes on industrial utilization of medicinal and aromatic plants. *Acta Hortic*, 333, 1993 47–54.

7. De Silva T and Atal CK, *Pressing, Refinement and Value Addition of Non-wood Forest Products*. FAO Report of the International Expert Consultation on Non-wood Forest Products, 1995, pp 167–193.

8. Doris MT, Christopher DG and William LH, Potential health benefits of dietary phytoestrogens: a review of clinical, epidemiological and mechanistic evidence, *J Endocrinol Metab*, 83(7), 1998, 2223 (phytoestrogens).

9. Edwards AM, Blackburn L, Townsend S and David J, Food Supplements in the treatment of primary fibromyalgia: a double-blind cross over trial of anthocyanidins and placebo. *J Nutr Environ Med*, 10, 2000, 189–199 (anthocyanins).

10. Fahey, JW, *Moringa oleifera*: a review of the medicinal evidence for its nutritional, therapeutic and prophylactic properties. Part I. Trees for Life J. Available at: www.TFLJournal.org (glucosinolates), 2005.

11. Farnsworth NR, and Soejarto DD, Potential consequence of plant extinction in the United States on the current and future availability of prescription drugs. *Econ Bot*, 39(3), 1985, 231–240.

12. Germany leads in branded phytomedicines. 1996, *OTC Bull* Jun 14: 15.

13. Gertjan S, The protein digestibility – corrected amino acid score, *J Nutr*, 130, 2000, 18658–18678.

14. Giovannucci E, Tomatoes, tomato-based products, lycopene and cancer: a review of the epidemiological literature, *J Natl Cancer Inst*. 91, 1999, 317–331 (lycopene).

15. Giovannucci E, Ascherio A, Rimm EB, Stampfer MJ, Codlitz GA, and Willett WC, Intake of carotenoids and retinol in relation to risk of prostate cancer, *J Natl Cancer Inst* 87, 1995, 1767–1776 (carotenoid).

16. Hasler CM, Functional foods: their role in disease prevention and health promotion. *Food Technol*, 52, 1998, 63–70.

17. Howell AB, Vorsa N, Marderosian AD, and Foo, LY, Inhibition of adherence of P-fimbriated *Escherichia coli* to uro epithelial-cell surfaces by proanthocyanidin extracts from cranberries. *N Engl J Med* 339, 1998, 1085–1086 (proanthocyanidins).

18. Huang MT, and Ferraro T Phenolic compounds in food and cancer prevention. In: Huang MT, Ho CT, and Lee CY (eds), *Phenolic compounds in food and their effects on Health II: antioxidants and cancer prevention*, American Chemical Society, ACS Symposium Series 507, Washington DC, 1992, pp 8–34 (flavanols).

19. International life sciences institute, Safety assessment and potential health benefits of food components based on selected scientific crit eria. ILSI North America technical Committee on food components for health promotion. *Crit Rev Food Sci Nutr*, 39, 1999, 203–316.

20. Jacobs DR, Meyer KA, Kushi LH, and Folsom AR, Whole grain intake mat reduce the risk of ischaemic heart disease death in post menopausal women: the IOWA Women's Health Study. *Am J Clin Nutr*, 68, 1998, 248–257.

21. Katan MB, Grundy SM, Jones P, Law M, Miettinen T, and Paoletti R, Stressa workshop participants. Efficacy and safety of plant stanols & sterols in the management of blood cholesterol levels, *Mayo Clin Proc*, 78(8), 2003, 965–978 (stanols and sterols).

22. Keevil JG, Osman HE, Reed JD, and Folts JD, Grape juice, but not orange juice or grape fruit juice, inhibits human platelet aggregation. *J Nutr*, 130, 2000, 53–56 (plant polyphenolics).

23. Khaw K and Barrett Connor E, Dietary fiber and reduced ischaemic heart disease mortality rates in men and women: a 12 year prospective study, *Am J Epidemiol*, 126, 1987, 1093–1102.

24. The Lancet, Pharmaceuticals from plants: great potential, few funds (Editorial). *Lancet*, 343, 1994, 1513–1515.

25. Lange D, *Untersuchengen zum Heilpflanzenhandel* in Deutschland. Bonn, Germa naturschutzny; Bunesamp fur, 1996.

26. Lewington, A. Medicinal plant and plant extracts: a review of their importation into Europe, Traffic International, Cambridge, UK, 1993.

27. Lovejoy JC, The influence of dietary fat in insulin resistance, *Curr Diab Rep*, 2(5), 2002, 435–440 (PUFA).

28. Lucy Horeau, and Edgar J Dasilva, Medicinal plants: a re-emerging health aid. *EJP Electron J Biotechnol*, 2(2), 1999, DOI: 10.2225.

29. Mares-Perlman, JA, Millen AE, Ficek TL, and Hankinson SE, The body of evidence to support a protective role for lutein and zeaxanthin in delaying chronic disease. Overview. *J Nutr*, 132, 2002, 518S–524S (lutein and zx).

30. Morand C, Dubray C, Milen Kovic D, Lioger D, Martin JF, Scalbert A, and Mazur A, Hesperidin contributes to vascular protective effects of orange juice: a randomized crossover study in healthy volunteers, *Am J Clin Nutr*, 93, 2011, 73–80.

31. Murkies F, Wilcox G, and Davis SR, Phytoestrogens, *J Clin Endocrinol Metabol*, 83, 1998, 297 (lignans).

32. Nakamura Y and Miyoshi N, Cell death induction by isothiocyanates and their underlying molecular mechanisms. *Biofactors*, 26(2), 2006, 123–134 (isothiocyanates).

33. Natural Medicine Marketing, Market Report – Traditional Chinese Medicine – the Chinese Market and International opportunities. Natural Medicine Marketing, London, UK, 1996.

34. Nutrition Business Journal, Functional Foods Report 2002. *Nutr Bus J*, San Diego, CA, 2002.

35. Park Y, Subar AF, Hollenbeck A, and Schatzkin A, Dietary fibre intake and mortality in NIH-AARP Diet and Health Study. *Arch Intern Med*, 171(12), 2011, 1061–1068.

36. Prajapati ND, Purohit SS, Sharma AK, and Kumar A, *Handbook of Medicinal Plants*, Agrobios, India, 2003.

37. Pratt DE, Natural antioxidants from plant material. In: Huang MT, Ho CT, and Lee CY (eds), *Phenolic Compounds in Food and Their Effects on Health II: Antioxidants and Cancer Prevention*, American Chemical Society, ACS Symposium Series 507, Washington DC, pp 54–71 (flavonols).

38. Qian MC, Fan X, and Mahattanatawee K, *Volatile sulfur compounds in food. ACS Symposium Series 1068*, American Chemical Society, 2011, doi: 10.1021/bk-2011-1068. ISBN: 978-0-08412-2616-6 (sulphides & thiols).

39. Satoshi F, Hamaguchi K, Seike M, Himeno K, Sakata T, and Yoshimatsu H, Role of fatty acid composition in the development of metabolic disorders in sucrose induced obese rats. *Exp Biol Med*, 229(6), 2004, 486–493 (MUFA).

40. Sloan AE, Top ten trends to watch and work on: the more things change the ore they stay the same. *Food Technol*, 48, 1994, 89–100.

41. Sloan AE, The top ten functional food trends: the next generation. *Food Technol*, 56, 2002, 32–58.

42. Tuley De Silva (Ed), A Manual On Essential Oil Industry, *Presentation at the 3rd UNIDO Workshop on Essential Oil and Aroma Chemical Industries, at Turkey*, UNIDO, Veinna.

43. Vinay T, *Camp Workshop: Plants under threat – New list forged Medicinal Plant Conservation, Vol 2. Newsletter of the IUCN Species Survival Commission*. Bonn, Germany; Bundesamt fur Naturschutz, 1996.

44. WHO, WHO Guidelines on Good Agricultural and Collection Practices (GACP) for Medicinal Plants, 2003, p 1, Geneva.

Chapter 4

1. (5 Jan 1990). Information Letter No.771, Health Protection Branch, Health and Family Welfare, Canada.

2. (13 August 1987). Information Letter No. 726, Health Protection Branch, Health and Family Welfare, Canada.

3. (1965). "Council Directive 65/65/EEC of 26 January 1965 on the approximation of provisions laid down by law, regulation or administrative action relating to proprietary medicinal products." Official Journal of the Eurpean Communities 22.

4. (1968). Medicines Act 1968, London HMSO.

5. (1975). "Council Directive 75/318/EEC of 20 May 1975 on the approximation of laws of Member states relating to analytical, pharmacotoxicological and clinical standards and protocols in respect of the testing of proprietary medicinal products." Official Journal of the European Communities 147.

6. (1975). "Council Directive 75/319/EEC of 20 May 1975 on approximation of provisions laid down by law, regulation or administrative action relating to proprietary medicinal products." Official Journal of the European Communities L 147.

7. (1977). The Medicines (Retail Sale or Supply of Herbal Remedies) Order, Statutory Instrument: SI 1977, London: HMSO. 2130.

8. (1991). "Commission Directive 91/507/EEC of 19 July 1991 modifying the Annex to Council Directive 75/318/EEC on the approximation of laws of Member states relating to analytical, pharmacotoxicological and clinical standards and protocols in respect of the testing of proprietary medicinal products " Official Journal of the European Communities 270/32.

9. (1998). Regulations for registration of herbal preparations, health and supplementary food, cosmetics and antiseptics that have medicinal claims, General Directorate of Medical and Pharmaceutical Licenses, Ministry of Health, Kingdom of Saudi Arabia.

10. (December 1995). A Guide to what is a medicinal product. Medicines Act Leaflet MAL 8. London, Medicines Control Agency.

11. (October1985). Review of Herbal Products under Medicines Act 1968 and EEC Directives, Medicines Information Sheet, DHSS Medicines Division.

12. Anderson, L. A. (1986). Pharm J 236: 303.

13. Atherton, D. J. (1994). "Towards the safer use of traditional remedies." British Medical Journal 308: 673-674.

14. Bieldermann, B. (1990). Phytopharmaceuticals - The Growing European Market? ESCOP Symposium "European harmony in phytotherapy. Brussels.

15. Braun, R. (1987). Aufbereitung wissenschaftlichen Erkenntnismaterials durch Kommissionen. Zulassung und Nachzulassung von Arzneimittein. B. Schneiders and R. Mecklenburg. Basel, Aesopus: 95-98.

16. Chakravarty, B. K. (1993). "Herbal medicines. Safety and Efficacy Guidelines." The Regulatory Affairs Journal 4: 699-701.

17. Jayasuriya, D. C. (1990). The regulation of medicinal plants - a preliminary review of selected aspects of national legislation.

18. Keller, K. (1992). "Results of the revision of herbal drugs in the Federal Republic of Germany with a special task force on risk aspects." Zeitschrift fur phytotherapie 13: 116–120.

19. Kishi, T. (1989). Standardization of Oriental (Kampo) medicine formulations. Regulations and Practices in Japan. New Drug Developments from Natural Products. I. R. Lee, H. S. Yun-Choi and I. Chang. Seoul, Korean Society of Pharmacognosy.

20. Marwick, C. (1995). "Growing use of Medicinal Botanicals Forces assessment by Drug Regulators." JAMA 273: 607-609.

21. McAlpine, D. (1992). Pharmaceutical marketing 4(4): 24.

22. Mukherjee, P. K., M. Venkatesh, et al. (2007). "ticAn Overview on the development in regulation and control of medicinal and aromatic plants in the Indian system of medicine." Bol Latinoan Caribe Plant Med Aromaticas 6(4): 129-136.

23. Phillipson, J. D. (1981). "Herbal medicines." Pharm J 227: 387.

24. Schwabe, U. and D. Paffrath, Eds. (1995). Arzneiverordnungs - Report 1995 Stuttgart, Gustav Fischer Verlag.

25. Silva, T. D. (2009). Regulation of Herbal Health Care Products. Traditional and Alternative medicine: Research and Policy Perspectives. T. B. Tuley De Silva, Manoranjan Sahu, Le Mai Huong. Delhi, Daya Publishing House: 35.

26. Tsutani, K., Ed. (1993). The evaluation of herbal medicines: an east Asian perspective. Clinical Research methodology for complementary therapies. London-Sydney-Auckland, Hodder and Stockton.

27. Wang, X. (1991). "Traditional Herbal medicines around the Globe: Modern perspectives. China: Philosophical Basis and Combining Old and New. Proceedings of the 10th General Assembly of WFPPM, Seoul, Korea, 16-18 October 1991." Swiss Pharma 13(11a): 68-72.

28. WHO (1991). Guidelines for the assessment of Herbal medicines. Geneva, World Health Organization.

29. WHO (1994). Guidelines for formulation of national policy on herbal medicines. Alexandria, World Health Organization.

30. WHO (1998). Regulatory situation of Herbal medicines: A Worldwide Review. Geneva, WHO.

31. WHO (2005). National Policy on Traditional medicine and regulation of herbal medicines - Report of a WHO Global survey. Geneva, WHO.

32. Yamada, Y. (1991). "Traditional herbal medicines around the Globe: Modern Perspectives. Japanese Traditional Medicines. Proceedings of the 10th General APPM, Seoul, Korea, 16-18 October 1991." Swiss Pharma 13(11a): 76-78.

Chapter 5

1. Seidl P R (2002) Pharmaceuticals from natural products: Current Trends. An Acad Bras Cienc, 74: 145-150

2. http://planningcommission.nic.in/aboutus/taskforce/tsk_medi.pdf

3. http://www.indianmedicine.nic.in/writereaddata/linkimages/7870046089-Ayush%20%20n%20 policy%20ISM%20and%20H%20Homeopathy.pdf

4. http://www.indianmedicine.nic.in/showfile.asp?lid=67

5. http://nmpb.nic.in/index1.php?level=0&linkid=74&lid=413

6. http://www.csir.res.in/External/Utilities/Frames/achievements/main_page.asp?a=topframe. htm&b=leftcon.htm&c=../../../Heads/achievements/CSIRMilestones.htm

7. http://www.cimap.res.in/cimapdev/index.php?option=com_content&view=article&id=123&It emid=157

8. http://www.iiim.res.in/acheive.html

9. http://www.dst.gov.in/scientific-programme/td-drugs.htm

10. http://dbtindia.nic.in/uniquepage.asp?ID_PK=20

11. http://www.icmr.nic.in/About_Us/About_ICMR.html

12. http://drdo.gov.in/drdo/English/index.jsp?pg=tech_lifesciences.jsp

13. Alok S, Shanker C, Lalit kumar T, Mhendra S, Rao Ch V (2008) Herbal Medicine for Market Potential in India: An Overview, Acad J Plant Sci, 1(2): 26-36.

14. Inamdar N, Edalat S, Kotwal V B, Pawar S (2008) Herbal drugs in Milieu of modern drugs, Int J Green Pharm, 2 (1): 2-8.

15. Dubey N K, Rajesh K, Tripathy P (2004) Global promotion of herbal medicine, India's opportunity, Curr Sci, 86: 37-41

16. Khan S N ( ) 4. DST-Promoting R&D in Ayurvedic Medicines: Government of India Initiatives, Health Administrator, 20 (1&2), 14-20

17. http://www.tkdl.res.in/tkdl/langdefault/common/Home.asp?GL=Eng

18. http://www.wbhealth.gov.in/wbsmpb/index.html?pass_file_id=

19. http://herbaluttarakhand.org/introduction.html

20. http://tripurabiodiversityboard.in/tbd/MPlants.aspx

21. http://www.smpborissa.org.in/

22. http://megforest.gov.in/activity_medic_plants.htm

23. http://www.smpbkerala.org/

24. http://karnatakaforest.gov.in/English/forest_glance/medical_plants.htm

25. http://haryanaforest.gov.in/Medicinal/StateMedicinalPlantsBoard.aspx

26. http://jkdism.in/docs/smpb_data.pdf

27. http://jkdism.in/docs/smpb_data.pdf

28. http://cgvanoushadhi.gov.in/

29. http://smpbassam.org/

30. http://www.apsmpb.org/

Chapter 6

1. WHO, *Quality Control Methods for Medicinal Plant Materials*, World Health Organization, Geneva, 1998b.

2. WHO, *Quality Control Methods for Medicinal Plant Materials*, World Health Organization, Geneva, 1992.

3. WHO, General Guidelines for Methodologies on Research and Evaluation of Traditional Medicine, World Health Organization, Geneva, 2002c.

4. WHO, The International Pharmacopoeia, General Methods of Analysis, 3rd edn. World Health Organization, Geneva, 1979, 1.

5. WHO, *The International Pharmacopoeia, Quality Specifications*, 3rd edn. World Health Organization, Geneva, 1981, 2

6. Wani MS, Herbal medicine and its standardization. Pharma info, 1, 2007, 6.

7. Houghton P, Establishing Identification criteria for botanicals, *Drug Information J*, 32, 1998, 461–469.

8. Gaedcke F, Steinhoff B, Quality Assurance of herbal medicinal products, In: Herbal Medicinal Products, Stuttgart: Medpharm GmbH Scientific Publishers, 37–66, 2003, 81–88.

9. Eskinazi D, Blumenthal M, Farnsworth N, and Riggins CW, *Botanical medicine: Efficacy, Quality Assurance and Regulation*, Mary Ann Liebert, New York, 1999.

10. EMEA, *Quality of Herbal Medicinal Products*, Guidelines European Agency for the Evaluation of Medicinal Products (EMEA), London, 1998.

11. De Smet PAGM, Overview of herbal quality control. *Drug Inform J*, 33, 1999, 717–724.

12. Bisset NG, *Herbal Drugs and Phytopharmaceuticals*. CRC Press, Boca Raton, FL, 1994.

13. Bauer NG, Quality criteria and standardization of phytopharmaceuticals: can acceptable drug standards be achieved? *Drug Inform J*, 32, 1994, 101–110.

14. Oluyemisi FK, Henry OE, and Peter OA, Standardization of herbal medicines – a review, *Int J Biodivers Conserv*, 4(3), 2012, 101–112.

15. Duke JA and Martinez, RV, *Handbook of Ethnobotanicals (Peru)*, CRC Press, Boca Raton, FL, 1994.

16. WHO, *Guidelines for the appropriate use of herbal medicines*, WHO Regional Publications, Western Pacific Series No. 3 WHO Regional Office for the Western Pacific, Manila, 1998.

17. Bradley P, *British Herbal Compendium*, Vol 2, British Herbal Pharmacopoeia, Dorset, UK, 2006.

18. The Ayurvedic Pharmacopoeia of India, Part 1, Vol I–V (1990–2006) Government of India, New Delhi.

19. The European Scientific Cooperative on Phytotherapy (ESCOP), ESCOP Monographs on Medicinal Uses of Plant Drugs, ESCOP Secretariat, UK, 1999.

20. Indian Pharmacopoeia, Ministry of Health and Family Welfare, Government of India, New Delhi, 1996.

21. Gupta AK, Tandon N, and Sharma M (eds), *Quality Standards of Indian Medicinal Plants*, Vol I–IV. Indian Council of Medical Research, New Delhi, 2003–2006.

22. Indian Herbal Pharmacopoeia, Regional Research Laboratory, Jammu-Tawi and IDMA, Mumbai, 2002.

23. Wallis TE, *Textbook of Pharmacognosy*, 5th edn, CBS, New Delhi, 98, 1985.

24. Evans WC, *Trease and Evans' Pharmacognosy*, 14th edn, Saunders, London, 105, 1996.

25. Rajani M and Kanaki NS, Phytochemcial Standardization of Herbal Drugs and Polyherbal Formulations, In: Ramawat KG, and Merillon JM (eds). *Bioactive Molecules and Medicinal Plants*, Springer, 2008.

Chapter 7

1. George Francis, Zohaentr Kerem, Harinder PSM, and Klaus B, The biological action of saponins in animal systems: a review, *Br J Nutr*, 88, 2002, 587–605.

2. Arctander S, *Perfume and Flavor Materials of Natural Origin,* Allured Publishing Corporation, Carol Stream, IL, 1994.

3. Guenther E, *The Essential Oils Volume One: History-Origin in Plants-Production-Analysis.* D. Van Nostrand Company, Inc. New York, NY, 1948.

4. Chrastil J, Solubility of solids and liquids in supercritical gases, *J Phys Chem*, 86, 1982, 3016–3021.

5. Bajaj YPS, *Medicinal and Aromatic Plants*, Vol 9, Springer, Berlin, 1996.

6. Braithwaite A and Smith FJ, *Chromatographic Methods*, Chapman and Hall, London, 1986.

7. Charlwood BV, and Banthorpe DV, *Methods in Plant Biochemistry*, Vol 7, Terpenoids, Academic Press, London, 1991.

8. Cordell GA, *Introduction to Alkaloids*, John Wiley, New York, 1981.

9. Gunstone FD, Padley FB, and Harwood JL, *The Lipid Handbook*, Chapman Hall, London, 1986.

10. Handa SS, Khanuja SPS, Longo G, and Rakesh DD, *Extraction technologies for medicinal and aromatic plants*, Trieste: ICS UNIDO, 2008.

11. Harborne JB, *Phytochemical Methods: A Guide to Modern Techniques of Plant Analysis*, 3rd edn, Chapman and Hall, London, 1973.

12. Haslam E, Vegetable tannins – Lessons of a phytochemical lifetime, *Phytochemistry*, 68(22–24), 2007, 2713–2721.

13. Heftmann F, *Chromatography: Fundamentals and Applications of Chromatographic and Electrophoretic Techniques*, 5th edn, Elsevier, Amsterdam, 1992.

14. Markham KR, *Techniques of Flavonoid identification*, Academic Press, London, 1982.

15. Sherma J and Zweig G, *Paper Chromatography*, Academic Press, New York, 1971.

16. Touchstone JC, and Dobbins MF, *Practice of Thin Layer Chromatography*, John Wiley, Chichester, 1978.

17. Wagner H, Bladt S, and Zgainski EM, *Plant Drug Analysis – A Thin Layer Chromatography Atlas*, Springer-Verlag, New York, 1984.

Chapter 8

1. Alvi M N, Ahmad S, Rehman K, Preparation of menthol crystals from mint (Mentha arvensis), *Int J Agri Biol*, 3(4), 2001.

2. Atal CK, Gupta OP, and Afaq SH, Commiphora mukul source of guggal in Indian systems of medicine. *Econ Bot* 29(3), 1975, 209–218.

3. Atanassova M and Bagdassarian V, Rutin content in plant products, *J Univ Chem Tech Met*, 44(2), 2009, 201–203.

4. Bajaj AG and Dev S, Chemistry of Ayurvedic crude drugs. V. Guggulu (resin from Commiphora mukul.). 5. Some new steroidal components and stereochemistry of guggulsterol-I at C-20 and C-22. *Tetrahedron* 38(19), 1982, 2949–2954.

5. Bernard RL, and Lee Huyck C, Comparison of extractive procedures for digitalis, *J Pharm Sci*, 52(9), 1963, 904–905.

6. Chao Yung Su S and Ferguson NM, Extraction and separation of anthraquinone glycosides, *J Pharm Sci*, 62(6), 1973, 899–901.

7. Chen KK, A Pharmacognostic and chemical study of Ma Huang (*Ephedra vulgaris* var. Helvetica). *J Am Pharm Assoc*, 14, 1925, 189–194.

8. Chauhan SK, Kimothi GP, Singh BP, and Agrawal S, A Spectrophotometric method to estimate piperine in piper species, *Anc Sci Life* 18(1), 1998, 84–87.

9. Eccles R, Menthol and related cooling compounds, *J. Pharm. Pharmacol.* 46, 1994, 618–630.

10. Gopinath V, Kokila L, Lavanya R, and Brindha P, Quality control studies on Panchatiktaka Guggulu Kwatha Curanam, *J Pharm Res*, 4(1), 2011, 229–232.

11. Hamrapurkar P D, Kavita J and Sandip Z, Quantitative estimation of piperine in *Piper nigrum* and *Piper longum* using high performance thin layer chromatography, *J Appl Pharmaceutical Sci*, 01(03), 2011, 117–120.

12. Hardin, A, Crandall PG, and Stankus T, Essential oils and antioxidants derived from itrus by-products in food protection and medicine: an introduction and review of recent literature. *J Agric Food Inf*, 11(2), 2010, 99–122.

13. Hirata A, Murakami Y, Shoji M, Kadoma Y, and Fujisawa S, Kinetics of radical-scavenging activity of hesperetin and hesperidin and their inhibitory activity on COX-2 expression. *Anticancer Res*, 25(5), 2005, 3367–3374.

14. Huggett Q, Physical properties of menthols. *Quart J Pharm Pharmacol*, 15, 1942, 218–228.

15. Ikan R, *Natural Products, A Laboratory Guide*, 2nd edn, Academic Press: New York, 1991.

16. Kanaze FI, Termentzi A, Gabrieli C, Niopas I, Georgarakis M, and Kokkalou E, The phyto-chemical analysis and antioxidant activity assessment of orange peel (*Citrus sinensis*) cultivated in Greece-Crete indicates a new commercial source of hesperidin. *Biomed Chromatogr* 23(3), 2009, 239–249.

17. Karisma S, Priti T, Shivprakash K, and Pundarikakshudu K, Spectrophotometric determination of andrographolide in *Andrographis paniculata* Nees and its formulation, *Indian J Pharm Sci*, 69(3), 2007, 457–458.

18. Komes D, Horžić D, Belščak A, Kovačević Ganič K, and Baljak A, Determination of caffeine content in tea and maté tea by using different methods, *Czech J Food Sci*, 27, 2009.

19. Krewson CF, and Couch JF, Production of rutin from Buck wheat, *J Pharm Sci*, 39(3), 1950, 163–169.

20. Nagababu E and Lakshmaiah N, Inhibitory effect of eugenol on non-enzymatic lipid peroxidation in rat liver mitochondria. *Biochem Pharmacol*, 43, 2393–2400.

21. Pavia, Lampman, Kriz, and Engel, *Introduction to Organic Laboratory Techniques: A Microscale Approach*. Saunders College Publishing, 1999.

22. Rajani M, Neeta S, and Ravishankara MN, A rapid method for isolation of andrographolide from andrographis paniculata nees (Kalmegh), *Pharm Biol*, 38(3), 2000, 204–209.

23. Rothrock JW, Hammes PA, and McAleer WJ, Isolation of Diosgenin by Acid Hydrolysis of Saponin, *Ind Eng Chem*, 49(2), 1957, 186–188.

24. Varsha MJ, Uttam SK, Sachin BG, and Vilasrao JK, Development and validation of HPTLC method for determination of glycyrrhizin in herbal extract and in herbal gel, *Int J ChemTech Res*, 1(4), 2009, 826–831.

Chapter 9

1. Abdin MZ, Israr M, Rehmann RU, and Jain SK, Artemisinin a novel antimalarial drug. Biochemical and molecular approaches for enhanced production, *Planta Med* 69, 2003, 289–289.

2. Abdul-Ghani AS and Amin R, Effect of aqueous extract of *Commiphora opobalsamum* on blood pressure and heart rate in rats, *J Ethnopharmacol* 57(3), 1997, 219–222.

3. Al-Harbi MM, Qureshi S, Raza M, et al. Anticarcinogenic effect of *Commiphora molmol* on solid tumors induced by Ehrlich carcinoma cells in mice. *Chemotherapy*, 40(5), 1994, 337–347.

4. Ali S, Ansari KA, Jafry MA, et al, *Nardostachys jatamansi* protects against liver damage induced by thioacetamide in rats, *J Ethnopharmacol* 71(3), 2000, 359–363.

5. Amroyan E, Gabrielian E, Panossian A, et al. Inhibitory effect of andrographolide from *Andrographis paniculata* on PAF-induced platelet aggregation. *Phytomedicine*, 6(1), 1999, 27–31.

6. Anonymous, *Wealth of India (Raw materials)*, Publications and Information Directorate, CSIR, New Delhi, Vol VII, 87, 1996.

7. Auer W, et al. Hypertension and hyperlipidaemia: garlic helps in mild cases. *Br J Clin Pract Suppl* 44(Suppl 69), 1990, 36.

8. Barrie SA, Wright JV, and Pizzorono JE, Effects of garlic oil on platelet aggregation, serum lipids and blood pressure in humans, *J Orthomolec Med*, 2, 1987, 1521.

9. Batkhuu J, Hattori K, Takano F, et al. Suppression of NO production in activated macrophages in vitro and ex vivo by neoandrographolide isolated from *Andrographis paniculata*, *Biol Pharm Bull* 25(9), 2002, 1169–1174.

10. Brosche T, Platt D, and Dorner H, The effect of a garlic preparation on the composition of plasma lipoproteins and erythrocyte membranes in geriatric subjects. *Br J Clin Pract Suppl*, 44(Suppl 69), 1990, 1219.

11. Chandan BK, Sharma AK, and Anand KK, *Boerhavia diffusa*: a study of its hepatoprotective activity. *J Ethnopharmacol* 31(3), 1991, 299–307.

12. Chatterjee A, Basak B, Saha M, et al. Structure and stereochemistry of nardostachysin, a new terpenoid ester constituent of the rhizomes of *Nardostachys jatamansi*, *J Nat Prod* 63(11), 2000, 1531–1533.

13. Deng R, Therapeutic effects of Guggul and its constituent Guggulsterone: cardiovascular benefits, *Cardiovasc Drug Rev* 25(4), 2007, 375–390.

14. Edwin R and Chungath JI, Studies in *Swertia chirata*, *Indian Drugs*, 25, 1988, 143–146.

15. Handa SS, Mundkinajeddu D, and Mangal AK, *Indian Herbal Pharmacopoeia*, RRL, Jammu, IDMA, Mumbai, 1998.

16. Jarald E, Nalwaya N, Sheeja E, Ahmad S, and Jamalludin S, Comparative study on diuretic activity of few medicinal plants in individual form and in combination form Indian Drugs, 47(3), 2010, 20–24.

17. Joshi P and Dhawan V, *Swertia chirayita* – an overview, *Curr Sci*, 89(4), 2005, 635–640.

18. Kirtikar KR and Basu BD, *Indian Medicinal Plants*, 2nd edn, vols 1–4. Periodical Experts, Delhi, 1935a, p 1659, 1660.

19. Manu KA and Kuttan G Immunomodulatory activities of Punarnavine, an alkaloid from *Boerhaavia diffusa*, *Immunopharmacol Immunotoxicol*, 31(3), 2009, 377–387.

20. Mueller MS, Karhagomba IB, Hirt HM, and Wemakor E, The potential of *Artemisia annua* L. as a locally produced remedy for malaria in the tropics: agricultural, chemical and clinical aspects, *J Ethnopharmacol*, 73(3), 2000, 487–493.

21. Sairam K, Rao CV, and Goel RK, Effect of *Convolvulus pluricaulis* Chois on gastric ulceration and secretion in rats. *Indian J Exp Biol*, 39(4), 2001, 350–354.

22. Sasmal S, Majumdar S, Gupta M, Mukherjee A, and Mukherjee PK, Pharmacognostical, phytochemical and pharmacological evaluation for the antipyretic effect of the seeds of *Saraca asoca* Roxb, *Asian Pac J Trop Biomed*, 2(10), 2012, 782–786.

23. Shishodia S, Harikumar KB, Dass S, Ramawat KG, and Aggarwal BB, The Guggul for chronic diseases: ancient medicine, modern targets. *Anticancer Res*, 28(6A), 2008, 3647–3664.

24. Sivarajan VV and Balachandran I, *Ayurvedic Drugs and their plant sources*, Pxford and IBH Publishing Co. Pvt Ltd., New Delhi, 1994, p 245.

25. Van Agtmal MA, Eggelte TA, and Van Boxtel CJ, Artemisinin drugs in the treatment of malaria: from medicinal herb to registered medication, *Trends Pharmacol Sci* 20(5), 1999, 199–205.

26. Warrier PK, Nambiar VPK, and Ramankutty C (eds), *Indian Medicinal Plants: A Compendium of 500 species*, Vol 2, Orient Longman, Hyderabad, 1994b, p 129.

27. WHO monographs on selected medicinal plants, Vols 1 and 2, WHO, Geneva, AITBS Publishers, India.

Chpater 10

1. Askinson GW, In: *Perfumes and Cosmetics*, 5th Edn, The Norman W Henley Publishing Company, New York, 1925, p 20.

2. Balsam MS and Sagarin E, In: *Cosemtics Science and Technology*, Vol 1, Wiley Inter Science, New York, 1972, p 108.

3. BHMA, The British Herbal Pharmacoepia, 1983.

4. Bouillon C, Shampoos and hair conditioners. *Clin Dermatol*, 6, 1988, 83–92.

5. Bruno B, Luisella V, Laura C, and Elisa BM, *Herbal Principles in Cosmetics*, CRC Press, 2010.

6. Calabrese V, et al. Biochemical studies of a natural antioxidant isolated from rosemary and its application in cosmetic dermatology. *Int J Tissue React* 22(1), 2000, 5–13.

7. Caldecott, Todd, *Ayurveda: The Divine Science of Life*. Elsevier/Mosby, 2006.

8. Evans WC, *Trease and Evans Pharmacognosy*, Balliere Tindall, 13th Edn, London, 1989.

9. Schneider G, Gohla S, Schreiber J, Kaden W, Schönrock U, Schmidt-Lewerkühne H, Kuschel A, Petsitis X, Pape W, Ippen H, and Diembeck W, *"Skin Cosmetics" in Ullmann's Encyclopedia of Industrial Chemistry*, Wiley-VCH, Weinheim, 2005.

10. Jellinek S and Fenton GL, In: *Formulation and Function of Cosmetics*, Wiley Inter Science, New York, 1970, p 108.

11. Kapoor VP, Herbal Cosmetics for skin and hair care, *Nat Prod Rad*, 4(4), 2005, 306–314.

12. Korac RR and Khambolja KM, Potential of herbs in skin protection from UV radiation, *Pharmacogn Rev*, 5(10), 2011, 164–173.

13. Maiti PC, Roy S, and Roy A, "Chemical investigation of Indian soapnut, *Sapindus laurifolius* Vahl." *Cell Mol Life Sci (Birkhäuser Basel)* 24(11), 1968, 1091.

14. Marriott RH, Cosmetics as a factor in Civilization, In: Middleton AW (Ed) *Cosmetic Science*, Buttersworth Scientific Publications, London, 1959, p 311.

15. Nadkarni KM, In: *Indian plants and drugs with their medicinal properties and uses*. Norton and Co. Madras, 1910, p. 120.15. Patkar KB, Herbal Cosmetics in India, *Ind J Plast Surg*, 41, 2008, S134–S137.

16. Patkar KB and Bole PV, In: *Herbal cosmetics in ancient India with a treatise on planta cosmetica*. Bharatiya Vidya Bhavan Mumbai, India Mumbai: World Wide Fund for Nature, 1997.

17. Roy RK, Thakur M, and Dixit VK, Hair growth promoting activity of *Eclipta prostrata* in male albino rats. *Arch Dermatol Res*, 300(7), 2008, 357–364.

18. San Philippo A and English JC, An overview of Medicated shampoos used in Dandruff treatment, P&T, 31(7), 2006, 396–400

19. Shweta KG, Rajan BM, Urvashi KP, Blessy M, and Hitesh NJ, Herbal plants: used as cosmetics, *J Nat Prod Resour*, 1(1), 2011, 24–32.

20. Srivastava JK, Shankar E, and Gupta S, Chamomile: a herbal medicine of the past with bright future, *Mol Med Rep*, 3(6), 2010, 895–901.

21. Wagner H, Hikino H, and Farnsworth NR (eds), In: *Economic and Medicinal Plant Research*, Vol 2, Academic Press, London, 1988, p 73.

22. Wagner H, Hikino H, and Farnsworth NR (eds), In: *Economic and Medicinal Plant Research*, Vol 3, Academic Press, London, 1989, p 106.

23. Watt G, In: *The Commercial Products of India-John Murray*. London, 1908, p. 68.

24. Wren RC, *Potter's New Cyclopedia of Botanical Drugs and Preparations*, C W Daniels, 1985.

Chapter 11

1. Berlin J, Formation of secondary metabolites in cultured plant cells and its impact on pharmacy, In: YPS Bajaj (ed), *Biotechnology in Agriculture and Forestry*, Vol 4, Medicinal and Aroamtic Plants I, Springer, Berlin, 1988, pp 37–59.

2. Bhojwani SS and Razdan MK, *Plant Tissue Culture: Theory and Practice*, a revised edition, Elsevier, Amsterdam, 2005, pp 537–562.

3. Brodelius P, Deus B, Mosbach K, and Zenk MH, Immobilized plant cells for the production and transformation of natural products, *FEBS Lett*, 103, 1979, 93–97.

4. Brodelius P and Nilsson K, Entrapment of plant cells in different matrices, *FEBS Lett*, 122, 1980, 312–316.

5. Davis DA, Tsao D, Seo JH, Emery A, Low PS, and Heinstein D, Enhancement of phytoalexin accumulation in cultured plant cells by oxalate, *Phytochemistry*, 31, 1992, 1603–1607.

6. Di Cosmo F and Towers GHN, Stress and metabolism in cultured cells. In: BA Timmermann et al. (eds), *Recent Advances in Phytochemistry*, Vol 18, Phytochemical adaptations to stress. Olenum, New York, 1984, pp 97–175.

7. Doaa ARM and Wafaa AH, Potential application of immobilization technology in enzyme and biomass production (review article). *J Appl Sci Res* 5(12), 2009, 2466–2476.

8. Eilert U, Elicitation: methodology and aspects of application. In: F Constabel and I K vasil (eds), *Cell Culture and Somatic Cell Genetics of Plants*, Vol 4, Cell Culture in Phyto chemistry, Academic Press, San Diego, CA, pp 153–188.

9. Fujita Y, Hara Y, Moromoto T, and Misawa M, Semisynthetic production of vinblastine involving cell cultures of C. *roseus* and chemical reaction. In: HJJ Nij Kamp et al. (eds), *Progress in Plant Cellular and Molecular Biology*, Kluwer, Dordrecht. 1990, pp 738–743.

10. Fujita Y, Tabata M, Nishi A, and Yamada Y, New medium and production of secondary compounds with two-staged culture method. In: A. Fujiwara (ed) *Plant Tissue Culture*. Jpn Assoc Plant Tissue Cult, Tokyo, 1982, pp 399–400.

11. Galun E, Aviv D, Dantes A, and Freeman A, Biotransformation by plant cells immobilized in cross-linked polyacrylamide-hydrazide, *Planta Medica*, 49, 1983, 9–13.

12. Lambie AJ, Commercial Aspects of the Production of Secondary Compounds by Immobilised Plant Cells in Secondary Product from Plant Tissue Culture, Charlwood, B. V. and Rhodes, M. J. C., (Eds), Clarendon Press, Oxford.

13. Misra SP, *Plant Tisue Culture*, Ane Books Pvt Ltd, New Delhi, 2009, 185–208.

14. Moreno PRH, van der Heijden R, and Verpoorte R, Cell and tissue cultures of C. *roseus*: a literature survey II, updating from 1988–1993, *Plant Cell Tissue Organ Cult*, 42, 1995, 1–25.

15. Rucker W, Digitalis spp.: in vitro culture, regeneration and production of cardenolides and other secondary products. In: YPS Bajaj (ed), *Biotechnology in Agriculture and Forestry*, Vol 4, Medicinal and Aromatic Plants I. Springer, Berlin, 1988, pp 388–418.

16. Scott CD, Immobilized cells: a review of recent literature. *Enzyme Microb. Technol.* 9, 1987, 66–73.

17. Tabata N, Mizukami H, Hiroaka N, and Konishima M, Pigment formation in callus cultures of *Lithospermum erythrorhizon*, *Phytochemistry*, 13, 1974, 927–937.

18. Tanaka A and Nakajima H, Application of immobilized growing cells. *Adv Biochem Eng Biotechnol* 42, 1990, 97–131.

19. Veeresham C (2006) *Medicinal Plant Biotechnology*, CBS Publishers, New Delhi.

20. Williams PD and Mavituna F, Immobilized plant cells, In: Fowler MW, Warren GS, Moo-Young M (eds). *Plant Biotechnology: Comprehensive Biotechnology, Second Supplement*, Pergamon Press, Oxford, 1992.

21. Zenk MH, El-Shagia H, Arens H, Stockgt J, Weiler EW, and Deus D, Formation of the indole alkaloids serpentine and ajmalicine in cell suspension cultures of C. *roseus*, In: Barz WRE et al (eds). *Plant Tissue Culture and its Biotechnological application*, Springer, Berlin, 1977.

Chapter 12

1. Vinod VS, *Managing Intellectual Property – The Strategic Imperative*, Prentice Hall of India Pvt Ltd, New Delhi, 2006.

2. Chandrasekaran A, *Intellectual Property Law*, C. Sitaraman and Co., Pvt Ltd, Chennai, 2009.

3. Jenne WK, *Intellectual Property Management*, Springer Verlag, US, 2004.

4. Chanda R, Intellectual Property Rights, *IIMB Manag Rev*, 14(3), 2005, 60–72.

5. Correa CM, *Intellectual Property Rights, The WTO and Developing Countries: TRIPS Agreement and Policy options*, Zed Books, New York, 2000.

6. The Indian Patent Act 1970 (Bare Act), Universal Publishing, New Delhi.

7. Gupta AK, Impact of WTO on Indian farmer's rights and a– a case of intellectual property rights and emerging biosafety protocol, In: *Impact of WTO Agreement on Indian Agriculture*, IIM, Ahmedabad, 1994, 10.1–10.51.

8. Biodiversity Bill insists on sovereign rights (2001), *The Hindu*, 8 March, 2001, Available at: http://www.ielrc.org/content/n0101.htm

9. Traditional Knowledge in Asia-Pacific Problems of Piracy and Protection (2002), *Genetic Resources Action International (GRAIN) and Kalpavriksh Environmental Action Group, Oct 2002*, Available at: http://www.grain.org/briefings/?id=97,www.grain.org/publications/tk-asia-2002-en.cfm

10. Kate K and Laird SA, *The Commercial Use of Biodiversity, Access to Genetic Resources and Benefit Sharing*, Earthscan, London, 1999.

11. Medicinal Plants, International Trade Forum, Published October 17, 2001, Available at: www.tradeforum.org/news/fullstory.php/aid/301/Medicinal_Plants.html

12. Declaration on Science and the Use of Scientific Knowledge and Agenda – Framework for Action, Available at: www.nature.com/wcs/1news/01-1a.html

13. Christopher A, The New World Trade Organization Agreements: Globalizing law through services and intellectual property, Cambridge University Press, Cambridge, 2000.

14. Jayunta B, *World Trade Organization: An India Perspective*, Eastern Law House, Calcutta, 2000.

15. Lionel B and Spyros M, *Intellectual Property and Ethics*, Vol 4, Sweet and Maxwell, London, 1998.

16. Michael B, *Intellectual Property aspects of Ethnobiology*, Sweet and Maxwell, London, 1999.

17. Chowdhury NK and Aggrawal JC, *Dunkel Proposals*, Vol II: Implications for India and the Third World, Shipra Publications, Delhi, 1994.

18. Vivekandan VC, *Law Shop on Intellectual Property Regime for Pharma Industry*, National Law School of India University, Hyderabad, 1999.

19. Erbisch FH and Maredia KM, Intellectual Property Rights in Agricultural Biotechnology, Universities Press (India) Ltd, Hyderabad, 1998.

20. Manoj V, Patents on life, India and the TRIPS mandate, *Econ Polit Wkly*, 33(4), 1998, 152–154.

21. Koshy S, Patents and the Pharmaceutical Sector, *Lawyers Collective*, 15(5), 2000, 11–12.

22. Khera HK, Patents and sui generis system for protection of plant varieties: A threat to food security and health care, *Central Indian Law Quarterly*, 13(2), 2000, 182–196.

23. Gopakumar GN, Impact of TRIPS on Indian Pharmaceutical Industry, *J Intellect Prop Rights*, 13, 2008, 432–441.

24. Rajshree C, Knowledge as property issues, In: *The Moral Grounding of Intellectual Property Rights*, Oxford University Press, New Delhi, 2010.

Chapter 13

1. Kakiuchi N, Hattori M et al (1986) Studies on dental caries prevention by traditional medicines. 8. Inhibitory effect of various tannins on glucan synthesis by glucosyl transferase from Streptococcus mutans, Chemical Pharmacology Bulletin, 34 (2): p 720–725.

2. Engel C (2002) In: Wild Health - How animals keep themselves well and what we can learn from them, Houghton Mifflin Company, New York.

3. Matthew E G, Anne M H (1993) Grooming with Trattinnickia resin: possible pharmaceutical plant use by coatis in Panama.

4. Philippe C, Anne O, Francesco B, Gregoire C, Michel C (2003) Evidence for collective medication in ants, Ecology Letters, 6, p 19–22.

5. Wimburger P H (1984) The use of green plant material in bird nests to avoid ectoparasites, Auk, 102, p 615–618.

6. Mazars G (1994) Traditional veterinary medicine in India, Rev.Sci Tech Off Int Epiz, 13 (2), p 443–451.

7. Clark L, Mason J R (1988) Effect of biologically active plants used as nest material and the derived benefit to starling nestling, Oecologia, 77, p 174–180.

8. Robles M, Aregullin M, West J, Rodriguez E (1995) Recent studies on the Zoopharmacognosy, Pharmacology and Neurotoxicology of Sesquiterpene lactones, Planta Med, 61, p 199–203.

9. Weldon P J, Aldrich J R, Klum J A, Oliver J E, Debboun M (2003) Benzoquinones from millipedes deter mosquitoes and elicit self-anointing in capuchin monkeys (Cebus spp), Naturwissenschaften, 90, p 301–304.

10. Deem S L, Emmons L H (2005) Exposure of free ranging maned wolves (Chrysochyon brachyurus) to infectious and parasitic disease agents in the Noel Kempff Mercado Naitonal Park, Bolivia, J Zoo Wild life Med, 36 (2) p 192–197.

11. Huffmann M A, Seifu M (1989) Observations on th eillenss and consumption of a possibly medicinal plant Vernonia amygdalina (Del) by a wild chimpanzee in the Mahale Mountains National Park, Tanzania, Primates, 30, p 51–63.

12. Baker M (1996) Fur rubbing: Use of medicinal plants by capuchin monkeys (*Cebus capucinus*), American Journal of Primatology, 38, p. 263–270.

13. Milton K (1979) Factors influencing leaf choice by howler monkeys: a test for some hypotheses of food selection by generalist herbivores, American Naturalist, 114, p 362–378.

14. Janzen D H (1978) Complications in interpreting the chemical defences of trees against tropical arboreal plant-eating vertebrates, The Ecology of Arboreal Folivores (Ed) Montgomery G, Smithsonian Press, Washington DC, pp 73–84.

15. Rodriguez E and Wrangham R (1993) Zoopharmacognosy, The use of medicinal plants by animals In: Kelsey RD, John TR, Helen AS (Eds), Recent Advances in Phytochemistry, Vol 27: Phytochemical Potential of Tropical Plants, Plenum Press, New York, p 89.

16. Wrangham RW (1995) Leaf swallowing by chimpanzees and its relation to a tapeworm infection, Am J Primatology, 37 (4), p 297–303.

17. Kruelen DA (1985) Lick use by large herbivores: A review of benefits and banes of soil consumption, Mammal Rev, 15, p 107–123.

18. Clayton DH and Wolfe ND (1993), The adaptive significance of self-medication, Trends Ecol Evolution, 8, p 60–63.

19. Valderrama X, Robinson JG, Attygale AB, Eisner T (2000) Seasonal anointment with millipedes in a wild primate: A chemical defense against insects, J Chem Ecol, 78, p 603–611.

20. Baker M (1996) Fur rubbing: use of medicinal plants by capuchin monkeys (Cebus capucinus) Am J Primatology, 38(3), p 263–270.

Index

A

A. acuminata 114
A. barbadensis 110, 111
A. belladonna 114
abscisic acid 374
Acacia catechu 294
acetyl value 210, 227
acevaltrate 106
acid value 227
acne 338
A. concinna 342
Acorus calamus 313, 352
acyclic monoterpenes 239
adaptogen 16, 103, 104, 358
Addison's disease 94
adulteration 66, 152, 204
Adverse Drug Reaction Monitoring System 143
A. ferox 111
affinity chromatography 252
aflatoxins 209
agar 373
Agave sisalona 99, 236
aged garlic extract 316
agnivesha tantra 35
agrobacterium 375, 381, 382, 389
agrochemicals 417
ahamkara 38, 39
ajmalicine 85
ajoenes 315
alchemy 3, 401
aldose reductase 261
aldrin 206
alfalfa 357
alginic acid 209
alkaloids 221, 296
allantoin 338, 359
allicin 315
alliin 315
alliinase 315
Allium sativum 153, 314
allyl sulfides 315
almond oil 354
Alochaka agni 46
aloe 109
Aloe barbadensis 109, 153
aloetic juice 111
Aloe vera 110, 340, 343

ama 49
amarogentin 333
amaroswerin 333
Amberlite XAD-7—a resin 389
amchi system 55
American ginseng 104, 349
American podophyllum 91
amla 346, 347
ammoniacum resin 244
ammonium molybdate 262
amoebic dysentery 97
amoebicide 98
A. mossambicensis 420
Anchusa officinalis 368
androgenic alopecia 350
Andrographis paniculata 279, 319
andrographolide 279, 321
aniseed 73
anthocyanins 81, 233
anthraquinone glycosides 229
anti-ageing 344, 347, 349
anti-amoebic 419
antibacterial 270
anti-carcinogenic 273
anti-cellulite 339
anticholinergic 112
anticonvulsant 273
anti-dandruff 345, 351
anti-inflammatory 273, 279
anti malarials 95, 270
ant imicrobials 341
anting 422, 423
anti-parasitic effect 422
anti-pruritic 270
anti-pyretic 279
anti-seborrheic 345
antispasmodic 106
anti-tyrosinase 355
Anubis baboons 421
apana vayu 45
A. perryi 111
aphrodisiac 103, 349
A. pluriseta 420
apradhana dravya 52
Arabic (Unani) medicines 32
arbutin 353, 380
Arctium lappa 352

Arnica montana 347
arogya 44
aromatherapy 361
arteether 331
artemether 331
Artemisia annua 10, 329, 330, 381
Artemisia chamomila 329
artesunate 331
arthropod juvenile hormone analogs 423
artimisinin 331
ascaricides 206
aseptic culturing 365, 375
Ashoka 321
ashtanga hridaya 2, 37
ash Values 204
ashwagandha 16, 152
aspergillus 209
A. spicata 109
Aspilia rudis 420
astanga sangraha 37
astringent 339
atharvana veda 17, 417
atherosclerosis 303, 316
atrial fi brillation 101, 102
Atropa 112, 113
attar 356
aurones 233
aushadhi sukta 34
Australian Register of Therapeutic Goods 131
Australian Regulatory Guidelines 132
automatic compulsory license 403
autoradiography 249
auxillary bud culture 368
Auxins 373
avalambaka kapha 46
Avicenna 4
Ayurveda 15, 32
Ayurvedic materia medica 307
Ayurvedic Pharmacopoeia 145
Ayush 155
Azadirachta indica 294, 351
Azelaic acid 339, 354
Azhadirachta indica 423

B

Babchi 359
badam 354
Bahlika 55
bahyakaranas 39
Baljet test 280, 284
balsamic acids 242
Balsamodendron mukul 317
Balsams 245
B. aquifolium 292
B. aristata 292
basil 298

batch culture 376
bath salts 361
Baudouin test 227
bdellium 11
bear-medicine 424
beauty aid 354
beggar's buttons 352
Belladonna 112
Beninca hispida 313
benzoin 243
berberine 291
Berne Convention 393
Beta-arbutin 353
Bhaisajya Vyakhyana 52
Bharadwaja 34
Bhava Mishra 55
Bhava Prakasha 37, 55, 308
Bhela Samhita 3, 37
Bhrajaka agni 45
Bhringraj 347
Bhuta-vaidya 53
bimaristan 4
binary vectors 382
bioautography 249
bioavailability enhancer 19
biodiversity 26, 408
biopesticides 384
biopiracy 152, 407, 413
bioreactors 376
biotechnological processes 15
biotrade 409
bio transformation 378
bird nesting 422
bitter almonds 354
bitter pith chewing 422
bitter plants 419
bitter tonics 96
blonde psyllium 115
Bodhaka kapha 46
boeravinones A, B, C, D 310
Boerrhavia diffusa 309
Bolar Provision 404
.Bonobo monkeys 422
Born Trager's test 232, 266
B. procumbens 309
Brahma 34
Brahmi 347, 349
breasted nuthatch 423
B. repens 309
Brhat Tryi 37
British Patent Act 402
bronchodilator 258
buckwheat 261
bulk laxative 117
B. verticillata 309
B. vulgaris 292

C

C$_{23}$ steroidal glycosides 101, 282
cabbage rose 356
Caesalpinia pulcherrina 423
Caesalpinia spinosa 294
caffeine 267, 339
Calabar bean 6
calamus 352
calcium sennosides 264
Calendula officinalis 343
callus 375
Camellia sinensis 267, 346
Canada turpentine 244
Cannabis sativa 15
Canon of Medicine 54
capsaicin 378
Capuchin monkeys 421
carbenecillin 373
cardenolide 101
cardiac arrhythmias 96
cardiac glycosides 101, 229
Carica papaya 107, 356
CARISM 171
carnivores 420, 426
carotenoids 81
carthamin 356
Carthamus tinctorius 355
casein hydrolysate 373
cashew pedicels (Anacardium occidentale) 421
Cassia acutifolia 115, 264
Cassia angustifolia 115, 264
Cassia auriculata 294
Casurina equistifolia 294
catechins 81
catechu-tannic acid 294
catharanthine 379
Catharanthus 379, 385, 387, 388
Cat's valerian 326
C. calisaya 96
celite 249
cell acclimatization 376
cell-based screening systems 172
cell culture 172, 376
cell permeabilization 389
cell proliferant 359
cell suspension cultures 371, 379
Centella asiatica 313
cephaeline 98
Cephaelis acuminata 97
chalcones 233
chamomile 344
Chamomilla recutita 344
Charaka Samhita 35, 37
chebulic acid 294
chemical markers 214
chemostat 376

Chen-Kao test 259
Chimpanzees 420
Chinese galls 295
Chinese ginseng 349
Chinese medicine 32, 55
Chinese Pharmacopoeia 139
Chirata 331, 332
Chitta 39, 40
chlordane 206
chlorinated hydrocarbons 206
chromatographic fingerprint analysis 214
chromatography 246
Chrysocyon brachyurus 424
chyawanaprash 311, 346
cichoric acid 361
CIMAP 166, 177
cinchinidine 271
cinchona 95, 270, 387
cinchonine 96
cinchotannic acid 271
cinnamon 298
citronella 73
Citrus aurantium 288
Citrus Limoni 354
Citrus sinensis 288
clay 424
C. ledgeriana 96, 375, 388
Clitorea ternata 311, 313
Clonal Propagation 368
cloning 382
closed continuous culture 376
clove 73
cocaine 6
coconut milk 373
Cocos nucifera 348
co-cultivation 382
codeine 378
coenzyme Q10 340
coffee 267
C. officinalis 97
co-integrating vector 382
cola nuts 267
Cola vera 267
colchicine 389
colophony 244
column chromatography 222, 246, 251
comfrey 359
Commiphora mukul 303, 317, 318
commons license 411
compulsory license 395, 405
conditioned medium 376
conditioners 341
confectionary 94, 285
conifer 421
continuous culture 376
conventional foods 79

Convention on Biodiversity 27, 409
Convolvulus microphyllus 311
Copaiba 244
Copyright Enforcement Advisory
    Council (CEAC) 397
corn kernel meal 357
corn silk extract 357
Corvus brachyrhynchos 423
cosmaceuticals 339
cosmetic 335
cosmetology 335
Costus speciosus 100
C. robusta 97
C. roseus 368, 389
crude fibre 205
cryopreservation 370
C. succirubra 96
Curacao aloe 111
Curcuma longa 358
cyanogenetic glycosides 229
cytokinins 373

D

Dakshaprajapati 34
damask 356
Daniel H Janzen 419
Daruharidra 291
Datura 112, 369
DDT 206
decaffeinated coffee 268
Defence Institute High Altitude
    Research (DIHAR) 175
Defence Research and Development Organisation 174
Dehydroandrographolide 321
De Materia Medica 3
Department of Agricultural Research and
    Education (DARE) 176
Department of AYUSH 145
Department of Biotechnology 171
Department of Horticulture and Cash Crops 191
Department of Indian Systems of Medicine and
    Homeopathy (ISM&H) 146, 155
Department of Science and Technology 170
dermatitis 338
dermatopharmaceuticals 336
Design Act 398
Designated National Repository (DNR) under the
    Biological Diversity Act 166
Detection of Hazardous Chemical Contaminants and
    Residues 206
determination of bitterness value 211
determination of moisture content 203
determination of Volatile Oils 204
Dhanwantri 34, 36
dianthrone glycosides 264
dieldrin 206

dietary fibre 84
Dietary Supplement Health and Education
    Act of 1994 (DSHEA) 77
dietary supplements 74, 75
differential retention 246
digital encyclopedia 413
Digitalis lanata 101, 282, 375
Digitalis orientalis 282
Digitalis purpurea 100, 101, 282, 375
digitoxigenin 102
Digitoxin 6, 102
digoxin 102, 379
D. innoxia 114, 115
Dioctophyma renale 424
Dioscin 69, 99
Dioscorea 98
Diosgenin 99, 236, 276, 378
diosmin 288
dioxin 206
D. lutea 101
DMARP 180
D. metel 113, 114
DNA isolation 382
dormancy 373
dosha 44
D. quercifolia 114
Dragendorff's reagent 223, 250, 275
dragon's blood 244
dravya 50
Dravya Guna 2, 37, 49
DRDO 174
dropsy 282
Drug Master Files 405
Drugs Controller General of India 147
D. stramonium 114
Duboisia 112
Dunkel's draft 394, 403
dusky footed wood rats 421

E

E- and Z-guggulsterones 304
E. angustifolia 360
Eclipta alba 347
Eclipta prostrata 347
ectoparasites 422
edible burdock 352
electrochromatography 248
ellagic acid 294, 346
Eloy Rodriguez 416, 420
E. macrorhyncha 261
E. major 257
Embelica officinalis 294
embryo culture 368
Emetine 97, 98
emolliency 339
emollient 341, 348–349, 354

endoparasites 419
endurance enhancer 103
enfleurge 219, 241
English lavender 349
enriched/fortified/superfortified foods 79
entrapment 377
E. pallida 360
Ephedra 257
Ephedra vulgaris var Helvetica 257
Ephedrine 6, 257, 258
epicatechins 81, 322
E. purpurea 360
Erdmann's reagent 259
erythroquinine test 272
Eschscholtzia californica 389
essential oil 70, 73, 151
ester value 210
ethical drugs 68
ethical phytomedicines 68, 309
ethnopharmacology 29
ethylene 206, 374
ethylene chlorhydrin 206
eucalyptus 261, 294
Eugenia caryophyllus 298
eugenol 238, 298, 325
European Scientific Cooperative of
    Phytotherapy (ESCOP) 129
European starlings 423
Evolvulus alsinoides 311, 313
Exclusive Marketing Rights (EMR) 403
explant 373
ex situ cultivation 161
E. youmani 261

F

Fagopyrum esculentum 261
False Daisy 347
FAO, UN 59
fenugreek 342
Ferric chloride test 290
fertility modulating plants 419
F. esculentum 261
fibre-rich plant foods 117
Ficus exasperata 420
field-raised ginseng 27
Fitelson test 227
flash chromatography 252
flavanones 81, 233
flavanonols 233
flavones 233
flavonoid 232, 261, 338, 340
flavonols 82
flavononones 233
foaming index 210
foam test 278
Food and Agriculture Organization (FAO) 410

Food and Drug Administration (FDA) 137
foraging 419
Forced-flow planar chromatography (FFPC) 213
Forest Productivity and Agroforestry Division 192
Formica paralugubris 421
Forsythia intemedia 379
fruit ripening 384
fufuryl aminopurine (kinetin) 374
functional fibres 84
functional food 74, 79
fungal toxins 209
fungicides 206
fur rubbing 423

G

GABA (γ-aminobutyric acid) 106
Galen 4
galenicals 66, 96
gall formation 367
gallic acid 294, 346
gallotannin 294
Garden heliotrope 326
garlic 314
gas chromatography 213, 246, 253
gastritis 104
G. biloba 355
gelatin 296
gel filtration chromatography 252
gelling agents 373
gerite 373
General Agreement on Tariff and
    Trade (GATT) 394
gene restructuring 382
gene transfer strategies 382
Geographical Indications of Goods 398, 413
geophagy 418, 424
germplasm storage 369
G. glabra var.glandulifera 93
gibberellins 374
ginkgo 18, 21, 355, 366
ginseng 16, 27, 103, 152
ginsenosides 104
glabranin 285, 340
glucosinolates 82, 378
glycyrrhetenic 94
glycyrrhetenic acid 285
glycyrrhiza 93, 285
glycyrrhizin 94, 285, 340
Goldbeater's skin test 296
golden root 361
Golden triangle partnership (GTP) 155
Gottlieb Haberlandt 365
grape seed 21, 362
greater burdock 352
greater triad 37
green chiretta 319

green tea 21, 340
grooming 418
growth inhibitors 374
Guaiacum 244
guggulipid 303
guggulu 303, 317
guggulusterols I 303
guggulusterones Z and E 318
Gulf of Mannar Biosphere Reserve
    (GOMBR) 191
guna 38, 44, 49–51, 307
Guru 43
guruparampara 307
gurvadi gunas 42
Gyanendriyas 39

H

Haberlandt 365, 368
habitual constipation 117, 264
Hager's reagent 223, 275
hair conditioners 343, 345, 347, 349, 356
hair darkeners 345
hair nourisher 348
hair rejuvenator 349
hair strength 352
hair tonic 345
hair wash 111
H. albus 113, 114
Hamadryas baboons 421
Hanig 365
haploid plants 369
Harita Samhita 3, 37
Hatch–Waxman exemption 404
H. aureus – Golden henbane 113
head lice 358
head space trapping 220
Health and Education Act (DSHEA) 138
health food categories 79
health foods 74
heavy metal 152, 296
hecogenin 100, 236
hemisuccinate carbenoxolone sodium 94, 285
hemolysis 235
henna 345
hepatic microsomal lipid peroxidation 279
hepatoprotectant 279
heptachlor 206
herbal hair colourants 347
herbalism 416
herbal medicine 120, 125, 130, 145
herbal nutritional supplements 151
herbal single ingredients 6
herbal tea 346
herbal tranquillizers 105
herb-drug interactions 28
herbicides 206

herbivory 425
Hesperidin 288
hibiscus 346
high performance liquid chromatography 213, 252
high performance thin layer chromatography 213
high-speed counter current chromatography
    (HSCCC) 214
Hildebrandt 366
Himalayan Mayapple 92
Himalayan yew 87
H. niger 114
hogweed 350
Holy Basil 324, 358
Homatropine 112
Honey Bee Network 414
horse-radish peroxidase enzyme 379
hot continuous percolation, 219
hot-pressed oil 226
house sparrows 423
H. reticulatus 113, 114
humectant 362
hybrid embryos 369
Hydrastis 292
hydrodistillation 219
Hyoscine 112, 114
Hyoscyamus 112, 386

I

Ilex paraguariensis 267
Imminex 168
immunostimulant 279, 360
Indian Bdellium tree 317
Indian Contract Act 399
Indian Copyright Act 397
Indian Council of Agricultural Research 176
Indian Council of Medical Research 173
Indian gooseberry 346
Indian Institute of Agricultural Research (IIAR) 166
Indian Institute of Integrative Medicine 166
Indian Institute of Science 414
Indian Institute of Technology 194
Indian lilac 351
Indian Medicine Practitioners Cooperative
Pharmacy and Stores Ltd (IMPCOPS) 192
Indian Medicines Development Corporation
    Bill, 2005 146
Indian Medicines Pharmaceutical Corporation
    Limited (IMPCL) 157
Indian Patent and Designs Act 396
Indian Patents Act 396
Indian pennywort 349
Indian Podophyllum 91, 93
Indian sandalwood 360
Indian senna 116
Indian snake root 80
Indian valerian 105

Indole Acetic Acid (IAA) 373
industrial phytochemicals 70
inert resins 243
insecticides 206
in situ conservation 161
intellectual property 391, 410
intestinal nematodes 420
Inula racemosa 318
iodine value 227
ion exchange resins 249, 252
ionic network formation 377
Ipecac 97
iridoid glycosides 98
Isabgol 115
isoborneol 380
isoflavanes 233
Ispaghula 115–117
IUCD-induced menorrhagia 311

J

Jane Goodall 419
Japanese peppermint oil 300
Japanese valerian 106
Japan wax 225
Jatamansi 328
jojoba oil 345
J. paniculata 319
Justicia latebrosa 319

K

Kalmegh 279, 319
Kalpana gnana 49, 52
Kalpavriksh Environmental Action Group 29
kampo drugs 142
Karl Fischer reagent 203
Kasyapa Samhita 37
Kaumarabritya 53
Kedde's test 284
Keller-Kiliani test 231, 284
kerapathite 271
khus 361
kidney worm 424
kieselguhr 249
kinetin 373
Kledaka kapha 46
knowledge network on medicinal plants 167
kojic acid 353
Krishnachura 423

L

Lafon's reaction 238
Laghu Tryi 37
lahsun 314
Laibach 365
Lavandula angustifolia 349, 388
lavender 349, 350

lawsone 340, 345
Lawsonia inermis 345
laxatives 115
leaf alkanes 226
leaf cutin acids 225
Legal's test 284
Leibermann burchard reagent 250
lemongrass 73
lemon oil 355
lemon peel bioferment 355
leopard's bane 347
leucoderma 359
license of right 403, 404
lighter triad 37
Ligusticum wallichii 424
Linsmaier and Skoog medium 387
Liquorice 93, 94
list of Essential Medicines 14
Lithospermum erythrorhizon 366, 368, 389
lobeira fruit 424
L. porteri 424
Lucerne 357
lupeol 236
Lupinus 367, 381
lycopene 81
Lythospermum erythrorhizon 386

M

maceration 204, 219
Machosma tenuiflorum 323
macroscopic evaluation 201
Ma Huang 257
Manchurian liquorice 93
Mandelin's reagent 293
mandukparni 349
maned wolf 424
marine pharmacognosy 29
marmesin 380
Mayer's reagent 223, 259
meat tenderizer 107
medhya rasayana 313
Medicago sativa 357
medicinal properties of water 17
Melaleuca alternifolia 357
melanin 353
melanocytes 353
melanogenesis 340
menorrhagia 291
Mentha piperita 300, 388
menthol 300, 338
methamphetamine 258
methi 342
Meyer's reagent 275
microdistillation 220
microelements 372
microencapsulation 377

micropropagation 171, 368
microscopic evaluation 202
microwave-assisted extraction 219
Mimamsa 38
Mitracarpus scaber 353
Modified Borntrager's test 232, 266
Molisch' test 231
molluscicides 206
Morinda anthraquinones 385
morphogenesis 373
morphological variation 368
Morus alba 353
Morus bombycis 353
motion sickness 112
mountain arnica 347
mukul myrrh tree 303
mulethi 95
Murexide test 223, 269
mycotoxins 209

N

nadi pariksha 48
Naphthalene acetic acid (NAA) 373
naphthaquinone dye 345
naphthaquinone glycosides 229
Naphthoxy acetic acid (NOA) 373
Nardostachys grandiflora 328
Nardostachys jatamansi 65, 106, 326, 327
natural laxatives 264
Neem 11, 351, 423
Neem oil 351
nematocidal activity 420
nematocides 206
Neotoma fuscipes 421
neuralgia 291
Nickell 366
Nicotiana 369
nifedipine 303
nut galls 294
nutmeg 298
nutraceutical 74, 75
Nutritional Labelling and Education
    Act (NLEA) 77, 138

O

oak (quercus sps) 294
O. album 323
Ocimum sanctum 323, 358
O. flexuosum 323
O. frutescens 323
O-glycosides 229
O. hirsutum 323
O. inodorum 323
O. monachorum 323
O. nelsonii 323
open continuous culture 376

organ culture 375
organic foods 74
organogenesis 381
Ornus Sanitatus 5
Orthosiphon aristatus 389
O. tenuifl orum 323
oushadi 52
oxytocic 270

P

pachaka agni 45
paclitaxel 87, 91
padartha 50
P. afra 115
palisade ratio 202
palmarosa 73
panaxosides 104
Panax quinquefolius 16
Panax quinquifolium 349
panchabhootas 40
pancheekarana 40
Panchkula 182
Pan troglodytes 422
papain 107–109, 356
Papaver somniferum 387, 389
papaya 356
paper chromatography 246, 266
Papio anubis 421
Papio hamadryas 421
Paris convention 393
partition coefficient 246
Passer domesticus 423
patchouli 73
patenting life forms 408
patent rights 395
Patents Act 402
Paullinia cupana 267
pepper 273
peppermint 73
percolation 204, 219
perfumery 298
permeabilization 389
peroxidase enzyme 379
peroxide value 227
Persian liquorice 93
Pesez's test 259
pharmacovigilance programme in India 308
Phenazone test 296
phospholipids 224, 225
phosphotungstic 259
photoequivalence 215
Phyllanthus emblica 346
physiological ash 205
physiological homeostasis 78
physostigmine 6
phytoalexins 385

phytoestrogens 83
Picea abies 421
piperanine 274
Piperidine 273, 274
Piper longum 273
plagiarism 407
Plantago ovata 115
plantago seeds 115
plant cell immobilization 377
plant cell transformation 383
plant resins 243
plant stanols/sterols 83
plant waxes 225
Plasmodium falciparum 270, 331
P. notoginseng 103
podophyllin 92
podophyllotoxin 92
Podophyllum 91, 244
Podophyllum hexandrum 91
Podophyllum peltatum 91
pollen culture in vitro 369
pollen grains 376
pollution 417
poly pharmacy 19
polyploidy 105
Polyunsaturated fatty acids (PUFAs) 83
P. ovata 115
P. psyllium 115
Prabhava 50, 51, 307
prakrti 48
Prakruti 38
pramana 44
Prana vayu 45
Prayogagnana 50
prebiotics 76
prepared resins 243
primary and secondary metabolites 418
primary metabolites 12
primates 420, 426
primitive cultivars 370
Prithvi 40, 43
proanthocyanidins 82, 385
probiotics 76
process patent 395
production of essential oils 73
production of mint oil 73
prokaryotic promoters 382
proprietary non-prescription products 74
prostaglandins 285
Protection of Plant Varieties and
    Farmers' Right Act 412
Proxmire Bill' of 1976 138
Prunus amygdalis 354
pseudoephedrine 258
P. somniferum 388
Psoralea corylifolia 359

pulse diagnosis 48
Punarnava 309
punarnavoside 310, 311
pungency 273
pure drugs 23
purified papain 109
purple foxglove 100
purslane 350
Purusha 38
pushkara guggulu 318
pusley 350

Q
Qesophagostemum 420
quality control of pure drugs 19
Quality Standards of Indian Medicinal Plants. 173
quantitative chemical evaluation 212
quantitative TLC 249
quercetin 261, 288, 346
Quingao 330
Quinghaosu 330
quinic acid 271
quinidine 96, 271
Quinine 96, 257, 270, 271, 423
quinine sulphate 271
quinoline alkaloid 270
quinones 265

R
radial PC 248
radioactive contamination 208
radionuclides 208
Rajas 38
raktha punarnava 310
Ranjaka agni 45
Rasa 40, 50, 307
Rasachikitsa 54
Rasayana 53, 54
rauffricine 380
Rauwolfia serpentina 6
Raymond's test 284
R&D of functional foods 79
recombinant DNA 15
Reetha 342
refractive index 227
Reichert Meissl value 210, 227
resin acids 243
resin alcohols 243
resin phenols 243
restriction endonuclease enzymes 367
resveratrol 340, 362
retardation factor (Rf) 215
retention time 253
retinitis 261
reusable biocatalysts 377
rhamnoglycoside 261

rhamnose 277, 289
rhinoplastic surgery 401
rhodamine dyes 249
rice-based wine 353
Richard Wrangam 416, 420
Rig Veda 3, 34
rodenticides 206
Roman Chamomile 344
root cultures 375
Rosa centifolia 356
Rosa damascena 356
rosemarinic acid 385
Rosemary 343, 344
rose oil 356
Rosmarinus officinalis 343
rotation planar chromatography (RPC) 213
rubefacient 344
rupa 40
Russian liquorice 93
rutin 261, 288, 340
rutinose 288

S

Sacred basil 324
Sadhaka agni 46
safflower 355
salad oil 348
Salkowski test 278
Salmonella 208, 209
Salvia officinalis 352
Samana vayu 45
Samgrahas 35
Samhitas 35
Sami Labs 196
Samkhya 38, 41
Samsara 41
Samyakyogagnana 50
Sandalwood 73, 360
Sange's test 238
Santalum album 360
Sapindus mukorossi 342
Sapindus trifoliatus 342
Saraca asoca 321
Sarangadhara Samhita 37
sarmentogenin 236
Sarpagandha 6, 80
sarsasapogenin 100, 236
Sattwa 38
Saunders 366
Sausserea lappa 313
saw palmetto 350
Schleiden and Schwann 365
Scopolia carniolica 113, 114
Scoville units 274
secondary metabolite 12, 425
sedative 106

seed dormancy 369
Semi Conductor Integrated Circuits
    Layout Design Act 398
Senna 115
sennosides 264, 265
Serenoa repens 350
serpentine 85, 378
Sesamum indicum 348
sesquiterpene 239, 422
Seydler 1
S-glycosides 229
Shalakya-tantra 52
Shallaki 168
Shalya-tantra 52
shampoos 341
Shankapushpi 311
sharira 43
shigella 209
shikakai 341
Shikonin 366, 386
Shinoda's test 234, 290
shoe flower 346
shoot meristem 369
shoot tip culture 367
shrink-proofing wool 107
Shuddha guggulu 303
Siddha 53, 145, 155
Simmondsia chinensis 345
Simon's test 259
single-cell culture 376
size exclusion chromatography phases 252
skin-borne parasites 423
skin cleansers 349
skin conditioning agent 348, 349, 352, 355, 362
skin moisturizer 348, 351
skin rejuvenators 360
skin whiteners 353
S. laciniatum 99, 375
Sleshaka kapha 46
Snigdha 43
soap berry 342
soap nut 342
soap pod 341
Solanum lycocarpum 424
solasodine 100, 235
solidifying point 227
solid-phase micro-extraction 220
soluble fibre 84
somaclonal Variation 368
somatic hybridization 370
Sophora japonica 261
sorbents 252
Sowa-Rigpa 55
Spanish liquorice 93
Spanish or French psyllium 115
spikenard oil 328

spreading hogweed 310
standardized extracts 67
standardized herbal formulation 172
standardized turmeric extract 21
State Forest Research Institute 178
stationary phase 251
Statute of Anne 392
S-thalidomide 14
stigmasterol 100
stilbenes 340
stimulant digestive 273
stimulant laxative 117
stinging nettle 344
stomachics 96
stomatal indices for leafy drugs 202
stomatal numbers 202
S. trifoliatus 342
Sturnus vulgaris 423
sublimation 219
sui generis 399
sunburn 338
sunscreen 347, 349
super critical fluid extraction 68, 219, 240, 241
surface immobilization 378
surfactant 235, 285
surgery 401
Sushruta 36, 37
suspension cultures 367, 376
sweet flag 352
sweet sagewort 330
sweet worm wood 330
swelling index/swelling factor 210
Swertia chirata 331
Swertia chirayita 331
swetha punarnava 310
Symphytum officinale 359
Synergism 18

T

Tabata 386
Tagara 105, 326
Takshashila 36, 37
tamarins 422
tamas 38
tanmatras 41
tannic acid 223
tannins 268, 294
taxanes 87
Taxus biomass in trade 90
Taxus brevifolia 87
tea tree 357
tenderizing meat 107
test for colophony 245
test for guaiacum resin 245
test for umbelliferone 245
tests for cyanogenetic glycosides 232

tetracyclic (steroidal) 235
tetracyclic triterpenes 104
tetraploid 327
TGA Approved Terminology for Drugs 132
T. globosa 88
Thalictrum minus 387
Thalictrum rugosum 389
Thalleioquin test 272
therapeutic index 282
thermal desorption 219
thermodistillation 220
thermogenic drug 21
thermogenic stimulant 316
The WHO guidelines 122
thiarubrine 420
Thidiazuron (TDZ) 374
thin layer chromatography 213, 246, 248, 269
Thiocyanate glycosides 229
THMP Regulations 2005 128
Thuja plicata 423
Tibetan medicine 32, 92
Tinnevelly Senna 115
tissue culture 368, 375
TLC 202, 215, 242, 248, 249, 269
Tollen's test 284
tomatidine 235
tomato juice 373
tonics 341
topoisomerase 93
total ash 205
total extracts 340
total sennosides 117
totaquine 96
totipotent 376
toxic benzoquinones 424
toxic metals and non-metals 206
toxic phenols 418
trademark 397
Trade Related Intellectual Property Subjects (TRIPS) 394
trade secrets 399
Traditional Chinese medicine (TCM) 131
Traditional Knowledge Digital Library (TKDL) 146, 155, 169, 413
transformed roots 387
transgenic plants 370
transgenic rice able 385
transgenic tobacco 370
Trattinickia aspera 424
Trianthema 310
tricyclic 239
tridoshas 307
Trigonella foenum-graecum 342
Trigunas 38
TRIPS Agreement 395
tropism 373
true waxes 225

Tulsi 323, 358
turbidostat 376
Turkish galls 294, 295
turmeric 298, 358
T. wallichiana 88
tyrosinase 353

U

Udana vayu 45
ultrasonication 219, 389
Umbellularia caifornica 421
Unani Pharmacopoeia of India 145
United Nations Bureaux 394
United Nations Commission on International
    Law (UNICITRAL) 394
United Nations Convention on
    Biological Diversity 121
United Nations Industrial Development
    Organization (ICS-UNIDO). 166
United States Patent and Trademark Office
    (USPTO) 169, 413
Universal Medicaments Pvt. Ltd. 196
UNO 27
Ursus arctos 424
Urtica dioica 344
Usna 43
US patent and Trademark Office 392
Uva ursi 353

V

vacuum liquid chromatography 252
vaidyas 52
Vaiseshika 38
Vajikarana 53
Valepotriates 106, 327
valerenic acid 327
valerenone 106
Valerian 325
Valeriana officinalis 105, 325
Valeriana wallichii 389
vanishing cream 338
variolation 11
Vayu 40
Vaz 352
V. diocia 106
Veda 34
Vedanta 38
Vedic 33, 416
vegetative propagation 373
velcro 420
venonioside B1 422
Vernonia amygdalina 422
Verticillium dahliae 388
Vesicular Arbuscular Mycrorrhizal 381
veterinary therapy in India 416
vetiver 73, 361

Vetivera zizanioides 361
V. excelsa 326
V. flaurei 326
V. hardwickii 326
Vicco Laboratories 195
vinblastine 379, 387
vincristine 379, 387
vindoline 379
Vipaka 50, 51, 307
virya 50, 51, 307
viscosity 227
Vitamin C 354
Vitamin P 288
vitamins 132, 340
Vitis vinifera 362
V. mexicana 106
Vochting's 365
V. officinalis 326, 375
Vyana vayu 45

W

Wagner's reagent 223, 259
Wagner's solution 275
wash nut 342
water chemistry 426
water memory 17
water or hydrodistillation 240
water-soluble ash 205
wattle (Acacia sps) 294
Western herbal medicine 131, 316
wheat germ 340
white chiretta 332
whitening agents 353
willow (Salix caprea) 294
wolf's bane 347
wood ants 421

X

xanthine alkaloids 339
Xanthydrol test 284

Y

yamogenin 99
yastimadhu 95
yeast extract 373
yew tree 87
Yoga 38, 155
yucca 236
Yukti vignana 49

Z

Zaire 97
Zanzibar aloes 110
Zea mays 357
zeaxanthin 81, 343
zoopharmacognosy 29, 416